SMALL ANIMAL EMERGENCY
and
CRITICAL CARE
for Veterinary Technicians

SMALL ANIMAL EMERGENCY and CRITICAL CARE
for Veterinary Technicians

Second 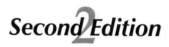Edition

Andrea M. Battaglia, LVT
Hospital Operations Director
Veterinary Medical Center of Central New York
Syracuse, New York

With 150 illustrations with 6 color plates

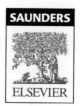

SAUNDERS

ELSEVIER

SAUNDERS
ELSEVIER

11830 Westline Industrial Drive
St. Louis, Missouri 63146

Small Animal Emergency and Critical Care for Veterinary
Technicians, ed 2
Copyright © 2007, 2001 by Saunders, an imprint of Elsevier Inc.

ISBN: 978-1-4160-2804-8

Notice

Knowledge and best practice in this field are constantly changing. As new research and experience
broaden our knowledge, changes in practice, treatment and drug therapy may become necessary or
appropriate. Readers are advised to check the most current information provided (i) on procedures
featured or (ii) by the manufacturer of each product to be administered, to verify the recommended
dose or formula, the method and duration of administration, and contraindications. It is the
responsibility of the practitioner, relying on their own experience and knowledge of the patient,
to make diagnoses, to determine dosages and the best treatment for each individual patient, and
to take all appropriate safety precautions. To the fullest extent of the law, neither the Publisher nor
the Author assumes any liability for any injury and/or damage to persons or property arising out or
related to any use of the material contained in this book.

The Publisher

Previous edition copyrighted 2001

Library of Congress Cataloging in Publication Data
Battaglia, Andrea M.
  Small animal emergency and critical care for veterinary technicians / Andrea M. Battaglia. -- 2nd ed.
      p. cm.
  Includes bibliographical references and index.
  ISBN 978-1-4160-2804-8
  1. Veterinary emergencies--Handbooks, manuals, etc. 2. Veterinary critical care--Handbooks,
manuals, etc. I. Title.
SF778.B38 2007
636.089'6025--dc22   2006052310

Publishing Director: Linda L. Duncan
Publisher: Penny Rudolph
Managing Editor: Teri Merchant
Book Production Manager: Linda McKinley
Project Manager: Stephen Bancroft
Designer: Kimberly E. Denando

Printed in The United States of America

Last digit is the print number: 9 8 7 6 5 4 3

To Audrey, Hannah, and Rhiana—dream big and reach high.
The possibilities are endless.

Contributors

Melissa Ambeau, LVT
Veterinary Medical Center of Central New York
Syracuse, New York

Amy N. Breton, CVT, VTS (Emergency and Critical Care)
Emergency and Critical Care Technician
Veterinary Emergency and Specialty Center of New England
Waltham, Massachusetts

Daniel L. Chan, DVM, Diplomate ACVECC, ACVN, MRCVS
Lecturer in Emergency and Critical Care
Veterinary Clinical Sciences
The Royal Veterinary College, University of London
North Mymms, Hertfordshire, United Kingdom

**Craig C. Cornell, BS, RVT, VTS
(Anesthesia, Emergency, and Critical Care)**
Animal Health Technician
Veterinary Teaching Hospital
University of California, Davis, California

Dennis T. Crowe, Jr., DVM, Dipl ACVS, ACVECC, FCCM, NREMT-I, NCFF
Chief of Staff, Pet Emergency Clinic, Inc.
Ventura, California;
President, Veterinary Surgery, Emergency and Critical Care Services and Consulting
Bogart, Georgia;
President, Integrated Health Technologies, Inc.
Carson City, Nevada

Amy Curran
Monitoring/Lab Equipment for the ER/ICU
Angell Animal Medical Center
Boston, Massachusetts

**Harold Davis, BA, RVT, VTS
(Emergency and Critical Care)**
University of California, Davis, California

Jennifer J. Devey, DVM, Diplomate ACVECC
Director of Emergency Service and Intensive Care Unit
Calgary Animal Referral and Emergency Centre
Calgary, Alberta, Canada

Pam Dickens, CVT
New Port Richey, Florida

Eric N. Glass, MS, DVM, ACVIM (Neurology)
Section Head, Neurology and Neurosurgery
Red Bank Veterinary Hospital
Tinton Falls, New Jersey

Tanya Jackson, BS, DVM
Veterinarian, Animal Ark Veterinary Hospital
Baldwinsville, New York

**Marc Kent, DVM, Diplomate ACVIM
(Neurology and Internal Medicine)**
Assistant Professor
Department of Small Animal Medicine and Surgery
College of Veterinary Medicine,
University of Georgia, Athens, Georgia

Marcie Marshall
Hospital Administrator
Veterinary Medical Center of Central New York
Syracuse, New York

**Lisa Moses, VMD, Diplomate ACVIM
(Small Animal Internal Medicine)**
Staff Veterinarian
Section of Emergency and Critical Care Medicine
Angell Animal Medical Center
Boston, Massachusetts

Donna A. Oakley, CVT, VTS (Emergency and Critical Care)
Director, Penn Animal Blood Bank
School of Veterinary Medicine
University of Pennsylvania, Philadelphia, Pennsylvania

Ed Park, DVM
Resident, Emergency and Critical Care
Advanced Critical Care and Internal Medicine
Tustin, California

**Richard W. Reid, DVM, Diplomate ACVIM
(Small Animal Internal Medicine)**
President and Chief Medical Officer
Sound VUE, Veterinary Ultrasound and Endoscopy, PC
Smithtown, New York

Ann Marie Ritchie, CVT, VTS (Emergency and Critical Care)
Hospital Manager
Ocean State Veterinary Emergency Services
Tiverton, Rhode Island

Nancy Shaffran, RVT, VTS (Emergency and Critical Care)
Senior Veterinary Nursing Specialist
Veterinary Specialty Team
Pfizer Animal Health, Erwinna, Pennsylvania

Don Shawver, CRTT, MS
New Buffalo, Michigan

Edward L. Spindel, MS, DVM
Animal Ark Veterinary Service
Baldwinsville, New York

Preface

I am excited to share the second edition of *Small Animal Emergency and Critical Care for Veterinary Technicians*. An amazing group of people who live what they write contributed to this book. A technician who was directly involved with helping during the September 11, 2001, terrorist attacks in New York City contributed a chapter on preparing for a disaster. Technicians and doctors with years of experience improving their skills in a clinical setting have provided how-to techniques. People who have dedicated their careers to saving the lives of our furred, feathered, and scaly friends have shared how to be successful and improve as an emergency critical care technician.

Veterinary technicians involved in emergency and critical care medicine must understand the vital role they play. Many times it is the veterinary technician who begins the life-saving procedures before the veterinarian on duty has a chance to join the team.

Small Animal Emergency and Critical Care for Veterinary Technicians provides a valuable resource for veterinary technicians and students interested in this specialized area. Many life-saving procedures are detailed through diagrams and step-by-step descriptions. Common drugs used to stabilize and maintain the critically ill or injured small animal are discussed, including information about the mode of action and dosage. Chapters dedicated to shock, cardiopulmonary resuscitation, and trauma introduce the emergency section and provide information on how to assess and stabilize the critically ill or injured small animal.

The book is divided into three sections. The first section focuses on critical care techniques. Many supportive therapies are discussed. A procedure is highlighted in each chapter and described in a Technical Tip. A new chapter in this section covers isolation techniques in emergency practice and stresses the importance of monitoring these isolated patients.

The second section focuses on specific types of emergencies. Each chapter details specific situations encountered in the emergency room. The type of emergency is defined. A checklist is provided with information on how to equip the emergency room with the proper drugs and items needed for the specific emergency. Clinical signs, most common treatment protocols, and Technical Tips are given for each emergency. A new chapter in this section covers avian and exotic patients, including basic restraint techniques, sampling techniques, and common emergencies.

The technician involved in emergency and critical care medicine often is required to work inconsistent hours and night shifts. Scheduling is a big challenge in any 24-hour facility. The final section provides scheduling solutions and suggestions for adapting to shift changes. This creates a healthier work environment and reduce staff turnover. This section also includes a new chapter on risk management, which involves understanding the liability risks that we take when we assume responsibility for the medical care of our patients. This chapter emphasizes the importance of good client communication and documentation.

My hope is for the reader to use this book as another tool in providing the best possible care for the critically ill or injured small animal. Veterinary medicine continues to evolve in all areas. No single resource should be considered the final word on any subject. Veterinary technicians should continue their educations on a daily basis through publications, continuing education seminars, and practical experience. The best resources for learning continue to be the animals we interact with and other members of our team. We must continue to learn more and be willing to share what we have learned. The animals we work with deserve our best effort.

This work will continue to be edited for years to come for the benefit of our profession so we can continue to provide the best patient care possible for our critically ill or injured small animals. Thank you for your dedication to improve your knowledge and skills for the many people who trust you with their pets and for the pets that will pass through your hands.

Andrea M. Battaglia

Acknowledgments

The year 2006 marks my 20th year as a licensed veterinary technician. I have had the opportunity of working in private hospitals, academia, industry, emergency clinics, and now a very progressive specialty, an emergency and critical care facility. Every experience has brought me new challenges, new lifetime lessons never forgotten, and an appreciation for the unique contributions each of us bring to our profession everyday.

Dr. Tim Robinson—you will always have my gratitude for creating a place where work as veterinary technician is challenging, satisfying, and fun.

Thank you to all the dedicated, skilled, professional doctors, veterinary technicians, and veterinary assistants working at the Veterinary Medical Center of Central New York—you keep me humble.

A special thank you to the girls, LeeAnn, Marcie, Heather, and Sharon, for all of your support and friendship. I look forward to becoming more successful, wiser, and better with you for many years to come.

Finally, thank you to the owners who trustingly hand me their critically ill or injured pets. I promise to continue to learn from each of my experiences so I will be able to improve my skills for future small animal patients that pass through my hands.

Contents

SECTION

I

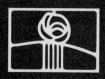

CRITICALLY ILL SMALL ANIMALS

This section introduces many technical skills needed to care for the critically ill small animal. Commonly used supportive therapies and procedures for maintaining the critically ill patient through anesthesia are included.

CHAPTER 1

Skill of Observation and Interpretation

ANDREA M. BATTAGLIA

Veterinary emergency and critical care medicine continues to evolve, providing higher levels of care. Many 24-hour emergency and critical care facilities have been established throughout the country, and many more are in various stages of planning and development. The veterinary technician involved in emergency care, critical care, or both must continue to educate him or herself to participate successfully in this ever-changing profession. Observation skills and the ability to interpret the observation and act upon it immediately are crucial in the care of the critically ill or injured patient (Color plates 1 to 3). For example, a slight change in the breathing pattern might indicate the necessity for quick intervention to save the life of the patient; a decreased response during a neurologic evaluation might indicate a need for change in the treatment plan to improve the patient's prognosis; a change in posture might indicate a need to implement a pain management program. Many possibilities in the form of equipment and procedures are available to provide optimal patient care; however, these tools will never take the place of a skilled veterinary technician. In this technologic age, it must not be forgotten that the "hands on" skills of observation, interpretation, and monitoring continue to play a crucial role in treatment.

When the critically ill or injured small animal patient arrives, the technician makes the initial assessment by checking the vital signs and obtaining a history from the owner. He or she should create and follow a triage form and questionnaire (Fig. 1-1). It is easy for owners to become sidetracked when talking about their pets; in an emergency, time cannot be wasted. Therefore it is important to know the normal parameters for the dog and cat to properly assess what is abnormal (Figs. 1-2, A and B, and 1-3). Variations in the normals may occur, depending on the breed, size, or age of the animal. On physical exam, an obvious problem may avert one's attention from something less obvious. For this reason, it is important to do complete physical exams on every patient when initial stabilization has been successful (Fig. 1-4).

1 2 3 4 5 6 7 8 9

Weight: _____
Date: _____   Triage time: _____   Initial: _____   Doctor exam: _____ (Time)

Client name: _____   Pet name: _____   Species: _____   Breed: _____

History:
Primary concern:
_____
_____
_____

Medications:
_____

Receiving aspirin therapy? Y/N

Exposure to potential toxins? Y/N

Indoor/outdoor

Kenneled/chained/allowed to roam freely/fenced in yard

Diet _____

Date of last vaccination _____

Date of last doctor visit _____

Other: _____
_____
_____

Examination:

Ambulatory? Y/N   If Yes: Normal   Weak   Ataxic   Lame _____

Mucous membrane color: Pink   Pale pink   Pale white   Brick red   Cyanotic

Respiratory rate: _____   Ventilatory nature: Eupneic   Increased effort   Tachypneic   Dyspneic

                   Lung sounds: Clear   Harsh   Crackles   Absent

Heart rate: _____   Heart sounds: Normal   Murmur   Muffled   Distant

Pulse rate: _____   Pulse quality: Strong   Fair   Weak   Poor   Bounding

Temperature: _____

Attitude: QAR   BAR   Lethargic   Semicomatose   Comatose   Anxious

Behavior: Blue   White   Red

Overall assessment: SAPT   Reassess   Immediate stabilization required

Fig. 1-1 Triage questionnaire.

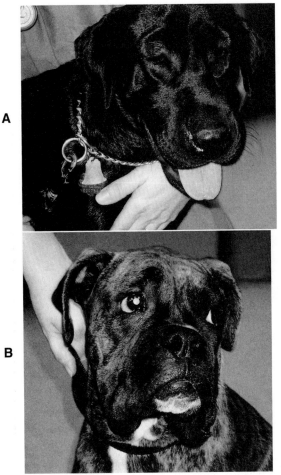

Figs. 1-2 A and **B** The skill of observation. The Labrador puppy and boxer are experiencing an anaphylactic reaction. Both had severe facial swelling and showed signs of respiratory difficulty as the condition progressed. Because of breed conformation, it was more difficult to assess in the boxer than the Labrador puppy; however, because of the history of recent vaccinations and observations of hives on other areas of the body a diagnosis could be made and treatment initiated.

When it is determined the animal needs to be admitted into the hospital and the owners have agreed to treat the condition, the owner needs to fill out the chosen forms completely. The time the owner takes to complete the forms will give the emergency critical care team the time to do the necessary procedures to stabilize the animal. A signed form giving the team consent must be obtained before treatment is initiated (Fig. 1-5).

Readiness is the key to efficient and successful stabilization. All stations and carts should be restocked during each shift, and equipment and oxygen sources must be fully functional and ready to be used (Box 1-1).

The veterinary technician should not hesitate to bring the owner into the hospital to alleviate any anxiety they may be experiencing as a result of separation from the pet. This action helps to develop mutual trust and generally fosters a positive working relationship and provides the staff with an opportunity to meet the owner. Visitations should be encouraged to convey the perception that the owner is a valued member of "the team." A hospital visitation protocol should be established to avoid unnecessary misunderstandings between the owner and staff (Fig. 1-6). The small animal patient is now recognized as a family member in everyone's mind.

It is important the client understands the procedures that may be performed, the risks involved, and the severity of the animal's condition before departure. A copy of the plan should be available for the owner to take home. The owner must also make a decision whether the animal is to be given cardiopulmonary resuscitation if an arrest occurs. The team is notified, the owner's wishes are recorded on the chart, and a code is placed on the cage card.

The treatment and monitoring of critically ill small animal patients often involves various drug and fluid therapies. Several staff members continually assess and note the animal's response to the treatment throughout the day. Verbal communication and record keeping play a very important role in the continuous monitoring of the critical small animal patient. Because veterinary technicians need to communicate throughout their shifts, they do so via written notes highlighting important changes that may have occurred. The information is then shared during shift changes. Making rounds after each shift ensures the important information is being passed on and assists in maintaining the best patient care possible (Fig. 1-7).

Location has long been considered the most important factor when selecting real estate and ensuring the success of a business. However, location must also be considered when treating the critically ill or injured patient. High visibility and accessibility is crucial in the successful treatment of patients.

Creating a section in the hospital for the high-maintenance patients can be accomplished by

Triage
The screening and classification of sick, wounded, or injured to determine priority needs for efficient use of medical and nursing power, equipment, and facilities. Use of triage is essential to maximize the number of lives saved during an emergency situation that produces more sick and wounded than the available medical care personnel can possibly handle at one time.

What to Bring with You
Stethoscope, thermometer, exam gloves, penlight, highlighter/pen, triage clip board

Mirror Check
We do not want to scare our clients! So remember to wash the blood off your hands and face.

Initial Contact
Greet owners with a hello and welcoming smile. Introduce yourself and include your position as the emergency triage nurse. Ask what brings (pet's name) here today. Remember—this is an unscheduled visit and most pet owners are feeling stress on many levels. Plans may have had to be changed, sitters for younger children arranged, financial concerns, and so on; you will hear it all unless you attempt to keep the focus on their pet.

History
History is very important but time does not allow for details of all other ailments the pet has had since birth. Please follow the format on the attached triage sheet.

Physical
Allow the pet to become acquainted with you. Many dogs are triaged in the waiting room. All cats are moved to an exam room or taken to the treatment area before being removed from their carrier.

Behavior
Examine the animal's status and behavior. Note behavior and highlight appropriate code on the sheet after completing the TPR. (*Blue*—usually reserved for the happy puppy and not often seen in the emergency room, *white*—normal behavior and no obvious sign of aggression, *red*—use Caution.)

Do not attempt to TPR/ask owners to assist with a timid or an aggressive dog in the waiting area. Take the pet to the treatment area for assistance.

Highlight line *immediate stabilization required* when appropriate.

Note the time on the chart once triage is completed, and highlight the order of priority. Communicate with the owner if there is a waiting time. Explain that the emergency room staff is stabilizing other patients in the treatment area. Remember to update the owner within 5 minutes if you have rushed their pet to the back for immediate stabilization. Remember that 5 minutes will seem like 20 minutes to them.

Hospitalizing Their Pet
Thank the owner for allowing the site to take care of (pet's name). Let them know the site is open every day, 24 hours a day, and they can call for an update at any time.

Fig. 1-3 Normal parameters form.

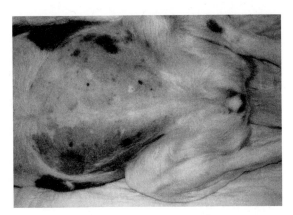

Fig. 1-4 A two-year-old female beagle arrived at the clinic with vomiting, lethargy, and anorexia. The triage team assumed she had ingested a foreign body (based on the history and initial assessment). Petechiae were discovered on the ventral part of the abdomen during the full physical, and the diagnostic plans were adjusted accordingly.

Case # _____

Your pet appears to have a severe medical emergency and requires immediate emergency treatment.

A doctor is examining your pet now: As soon as your pet's condition allows, the doctor will give you a medical recommendation and a cost estimate for further care.

Payment information: There are no payment plans or billing options for emergency care at the _____ . Payment is required at time of service.

Cost of immediate life-threatening treatment:
Charges can run _____ to _____ for the first 30 minutes but may be higher in very critical emergencies.

Emergency Radiographs $ _____
Emergency Injections $ _____
Emergency Parvo Test $ _____
Other _____ $ _____

I give consent for immediate treatment and *accept payment conditions* outlined above.

I do not give consent for treatment and wish to speak to a doctor first—even though the delay in treatment may be detrimental to the health of my pet. I will not hold the Veterinary Medical Center or its staff responsible for any adverse outcome that this delay might cause.

Signature _____ Date _____

Fig. 1-5 Emergency treatment consent form.

BOX 1-1

Checklist for Restocking Emergency Station

Two 24-gauge IV catheters
Two 22-gauge IV catheters
Two 20-gauge IV catheters
Two 18-gauge IV catheters
Two 14-gauge IV catheters
Clippers
Scrub solution
Triple antibiotic ointment
Four 20-gauge needles for minicutdown
One roll of 1-inch tape for stabilization
Bag of 1-L crystalloid solution—regular drip (10-drop/ml set)
Bag of hetastarch
Bag of 500-ml crystalloid solution—minidrip (60-drop/ml set)
Heparinized capillary tubes

Ethylenediaminetetraacetic (EDTA) acid tube
Clot tubes
Vacutainer tube containing lithium heparin
Oxygen delivery system
Suction unit
Warming system
Easy access to monitoring equipment
Laryngeal scope
Light for assessing pupillary light response (PLR)
Endotracheal tubes with stylet
Cart with materials for quick wraps to control hemorrhage
Sterile KY Jelly
Crash cart with appropriate drugs for CPR
Sheets for documentation of stabilization procedures
Pen

Your pet has been admitted to our hospital for diagnostics, treatment, or surgery. You can rest assured that we will dedicate ourselves to providing your pet with the best care available.

We believe that other factors can contribute toward your pet's successful recovery besides high quality medical care. Among these factors are your pet's security and comfort. Thus we would like to encourage you to visit your pet if he/she is going to be hospitalized for over a 24-hour period.

Please be advised that though we encourage visitors, we must protect the security and comfort of all our patients while not allowing interference with our doctors and staff in their attempt to provide care to other patients. The following visitation regulations apply:

- Please call ahead.

- Patients housed in our Environmental Oxygen Therapy Unit—a maximum of 5-minute visitation no more than every 12 hours: Please understand that environmental oxygen delivery is critical to your pet's condition and we may not be able to allow you to hold your pet.

- Cage side visitations—no more than two people at one time for a maximum of 10 minutes every 12 hours.

- Exam room visitations—up to 30-minute visitation (depending on therapy/treatment schedule) no more than every 12 hours.

- For their own safety, no small children are allowed in the treatment area.

- To protect the privacy of our other clients, please limit questions to your own pet's condition only.

- For their own comfort and security and your safety, please do not attempt to pet or touch other hospitalized patients.

Visitation may not be possible at times because of case load of emergency patients, procedures being performed in treatment/surgery, or the critical nature of your own pet. Your patience is appreciated, and we will do our best to offer you an alternative time to visit. Your cooperation in the above regulations is appreciated. As always, if you have any concerns or questions, do not hesitate to call.

To schedule a visitation with your pet please call:

Fig. 1-6 Hospital visitation policy.

- Why is the patient here? What is the complaint/condition?
- What is the diagnosis/suspected disease?
- What is the typical behavior and response to treatment?
- Review the parameters of TPRs: urinating/defecating?
- Discuss special instructions with the staff.
- Demonstrate special procedures (CVPs, trach tube care).
- Is the patient post-op? Are there any anesthetic complications?
- Is the animal an orthopedic post-operative patient? What are the special handling instructions? Are there non–weight-bearing instructions?
- What is the response to pain control being used?
- Nutrition—Is the patient NPO? If NPO, how long? Is PPN being considered? Has the patient been offered food? Is the patient eating? If the patient is not eating has syringe feeding started?

Overall view of the patient:
- Check IV fluids. What is the rate? What are the additives?
- Check IV catheter wrap and palpate above leg. Has catheter care been performed?
- Check the respiratory pattern of the patient.
- Check the position of the patient. Note on record how the patient is positioned and begin repositioning every 4 hours if necessary.
- Check the response of the patient to the sound of your voice.
- Check the position of the blankets for comfort of the patient.
- Check the treatment flow chart. Is it complete?

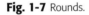

Fig. 1-7 Rounds.

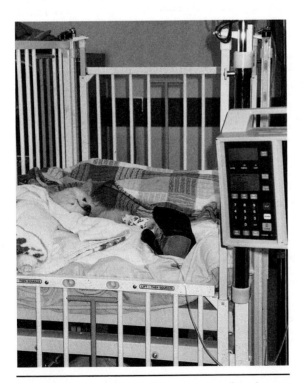

Fig. 1-8 The Pet Bed by Hard Manufacturing allows for easy access to the patient and high visibility.

relocating a bank of cages. Large breed dogs can be placed on mats and blankets in an area sectioned off with baby gates. All patients should be elevated above the floor to help prevent nasocomial infections. In these situations, special care needs to be taken to keep fluid lines and closed collection systems clean.

The PetBed manufactured by Hard Manufacturing allows full access to the patient. The bed can be moved to any area of the hospital. Poles are attached to the corners for monitoring equipment and fluid pumps (Fig. 1-8).

Veterinary technicians can help to create an optimum emergency and critical care center by acting as team players. To accomplish this goal, they must educate themselves and share new information they have obtained through continuing education, seminars, and journals with the entire staff. Maintaining good communication skills (verbal and written) is essential for establishing a solid network to accomplish the main goal—providing the best nursing and medical care for the critically ill or injured small animal patient.

CHAPTER 2

Basic Monitoring of the Emergency and Critical Care Patient

LISA MOSES, AMY CURRAN

Accurate and continuous monitoring is central to the care of critically ill animals. Although this chapter reviews the techniques of equipment- and machine-based monitoring, the importance of observation, palpation, and auscultation as basic nursing practices cannot be overstated. Because technicians often spend more time with critically ill patients than doctors can, their observations fill gaps in knowledge crucial for successful treatment decision making.

Without standardized record keeping, monitoring is not useful for patient care and can lead to erroneous conclusions. Records for emergency or critical patients should be in table or flow sheet form, with labeled spaces for listing monitoring values, time when the monitoring was done, and the name or initials of whoever did the monitoring (this will allow trends to be noted at a glance). Space should also be provided on the record to list which pieces of equipment were used and any notes regarding the patient that will allow consistency in monitoring between different shifts.

This chapter is divided into two sections. The first part will review basic laboratory practices and interpretation of results needed to care for the emergency and critical care patient. The second will discuss intensive care unit (ICU) monitoring equipment and techniques of use.

Blood Tests Using Centrifuges and Analyzers

Sample collection is as important to accurate results as the function of the analyzers. Hemolysis, which can interfere with a number of blood tests, can be avoided by proper technique. A clean venipuncture, use of the largest needle possible and light suction on the syringe will minimize hemolysis. Use of vacutainer needles and vacutainer butterfly collection systems will also help minimize hemolysis and premature activation of blood clotting.

Animals in the critical care setting usually need multiple blood sample evaluations. Long, large-bore catheters placed in central veins

9

(e.g., jugular, medial saphenous, or lateral saphenous) can provide the technician with a sampling port. These central lines can be maintained for many days or indefinitely, depending on the type of catheter, and avoid the discomfort and complications associated with multiple venipunctures.

Processing Blood Samples

Before a blood sample is collected, a laboratory reference should be consulted to make sure the proper container and sample handling will be used. Specific tests have exact requirements for sample handling and containers, and these protocols must be followed. Collection of the appropriate amount of blood is important. For example, if an ethylenediaminetetraacetic acid (EDTA) tube is not filled by vacuum suction and too little blood is used, then the ratio of anticoagulant to blood will be too high and some values will be erroneous.

Once the sample is placed in the tube, it should be rotated gently approximately 10 times to mix the anticoagulant with the blood. Serum or plasma should be removed from spun red blood cells (RBCs) within 30 minutes and refrigerated (or frozen if the particular test requires it). Blood for packed cell volume (PCV) and total solid measurement should be transferred to capillary tubes immediately. For certain tests, such as PCVs and tests run on serum or plasma, the blood sample must be spun in a centrifuge. The centrifuge should always be balanced by a sample of similar volume on the opposite side to prevent uneven wear on the motor, which eventually will cause vibration. The correct speed should be selected depending on the sample being spun. Samples should not be removed from the centrifuge until it has come to a complete stop. The brake should not be used when the head is still rotating at high speeds to avoid excessive wear.

Serum or plasma color and clarity should always be evaluated and the results recorded in the patient record. This information can give important clues about the patient's disease process. Normal serum is clear and colorless. Common changes in serum color and clarity include the following:

- Lipemic (white, turbid)—Lipemic serum indicates high levels of fat in the blood and can occur if the animal has eaten recently. It can also be associated with various diseases such as acute

pancreatitis, diabetes mellitus, hypothyroidism, and primary lipid disorders. The technician may need to repeat the test after withholding food for 12 hours (if appropriate).
- Icteric (yellow)—Icteric serum occurs most commonly in patients with liver disease or hemolytic anemia.
- Hemolyzed (red)—Hemolyzed serum occurs usually as a result of poor sampling technique and handling; however, it can also indicate intravascular hemolysis associated with hemolytic anemia.

Reference Ranges

The reference values for the individual machine should be used, because machines vary significantly and reference values for each machine are established separately. The appendix of *Kirk's Current Veterinary Therapy XIII Small Animal Practice* (Bonagura JD, 2000) contains reference ranges for commonly used hematology and chemistry analyzers.

Packed Cell Volume and Total Plasma Proteins Measurements

The PCV or hematocrit (HCT) and total plasma protein (TP) are important tools in the emergency and critical care patient. They are quick and simple to perform and give a lot of information. The two tests should always be run together for more accurate interpretation of the patient's status.

Indications

Any patient arriving at the emergency department or ICU, especially those animals who may have the following:

- Dehydration
- Anemia
- Trauma
- Shock

Equipment

- Micro-HCT centrifuge
- Capillary tubes with or without anticoagulant, depending on the sample type

- Clay trays to seal the capillary tubes
- Card or slider tray tube reader to measure the PCV
- Refractometer to measure the TP

Technique

Whole blood, either put directly into anticoagulant-containing capillary tubes or removed from a properly filled EDTA tube or heparinized syringe placed in a plain capillary tube, may be used. Capillary tubes must be sealed with clay after the sample is inserted and before they are placed in the centrifuge. The clay end should face outward. At least two to three capillary tubes should be filled in case of breakage within the centrifuge.

After the sample is spun, three layers will be evident. The red cell column or PCV is closest to the clay. The buffy coat is a white or turbid layer just above the PCV and is composed of white cells and platelets. The third layer is the plasma protein layer.

Once the plasma is evaluated, the PCV is read using a micro-HCT tube reader—a slide rule used to estimate the PCV volume by percentage of total blood volume. The simplest type is a card with markings on it that are lined up with the red cell column to determine the PCV. In addition, wheeled micro-HCT readers are available in which the capillary tube is inserted in a groove and marked wheels are rotated under the sample to provide the PCV. Both types have instructions on them. The buffy coat percentage also should be read and recorded.

A refractometer is a device used to determine the TP. The capillary tube is split above the buffy coat, and the plasma protein is blown onto the surface of the refractometer. The technician reads the refractometer by looking into the instrument and looking at the column on the grid labeled *g/dl*. The line where the shaded area meets the light area is the TP. The refractometer should be calibrated regularly using distilled water, which has a specific gravity of zero.

Spun capillary tubes from each reading may be kept taped to a white piece of paper and labeled with patient information along with the date and time of collection. This provides a visual record of changes in the plasma protein color and clarity over time, which may provide valuable information on the patient's clinical course.

Troubleshooting

Erroneous readings can be made if the blood is clotted. Lipemia and hemolysis will falsely increase the TP. Administration of oxyglobin hemoglobin (Hb)

solution within 3 to 4 days will cause changes in the PCV that make it inaccurate.

The machine-calculated PCV (from a hematology analyzer) may be 1 to 3 points higher than a measured PCV from a spun micro-HCT tube as a result of trapping of plasma in the red cell column. Proper centrifuge speeds and at least 3 minutes of spinning will help minimize this artifact.

Interpretation

Normal adult canine PCV is 37% to 54%, with lower values in puppies and higher values in sighthound breeds such as greyhounds. Normal adult feline PCV is 30% to 47%, also with lower values in young kittens. TP normal ranges are 6.0 to 7.8 g/dl in dogs and 6.2 to 8.0 g/dl in cats. These values also vary with age.

Anemia is defined as PCV below the reference range. The PCV should always be interpreted along with the TP, because dehydration and splenic contraction (especially in dogs) affects the PCV. The TP can give important clues to whether dehydration or splenic contraction is affecting the PCV measurement. Dehydration will cause rises in the PCV because it is measured as a percentage of the blood volume. With dehydration, less water is found in the blood and the relative percentage of the PCV will increase without an actual increase in the red cell number. The TP will also rise in this situation because relatively more proteins and less water are found in the plasma. Conversely, the PCV and TS are good tools to gauge the effects of IV fluids and rehydration because they are expected to drop when diluted with IV fluids.

In dogs and cats, the spleen acts as a reservoir for RBCs and can expand and contract. It will contract in response to exercise or blood loss and expand under the influence of sedation and anesthesia. This causes increases and decreases in the PCV, respectively, but does not change the TP measurement.

General Guidelines for Interpretation of Packed Cell Volume and Total Plasma Protein

- High PCV with the following:
  - Normal TP implies splenic contraction or breed-related high normal.

- Low TP implies protein loss or decreased production with splenic contraction and dehydration (commonly seen in hemorrhagic gastroenteritis)
- High TP implies dehydration.
- Low PCV with the following:
  - Normal TP implies anemia from erythrocyte destruction or decreased production.
  - Low TP implies blood loss or dilution from IV fluids.
  - High TP implies protein overproduction with anemia as in bone marrow diseases or other chronic illnesses such as feline infectious peritonitis.
- Normal PCV with the following:
  - Low TP implies decreased protein production or increased loss from the gastrointestinal or urinary tract.
  - High TP implies dehydration with anemia or increased globulin production as in feline infectious peritonitis or other infectious diseases.

(Note: These guidelines only mention the most basic and common interpretations.)

Electrolyte and Chemistry Analyzers

Electrolyte and chemistry analyzers are now available as point-of-care (POC) instruments that allow near immediate results in an emergency room and ICU setting. Rapid assessment of electrolyte levels and blood chemistry provide vital information that guides immediate therapy.

Indications

Most patients entering the critical care unit will benefit from POC testing of electrolytes and, if available, blood chemistry analysis.

Common emergencies that would cause electrolyte derangements include the following:

- Vomiting, diarrhea, or both
- Diabetes mellitus
- Urinary tract disease
- Toxin ingestion
- Eclampsia

Patients with any potentially serious illness or trauma could benefit from blood chemistry testing to assess organ function.

Equipment

POC testing has become more affordable and common in veterinary practices that see emergency and critical cases. A variety of either portable or smaller bench top instruments have been developed for veterinary practices. Some sophisticated instruments developed for human medicine, like the Nova Critical Care Xpress, have been adapted for use in busy veterinary hospitals. Many instruments that analyze electrolytes and some blood chemistry also can be used to perform blood gas analysis. Instruments like Heska's iStat use cartridges that come in various configurations to allow the user to choose between single analytes such as glucose or creatinine and combination panels.

The main function of any critical care laboratory's electrolyte analyzer is to provide rapid and accurate electrolyte results at a reasonable cost. The buyer must take all of this into account before making a purchase. It is important to research not only the unit itself but also its associated costs such as reagents, standards, electrodes, annual maintenance, cleaning solutions, and conditioning solutions. Certain types of analyzers require more labor-intensive maintenance and may be more prone to technical difficulties. Opinions of current users of the same equipment may be helpful in decision making. Internet message boards on sites like the Veterinary Information Network have discussions on various pieces of POC equipment.

After the final decision is made regarding what type of electrolyte analyzer to use, a technical manual should be acquired and read thoroughly. A maintenance protocol and cleaning schedule should be established. The staff should keep a technical support number close to the unit in plain view for unfamiliar users. All the unit's maintenance records must be kept, as well as detailed notes of technical support remedies to problems that arise, so that the next time the problem occurs it can be dealt with more rapidly. When purchasing an electrolyte analyzer, one should consider buying a yearly maintenance contract to ensure the analyzer can be repaired quickly if a major malfunction occurs. This purchase will increase the initial costs but will be insurance for the times when the machine experiences problems and is unable to be fixed by the staff. Having a second, less expensive, bedside analyzer for backup should also be a consideration.

Additional factors that influence the choice of analyzer include anticipated number of panels, whether individual chemistries or full panels are needed, reagent shelf life, and overall costs.

Technique

The sampling needed for most electrolyte analyzers is heparinized blood or serum. Some pieces of equipment allow testing of body fluids other than blood, which is useful in emergency practice. The sampling requirements for each individual electrolyte analyzer must be referred to consistently, and good sample handling techniques must be practiced. Good sample handling techniques are essential to avoid artifacts or damage to the analyzer, such as destruction of an electrode.

A chemistry panel usually requires a serum sample. The blood sample should be collected into a serum-separating vacutainer tube and spun within 30 to 40 minutes of collection. The sample should be kept refrigerated until it is run unless otherwise indicated by the instructions provided by a reference lab or the manufacturer of the particular equipment.

Troubleshooting

As with all analyzers, it is optimal for the entire technical staff to be trained in its use. One or two well-trained technicians should be responsible for the day-to-day and general maintenance of the machine. Quality control for POC testing equipment (or any laboratory equipment) makes the difference between getting accurate and dangerously misleading, erroneous results. Unexpected results or results that are significantly different from past data, as well as possible artifactual problems, should prompt critical analysis of potential changes in the patient's condition. Each piece of equipment has its own list of sample factors that can interfere with the accuracy of results. Staff members must be familiar with this list. For example, some analyzers will produce erroneous results if the sample is lipemic.

Blood samples should be run in a timely manner to avoid postcollection changes in values that will confuse interpretation of results. For example, blood glucose levels will drop within the tube over time because of the RBCs' continued metabolism of the glucose after the sample is taken.

Sample requirements can be significant in small patients, patients with anemia, or patients who require frequent sampling. The total amount of blood drawn during the day or hospital stay should be tracked in these patients to avoid iatrogenic anemia.

Interpretation

The goal of these two kinds of blood tests is to narrow down which organ system or systems are being affected by the patient's disease process. A general chemistry profile gives an indication of liver and kidney function, acid-base status, and plasma protein levels. Electrolyte analysis may reveal surprising changes, considering the patient's signs, or may greatly aid in ruling in or out certain diseases. The technician should be familiar with life-threatening electrolyte abnormalities that require immediate attention. These include the following:

- Hyperkalemia, often seen with urethral obstruction, acute renal failure, or hypoadrenocorticism (Addison's disease)
- Hypocalcemia, often seen with eclampsia or hypoadrenocorticism
- Severe hypernatremia, often seen with nonketotic hyperosmolar diabetic crisis

The blood chemistry can also reveal life-threatening abnormalities that the technician should recognize. These include the following:

- Hypoglycemia, commonly seen in neonatal animals, toy breed puppies, and animals with sepsis
- Severe azotemia (elevations in blood urea nitrogen and creatinine, indicating kidney failure)

Just as one panel will show one snapshot in time, a series of panels will show the effect of the clinician's treatment plan. As with all emergency and critical care monitoring, serial monitoring is most informative. The progress of the patient and the particular disease process will dictate the frequency of electrolyte and chemistry analysis.

Hematology Analyzers

Hematology analyzers provide complete blood counts, which typically include at least RBC, white blood cell (WBC), and platelet counts along with

WBC differential counts, and RBC indices (which are indicators of variations in size and color of RBCs [which relates to RBC regeneration]). A variety of automated hematology cell counters are available, and recently some POC instruments for veterinary use have been marketed.

Indications

Most patients arriving at the emergency department or ICU are likely to have problems that may cause complete blood count abnormalities. The following types of patients are particularly vulnerable:

- Patients with possible blood loss or anemia
- Patients with infectious or inflammatory conditions, such as fever and sepsis
- Patients with petechia or ecchymoses suggesting platelet abnormalities

Equipment

A blood smear is a very useful, inexpensive, and quick way to gain large amounts of information about an emergency patient. The only equipment needed is a drop of fresh blood, microscope slides, standard Diff-Quick stains, and a microscope.

POC testing for hematology is available from multiple companies and is sometimes combined with chemistry analyzer functions. Some machines just provide WBC counts; however, others also provide RBC counts and platelet counts. Some provide numeric results only; others provide graphic results. The equipment should be well researched before purchase, because each machine offers something different. Veterinary machines are recommended over human machines because the variation in cell sizes can alter machine readouts significantly if they are not calibrated for that species. No machine currently can replace a manual examination, and blood smears always should be evaluated.

Technique

Blood smear evaluation begins with a low-power scan of the smear to look for platelet and RBC clumps and to see whether WBCs are disproportionately clustered at the feathered edge. If RBC clumps are present, then a slide agglutination test using fresh whole blood or blood from an EDTA tube diluted 1:10 with saline on a slide should be performed. This will help the technician to distinguish between rouleaux formation and autoagglutination, which indicates an antibody attached to RBC membranes (characteristic of immune-mediated hemolytic anemia).

At 40× magnification, the smear should be examined where the cells are in one layer, not touching each other. The technician should estimate the WBCs by multiplying the number of cells in one field by 1600. He or she should count several fields to ensure a representative sample. If the white cells are clustered at the feathered edge, then this estimate will be falsely lowered.

At 100× magnification, the platelet count can be estimated by multiplying the number of platelets in a field by 15,000. RBC and WBC morphology should be evaluated at this field. Spherocytosis and inclusion bodies are some of the features that are important to notice.

For automated hematology analyzers, the technician should refer to specific instructions for specimen collection, handling, and processing. Most analyzers use blood collected into an EDTA (lavender top) tube that has been completely filled to ensure appropriate dilution of the blood in the anticoagulant.

Troubleshooting

Inappropriate smearing and staining can affect estimations of cell counts from blood smears. The blood must be evenly smeared in a monolayer, allowed to dry entirely, and stained within 2 hours of smearing. Stains are affected by dilution from water, contamination, and exposure to formalin vapors. Stains should be discarded and changed regularly, as recommended by the manufacturer or a reference lab. Additionally, clumping of cells and counting from thick areas of the smear will cause errors in cell counts.

If EDTA anticoagulated whole blood is used, then partially filled tubes will overdilute the blood and change cell counts.

Interpretation

The technician should refer to a hematology atlas for pictures of cell morphology changes that are significant in emergency patients (e.g., spherocytes).

- Normal WBC counts in adult dogs are approximately 6000 to 17,000 cells.
- Normal WBC counts in adult cats are approximately 5500 to 19,000 cells.

- Normal platelet counts in adult dogs are approximately 160,000 to 430,000 cells.
- Normal platelet counts in adult cats are approximately 300,000 to 800,000 cells.

The technician should refer to the reference lab used by the hospital or manufacturer of an automated hematology analyzer for specific reference ranges.

Blood Gas Analysis

Blood gas analysis provides information about the acid-base status of a patient and oxygenation and ventilation. Acid-base and oxygenation disturbances are frequent occurrences in patients in the emergency department or critical care unit; consequently, blood gas analysis is common. The blood (and whole body) is normally maintained within a narrow pH range. Most cellular systems are dependant on this homeostasis and do not function normally when out of the normal pH range. Either venous or arterial blood can be used for blood gas analysis. Only arterial samples give information about oxygenation. Arterial blood has passed through the lungs and should be saturated with oxygen given normal lung function. If a problem exists with gas exchange in the lung, then this will be reflected in the amount of oxygen that binds with the RBCs. The partial pressure of oxygen in arterial blood (Pao_2) will reflect the patient's oxygenation status. Venous samples can be used to give information about acid-base status and ventilation.

Most commonly available "bedside" blood gas analyzers also measure electrolytes and may provide some other serum chemistry information, such as blood glucose or creatinine. This information is very useful in the immediate assessment of an unstable patient.

Indications

Any patient arriving at the emergency department with a potentially serious illness or trauma may benefit from blood gas analysis. A blood gas analysis is particularly helpful in patients with the following:

- Respiratory emergencies including the following:
  - Pulmonary thromboembolism
  - Pneumonia
  - Congestive heart failure
- Metabolic emergencies including the following:
  - Urethral obstruction

- Diabetic ketoacidosis or nonketotic hyperosmolar crisis
- Eclampsia
- Hypoadrenocorticism (Addison's disease)
- Ethylene glycol toxicity
- Any form of shock

Equipment

When considering blood gas equipment, reliability and ease of use are the first priorities. Both hand-held and larger machines are available. Most are easy to use, but among electrolyte analyzers, more maintenance is needed for the larger machines than for hand-held units. However, hand-held units tend to be less cost effective than the larger units if a large number of samples are being run. Different machines may analyze only blood gases, or they may analyze blood gases and electrolytes, or blood gases, electrolytes, and chemistries, on a single blood sample.

All users should be instructed in the sampling and sample input procedures for the machine. If a larger machine is in place, one person should be assigned to be in charge of blood gas equipment maintenance. This can be done only by reading the technical manual and developing a close relationship with the provider's technical support branch. All maintenance instructions should be followed precisely; if calibrations are needed, these must be done daily.

One of the most popular blood gas analyzers is the iSTAT Blood Gas Analyzer made by the Heska Corporation. It is a small, hand-held unit with an available printer attachment that allows a clinic to choose from several cartridges to tailor the results to the patient's needs. Individual cartridges are easy to use and require less than 0.1 ml of anticoagulated blood.

An alternative blood gas analyzer in use is the Critical Care Xpress made by the Nova Corporation. This machine is a larger tabletop unit that requires quite a bit of maintenance; however, it can provide more values with a 0.15 ml blood sample. Although this analyzer carries a larger price tag, it is more versatile.

Technique

Blood for blood gas analysis should be collected into syringes or containers coated with 1:1000 diluted heparin. The preferred collection containers are commercially available syringes preloaded with a dehydrated heparin pellet or arterial sampling "pens" that fill heparin-coated capillary tubes via arterial pressure.

If these are not available, then manually heparinized syringes can be made. The syringe is filled with heparin (1000 U/ml) and the heparin is expelled. The blood sample can then be drawn. Commercially available blood gas syringes and arterial samplers have minimum sample requirements to ensure the correct ratio of blood to anticoagulant. The machine may only require 0.125 to 0.3 ml of blood even though more may need to be drawn for the specific container. If using a heparinized syringe, the sample must be gently rolled in the hands to ensure mixing of the heparin with the blood.

Venous samples may be drawn from any peripheral or central vein. The status of the tissues in the area from which the blood was sampled can affect results. For example, a sample taken from a vein in a traumatized limb will be different from a sample taken from a vein that has more normal blood flow.

Arterial sampling should be done via an arterial puncture or arterial catheter using a 25- or 26-gauge needle. Arterial samples are most often collected from the femoral artery and the dorsal pedal artery. To puncture an artery, the technician should first feel for a good pulse. Positioning for the sample is with either one or two fingers on the pulse. If using the one-finger method, then the technician should feel for the pulse, visualize the artery under his or her finger, and aim the needle at a 45-degree angle toward the pulse. The needle should enter the artery, and blood will travel into the self-filling syringe or into the capillary tubes in a specialty arterial gas pen until the desired amount is reached. If using the two-fingered method, then the technician should feel for the pulse with two fingers spaced about one inch apart. The needle should be positioned at a 90-degree angle, halfway between the two fingers. On entering the artery, the blood should pulse up the syringe barrel. After the sample is drawn, any air bubbles should be expelled and the syringe capped tightly. If using an arterial capillary sampler, the blood should be allowed to fill the capillary tubes inside the sampler completely; then the needle should be removed and capped tightly. Ideally, samples should be analyzed immediately or within 15 to 30 minutes if stored at room temperature. If a sample cannot be analyzed right away, then the technician should place the tightly capped syringe into an ice bath and analyze within 1 hour. Most analyzers will require additional information, including the patient's identification number, temperature, and the percent of inspired oxygen the animal is breathing at the time of sampling (FiO_2). The percentage of oxygen in room air at sea level is 21%. For optimal results, a core temperature should be taken no more than 5 minutes before drawing the blood. All of this information should be acquired and recorded before drawing the sample.

An arterial catheter can be placed in a dorsal pedal artery using aseptic technique. It is recommended to have a three-way stopcock on the line to draw blood and flush the catheter well. These catheters should be labeled as an arterial line and must be monitored frequently. An arterial line must also be flushed with heparinized saline (150 IU/150 ml 0.9 sodium chloride) and optimally heparin locked.

Troubleshooting

Acquiring a blood gas is fairly straightforward. A venous blood gas uses the same technique as drawing a venous blood sample for other blood tests. An arterial blood gas is trickier, but the pulsitile action of the blood in a syringe or capillary tube helps indicate the accuracy of the arterial puncture. Anatomically, a vein lies in close proximity to an artery, and a great chance exists that the vein may be punctured instead. Looking at the values and the clinical picture of the patient is the best way to gauge which sample has been drawn. If the patient appears to be clinically stable and the technician is confident in the accession, then he or she can look to the partial pressure of oxygen (PO_2) and partial pressure of carbon dioxide (PCO_2) to help make the decision. If the patient is in respiratory distress and the PO_2 and PCO_2 numbers are within venous ranges, then a great possibility exists that the accession was executed properly. However, if the patient looks clinically stable and the bloodwork indicates more of a venous sample, then taking a known venous sample may be beneficial to compare numbers. If the PO_2 and PCO_2 of both samples are comparable, then it is highly likely a vein was punctured in both accessions.

An arterial catheter is the optimal way to be consistent in accessions, although a risk of a significant bleed exists if the catheter apparatus is dislodged. The placement of arterial catheters requires more skill than a venous catheter, but technicians can become proficient with practice. After multiple attempts to access the artery without success, the artery can begin to spasm and rendered temporarily useless.

Other problems with a blood gas revolve around the blood gas analyzers. The more complex machines require more calibration and maintenance than some of the hand-held machines. There should be one person designated for all maintenance of this equipment.

Interpretation

This discussion focuses on the components of a blood gas analysis that examines the patient's acid-base and respiratory status (Table 2-1). Electrolytes are addressed in detail in their own section of this chapter.

Definitions. The following definitions should be noted:

- Pao_2 is the partial pressure of oxygen in the blood. This value indicates how well the blood is being oxygenated. This number is looked at to try to ascertain how well the lungs and pulmonary circulation is functioning.
- pH is a measure of the acidity or alkalinity of the blood. In general, pH measures the amount of hydrogen ions in the blood. The pH value has a narrow window of normalcy. If the value strays beyond normal, the buffering system is triggered to help compensate for the abnormal value. This value is affected by both metabolic and respiratory factors. Technicians use the rest of the arterial blood gas values to sort out where the patient is failing and compensating.
- $Paco_2$ is the partial pressure of carbon dioxide (CO_2) in the circulating blood and is an indicator of ventilation. Because CO_2 acts as an acid, excess CO_2 may cause acidosis or the body may hypoventilate to raise CO_2 levels to compensate

for akalosis. $Paco_2$ is considered the *respiratory component* of a blood gas.
- HCO_3 (or bicarbonate ion) is the major buffer in the body. The level of bicarbonate ion determines the "metabolic component" of a blood gas.
- BE is the base excess (the amount of base above or below the normal buffer level). A base *deficit* is how far away from zero a patient is to the *negative* and describes how many units of base are needed to return the patient to neutral. A base *excess* describes how far from zero to the *positive* a patient is. A base excess or deficit indicates a *metabolic* disturbance or compensation in the patient's blood chemistry.

Simple Blood Gas Analysis. The following information should be noted:

- A simple acid-base disturbance is one with a primary disorder and the appropriate compensation.
- A mixed acid-base disturbance has at least two separate, simultaneous disturbances.
- The technician should begin by determining whether an acid-base disturbance is present by comparing the pH to the normal range. If the pH is normal, usually an acid-base disturbance is not present. In certain circumstances, the pH may be normal, but the bicarbonate ion, $Paco_2$, or base excess (or a combination of these factors) may be abnormal, indicating a compensated acid-base disturbance. If the pH is less than normal, the blood is acidemic. If the pH is greater than the normal range, the blood is aklalemic.

TABLE 2-1 🔬

Normal Blood Gas Values*

Sample	pH	Pco$_2$ (mm Hg)	HCO$_3$ (mm Hg)	Po$_2$ (mm Hg)
Dog venous	7.32-7.40	33-50	18-26	
Dog arterial	7.36-7.44	36-44	18-26	85-100
Cat venous	7.28-7.41	33-45	18-23	
Cat arterial	7.36-7.44	28-32	17-22	85-100

From Willard MD, Tvedten H, Turnwald GH: *Small animal clinical diagnosis by laboratory methods,* ed 3, Philadelphia, 1999, WB Saunders, p 103.

*In-house normal values should be established if the machine does not come with a published reference range.

- Next the technician should examine the base excess and the bicarbonate ion level. If they are above normal, then either primary or compensatory metabolic alkalosis is present. Metabolic acidosis is a common disturbance and can be caused by condition such as diabetic ketoacidosis or kidney failure. If the base excess and the bicarbonate ion level are low, then either primary or compensatory metabolic alkalosis exists. Metabolic alkalosis is less common in small animal species but can be seen with vomiting.
- Then the technician should compare the $Paco_2$ with normal ranges. If it is high, then either a primary or compensatory respiratory acidosis exists. If it is low, then either a primary or compensatory respiratory alkalosis exists. A high $Paco_2$ is the definition of hypoventilation and commonly occurs in patients with respiratory depression for any reason, including anesthesia. Respiratory alkalosis can occur with hyperventilation, occasionally pulmonary disease, or more commonly as a compensation for metabolic acidosis.
- The Pao_2 should be between 90 and 100 mm Hg with normal lungs while the patient is breathing room air (Fio_2). The expected Pao_2 for patients breathing different Fio_2 should be approximately $5 \times Fio_2$. For example, an anesthetized patient breathing 100% oxygen should have a Pao_2 of about 500 mm Hg. Values less than these are indicative of hypoxemia, and oxygen therapy is generally indicated below 60 mm Hg.

Colloid Osmotic Pressure

The definition of colloid osmotic pressure (COP) is the pressure exerted by colloid particles dissolved in a solution on a semipermeable membrane. To understand this concept, one should picture a bucket of fluid that is separated in the middle by a semipermeable membrane. This membrane will let smaller particles and water pass through to either side easily, but larger particles are forced to stay in their original compartments. Crystalloids are the smaller particles; colloids are the larger particles. If more colloid particles are found on one side compared with the other, the fluid and crystalloid particles will move from the side with the lower number of colloids (i.e., lower concentration) to the side with the higher number of colloids (i.e., higher concentration) to even out the pressure on the membrane. COP is the measurement of the pressure exerted on the capillary membrane by the colloid particles. COP helps technicians compare the concentration of one colloid solution with another. COP also determines the fluid flux among the various body fluid compartments. Importantly, it is the number of particles (not the size of the particles) that determines the COP. However, the size of the particle is what determines how long it is retained within the intravascular space.

Natural colloids are the proteins found in plasma. They consist of albumin, globulin, and fibrinogen. Synthetic colloids are water-based solutions that contain particles of several different sizes. Some examples are Dextran 70, hetastarch, pentastarch, and Hb solutions (Hb-based oxygen carriers).

Indications

Blood COP is important to help determine whether the vasculature is allowing too much of the plasma proteins to leak into the interstitium or the compartment outside the vessel. If fluid is allowed to leak outside of the vasculature, then edema or swelling will appear. Vasculitis or systemic inflammatory response syndrome are disease processes that will cause leaky vessels and low protein levels. In cases where hypovolemia is present, such as blood loss and shock, a low COP may indicate the need to rapidly expand the intravascular space. Colloid administration will draw water and electrolytes into the vasculature to help expand the circulatory system.

COP helps technicians determine the concentration of plasma proteins in the blood. A lack of plasma proteins is an indication for the clinician to administer some kind of colloid, whether in plasma, hetastarch, or in the form of dextrans, to help restore fluid pressure balance. The large colloid particles will help draw fluid back into the vessels. Keeping the blood proteins at a consistent level helps maintain the proper fluid balance to allow the body to function properly. On the other hand, if the COP is normal, indicating adequate plasma proteins, but other clinical factors such as a high total protein reading arise, then this would indicate to the clinician that he or she may need to administer crystalloids to restore fluid balance.

Equipment

A colloid osmometer measures the COP of blood, plasma, or serum. The machine uses a semipermeable membrane that separates the plasma entry port from a protein-free solution. It is recommended to use heparinized whole blood samples for clinical ease. The machine must be well maintained to ensure accurate results. It must be calibrated every day with solutions of a known COP, and it must be flushed with saline daily and zeroed with saline before and after each use.

Technique

The technician should draw a sample of whole blood into a heparinized syringe or vacutainer tube treated with lithium heparin. He or she should check for clots by carefully rolling tube in between two hands and expel a small amount of blood from the syringe (or insert a thin wooden stick into the blood in the tube and drag along the side). If no evidence of clotting is seen, the technician should proceed with sampling.

Troubleshooting

Once synthetic colloids are administered, one cannot correlate the total solid measurement to the COP. The solids reading may not take into account the amount of particles added from the synthetic colloids; therefore the COP reading is the more appropriate number to extrapolate information from.

Interpretation of Results

Normal values of whole blood range from 15.3 to 26.3 (mean 19.95) mm Hg in dogs and 17.6 to 33.1 (mean 24.7) mm Hg in cats.

Lactate

Lactate is a byproduct of the breakdown of glucose in anaerobic conditions (when tissue oxygen delivery is inadequate). It is normal to have some lactate circulating in the bloodstream. The liver is responsible for clearing lactate from the body by converting it back to glucose or oxidizing the molecule to CO_2 and water. Elevated lactate concentrations can serve as a marker for a diverse group of serious underlying conditions.

Indications

Lactate concentrations are usually considered to be accurate indicators of inadequate tissue perfusion. Therefore any patient at risk of poor perfusion

should have lactate levels monitored. This includes patients with the following:

- Animals in shock or any patient suspected of being in shock
- Animals with circulatory disturbances as in heart failure, thrombosis, or gastric dilation volvulus
- Animals with trauma, especially crush injuries

Equipment

Both hand-held and bench top machines are available to measure lactate levels. The iSTAT analyzer and the Critical Care Xpress analyze lactate on specifically ordered panels. For the Nova Critical Care Xpress, a minimum of 0.15 ml whole blood must be collected in a lithium heparin tube. Several hand held lactate analyzers are marketed toward athletes. The AccuCheck hand-held model requires a drop of whole blood. Each machine uses specify sample types; therefore checking with the manufacture for the particular machine is important.

Technique

Lactate can be measured using venous or arterial blood samples. The samples must be analyzed within 30 minutes. The method of analysis varies by machine type.

Troubleshooting

As with any equipment, a certain amount of maintenance is to be expected. The smaller, hand-held machines simpler. The technician must handle the calibrations and codes, but otherwise the machines are easy to set up and use. As mentioned earlier, the larger tabletop machines require far more maintenance and should be monitored and maintained by one or two individuals.

When preparing any blood for sampling, the blood should be tested for clots before insertion into the machine. The sample should also be mixed before sampling for uniformity.

Interpretation of Results

- Normal lactate levels: <2.5 mmol/L (dog), <1.5 mmol/L (cat)
- Mild increase: 3 to 5 mmol/L
- Moderate increase: 5 to 10 mmol/L
- Severe increase: >10 mmol/L

Increased lactate levels fall into one of two types of lactic acidosis: Types A and B. Type A lactic acidosis is the result of tissue hypoxia, poor tissue perfusion, and shock. Gastric dilation volvulus or septic abdomens caused by intestinal perforation are two examples where lactic acid concentrations will be elevated.

Type B lactic acidosis can be categorized in one of four groups:

1. Systemic illness (diastolic murmur, rheumatic fever, infection, leukemia)
2. Drugs and toxins (ethanol, salicylates, methanol)
3. Heredity and congenital errors in metabolism (glucose 6-phosphatase deficiency)
4. Miscellaneous

The most important aspect of lactate analysis to consider is that one sample is only a snapshot of the patient's condition. Serial lactate levels provide a more accurate picture of a disease process. To correct the abnormality, the underlying cause of the lactic acidosis must be treated. For example, poor tissue perfusion and shock require boluses of fluids, either crystalloids, colloids, or both. Oxygen support may be needed to reverse hypoxia. The inability to reduce plasma lactate concentrations may be a poor prognosticator of survival.

Treating lactic acidosis quickly and effectively will increase the patient's chances for survival. In general, tissue perfusion and oxygenation should be improved by aggressive fluid therapy +/− oxygen support, provided spontaneous ventilation is adequate.

Coagulation Tests

Coagulation abnormalities are common in patients who are critically ill. Coagulopathies can be associated with trauma and sepsis, as well as autoimmune, congenital, or idiopathic disease conditions. Determining the coagulation status of patients is imperative to assess the risk associated with diagnostic procedures and surgeries. For patients at substantial risk of bleeding, coagulation status should be determined before routine procedures such as IV catheter placement and cystocentesis are performed.

Tests of the patient's coagulation status that can be performed on site in the veterinary hospital include one-stage prothrombin time (PT), activated partial thromboplastin time (aPTT), activated clotting time (ACT), buccal mucosal bleeding time (BMBT), and platelet counts. Samples must be taken correctly for accurate coagulation tests. These tests determine whether deficiencies exist in different parts of the coagulation cascade. By identifying what part of the coagulation system is abnormal, specific treatment including blood component therapy can be tailored to the exact problem.

Indications

Many patients in the critical care setting should have clotting function assessed either at presentation or during their treatment. Patients with diagnoses or possible diagnoses listed are especially at risk of coagulopathies:

- Rodenticide toxicity
- Thrombocytopenia
- Immune-mediated hemolytic anemia
- Sepsis
- Disseminated intravascular coagulopathy
- Protein-losing nephropathies
- Liver disease
- Immune suppression as the result of drug therapy
- Receipt of large-volume blood transfusion

Equipment

POC testing for coagulation function is available for veterinary patients. At least two automated, tabletop devices are now in use. These analyzers use fresh whole blood or citrated blood and are most often used to analyze the PT and aPTT; however, they can also can measure ACT.

The ACT test can also be run using special vacutainer tubes filled with diatomaceous earth. The only other equipment needed is a heating block and a timer.

The BMBT requires a spring-loaded device that cuts two uniform incisions. The Simplate is one of these devices. Gauze squares or coffee filter paper and a timer are also required to perform the test.

Manual platelet counts can be done from a blood smear, or automated counts can be performed using an automated hematology analyzer calibrated for veterinary species.

Technique

In patients with possible coagulopathy, blood samples should be collected from peripheral veins rather than central veins in case of excessive bleeding as a result of venipuncture.

A straight vacutainer collection system or a vacutainer tube holder with a vacutainer butterfly line is used to draw 1 ml of blood into a dummy tube and discarded. The sodium citrate tube is filled with the correct amount of blood to avoid dilution. The tube is checked for clots by placing a wooden dowel in and drawing it up the side of the tube. If no clot is present, then the sample is ready for analysis. The technician should follow directions for the particular POC analyzer to complete the process. If fresh whole blood is to be used, then the blood must be placed immediately into the warmed cartridge after venipuncture.

A manual ACT is run using 3 ml whole blood. The venipuncture must be clean and blood must flow readily into the syringe. A venipuncture is performed and the first 1 ml is drawn and discarded. A new syringe is attached to the needle and 2 ml is drawn and placed directly into the ACT tube. Alternatively, a straight vacutainer collection system or a vacutainer butterfly set with the tube holders can be used. A dummy tube is filled with 1 ml of blood and discarded. The sample is then collected in an ACT tube. If the technician is concerned about iatrogenic blood loss, then the first 1 ml of blood does not need to be collected. The tube is rotated five times to ensure that the sample is mixed well. The tube is then placed in heating block at 37° C, and the time to formation of a clot is noted. The first reading is taken at 60 seconds. The technician does this by rotating the tube and doing a visual check for clot formation. If a clot is not present, then the tube is replaced in the heating block and checked every 5 seconds until a clot is noted.

The BMBT is performed using a spring-loaded device to standardize the size of the incision. The Simplate (a disposable device with a retractable blade) is used to cut two uniform incisions. The site used is the labial mucosa, which is exposed by folding the dorsal lip upward. A piece of gauze tied lightly around the muzzle can hold the lip back and increase venous hydrostatic pressure. The Simplate is placed over the site and the trigger is released. Timing of the test begins at this time. Coffee filter paper or gauze is held close to the incision site to absorb the blood. The actual incision site should not be touched because this will interfere with the test results. Timing is stopped once the flow has stopped and a clot is present. This value, reported in seconds, is the BMBT.

The technician calculates manual platelet estimates by counting the mean number of platelets in 5 to 10 microscope fields under 100× oil magnification and multiplying this number by 15,000. This estimates platelets/μl. The smear should be examined for clumping and examined in an area of a thin uniform layer.

(The reader should refer to the hematology section for information on analyzers for automated platelet counts.)

Troubleshooting

The patient's disease process needs to be taken into consideration any time a blood sample is drawn. The patient with anemia can only afford to give enough blood that avoids dilution within the vacutainer tubes to prevent iatrogenic blood loss. The area of venous access should be clipped and swabbed with a cotton ball soaked in alcohol. This helps prevent sample artifact.

The most consistently accurate samples are those taken in one venipuncture. This will help prevent excess bleeding, hematoma, and clot formation, and it provides the sample most representative of the circulating blood.

Pressure bandages should be applied over the venipuncture site for no less than 5 minutes to minimize bleeding. If a patient has a known coagulopathy, then a pressure bandage may need to stay on the site for a longer period of time. The site and surrounding tissue needs to be monitored closely for extraneous swelling.

Platelet clumping may occur if a sample is not collected using a vacutainer or if the sample is not analyzed soon after collection. If this happens, the platelet count may be falsely read as low. The blood sample should always be mixed gently and well in the EDTA tube for best results.

Interpretation

The PT and partial thromboplastin time (PTT) tests evaluate the extrinsic (external) and intrinsic (internal) and common portions of the clotting cascade. The coagulation cascade is made up of many clotting factors that work in conjunction with each other and with vitamin K to maintain the body's ability to clot. Normal ranges for PT and PTT will vary between analyzers. Normal values need to be established for individual machines. Prolonged results indicate a disruption in the coagulation cascade. If either the PT or the PTT is normal, and the other prolonged, several clotting factors can be ruled out. This is important when a question exists as to which of the plasma products available need to be administered.

Both the BMBT test and the platelet count are two diagnostic tests to determine bleeding disorders caused by a *primary hemostasis*. Primary hemostasis problems are related to platelet or vessel disorders. These disorders include von Willebrand's disease, thrombocytopenia, thrombocytopathia, and vasculopathies. The BMBT is a good test to perform for possible vasculitis or thrombocytopenia (low platelets). A platelet count is directly related to clot formation function. If an animal has low platelets, it will have a diminished ability to form a clot. The platelets start the clotting process. If the platelets are not there or do not work properly, then a clot cannot form. If the clot cannot form and unless pressure is applied to this area, then continual bleeding will occur. This animal is now predisposed to bleeding even with the minimal amounts of trauma.

ACT is a simple screening test for severe abnormalities in the intrinsic and common pathways of the coagulation cascade. It measures the time for the fibrin clot to form after activation by the diatomaceous earth in the tubes. PT, PTT, and ACT are some of the diagnostics for determining whether a *secondary hemostasis* exists, or formation of a secondary clot is present. Bleeding disorders related to secondary hemostasis are related to problems with the coagulation cascade. These are circumstances such as rodenticide ingestion, drug toxicity, and liver disease.

- Normal ACT time is 90 to 120 seconds for dogs and 60 to 90 seconds for cats.
- Normal BMBT range is 1.7 to 4.2 minutes for dogs and 1.0 to 3.2 minutes for cats.
- Normal platelet count is 160 to 525 × 10³ cells/μl for dogs and 160 to 660 × 10³ cells/μl for cats.

Basic Tools for Monitoring in the Intensive Care Unit

Patient monitoring can be artificially divided between traditional, physical examination–based monitoring and mechanical equipment–based techniques. As more complex monitoring equipment becomes affordable and consistently available in animal hospitals, it is important to remember that hands-on monitoring, such as observation of respiratory effort or body temperature, provides essential information about a patient that is as important as equipment-derived data.

Monitoring equipment can be obtained as new or used pieces. Because of the expense involved and how dependent medical care becomes on the results of monitoring, warranties and service contracts should be carefully scrutinized. Easily accessible, 24-hour technical service should be provided by the companies either supplying the machines or by the service contract provider.

One or two people should be appointed to maintain these machines, but all staff members should have the manuals available to them in case of breakdowns. Because each piece of machinery is different, staff training should include how to work and maintain all monitoring equipment.

Nothing can replace the human being in patient monitoring. Tools and machines may provide information that a physical examination or laboratory parameter cannot, but it is the human being who assesses the information, determines its validity, and develops a diagnostic or treatment plan based on the findings. Machines can err, and all unexpected abnormalities should be confirmed before treatment is adjusted. Confirming results may be as simple as getting another reading, but confirmation may also involve performing a second test. For instance, if the pulse oximeter is reading 75% but the patient has pink mucous membranes and is breathing normally, then the probe position should be checked before the patient can be assessed as being severely hypoxic.

A thorough physical examination is irreplaceable as a monitoring tool. Temperature monitoring is important. An elevated temperature may indicate hyperthermia, infection, or inflammation. A subnormal temperature may indicate environmental hypothermia, poor perfusion, or a decreased metabolic rate secondary to medications (e.g., opioids) or disease (e.g., hypoglycemia, hypothyroidism). Because metabolic rates are associated closely with temperature, it is vital to know the patient's temperature at all times. This can be especially important in shock states or in anesthetized patients in whom vital organs systems such as cardiac function and coagulation can be adversely affected by hypothermia. Continuous temperature monitoring should be performed in anesthetized patients. Temperature can be taken using aural, esophageal, or rectal thermometers. Ear infections, long ear canals, and environmental temperature can reduce the accuracy of aural thermometer readings. Rectal temperature may not reflect core temperature in poorly perfusing patients. Continuous core temperature probes are often part of multifunction monitors.

The stethoscope is a vital extension of the technician's ears and eyes. Abnormal breathing patterns, abnormal audible sounds, and coughing are indications for auscultation of the larynx, trachea, lungs, and heart. Baseline values should be obtained at the time of admission or at the beginning of each shift to assess changes in the patient's condition. If gastrointestinal function is abnormal, then gut sounds should be ausculted regularly. A lack of sounds indicates the possibility of ileus. An esophageal stethoscope is a useful tool in the anesthetized patient or a patient with long-term ventilator use. It allows clear auscultation of the lungs and heart and may allow early detection of abnormalities such as pulmonary cackles and heart murmurs.

Electrocardiogram Monitoring

The electrocardiogram (ECG) is a record of the electrical activity of the heart muscle used to monitor heart rhythm. Changes in the size or structure of the heart are also reflected in the ECG because those changes affect the direction and speed at which electrical impulses travel through the heart.

Indications

ECGs are used as diagnostic and monitoring tools. Many patients arriving at the emergency department or being treated in an ICU should have ECG tracings recorded at some point during the assessment or treatment, because heart function can be affected by many conditions other than primary cardiac disease. An ECG is often used to confirm arrhythmias ausculted using a stethoscope. Many arrhythmias are too subtle to be heard on auscultation or are intermittent, so normal auscultation does not negate the importance of ECG monitoring. In critically ill animals, continuous or serial intermittent ECG monitoring provides important information about trends in cardiovascular function.

Specific indications for ECG monitoring are the following:

- Trauma (especially with significant hemorrhage or possible thoracic cavity trauma)

- Shock (cardiogenic, hypovolemic, and distributive)
- Possible systemic inflammatory response syndrome or multiple organ dysfunction syndrome
- Syncope or collapse
- Anesthetized patients
- Poisoning or intoxication
- During cardiopulmonary cerebral resuscitation
- Cardiac or pulmonary disease
- Any ausculted arrhythmia
- During the IV bolus administration of drugs (i.e., potassium gluconate, sodium bicarbonate) that can produce arrhythmias

Equipment

ECG machines can provide results using a continuous display screen, a printout, or both. Because the technician can only gather accurate measurements by measuring waveforms and distances, printing capability is necessary for full assessment. A continuous display is important for monitoring of critical patients because their heart rhythms are expected to change over time.

ECG monitors also vary in the way they are connected to the patient. Traditionally, lead wires were connected to both the patient and the machine, limiting mobility of the patient. Telemetry units have leads attached to the patient along with a battery pack, usually slung around the patient's neck or taped to the body, which wirelessly transmits an ECG signal to monitors placed in convenient locations. Hand-held monitors, without leads, are available. These small devices are held against the patient's chest and a tracing is obtained. Most models have some memory capabilities to store tracings and some have printout capabilities. Although the quality of these tracings often is not equal to that obtained with regular ECG leads, the quality of the machines is improving; the major advantage is that a quick rhythm strip can be obtained in the examination room or at the patient's cage. Esophageal ECG devices are available for use in anesthetized patients. These devices tend not to be affected by other electronic monitoring equipment, as are external devices. They should not be used in combination with electrocautery units.

Technique

The technician should place the patient in right lateral recumbency, on the floor or a table covered with paper or a nonconducting material (metal tables should be avoided). Dyspneic or fractious animals can have ECGs recorded in any position. These tracings cannot be compared with standardized measurements but may still be useful to provide rhythm information.

The electrodes may be attached to the skin by alligator clips, wire, or adhesive patches. The alligator clips may be less traumatic if the teeth are filed, the spring is loosened, or a gauze or paper towel patch protects the skin inside a clip. If clips or wires are placed, then the technician should saturate the area with alcohol or ECG paste to provide good contact. For long-term attachment of traumatic alligator clips, wire suture may be preplaced and the clips attached to the wire. To do this, a 20- or 22-gauge hypodermic needle is passed through the skin in the desired location and the wire is threaded through the needle. The needle is removed, leaving the wire in place. The ends of the wire are twisted together to prevent inadvertent removal. It is advisable to place tape around the ends of the wire for safety and as a visual reminder that wires have been placed. The ECG clips then are attached to the wires.

Alcohol should not be used if the leads are being attached during CPR and, potentially, defibrillation because doing so is a fire hazard.

Alternatively, ECG patches can be applied to the skin. To improve adhesion, the skin should be well shaved, cleaned with alcohol, and dried before patch placement. Tissue glue can be used sparingly if needed. In recumbent patients the patches can be placed on the metacarpal and metatarsal pads and held in place using tape placed circumferentially.

The standard lead II or six-lead ECG is recorded using four electrodes that are attached to the patient. In most cases the unit has five leads or electrodes that are color coded and labeled on the basis of the human anatomy: right foreleg (RA), white lead; left foreleg (LA), black lead; right hind leg (RL), green lead; left hind leg (LL), red lead; and the V lead (C), which is an exploring lead and is brown. In most emergency situations, the four limb leads are attached and the V (brown) lead is not. The limb leads are attached just proximal to the point of the elbow and just proximal to the cranial point of the stifle joint.

A strip should include at least 1 minute's worth of tracing at both 50 mm/sec and 25 mm/sec speeds. The strip should be labeled with patient information and the date and time of the tracing, if the machine does not automatically do this.

Troubleshooting

Electrical interference, movement of the patient, and respiratory motion all commonly cause problems with obtaining a clear ECG tracing. Check the electrodes to make sure good contact is achieved with the skin by both placement and enough alcohol or paste. Respiratory motion is usually seen as a regular undulation of the baseline as the chest rises and falls. As long as this is regular, it will not unduly interfere with interpreting a rhythm strip. Conversely, shivering or 60-Hz cycle interference from other electrical equipment attached to the patient or nearby can cause unreadable ECG tracings. This type of tracing will look like a rough or fuzzy baseline, or the whole tracing will irregularly move up and down on the paper. If this happens, then the technician should remove or move other electrical equipment, try moving the electrodes to more peripheral locations on the body, or do both to reduce the interference.

Interpretation of Results

A normal tracing shows a P wave, QRS complex, and T wave, which correspond to atrial depolarization (P wave), ventricular depolarization (QRS complex), and ventricular repolarization (T wave). When reading an ECG rhythm strip, the fundamental principles are to calculate the heart rate, look for overall regularity of rhythm, make sure a P wave is present for every QRS complex (lack of P waves implies atrial fibrillation), and look for abnormally shaped complexes such as ventricular premature contractions.

In an emergency or arrest situation, it is important to confirm that electrical activity (i.e., an ECG waveform) has an associated heartbeat and pulse. Electrical activity does not necessarily mean that the heart is beating. Additionally, electrical complexes and ausculted heartbeats may not produce enough heart function to generate a pulse pressure. This is called a *pulse deficit* and is commonly seen in emergencies such as primary or secondary ventricular tachycardia. A pulse deficit represents a serious condition that must be addressed.

Each wave has a normal duration (milliseconds) and height (millivolts), as well as a normal interval between waves. These measurements are useful in determining the health of the electrical conduction system. Abnormalities are associated with conduction disturbances and can be associated with changes in the heart muscle or pericardial space.

Pulse Oximetry

Pulse oximetry noninvasively calculates oxygen saturation of Hb using spectrophotometry. This gives information about arterial oxygen content and, consequently, tissue oxygen delivery. The saturation of Hb in the arterial blood is usually referred to as Sao_2; however, when measured by pulse oximetry rather than an arterial blood gas, Hb saturation is referred to as SpO_2 and expressed as a percentage. Adult Hb molecules can exist in four forms: (1) oxyhemoglobin (oxygen bound to Hb), (2) deoxyhemoglobin, (3) carboxyhemoglobin (carbon monoxide bound to Hb), and (4) methemoglobin (an irreversible change in the shape of Hb that does not allow it to carry oxygen molecules). The pulse oximeter measures the amount of deoxyhemoglobin and oxyhemoglobin and calculates the relative percent of Hb that is saturated with oxygen.

The basic principle behind this technology is that deoxyhemoglobin absorbs red light but not infrared wavelengths, whereas oxyhemoglobin absorbs infrared wavelengths but not red light. A probe is applied to skin or mucous membrane, across an arterial bed, which emits lights at both red and infrared wavelengths. The relative amounts of each wavelength that are detected by the probe, after the blood absorbs some of each wavelength, allow the saturated proportion to be calculated. The probe will only read pulsatile flow so that the SpO_2 is based on arterial blood levels.

Pulse oximeters display the strength of the pulsatile signal either in a waveform or as a bar code. This signal must remain strong because the accuracy of the oximeter decreases when pulsatile flow is not detected or is poorly detected. Most oximeters give a continuous display of the pulse rate. This should correspond to the palpable pulse and ausculted heart rate to ensure accuracy.

Indications

- Animals at risk for hypoxemia
  - Patients with tachypnea or dyspnea
  - Patients who are anesthetized
  - Patients who are critically ill
  - Patients in rapidly deteriorating conditions
- Animals being monitored because they are receiving oxygen therapy or mechanical ventilation

Equipment

Pulse oximeters come as hand-held portable monitors or tabletop monitors. They are also often part of multifunction monitors. Tabletop monitors display a waveform and a digital readout to help confirm an arterial signal and accurate reading.

The probe can either be a transmittance type (the probe has two pieces; one side of a clip contains an light-emitting diode [LED] that shines across tissue to a second piece that acts as a photodetector) or reflectance type (both the LED and the photodetector are contained in a one-piece probe; the light is reflected off hard tissues back to the probe). Both types of probes are used, but clip type transmittance probes are most common in veterinary practice.

Technique

The probe is placed on skin and must remain in place for at least 30 seconds to obtain an accurate reading.
Probe placement options include the following:

- Tongue
- Lip
- Ear
- Prepuce and vulva
- Toe and toe web
- Metacarpus
- Ventral surface of the tail
- Axillary or inguinal skin fold
- Gastrocneumius tendon

Pigmented areas may not produce accurate readings. Haired areas may need to be clipped and cleaned to allow readings.

Troubleshooting

Potential sources of difficulty in obtaining pulse oximetry readings or accuracy include the following:

- Patient motion
  - Shivering or tremors
  - Seizure activity
- Poor perfusion states
  - Hypothermia
  - Hypovolemia
  - Vasoconstriction for other reasons
- Severe anemia
- Environmental light interference

- Pigmentation in skin, both natural and acquired, as in the following:
  - IV dyes used for diagnostic procedures (Note: Oxyglobin administration does not interfere with pulse oximetry; icterus may or may not interfere with it.)
- Abnormal Hb
  - Methemoglobinemia
  - Carboxyhemoglobin or carbon monoxide toxicity

To help obtain an accurate reading, the area may need to be clipped and cleaned (if appropriate) or warmed. If ambient light is interfering, then the probe can be covered. If the probe has been in position for more than 30 seconds and a strong signal is not obtained, then it can be repositioned.

If the probe is on the tongue of an anesthetized or unconscious patient, it should be repositioned every 5 to 10 minutes because the clips can occlude flow to the area. Whenever low readings are obtained but the reading does not match the patient's clinical status, an arterial blood gas should be evaluated.

Interpretation

A patient with normal lung function breathing room air (or 100% oxygen) should have a SpO_2 above 94%. Pulse oximetry cannot replace direct measurement of Pao_2 using arterial blood gases because SpO_2 does not correlate with Pao_2 in a linear relationship. At approximately 92%, the SpO_2 correlates to a Pao_2 of 60 mm Hg. Below this SpO_2 value, the Pao_2 rapidly declines to life-threatening levels. Patients with SpO_2 levels below 94% should be given supplemental oxygen.

Once the SpO_2 is in the normal range, pulse oximetry cannot detect changes in arterial oxygenation until a significant change has occurred. This can be a serious limitation when the patient is being supplemented with high levels of oxygen. For instance, during general anesthesia when a patient is breathing 100% oxygen, the Pao_2 should be approximately 450 to 500 mm Hg. The oximetry reading will not drop until the Pao_2 has decreased below approximately 100 mm Hg, which is a very significant decline. Therefore pulse oximetry should not be the only method of monitoring respiratory function during general anesthesia or mechanical ventilation. Despite these limitations, it is considered a minimum standard of monitoring human patients under anesthesia and is a very useful noninvasive technique.

End-Tidal Carbon Dioxide Monitoring

Capnometry is the measurement of CO_2 in a gas using spectrophotometry. Using this technology to record the concentration of CO_2 in a single end exhaled (end-tidal) breath is called *capnography*. Capnography provides a noninvasive means of assessing CO_2 levels in the body. Because CO_2 is the major byproduct of tissue metabolism, assessment of body levels give important information about perfusion, metabolism, and ventilation. End-tidal carbon dioxide ($ETCO_2$) monitoring is a reasonable alternative to measuring the $Paco_2$ using arterial blood gas analysis. All general anesthetic agents and many analgesics such as narcotics cause respiratory depression. This leads to a buildup of CO_2 or a respiratory acidosis. Because of this, $ETCO_2$ monitoring is always indicated in an anesthetized patient or for one in which respiratory depression or hypoventilation is a potential problem.

Indications

- Monitoring of ventilation in spontaneously breathing anesthetized or comatose, intubated patients
- Confirmation of endotracheal and feeding tube placement
- Monitoring of cardiopulmonary cerebral resuscitation
- Monitoring of patients undergoing mechanical ventilation

Equipment and Technique

Capnometers are either hand-held monitors or larger tabletop monitors. A sensor or sampling tube is attached between the breathing circuit and the endotracheal tube or on the open end of the endotracheal tube if it is not attached to a circuit. $ETCO_2$ can be measured with the sensor placed on the end of a tightly fitting face mask, although this technique is less accurate that in an intubated patient.

In sidestream type monitors, a sample of gas is sent down a small-bore tube that exits near the end of the endotracheal tube. The sample is measured away from the end of the tube. In mainstream type monitors, the measurement takes place right at the end of the tube. (The reader should refer to the troubleshooting section for more information on the difference between the two types.)

Both types of monitors display a numeric value, and most monitors also display a waveform. The waveform, or capnogram, is a graphic display of the changes in $ETCO_2$ over time. The shape of the capnogram provides important information about respiratory patterns, technical problems such as endotracheal tube occlusion or excessive rebreathing, and patient perfusion. Hand-held monitors do not provide capnograms. Some monitors will provide printouts of capnograms. Most multichannel monitors also include capnometry. (The reader should refer to the end of this chapter for more information about mutichannel monitors.)

Troubleshooting

Both sidestream and mainstream monitors have problems that may interfere with their accuracy and ease of use. With sidestream sampling, the small size of the sampling tube can lead to occlusion with secretions. Sidestream capnographs draw off a portion of the gas flow and may require increased oxygen flow rates (especially in small patients on low-flow closed circuit systems). Mainstream capnographs have heated sensors to prevent condensation of moisture from the exhaled gases. With long-term use, the inhaled gases can be heated enough to pose a risk of burns to the respiratory mucosa. Additionally, the larger device attached to the breathing circuit in a mainstream sampler adds significant dead space and weight to the tubing. Leakage of any portion in the breathing circuit (from the sidestream sampling tube) or at the level of a mainstream sensor can falsely lower readings. Mainstream monitors also require longer warm-up time and more frequent calibration that may make them unsuitable for use in an emergency or arrest situation.

Moisture can interfere with readings in both types of monitors. For this reason, the sensor should be positioned above the level of patient so that moisture in the endotracheal tube does not accumulate in the sensor or tubing. Sampling tubing and sensor devices should be checked regularly for accumulations of respiratory secretions or condensation, especially if readings do not correlate with the status of the patient based on other monitoring values. If the patient is stable enough to permit disconnection of the device, then exhaling into the sensor will easily rule out mechanical failure of a capnograph.

Interpretation

Normal arterial CO_2 values for an anesthetized patient with normal perfusion and pulmonary function are about 35 to 45 mm Hg. The $ETCO_2$ is 2 to 5 mm Hg less than the arterial value. The waveform or capnogram produced by exhaled CO_2 has a unique shape. Changes in the shape of the waveform give information about respiration and anesthesia technical problems. Basic analysis of the capnogram should include the following:

- Presence or absence of a waveform:
  - Absence of a waveform may indicate cardiac or respiratory arrest, apnea, disconnection of the breathing circuit, esophageal intubation or extubation, complete obstruction of the endotracheal tube, or malfunction of the monitor.
- Noting the actual $ETCO_2$ and comparing it with normal reference ranges:
  - Elevated CO_2 can result from either increased CO_2 production (usually from increased metabolism as in fever or seizure activity) or decreased elimination (i.e., hypoventilation).
  - Low CO_2 may indicate either decreased metabolism as in hypothermia or increased elimination with hyperventilation.
- Examination of the shape of the waveform:
  - If the baseline is above zero, then it usually indicates rebreathing of exhaled gases from exhausted soda lime or low fresh gas flow.
  - Gradual rise in the $ETCO_2$ without a normal plateau may indicate airway obstruction or kinked endotracheal tube.
  - A sharply peaked wave may be caused by tachypnea or a leak in the circuit.
  - A sudden drop in the wave to very low or zero can indicate disconnection or large leak, airway obstruction, extubation, or arrest.

Central Venous Pressure

Central venous pressure measurement (CVP) estimates the blood pressure (BP) within the right atrium by measuring pressure in the cranial or caudal vena cava. Right atrial pressure is a good indicator of vascular volume, so CVP is useful for monitoring fluid therapy in hypovolemic patients or patients at risk for volume overload.

Indications

Indications for CVP measurement include monitoring fluid therapy in patients who may be hypovolemic, such as in the following cases:

- Patients who have experienced trauma
- Patients with gastric dilation volvulus
- Patients with hemoabdomen

CVP measurement may also be indicated for monitoring patients at risk of volume overload such as in the following cases:

- Patients with preexisting heart disease who require IV fluid therapy
- Patients with right ventricular congestive heart failure
- Patients requiring high-volume IV fluid diuresis

Equipment

To measure CVP a central venous catheter must be placed in either the jugular, femoral, or saphenous vein. When placing a jugular catheter, the tip must be positioned at the entrance to the right atrium. For femoral or saphenous catheters, the tip should be positioned at the junction of the vein with caudal vena cava. If the catheter tip is proximal to either of these locations, then the measurements do not accurately reflect pressures in the right atrium. These measurements may still be used as trend measurements for intravascular volume estimates.

CVP measurements can be obtained using either a water manometer or an electronic pressure transducer. Water manometers are sold as disposable kits and consist usually of a clear plastic column that is marked in centimeters. Alternatively, a piece of plastic tubing can be taped to the wall of the cage with a metric ruler next to it for a "homemade" water manometer. The manometer is connected to the central venous catheter by extension tubing and a three-way stopcock. The setup is filled with heparinized saline from a syringe or fluid bag attached to the three-way stopcock. Vitamin B complex can be added to the fluids for better visualization of the fluid column. Single measurements are taken with

a water manometer. Electronic pressure transducers are often part of multifunction monitors but may be stand-alone monitors also. These monitors are attached to the patient's catheter using special extension tubing and the transducer. A display screen shows a pressure waveform and gives a continuous readout of the CVP.

Technique

For all techniques, a freely flowing catheter without occlusions is essential. The patient must be in the same position for each reading to allow the technician to compare readings and record patient position at each measurement. Lateral recumbency is ideal, but sternal recumbency is also used. A reference or zero point must be established by one of two methods. In the most widely used method, the three-way stopcock and bottom of the manometer is positioned at the level of the right atrium to establish a zero point. This level is at the height of the manubrium in a lateral patient or the scapulohumeral joint with the patient in sternal recumbency. The manometer may be taped in place on the wall of the cage so that the reference point is kept constant. Alternatively, the manometer and stopcock may be held on a stable surface next to the down shoulder in a lateral patient or the elbows in a sternal patient. An imaginary line from the level of the right atrium to the manometer is drawn, and whatever value in centimeters this corresponds to is set as the zero point and recorded for use in subsequent measurements. This value is subtracted from the final measurement to give an absolute CVP.

To obtain a measurement using a water manometer, the stopcock is turned off to the patient and the manometer is filled with saline. The stopcock is then turned off to the fluid bag or syringe, and the fluid level is allowed to equilibrate with the patient. The level of the meniscus is the CVP. This level will fluctuate with respiration because this changes intrathoracic pressure.

When using an electronic pressure transducer, a reference point is also established by placing the tranducer in a set location. This may vary depending on the system used. Once the setup is in place, it can be left connected to the patient for continuous readout. The system and catheter should be flushed with heparinzed saline every 4 to 6 hours or as directed by the manufacturer.

Troubleshooting

Inaccurate readings will be obtained if the following occur:

- Linking or thrombi occludes the catheter.
- Tip of the catheter is not appropriately placed.
- Catheter is moved in or out of the vessel among readings.
- Reference point is not kept constant among readings.
- Patient positioning changes among readings.

Interpretation

Normal CVP ranges from 0 to 5 (or 10, depending on the source) cm water. Values less than this suggest hypovolemia, and values above 10 suggest volume overload. Serial measurements are more useful to gauge response to therapy and trends in intravascular volume than are single numbers. Frequency of measurements depends on the stability of the patient and the potential for rapid deterioration. For example, a patient who has oliguric renal failure and is being given IV fluids may need CVP readings hourly to detect early signs of volume overload. Serial CVP measurements are often useful to guide treatment decisions in unstable patients. For example, IV fluid volumes given can be tailored to responses in the CVP in a patient with traumatic hypovolemic shock.

Blood Pressure

Measurement of arterial BP provides important information about tissue perfusion and overall cardiovascular function. Arterial BP consists of three values: (1) systolic, (2) diastolic, and (3) mean arterial pressures. Systolic pressure is the pressure in the arteries generated by ventricular contraction, and diastolic pressure is the pressure between contractions. Mean arterial pressure is the average pressure during the cardiac cycle. The pulse pressure equals the systolic minus the diastolic pressure and is palpated at the femoral, dorsal pedal, lingual, or other arteries. BP measurements and pulse quality are important monitoring tools in an ICU because organ function declines and cell death can occur at BPs above and below critical values. Therefore changes in BP dictate many therapeutic interventions in patients.

Indications

- Patients with possible cardiovascular abnormalities of any cause including the following:
  - Shock
  - Heart disease
  - Systemic inflammatory response syndrome or multiple organ dysfunction syndrome
- Patients with a rapidly changing clinical status
- Patients who have received anesthesia
- Patients being mechanically ventilated
- Patients with primary diseases that are associated with hypertension including the following:
  - Chronic renal failure
  - Hyperthyroidism
  - Hyperadrenocorticism (Cushing's syndrome)

Equipment

BP can be monitored using direct or indirect techniques. The technician makes direct BP measurements via an arterial catheter, most commonly by an electronic pressure transducer. This is the same equipment that can be used for CVP measurement; however, the system may use special tubing for arterial systems and may be connected to the patient through a fluid-primed pressure dome. Additionally, the system may be kept patent using a unidirectional flushing device that continuously infuses pressurized saline. Manufacturers of electronic pressure tranducers provide detailed information about this specialized equipment. The display will give values for systolic, diastolic, and mean pressure and preferably generates a continuous pressure wave.

Indirect or noninvasive BP can be measured in veterinary patients by automated oscillometric or ultrasonic (Doppler) techniques. Both work by occluding arterial pressure under a cuff. In oscillometric equipment, the machine inflates the cuff to pressures above systolic levels, then cuff pressure is automatically gradually decreased and the microprocessor detects oscillations that change at systolic, mean, and systolic BP. Those values are reported on a display screen. The entire process is automated. Models are manufactured specifically for veterinary use.

In ultrasonic techniques, a manually inflated cuff is attached to an aneroid sphygmomanometer so that readings may be obtained. A small ultrasound probe placed directly over the artery transmits an audible signal of the pulse when the cuff pressure decreases enough to allow flow to return to the artery. Depending on the model, the cuff may either be separate from the ultrasound crystal or attached to it. If separate cuffs are used, then human pediatric BP cuffs of varying sizes are usually used. They are modified for use with a Doppler system by tying a knot in one of the two lengths of tubing on the cuff (the other is connected to the sphygmomanometer). The probe is connected to a receiver-amplifier-speaker unit that is powered by a rechargeable battery. If background noise is significant or the noise of the probe disturbs the patient, then earphones may be connected to the receiver. The piezoelectric crystal in the probe is delicate and can be easily damaged. It should be wiped clean and covered with a manufacturer-supplied cover or a piece of gauze or foam (taped on the unit) when not in use. The cable that attaches the crystal to the receiver may also become worn with heavy use, leading to noise interference or poor performance. To help extend their life, the wire cables should not be bent or kinked.

Technique

Direct Arterial Pressure Monitoring. Direct arterial pressure monitoring is the gold standard for BP measurement. It is underused because of perceived technical difficulties in placing and maintaining arterial catheters, as well as lack of equipment. Arterial catheterization can become routine with practice. The availability of used monitoring equipment and transducers has substantially reduced costs and makes it affordable for any hospital dealing with critically ill or injured patients.

An arterial catheter can be placed in any artery; however, the most commonly used are the dorsal pedal and the femoral arteries. Femoral artery catheters may be harder to maintain because of the difficulties involved in wrapping and stabilizing that location. If a risk of bleeding exists, then it will be easier to maintain hemostasis if a more peripheral artery is catheterized.

Special arterial catheters are available, but commonly available IV catheters may be used (especially for short-term use). The area should be anesthetized with 1 to 2 ml of 2% lidocaine hydrochloride (which can be diluted with saline), injected subcutaneously 10 minutes before the procedure. Percutaneous methods or cutdown methods can be used to place the catheters. Short (1.5 to 2 inch) over-the-needle catheters tend to be difficult to maintain for longer periods of time because they tend to kink. Longer catheters (arterial, through-the-needle, or those placed by Seldinger technique) may last longer. Once the catheters are placed, they must be secured

well to prevent inadvertent dislodging and kinking. Aseptic technique should be observed during placement and maintenance of arterial catheters.

Arterial catheters are prone to thrombosis. Flushing can be accomplished manually by flushing with heparinized saline every hour. Alternatively, the catheters can be connected to a low constant rate infusion of heparinized saline delivered by an infusion pump or a pressurized bag. Electronic pressure transducer systems work with disposable pressurized unidirectional flushing devices that are connected directly to the system. If a transducer system is not available, then BP can be measured directly using the same manometer method as for measuring CVP.

Direct measurements can also be made as single readings using a needle introduced into the femoral artery attached to a pressure tranducer. This is most often performed in dogs. The area should be anesthetized as previously described.

Indirect Blood Pressure Monitoring. BP is measured indirectly using either an oscillometric device or a Doppler ultrasound flow detector. Indirect techniques are less accurate but are noninvasive and require less skill than direct BP monitoring.

Both methods entail placing a pressure cuff over an artery on the limbs or tail. Appropriate cuff size is important for accuracy of readings. The cuff width should be approximately 40% of the circumference of the limb or tail, and the length should be enough to encircle at least 60% of the appendage. Many cuffs have markings on them to indicate whether the fit is appropriate as the cuff is being placed. Some cuffs have markings on them indicating where the artery must come in contact with the cuff. A cuff that is too large can lead to artificially low readings, and a cuff that is too small can lead to artificially elevated readings. A piece of tape should be loosely applied to the cuff to prevent it from popping off when inflated.

Oscillometric devices. The technician should place an appropriately sized cuff distal to the elbow, around the midmetatarsal, or around the base of the tail. A lateral or sternal position gives more accurate readings, because the cuff should be near the level of the heart. The machine can be programmed to provide a single reading or repeated measurements over set time intervals. Most accurate readings in a conscious patient will be obtained with minimal restraint and minimal movement. Five readings should be obtained and averaged, discarding obviously different numbers. Weak pulse signals from poor flow, small arteries, shaking, and movement will interfere with the accuracy of the oscillometric device. Because of these limitations, it may be difficult to obtain readings using this method in very small dogs or cats, conscious animals, or animals in shock. It is very useful in anesthetized patients.

Doppler ultrasound flow detectors. Doppler ultrasound flow detectors use an ultrasonic probe placed over an artery and an occluding cuff placed proximal to the probe. The area over the artery is clipped (usually just proximal to the palmar metacarpal pad or plantar metatarsal pad or the ventral surface of the tail base). The probe is covered with ultrasound coupling gel (or the skin over the artery is covered), and it is placed over the vessels and adjusted until a pulse is audible. The probe can then be secured in place with tape. If the patient has a very deep groove in the location of the arch, then the probe can be secured better by placing a gauze square or cotton ball over the top of the probe before taping it in place. If the tape is placed too loosely, then the signal may be weak. In small patients the lack of a signal may indicate that the tape has been placed too tightly.

A BP cuff is placed just proximal to the ultrasonic probe and inflated using a sphygmomanometer. The cuff should be held at the approximate level of the heart; then the cuff is allowed to deflate slowly. The measurement at which the sound of the blood flow first is audible is the systolic pressure. The level at which the sound changes is the diastolic pressure. The diastolic pressure is not always heard using this method.

Lack of perfusion or very poor pulses, severe vasoconstriction, and poor probe contact can lead to an absent or very weak signal. During anesthesia the concurrent use of other electrical equipment, especially electrosurgical equipment, can interfere with the flow signal.

One of the significant advantages of the Doppler ultrasound flow detector over an oscillometric device is that the flow through an artery is transmitted by an audible signal. This allows use of the Doppler ultrasound probe for applications other than BP measurement. The quality and intensity of the audible pulse can be used to monitor blood flow. This can be done continuously in anesthetized or unconscious patients, allowing subjective but immediate detection of changes in cardiac output or heart rhythm. Doppler flow detectors can be used to determine the presence of flow in distal limbs whenever the technician is concerned about circulatory disturbances. This may be the case in patients with severe trauma to a limb or possible thromboembolic disease blocking blood flow. For example, cats with possible saddle thrombi

can have lack of blood flow confirmed by placing the Doppler probe over each femoral artery. This is a more sensitive indicator of flow than digital palpation.

The Doppler flow probe can be placed on the surface of the cornea (after placing ultrasonic gel) to monitor for the presence of blood flow to the head. This may be used in patients who the technician believes may have suffered cardiac arrest and can signal the need for cardiopulmonary cerebral resuscitation. This technique can also be used to monitor the success of resuscitative efforts during cardiopulmonary cerebral resuscitation.

Interpretation

Hypotension is defined as BP readings less than 80 mm Hg (systolic) or 60 mm Hg (mean) and always warrants treatment of underlying cause and continued monitoring. Below this level, shock (inadequate tissue perfusion and oxygen delivery leading to cellular death and organ damage) is expected. Controversy continues over what level of hypertension should prompt treatment, and often the decision to treat will be based on concurrent clinical signs of hypertension. In general, patients with systolic BP readings equal to or greater than 160 mm Hg are at risk for end organ damage.

In anesthetized and critically ill patients, BP trends are often more important for assessment of patient status than individual readings. Knowledge of a patient's BP trends, like other methods of monitoring discussed in this chapter, is an integral part of critical care treatment decisions.

Troubleshooting

The reader should review the individual method techniques for the specifics of troubleshooting. For indirect methods, localized poor flow, patient motion, inappropriate cuff size, and lack of consistent technique between readings will all lead to inaccurate or unobtainable readings. For Doppler ultrasound and direct arterial monitoring, operator skill will significantly affect the success of the method chosen, but both methods can be readily learned with practice.

Multifunction Monitoring Equipment

Monitors are available that combine most of the functions discussed previously. These multichannel or multifunction combination monitors are either created for human medical applications and adapted for veterinary use or designed specifically for the veterinary market.

Many combinations of features are available, although most combine at least ECG and heart rate, pulse oximetry, and respiratory rate (provided by a plethysmograph). Other commonly available parameters include noninvasive BP, core body temperature, and ETCO$_2$. These monitors are often intended as anesthesia monitors but are useful for emergency and critical patients in other settings.

Combination monitors provide at-a-glance information about many body systems all on one screen, take up less shelf or storage space than separate monitors, and often add features that may not be available when separate monitors are used (e.g., continuous core temperature readings). Disadvantages include cost, and certain features may not be as well adapted to veterinary species as others. For example, the pulse oximetry sensors included on some monitors may not be sized appropriately for veterinary patients. Additionally, combination monitors that provide noninvasive BP monitoring use oscillometric technology may not function appropriately for very small patients. Cardell combination monitors are the only ones that use Criticon oscillometric technology, which has been validated for veterinary species.

When considering purchasing a combination monitor, it is important to decide which features will be useful for the practice and investigate the technology of each feature. Warranty and service contracts are also important variables. Besides the equipment issues previously mentioned, warm-up time and calibration needs may affect a monitor's usefulness in an emergency situation and make it more suitable to the relatively controlled situation of an anesthetized patient.

The combination monitors can be mounted on a pole for portability or placed on a shelf for ease of monitoring. The technique of use and troubleshooting is similar to that mentioned in each monitoring section of this chapter.

Manufacturers of Equipment Listed in The Text

Blood Gas, Chemistry, Hematology POC Analyzers

I-stat Analyzer, Heska Corporation, Fort Collins, CO
Vet Stat, Vet Test, Lasercyte, Idexx Laboratory, Westbrook, ME

Lactate POC analyzer:
Accusport, Boehringer Mannheim Corporation, Indianapolis, IN
Osmometer:
Wescor 4400 Colloid Osmometer, Wescor, Logan, UT
Coagulation testing equipment:
SCA 2000, Symbiotics Corporation, San Diego, CA
Simplate, Organon Teknika Corporation, Durham, NC

Blood Pressure Monitoring Equipment

Dinamap Veterinary Blood Pressure Monitor, Critikon Incorporation, Tampa, FL
Doppler Ultrasound, Parks Medical Electronics, Aloha, OR
Mutifunction monitors:
Cardell Monitors, Sharn Veterinary Incorporated, Tampa, FL
Advisor Vital Signs Mutiparameter Monitor, Surgivet, Waukesha, WI

Suggested Readings

Anderson-Wessberg K: Electrocardiographic techniques. In Ettinger SJ, Feldman EC: *Textbook of veterinary internal medicine*, ed 6, St Louis, 2005, Elsevier Saunders, pp 326-327.

Baldwin K: Ideal sample taking and an investigation of the coagulation panel. Proceedings of the 21st Annual ACVIM Forum, Charlotte, NC, 2003, pp 843-844.

Crowe DT, Spreng DE: Doppler assessment of blood flow and pressure in surgical and critical care patients. In Bonagura JD: *Kirk's current veterinary therapy XII*, Philadelphia, 1995, WB Saunders, pp 113-119.

de Laforcade AM, Rozanski EA: Central venous pressure and arterial blood pressure measurement, *Vet Clin North Am Small Anim Pract* 31:1163-1174, 2001.

Hansen B: Blood pressure measurement. In Bonagura JD: *Kirk's current veterinary therapy XII*, Philadelphia, 1995, WB Saunders, pp 110-112.

Marshall M: Capnography in dogs, *Compend Cont Ed Prac Vet* 26:761-778, 2004.

Shaffran N: *Blood gas interpretation*. Proceedings of the 21st Annual ACVIM Forum, Charlotte, NC, 2003, pp 845-847.

Stepien RL: Diagnostic blood pressure measurement. In Ettinger SJ, Feldman EC: *Textbook of veterinary internal medicine*, ed 6, St Louis, MO, 2005, Elsevier Saunders, pp 282-285.

Wright B, Hellyer PW: Respiratory monitoring during anesthesia: pulse oximetry and capnography, *Compend Contin Educ Prac Vet* 18:1083-1096, 1996.

Wingfield WE, Raffe MR: *The veterinary ICU book*, Jackson, WY, 2002, Teton New Media.

CHAPTER 3

Patient's Lifeline: Intravenous Catheter

ANDREA M. BATTAGLIA

In the critically ill or injured small animal patient, an IV catheter must be properly placed and secured to function properly. It can be used to introduce drug and fluid therapies, blood products, and nutrition. The IV catheter can also be used to obtain multiple blood samples from a patient. This reduces the stress for the animal by avoiding frequent venipuncture and saves the technician time by providing a readily available port for blood sampling without the need for assistance.

Small animal patients in an emergency or critical care unit have diverse needs. Accessible vessels, size, species, and clinical presentation vary. The veterinary technician must become familiar with the various types and sizes of IV catheters available, the common venous access points on the animal, and the various procedures for placing IV catheters.

Types of Intravenous Catheters

Many types of IV catheters are available. Through-the-needle catheter units and over-the-needle catheters are most commonly used in veterinary practice. Animals requiring long-term fluid therapy, drug therapy, or both will benefit from peripherally inserted central catheters or central catheters designed for the jugular vessel.

Through-the-needle catheters usually are placed in the jugular vessels but also can be placed in the medial saphenous vein on cats and the medial and lateral saphenous veins on dogs. This type of catheter is most commonly available in 8- and 12-inch lengths and in 18 or 20 gauge.

The over-the-needle catheters usually are placed in peripheral vessels but can also be used in the jugular vessels of smaller patients, including neonates. They are available in multiple gauges and lengths, ranging from 10 to 24 gauge in diameter and ¾ to 5½ inches in length.

Multilumen catheters are available for delivering multiple fluid or drug therapies. Incompatible solutions can be administered simultaneously through this type of catheter. The lumens have separate entrance and exit ports to prevent any mixing of compounds. It is still important to understand the pharmacokinetics of the drugs being used to determine which drug is infused through the distal port. Some drugs will change the pH of the environment, which can inactivate or change other drug's action within the body.

Multilumen catheters are available in double, triple, or quadruple varieties, with a large selection of lengths and sizes. These catheters are placed using a guidewire or an introducer that peels or breaks away. Arrow International manufactures the Twin Catheter. It is a double-lumen catheter with an over-the-needle introduction design; these work very well in the peripheral vessels.

Antimicrobial impregnated central venous catheters are used most commonly in humans, but studies of their use in animals are under way. These catheters are impregnated with minocycline and rifampin or chlorhexidine and silver sulfadiazine. They significantly reduce the microbial colonization and bloodstream infection that can occur with long-term indwelling catheter use in humans. Antimicrobial impregnated central venous catheters are available as single-lumen or multilumen catheters in a variety of lengths and gauges. A guidewire or sheath that peels or breaks away is used for introduction.

Vascular access ports were introduced in the 1980s and were used most commonly in research animals and in people receiving chemotherapy. Universities and veterinary referral centers have found them to be very beneficial for patients on long-term cancer chemotherapy and for patients with chronic renal failure who need long-term fluid therapy.

The port is surgically placed subcutaneously. The catheter is surgically placed into the jugular vessel inserted into the port. The catheters are most commonly polyurethane or silicone; the ports are made of metal or plastic. The port has an inner diameter (septum) where injections are performed. This port can be located easily by palpating the septum and is accessed by puncture with a noncoring needle after the area is aseptically prepped. To avoid damaging the port, the technician should use only the needles recommended by the manufacturer.

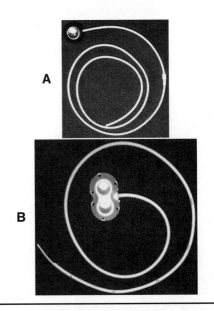

Fig. 3-1 Vascular access ports. **A,** Single-chambered vascular access port. **B,** Dual-chambered vascular access port.

Vascular ports are available in a variety of sizes, and single- and dual-chamber ports are available (Fig. 3-1).

Choosing the Right Catheter

Material

Critically ill small animals commonly need an IV catheter long term. It is necessary to be aware of the animal's treatment plan to choose the most appropriate catheter type.

A variety of compounds are used to make indwelling catheters. Polyvinyl chloride, polyethylene, polypropylene, polyurethane, silicone elastomer (Silastic), tetrafluoroethylene (TFE Teflon), fluoroethylenepropylene (FEP Teflon), elastomeric hydrogel, and blends of these materials (e.g., Vialon, a polyurethane blend) are the most common. Some compounds are more reactive than others (depending on the type and rigidity of the compound). Researchers believe that leaching of plasticizers and stabilizing agents may contribute to the adverse reactions some animals have to catheters.

Catheters made out of silicone and polyurethane are less thrombogenic than those made of other materials. Catheters made of polyvinyl chloride, polypropylene, and polyethylene are the most reactive.

Size

The preferred gauge and length of catheter used in a patient depend on the purpose of the IV catheter and the size of the patient. Critically ill patients often need large volumes of fluids. Therefore the technician would use the largest-gauge catheter that can be placed.

Catheter length is very important in animals needing central venous pressure monitoring, a procedure used to monitor fluid therapy. The catheter is placed in the jugular vein and must be long enough that the tip reaches the junction of the cranial vena cava and right atrium. In the cat or small dog, the technician can access the caudal vena cava by placing a catheter in the medial saphenous vessel. Radiographs should be taken to confirm proper placement when using the catheter for central venous pressure monitoring purposes.

Vascular Access Points

The best vascular access point to use on the small animal patient depends on many factors. The treatment plan and accessibility are primary concerns. The most common access points are the right and left cephalic, right and left lateral saphenous, right and left medial saphenous, and right and left jugular veins.

The jugular vessels are the best site if a patient needs prolonged fluid therapy or if multiple blood samples must be drawn. The technician should avoid placing catheters in the jugular vessels of animals with possible coagulopathies (it is very difficult to control hemorrhage at the insertion site).

Peripherally inserted central catheters are available for those situations when a central line is necessary but the jugular vessel is not an option for access. Long lines should be avoided in the animals that may be hypercoagulable because of the risk of intravascular clotting.

Placement

Correct placement of IV catheter units entails an understanding of catheter mechanics. All materials, including the catheter unit, heparinized saline, triple-antibiotic ointment to cover the insertion site,

and the materials needed to stabilize the unit, are readily available.

Placing over-the-needle catheters involves a four-step process after the site is shaved and surgically scrubbed. If the catheter is being placed in a limb, then it is important to create a sterile field in which to work. This is accomplished by wrapping a sterile bandage around the distal portion of the catheter site. The unit is placed into the vessel. Once a flashback is observed, the entire unit is advanced into the vein slightly to ensure that the stylet is placed in the vessel properly. The catheter is then advanced off the stylet into the vein. The stylet must be stabilized and not allowed to advance with the catheter. The stylet is then removed and the catheter is capped and flushed with heparinized saline (unless IV fluid therapy is started immediately through this catheter).

Placing a catheter into the jugular vessel is a team effort. The person restraining and positioning the animal must work with the person placing the catheter. The animal usually is placed in lateral recumbence for this procedure, with the neck extended. A rolled towel placed under the neck can assist in visualizing the vessel. It may be necessary to try different angles of the head and extensions of the neck before the vessel can be visualized or palpated. A cat's vessels can be palpated and visualized easily when the neck is extended and the head rotated outward.

Placing obese animals or breeds with thick necks in a sitting position, with the head slightly elevated and turned away from the venipuncture site, facilitates access to the jugular vessel.

Technical Tip Box 3-1 illustrates a six-step process that involves the use of a peel-away sheath needle.

Technical Tip Box 3-2 illustrates a six-step process called the *guidewire technique* (also called the *Seldinger technique*). An introducer (hypodermic needle), stylet, dilator, and catheter are used.

Technical Tip Box 3-3 illustrates a six-step process that involves the use of a catheter placement unit (through-the-needle catheter) that is contained in a sterile covering.

Technical Tip Box 3-4 describes a technique that uses a feeding tube and an over-the-needle catheter.

Stabilization

Once the catheter is in place, it must be stabilized properly. The wrap should provide additional catheter stabilization, increase patient comfort, and protect the

Box 3-1

Technical Tip: Peel-Away Sheath Technique*

Items needed:

- Items for prepping, drape, and sterile surgical gloves
- Peel-away sheath introducer with catheter
- Heparinized saline
- Injection cap with extension line
- Triple-antibiotic ointment
- Materials needed for stabilization

   Shave and surgically prep the site. Drape around the site. Sterile surgical gloves must be worn. Perform a small skin nick incision.

1. Insert the over-the-needle sheath through the small nick in the skin into the vessel.

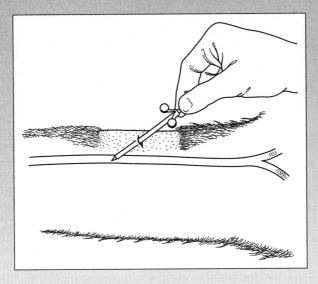

2. Advance the needle sheath slightly to ensure that the sheath and the needle are seated in the vessel.
3. Stabilize the needle and advance the sheath (slightly rotating it back and forth) into the vessel.

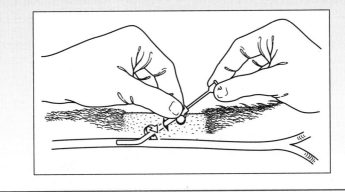

*Gloves and surgical drapes were omitted from illustrations so that positioning of hands and catheter could be shown. Gloves must be worn and a sterile field provided.

BOX 3-1

Technical Tip: Peel-Away Sheath Technique—cont'd

4. Remove the needle and place a finger over the opening to prevent excessive hemorrhage.

5. Insert the catheter through sheath.

6. Cap and flush the catheter with heparinized saline. Pull up and out on the tabs of the sheath. Slight hemorrhaging will occur around the site.

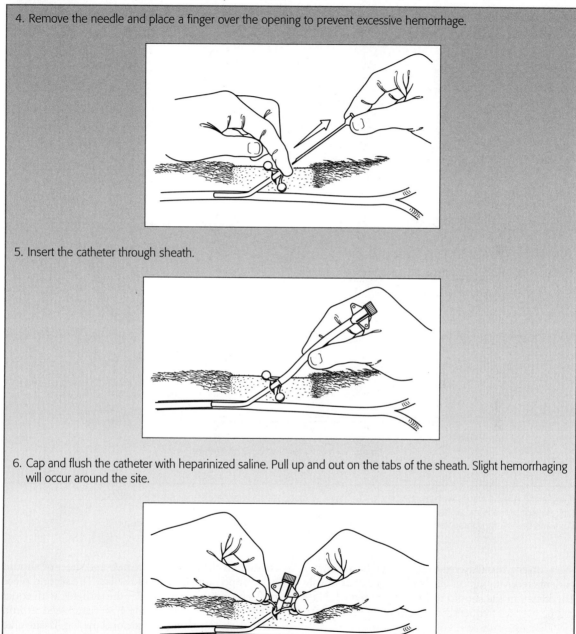

BOX 3-2

*Technical Tip: Guidewire (Seldinger) Technique**

Items needed:

- Items for prepping, drape, and sterile surgical gloves
- Hypodermic needle†
- Guidewire
- Dilator
- Polyurethane IV catheter
- Heparinized saline
- Injection cap with extension line
- Triple-antibiotic ointment
- Materials for stabilization

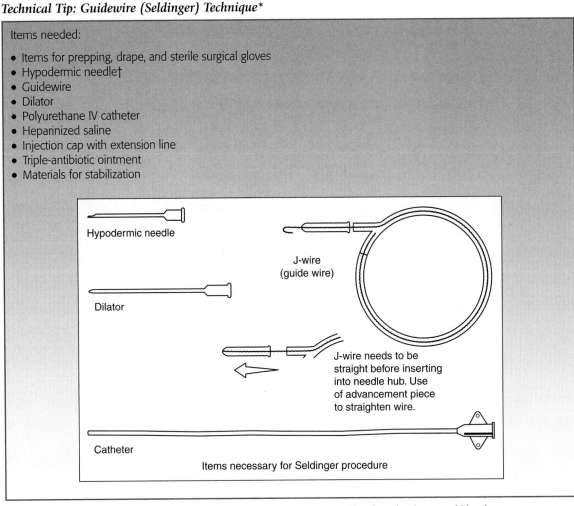

Hypodermic needle

J-wire
(guide wire)

Dilator

J-wire needs to be
straight before inserting
into needle hub. Use
of advancement piece
to straighten wire.

Catheter

Items necessary for Seldinger procedure

*Gloves and surgical drapes were omitted from illustrations so that positioning of hands and catheter could be shown. Gloves must be worn and a sterile field provided.
†This and the following three items are available in kits made by Arrow, Mila, and Cook Veterinary Products.

insertion site. Multilayered wraps should be avoided in patients receiving cancer chemotherapy intravenously. The insertion site should remain uncovered so that it can be checked frequently throughout the treatment.

Peripheral Catheters

Two ½-inch wide pieces of tape, long enough to go around the leg, are used for initial stabilization. The first is placed at the base of the hub. Tabs should be created on either side of the hub and the tape should be wrapped firmly around the leg. The second piece is placed, adhesive up, under the catheter, with equal lengths of tape on either side. It is crisscrossed around the catheter and wrapped around the leg. Tissue glue can be used to further stabilize the catheter. A small drop on either side of the hub is sufficient. Because some animals may have a severe tissue reaction to the ingredients in tissue glue, it should be used sparingly. This technique is very useful for active patients

BOX 3-2

Technical Tip: Guidewire (Seldinger) Technique—cont'd

Shave and surgically prep the site. Drape around the site. Sterile surgical gloves must be worn. Maintain sterility throughout the procedure.

1. Insert the needle into the vessel.

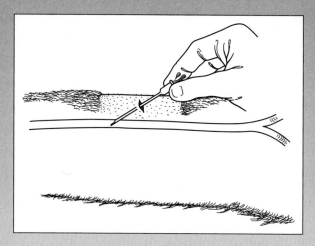

2. Place a guidewire into the vessel through the needle. For smaller animals, cats, and dehydrated patients, insert the straight end first.

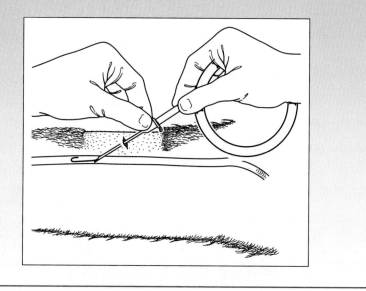

Continued.

Technical Tip: Guidewire (Seldinger) Technique—cont'd

3. Remove the needle from the vessel and off the wire.

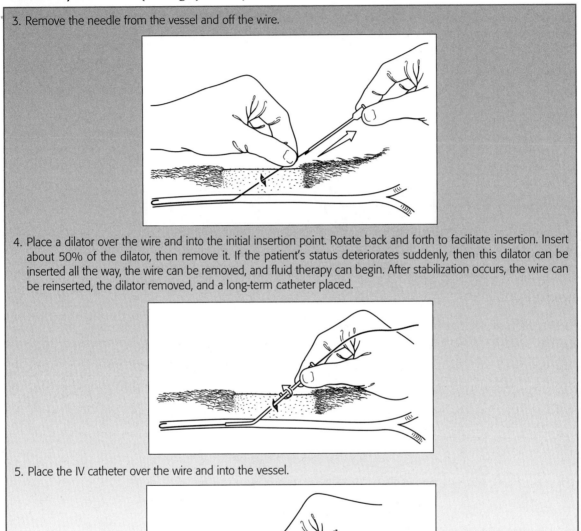

4. Place a dilator over the wire and into the initial insertion point. Rotate back and forth to facilitate insertion. Insert about 50% of the dilator, then remove it. If the patient's status deteriorates suddenly, then this dilator can be inserted all the way, the wire can be removed, and fluid therapy can begin. After stabilization occurs, the wire can be reinserted, the dilator removed, and a long-term catheter placed.

5. Place the IV catheter over the wire and into the vessel.

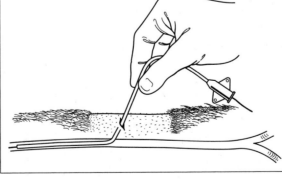

BOX 3-2

Technical Tip: Guidewire (Seldinger) Technique—cont'd

6. Remove the wire, cap the catheter, and flush it with heparinized saline.

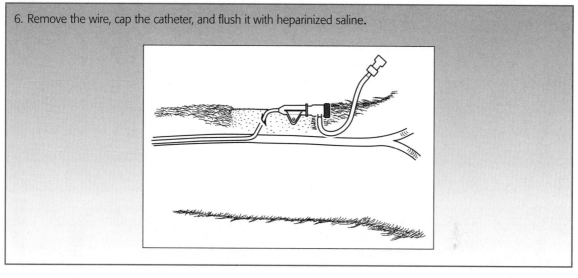

BOX 3-3

Technical Tip: Through-the-Needle Catheter Unit

Items needed:

- Through-the-needle catheter unit
- Injection cap with extension line
- Heparinized saline
- Triple-antibiotic ointment
- Materials for stabilization

1. Insert needle through the skin and into the vessel.

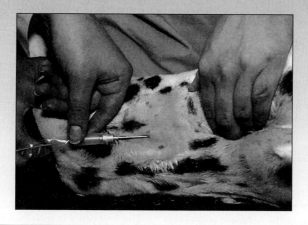

Continued.

BOX 3-3

Technical Tip: Through-the-Needle Catheter Unit—cont'd

2. Advance the catheter into the vessel and lock it into the needle hub.

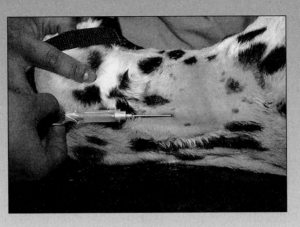

3. Remove the needle from the site.

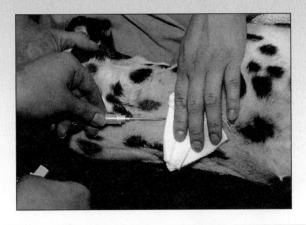

(especially fractious cats) or when quick stabilization is necessary.

A gauze pad with triple-antibiotic ointment is placed over the catheter insertion site. Cast padding is placed underneath the proximal portion of the hub to create padding between the leg and the catheter. It is wrapped around the leg to provide additional support.

Rolled gauze is used for additional support and for securing extended injection ports. Adhesive wrap (Vetwrap or Elastikon works well) can then be used to cover the entire bandage. Injection ports should always remain uncovered for quick venous access. Occasionally, it is necessary to extend the wrap to the toes to assist circulation. Cats usually need this extended wrap.

Jugular Catheter

Three pieces of tape long enough to go around the patient's neck are needed for initial stabilization. The first piece is split 2 inches down the middle and placed so that the small strips go along either side of

BOX 3-3

Technical Tip: Through-the-Needle Catheter Unit—cont'd

4. Place the needle guard over the needle.

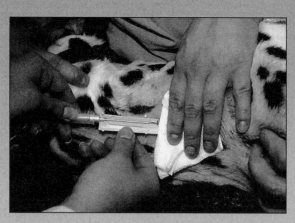

5. Apply pressure to the insertion site and remove the stylet.

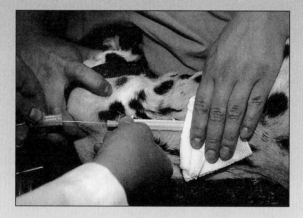

6. Cap and flush the catheter.

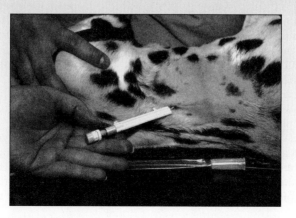

BOX 3-4

Technical Tip: Using an Over-the-Needle Catheter Unit and Feeding Tube for Jugular Catheter Placement

Items needed:

- 14-gauge over-the-needle catheter with a 5-French feeding tube or 16-gauge over-the-needle catheter with a 3.5-French feeding tube*
- Injection cap with heparinized saline
- Materials for stabilization

  Before performing this technique, confirm that the materials are compatible. Some catheters are tapered differently on the distal end, and feeding tubes cannot pass through them.

1. Shave and surgically prep the site.
2. Insert a 14-gauge over-the-needle catheter through the skin, into the vessel.
3. Advance the catheter off the stylet into the vessel.
4. Introduce a 5-French feeding tube through the catheter, into the vessel. A drop of 50% dextrose at the catheter hub may facilitate feeding tube introduction.
5. Cap and flush the catheter with heparinized saline. Remove the over-the-needle catheter from the vessel up to the initial insertion point. Loop the line and stabilize it to the patient.

*For smaller patients, a 16-gauge over-the-needle catheter with a 3.5-French feeding tube can be used.

---

the catheter. It is wrapped around the neck, incorporating the small strips for the final connection. The other pieces are placed on either side of the catheter and wrapped around the neck. (For additional stabilization, a piece of tape with tabs placed at the base of the catheter or needle guard and a drop of tissue glue [or sutures] is put on each tab of the butterfly so that it adheres to the neck. This is done before the tape is placed.) Cast padding is placed over the tape to provide additional support. Rolled gauze is placed over the cast padding. Adhesive wrap is placed to secure the entire bandage to the patient's neck. It is very important to check the tightness of the bandage around the neck after each layer is placed. If the patient shows any signs of discomfort or difficulty breathing, then the bandage should be removed immediately and rewrapped more loosely, using less material. Leashes should be placed around the shoulder, or a harness can be used (Figs. 3-2 and 3-3).

Through-the-needle catheters that are placed in the lateral saphenous veins of dogs can be secured using the following technique. The catheter is pulled out ½ inch and the needle guard placed pointing upward. A small piece of tape is placed on the catheter loop, with tabs on either side. The tabs are secured to the leg with tissue glue. This prevents the catheter from dislodging. Tape is used to secure the needle guard to the leg. A piece of cast padding is placed between the needle

guard and the leg to provide a cushion. The entire needle guard and catheter site can then be wrapped. Rolled gauze is used for more stabilization. Then adhesive wrap is placed over the entire bandage.

Through-the-needle catheters placed in the medial saphenous veins of cats or small dogs can be secured using the following method (the patient remains in lateral recumbence for this step). The catheter is pulled out far enough to loop around the stifle. Two inches usually is sufficient. (When the catheter is looped out, bleeding should be expected.) A piece of tape is placed around the catheter (with tabs on either side), and tissue glue is used for further stabilization. A gauze pad with triple-antibiotic ointment is placed at the insertion site, with tape to keep it in place. The patient is turned over carefully. The needle guard is placed along the lateral aspect of the patient's thigh and secured with tape. The catheter is secured using the same method and materials as previously mentioned.

Catheters placed in the medial aspect of the leg can also be wrapped without looping the catheter and leaving the needle guard on the medial side of the leg. The advantages of this method are less manipulation of the patient and a decreased risk of dislodging the catheter. The disadvantage (especially in cats) is the discomfort of the wrap. It extends to the toes, and a splint is needed, making it difficult

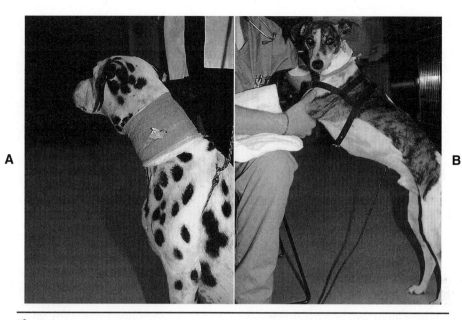

Fig. 3-2 A, Leash should be placed around shoulder to prevent additional stress to jugular catheter site. **B,** A harness can be used.

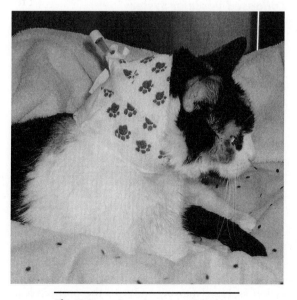

Fig. 3-3 Jugular catheter in a diabetic cat.

for the patient to ambulate. It also must be changed frequently during the day because it is soiled easily.

Challenges

Specific Breeds

Placing catheters in basset hounds and dachshunds is very challenging because their limb structure and loose skin make it difficult to place and stabilize IV catheters. Other breeds with loose skin can also be a challenge.

Visualizing and palpating the vessel is easier for the person placing the catheter when the skin is stretched and rotated upward by the restrainer. The technician should be very cautious about the degree of rotation. When the skin folds are released, the catheter port should be easy to access.

A small nick incision facilitates a smoother introduction of the catheter unit into the vessel. The catheter should be made of a rigid material such as Teflon, because it is less likely to kink while being advanced and will not migrate out of the vessel if stabilized properly.

Elastikon works well in stabilizing catheters in animals with loose skin folds. It is strong enough to hold the layers of skin back in most cases.

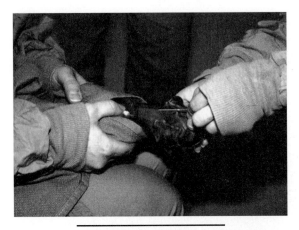

Fig. 3-4 Restraining the neonate.

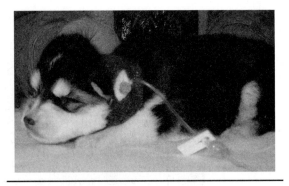

Fig. 3-5 Jugular catheter in a neonate with a low-flow extension set attached.

Neonates

Restraint is very important in facilitating a successful venipuncture in these animals. The jugular vessel is the most accessible vein.

The neonate should be cradled in the palm of the hands, using its arms as a support for the body. The animal should then be placed on its back, head toward the technician's fingers. Forelimbs must be held firmly to the chest. (Wrapping the patient in a towel sometimes works but can limit the technician's ability to monitor the animal during this procedure.) The person placing the catheter extends the head back and rotates it slightly until the vessel can be visualized. Using the other hand, the over-the-needle catheter is introduced into the jugular vessel. The animal should be held in an upright position when securing the catheter (Figs. 3-4 and 3-5).

Fractious Feline and Cantankerous Canine

The restraining tools and the restrainer are the keys to successful IV catheter placement in aggressive animals. Risks should not be taken with animals that show any signs of aggression, and the supplies available for protection should always be used. Restraining tools include muzzles, cat bags, towels, and sedation. Taking these precautionary measures prevents injury to the animal and staff.

The use of a catheter that acts as a multipurpose unit and has a long indwelling time is important. The following setup works well in the fractious animal. An 18-gauge, 12-inch through-the-needle catheter or a long, polyurethane catheter is placed in the lateral saphenous vein in the dog and the medial saphenous vein in the cat. A low-volume extension set is connected to the catheter. This setup allows access to a vessel at a distance. (Medex Inc, Hilliard, Ohio, makes a low-volume extension set with a 60-inch 1 ml line.) The technician is then free to draw blood or administer drug and fluid therapies through the extension set (Fig. 3-6).

Putting an Elizabethan collar on the animal blocks its vision and makes it more difficult for the animal to bite. A leash is left around the animal's neck and the end placed outside the cage.

Collapsed Vascular System

A minicutdown should be performed if an IV catheter cannot be placed quickly in an emergency situation. A hypodermic needle is used instead of a blade. The technician should hold a 20-gauge hypodermic needle like a pencil and, using the cutting edge of the bevel, make an incision through the skin, horizontally across the leg, to expose the vessel (the incision should begin distally). If the catheter placement is not successful, then incisions can be made parallel to the vessel, up the leg, until placement is successful.

Intraosseous cannulization also can be performed in an emergency. Intraosseous needles are available for this procedure. The most common sites include the medullary canal of the femur or humerus. Once the area is prepped with a local anesthetic, the needle is inserted into the greater tubercle of the humerus or the greater trochanteric fossa of the femur. Aspiration of bone marrow confirms the proper placement, or a radiograph can be taken.

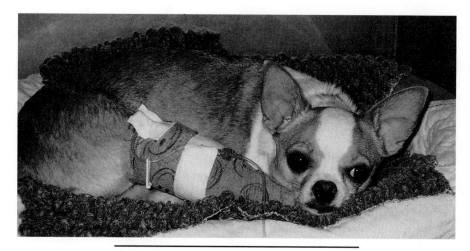

Fig. 3-6 Long line in lateral saphenous vessel of a dog.

Maintenance

Proper placement technique, catheter choice, and site maintenance all play an important role in determining the indwelling time of an IV catheter. The IV catheter site should be assessed during treatment times and every 2 hours if the animal is receiving fluid therapy. Visual checks and palpation of the area above the catheter are performed throughout the day. Bandages should be changed every 24 hours or if they become wet or soiled. IV catheters must be flushed with heparinized saline every 6 to 8 hours if a continuous IV drip is not being administered.

Once the bandage is removed, the site is evaluated for signs of redness or swelling. Phlebitis is one complication that can occur with an indwelling IV catheter. It is the inflammation of the vessel that results from an infection. The animal may show signs of discomfort when the catheter is flushed or palpated. The site may be hot and swollen. The catheter must be removed and the leg warm-packed every 4 hours until the swelling subsides (if this is observed). Culturing the catheter tips will assist in determining the cause and type of infection.

The catheter should be flushed to check for any leakage around the site. Once it has been determined that the catheter will be used for another day, it should be rewrapped and triple-antibiotic ointment replaced.

The Centers for Disease Control and Prevention do not recommend routine application of antimicrobial ointment to venous catheter insertion sites because it macerates the site in humans. Chlorhexidine patches are used as an alternative. The patch slowly releases chlorhexidine, which is the only solution known to maintain its bactericidal effects in the presence of bodily fluids over a 7-day period.

If the catheter must be replaced, then the old one should be left in place (if still functional) until a new line has been established. It is important to maintain venous access at all times in the critically ill small animal. All fluid administration sets and fluid bags are changed along with the IV catheter.

The IV catheter is the patient's lifeline in many situations. The veterinary team must work together to place and maintain IV catheters properly. The entire staff must understand IV catheter placement, stabilization, and maintenance protocols to provide optimal patient care.

Suggested Readings

Hanson B: Technical aspects of fluid therapy. In DiBartola SP: *Fluid therapy in the small animal practice*, Philadelphia, 1992, WB Saunders.

Manchon R, Raffe M, Robinson E: Central venous pressure measurements in the caudal vena cava of sedated cats, *J Vet Emerg Crit Care* 5(2):121, 1995.

Mathews K, Brooks M, Valliant A: A prospective study of intravenous catheter contamination, *J Vet Emerg Crit Care* 6(1):33, 1996.

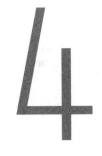

CHAPTER 4

Fluid Therapy

ANN MARIE RITCHIE

Fluid therapy is a vital tool in the veterinary hospital. It is used daily to treat various illnesses, to assist in stabilization, and to help recovery of emergency and critical care patients. Knowledge of why and how fluids are used is essential to increase the veterinary technician's value and competence. Fluid therapy in clinical medicine is used to replace hydration deficits, maintain normal hydration, correct hypovolemia, replace essential electrolytes and nutrients, and serve as a vehicle for infusing certain IV medications.

The editor and publisher acknowledge and appreciate the original contribution of Linda Katchatoorian and Kenneth Kalthoff, whose work has been incorporated into this chapter.

Fluid Types

Crystalloids

Crystalloids are water (H_2O)-based solutions containing electrolyte and nonelectrolyte solutes that are permeable to the capillary membrane and are used for rehydration and maintenance needs. Crystalloids are also commonly first-choice agents used for fluid resuscitation. Crystalloids are broken down into further categories based on their tonicity.

Hypotonic. Most of the fluids in this category are prepared as isotonic solutions. Dextrose is added or is already contained in the solution, which results in a hypotonic solution when it is metabolized. A hypotonic solution has a lower osmotic pressure relative to the fluid to which it is being compared. An example of this type of fluid is 2.5% dextrose in sodium chloride.

Hypotonic solutions are excellent maintenance fluids when supplemented with potassium chloride. They are the fluid of choice in patients who are predisposed to sodium retention, such as those with congestive heart failure or liver disease.

Hypotonic solutions are not to be used for shock treatment because H_2O will redistribute rapidly. They also could be detrimental in patients with acute renal failure or with cerebral injuries (Table 4-1).

TABLE 4-1

Comparison of Commonly Used Parenteral Fluids in the Dog and Cat

Solution	ELECTROLYTE CONTENT (mEq/L)						Glucose (g/L)	Calories (kcal/L)	Tonicity	Osmolality (mOsm/L)
	Na+	K+	Ca++	Cl−	Lactate	Acetate				
Lactated Ringer's	130	4	3	109	28				Isotonic	273
Acetated Ringer's	131	4	3	109		28			Isotonic	275
Ringer's	147	4	4	155					Isotonic	309
Sodium chloride 0.45%	77			77					Hypotonic	155
Sodium chloride 0.9%	154			154					Isotonic	310
Dextrose 2.5%							25	85	Hypotonic	126
Dextrose 5%							50	170	Hypotonic	253
Dextrose 10%							100	340	Hypertonic	505
Dextrose 50%							500	1700	Hypertonic	2525
Dextrose 2.5% in half-strength lactated Ringer's	65	2	1	55	14		25	85	Isotonic	265
Dextrose 5% in lactated Ringer's	130	4	3	111	28		50	170	Hypertonic	525
Dextrose 2.5% with 0.45% sodium chloride	77			77			25	85	Isotonic	280
Dextrose 5% with 0.45% sodium chloride	77			77			50	170	Hypertonic	405
Dextrose 5% with 0.9% sodium chloride	154			154			50	170	Hypertonic	560

Data from Covington TR, Dipalma JR, Hussar DA et al, eds: *Drug facts and comparisons*, 1985 edition, Philadelphia, 1984, JB Lippincott.

Isotonic. These fluids have a similar osmotic pressure to the fluid to which it is being compared. Isotonic solutions distribute evenly in the extracellular space when administered intravascularly. Only 25% of the administered crystalloid fluid remains in the intravascular space of the extracellular fluid (ECF) compartment after 1 hour. Examples of this type of fluid are 0.9% sodium chloride, lactated Ringer's solution, and Normosol-R.

Isotonic solutions are inexpensive, readily available, and a good replacement fluid for dehydration. They are also good resuscitative fluids for small animals that need rapid volume expansion.

Fluid redistributes rapidly, so infusion must be continued to maintain volume expansion. Isotonic solutions are not used for maintenance because of their high sodium and chloride content, osmolality, and inadequate potassium. They can also cause peripheral edema, because muscle and subcutaneous capillaries are less permeable to proteins.

Lactated Ringer's Solution. Lactated Ringer's solution is probably the most familiar and widely used crystalloid fluid in veterinary medicine. This solution provides a source of H_2O and isotonic concentrations of electrolytes (such as sodium chloride, NaLactate, potassium chloride, and $CaCl_2$). Lactated Ringer's solution is an alkalinizing solution, because the liver converts the lactate to bicarbonate.

Lactated Ringer's solution is best suited for ailments such as shock, diuresis, rehydration, volume expansion, acidosis, and it can be used for maintenance when supplemented with potassium chloride. Use of lactated Ringer's solution should be avoided in patients with alkalosis, hypercalcemia, severe hypekalemia, and (according to some researchers) liver disease and cancer. The debate as to the use of lactated Ringer's solution in patients with liver disease and with cancer is ongoing (the liver needs to be functional to convert the lactate, and cancer may cause high levels of lactate as a result of anaerobic metabolism). Because it is a balanced solution, it is also a good first choice for fluid therapy while awaiting laboratory results.

Hypertonic. Hypertonic fluids have a higher osmotic pressure to the fluid to which it is being compared. An example of this type of fluid is 7% sodium chloride. These solutions help draw fluid into the vascular compartment for rapid resuscitation. This effect is transient but may be prolonged when combined with a colloid such as hetastarch.

Hypertonic solutions are used for rapid volume expansion. These solutions are also used for treating head injury, cerebral edema, or increase intracranial pressure because they are highly effective at drawing H_2O out of the brain.

Caution should be used when administering hypertonic solutions, because they may cause hypernatremia, hyperosmolality, and increased bleeding. If infused too quickly, then hypotension, bradycardia, bronchoconstriction, and rapid shallow breathing may occur.

Synthetic Colloids

The term *colloid* refers to high-molecular weight substances that do not pass readily across capillary membranes. These macromolecules are negatively charged, and their presence in the vasculature pulls additional H_2O from the interstitium. Although large volumes of crystalloids will decrease the colloidal oncotic pressure, colloids actually increase oncotic pressure. Fluid will remain in the intravascular space as long as the colloidal pressure is greater than in the tissue. Normally, albumin provides this oncotic pressure. Albumin blood levels can be decreased dramatically in diseases associated with vomiting, diarrhea, fever, or excessive urination. Administering colloids along with crystalloid therapy during resuscitation and maintenance fluid therapy restores and maintains intravascular oncotic pressure.

These solutions are commonly described according to their molecular weight. The molecular weight of albumin is 69,000 Da (deka), and under normal circumstances albumin cannot cross vascular membranes. The colloidal solutions available vary in molecular weight and duration time for maintaining oncotic pressure.

Hydroxyethyl Starch. The most common products are hetastarch and pentastarch. They are synthetic polymers of glucose resembling glycogen (a large polysaccharide that is the chief storage form of carbohydrates in the body). Hetastarch has an average molecular weight of 450,000 Da; pentastarch has an average molecular weight of 264,000 Da. The metabolism of these products depends on their absorption by tissues (liver and spleen). The half-life of concentration in the blood is about 25.5 hours for hetastarch and 2.5 hours for pentastarch. A new hyroxyethyl starch (Voluven) is being introduced in Europe and has an average molecular weight of 130,000 Da with less coagulation effects.

Dextrans. Dextrans are high molecular weight polysaccharides composed of linear glucose residues that are isotonic. The polysaccharides are produced from sucrose-containing media when the enzyme dextran sucrase is produced while growing various strains of leuconostoc bacteria. Dextrans come in high and low molecular weight forms. The most commonly used are dextran 40, with an average molecular weight of 40,000 Da, and dextran 70, with an average molecular weight of 70,000 Da. In animals with normal renal functions, 40% to 70% of dextran is filtered by the kidneys and excreted in the urine producing mild diuresis. The remaining molecules are metabolized by dextranase into glucose in the liver. The half-life of dextran 40 is 2.5 hours, and the half-life of dextran 70 is about 25.5 hours (dextran has fewer large molecules than hetastarch).

Gelatins. Modified fluid gelatins are available in veterinary medicine. An example of this type of fluid is Vetaplasm. It is produced from cattle bone gelatin, prepared by a gradual controlled heating and chemical hydrolysis of raw material. Very few published clinical studies are available. The average molecular weight of the molecules is 30,000 Da. The duration of oncotic effect is about 4 to 6 hours. Little is known about the overall degradation of gelatins in blood.

Synthetic Colloid Pros

- Synthetic colloids provide a longer effect on colloidal oncotic pressure. They can be used as resuscitative and replacement fluids and are safe to administer as boluses to the animal with poor perfusion to correct hypovolemia.
- Synthetic colloids can be used safely to increase intravascular volume in animals with congestive heart failure. Underlying heart disease must be addressed and the afterload reduced.
- Fewer instances of peripheral edema result than when crystalloids are used exclusively.
- The need for positive inotropes or vasopressors (i.e., dopamine infusion) for blood pressure support is less common.
- Synthetic colloids can reduce the volume of crystalloids needed by 40% to 60% when used concurrently with colloids.

Synthetic Colloid Cons

- Synthetic colloids are expensive and can nearly equal that of natural colloids.
- In disease processes in which albumin leakage is already a problem, products with a molecular weight equal to or less than albumin should not be used because they will also leak into the interstitial space. Because of their larger molecules, hetastarch and pentastarch are recommended in these instances.
- Hetastarch and pentastarch can raise serum amylase levels without changing pancreatic function.
- Anaphylaxis has been reported in a very small percentage of cases.
- Dextrans have been associated with acute renal failure and interfering with platelet function. They can also alter cross matching results. Blood glucose and bilirubin levels can be falsely increased.
- Synthetic colloids can falsely elevate coagulation profiles.

Hemoglobin-Based Oxygen Carriers

Hemoglobin-based oxygen carriers such as oxyglobin can be used as an alternative to blood for animals with any type of anemia. Oxyglobin (hemoglobin glutamer-200 [bovine]) is an ultrapurified polymerized hemoglobin solution of bovine origin in a modified lactated Ringer's solution. Because of oxyglobin's oxygen-carrying capacities, it is useful for animals with hemolytic anemia, blood loss secondary to surgery or trauma, hypovolemia and other causes of shock, and any other condition involving poor tissue perfusion.

The oxygen delivery system of oxyglobin differs from the oxygen delivery system of blood. Hemoglobin, the protein that is encapsulated in the red blood cell, transports the oxygen from the lungs to the tissues through microcirculation. In a healthy animal, hemoglobin carries about 98% of the body's oxygen. When an animal is anemic, not enough red blood cells are available to oxygenate the tissues adequately. Oxyglobin's polymerized hemoglobin molecules provide the animal with the substitute oxygen transporting system by circulating in the plasma and transporting oxygen from the lungs to the tissues upon infusion. In addition, the hemoglobin molecules may perfuse to areas that red blood cells cannot reach.

The recommended dose of oxyglobin is 30 ml/kg of body weight at a rate of 10 ml/kg/hr. Blood typing and cross-matching are not necessary before administration.

Oxyglobin can be stored at room temperature or refrigerated for 24 months. It should not be frozen; once the overwrap is removed, oxyglobin should be used within 24 hours. Reconstitution or filters are not required for infusion. Oxyglobin is approved in dogs.

Rapid administration may result in circulatory overload and it is contraindicated in animals with advanced cardiac disease (e.g., congestive heart failure). The animal's central venous pressure (CVP) can be monitored during and after the administration to prevent overload from occurring.

Oxyglobin can interfere with serum chemistry tests, so blood samples should be obtained before administration. Transient discoloration (yellow) of

TABLE 4-2

Distribution of Body Water

	EXTRACELLULAR FLUID	
Intracellular Fluid	**Interstitial (¾)**	**Plasma (¼)**
40% of body weight is intracellular water.	15% of body weight is interstitial water.	5% of body weight is plasma water.
⅔ body water	⅓ body water	

the mucous membranes, sclera, urine, and skin may also occur.

Human Albumin

Human albumin is a natural colloid made from pooled human venous plasma that has been screened and treated to protect against the possibility of transmitting human disease. Albumin is used primarily as a volume expander and contains no clotting factors. Wearing gloves and a mask is recommended when handling this product.

Albumin is an important protein that is synthesized in the liver. It maintains colloid osmotic pressure, participates in intermediary drug metabolism, and is a free radical scavenger.

Human albumin is available in 5% and 25% solutions. The 25% albumin should be diluted in normal saline (added to a 250 ml bag to make a 10% solution). It can be given at no more than 1 ml/min, over 4 hours (because it contains no preservatives) and should not exceed 2 g/kg/day.

Albumin is indicated in patients suffering from cases of severe hypoalbuminemia including sepsis, systemic inflammatory response syndrome, and burns.

Circulatory overload can occur (and albumin is contraindicated) in patients with cardiac failure or that are severely anemic or dehydrated. The use of human albumin in veterinary patients is experimental, and more research is needed on the effects of this product.

Body Fluid and Electrolytes

The primary sources for body fluid intake are ingested H_2O, food that contains H_2O, and H_2O produced from the oxidation of carbohydrates, proteins, and fats. H_2O output occurs (healthy normal patient) through losses in urine and feces, as well as from evaporation from the skin and respiratory tract.

Total body water (TBW) accounts for approximately 60% of the adult patient's body weight. In the neonate patient, TBW is approximately 75% to 80% body weight, which decreases with increasing body fat levels.

This fluid is further broken down into intracellular fluid (ICF) and ECF. The ICF constitutes 40% of body weight or two thirds of TBW. Potassium and phosphorus are found in high concentrations within the cells in ICF. ECF (20% of body weight or one third of TBW) is further divided into interstitial (15% of body weight or 75% of ECF) and intravascular (5% of body weight or 25% of ECF). Sodium and chloride exist in high concentration in serum in ECF. Depending on the patient's condition, one area (ECF or ICF) may be affected more than another. Sodium, potassium, and chloride are the main electrolytes and are responsible for maintaining normal cellular function. Fluid therapy is intended to maintain these areas in equilibrium (Table 4-2).

Patient Assessment

Shock

If upon admittance it is determined that the patient is in shock, the main goal of fluid therapy should be directed at expanding intravascular volume. Fluid therapy is the primary method of treating all types of shock. Every injury is accompanied by some degree of shock and should be treated appropriately.

All types of fluid mentioned here can be used to treat shock. Crystalloids are the most commonly reached for shock therapy fluid in the emergency room. As mentioned earlier, although crystalloids have inadequacies (including limited intravascular time before redistribution), their easy availability and cost effectiveness make them hard to resist. Colloids and hypertonic saline solutions, especially when combined with crystalloids, may provide a more effective shock management. The crystalloid dose should be reduced by 40% to 60% when combined with the use of colloids (Table 4-3).

Dehydration

Before a fluid therapy regimen can be initiated, hydration status must be evaluated. Dehydration is often a sequela to a number of disease processes, and it can be subtle or obvious, depending of the duration and severity of the disease affecting the patient. The changes associated with dehydration are progressive.

- <5%—History of fluid loss (vomiting, diarrhea) but no abnormalities upon physical examination
- 5% (mild)—Mild loss of skin turgor, dry mucous membranes but not panting or pathologic tachycardia
- 7% (moderate)—Mild to moderate decreased skin turgor, dry mucous membranes, slight tachycardia, normal pulses
- 10% (severe)—Moderate to marked decrease in skin turgor, dry mucous membranes, tachycardia, weak rapid pulses, moderate mental depression
- 12% (critical)—Marked loss of skin turgor, sunken eyes, dry mucous membranes, slow capillary refill time (CRT), marked mental depression, shock

Dehydration is best corrected using the appropriate crystalloid solution because fluid from all of the body spaces is affected and must be replaced.

Body Weight

Body weight is the best means of assessing fluid volume loss and response to treatment. Upon admission, body weight is checked and the patient's baseline body weight is used as a quantitative guide. Weight is checked daily to document adequate hydration. Acute changes in weight are generally the result of changes in fluid status. An acute gain of 1 lb is equivalent to 500 ml in body H_2O. Losses of lean body mass are never rapid.

Skin Turgor

Skin turgor or pliability may approximate hydration status. This technique should be used in a consistent manner and location. The technician tests skin turgor by pinching up a fold of skin, quickly releasing it, and assessing the time it takes for the skin to return to its normal position. Skin that has a slight delay in return to normal may be approximated as 5% to 6% dehydrated. Skin that has a pronounced tenting effect with little or no return to normal may be approximated as 10% to 12% dehydrated.

This is a subjective evaluation. Skin turgor can by misleading in the obese patient because adipose tissue replaces subcutaneous interstitial H_2O and maintains elasticity despite a negative H_2O balance. In addition, a false impression of marked dehydration may be present in older, cachetic patients because of the loss of skin resiliency.

Mucous Membranes and Capillary Refill Time

Normal, nonpigmented mucous membranes are pink. Mucous membrane color depends on peripheral capillary blood flow, hemoglobin concentration, and tissue oxygenation.

The buccal mucous membranes are the most commonly evaluated tissue; however, the vulva, penis, and conjunctiva of the eye may also be used. Color may vary with disease states (pale, white for shock, anemia, or blood loss; injected, highly vascular red for sepsis; yellow or icteric for liver disease; cyanotic, blue for hypoxia). Normal membranes are also moist. Tacky, dry membranes may indicate dehydration. However, persistent panting, which may dry the mucous membranes, can give a false impression of dehydration.

CRT is a good indicator of peripheral perfusion. Digital pressure applied firmly to the mucous membranes reduces the capillary blood flow, resulting in a blanching of the tissue. In a healthy patient, the time for blood flow to return to the area is normally 1 to 2 seconds (depending on vascular tone and cardiac output). Prolonged CRT is an indicator of reduced peripheral blood flow as seen in the late stages of shock, heart failure, severe vasodilation, vasoconstriction, or pericardial effusion. A rapid CRT of less than 1 second is indicative of compensatory

TABLE 4-3

Comparison of Fluid Therapies in Shock

Fluid Type	IV Dosage	Indications for Use	Benefits	Potential Complications	Miscellaneous Data
Isotonic crystalloids Lactated Ringer's Normal saline solution	Initial dog: 40-90 ml/kg Initial cat: 20-60 ml/kg	Intravascular volume expansion	Readily available Inexpensive Easy to use Help correct electrolyte imbalances	Dilutional anemia Hypoproteinemia Pulmonary and peripheral edema Stay in intravascular space only a short time	Lactate in lactated Ringer's does not potentiate lactic acidemia
Hypertonic crystalloids Hypertonic saline (3%, 7%)	3%: 5-20 ml/kg 7%: 4-8 ml/kg Infusion: 1 ml/kg/min	Intravascular volume expansion	Small volume needed Rapid improvement of cardiovascular function Positive inotropic effect	Reflex bradycardia, hypotension Potential hypokalemia, hypernatremia	Contraindicated in hyperosmolar or hypernatremic states, heart failure, dehydration
Colloids Dextrans 40, 70	10-20 ml/kg/ day Infusion: 2 ml/kg/hr	Intravascular volume expansion Promotion of peripheral blood flow	Small volume needed Osmotically active Holds fluid in vascular space Remains in vascular space longer than crystalloids Volume expansion may persist for 4-8 hr Protentiates microcirculatory blood flow; coats endothelial surfaces Reduces incidence of thromboembolism	May decrease platelet function Renal failure possible if animal is oliguric and hypovolemia not corrected because of renal tubular obstruction Anaphylaxis (rare) Osmotic diuresis May interfere with crossmatching of blood May temporarily decrease immune competence Expensive	Contraindicated in thrombocytopenia, oliguric or anuric renal failure, heart failure

TABLE 4-3

Comparison of Fluid Therapies in Shock—cont'd

Fluid Type	IV Dosage	Indications for Use	Benefits	Potential Complications	Miscellaneous Data
Dextran 70 + hypertonic saline (3%, 7%)	4 ml/kg over 5-10 min	Intravascular volume expansion in hypovolemic and septic shock	Longer dwell time in intravascular space than hypertonic saline alone Other benefits as listed above	As above for hypertonic saline, dextrans	As above for hypertonic saline, dextrans
Hydroxyethyl starch (Hetastarch)	20 ml/kg/day	Intravascular volume expansion	Small volume needed Remains in intravascular space longer than crystalloids Osmotically active	Expensive Rarely: anaphylaxis Rarely: coagulopathy at high dosages (>20 ml/kg/day) Pulmonary edema if volume overload occurs	Increases serum amylase but does not alter pancreatic function
VetaPlasma (Marshalton Veterinary Group)	5 ml/kg every 4-6 hr as needed Infusion: 2-4 ml/min	Intravascular volume expansion Hypoproteinemia	Remains in vascular space longer than crystalloids Less coating of platelets than dextrans Can be repeated frequently	Expensive Not for use in dehydrated animals	Approved for use in dog and cat
Blood products				Osmotic diuresis	

shock, fever, pain, excitability, and systemic inflammatory response syndrome.

Corrective fluid therapy should improve perfusion, mucous membranes should moisten and improve to pink, and the capillary refill time should return to less than 2 seconds.

Third-Space Losses

The patient should be assessed for any third-space losses. Accumulation of large volumes of fluids in cavities such as pleural, peritoneal, or interstitial spaces can occur with different disease states and trauma. Fluid accumulation in interstitial spaces (e.g., inflammation around a trauma or fracture site, edema) should also be considered. Fluid lost to third spacing does not decrease body weight.

Lab Findings

A baseline set of blood values should be obtained and evaluated before any fluid regimen is started. The baseline values not only assist in choosing the proper fluid and blood volume replacements to be administered but also act as a reference point to determine any changes in the therapy plan. It is often helpful to obtain all possible blood samples before fluid administration, even if a treatment plan has not yet been implemented. The samples can always be discarded if not needed.

Packed Cell Volume or Hematocrit. The packed cell volume (PCV) should be closely monitored during fluid administration. Whether treating for shock, dehydration, or simply administering supportive care, the PCV should be checked once per day. A normal PCV is 39% to 55% in a healthy dog and 24% to 45% in a healthy cat. If the PCV drops abruptly below 20%, then a blood transfusion should be administered.

Total Plasma Protein. Total plasma protein (TP) relates to the relative serum oncotic pressure. If the serum oncotic pressure falls, then more fluid will enter the interstitium. This edema can create life-threatening disease. TP (and more importantly albumin) levels can decrease rapidly in disease and rehydration. Normal TP levels should be maintained above 3.5 g/dl and albumin levels above 2.0 g/dl. Plasma is the best fluid source for TP replacement therapy in the patient. Alternatively, colloids can also be used to help maintain serum oncotic pressure.

Urine Specific Gravity. Monitoring the patient's urine specific gravity can assist in monitoring the its hydration status. Obtaining a urine sample before fluid administration can help determine renal function. If renal function is normal, then the urine specific gravity should be elevated (>1.050) in a dehydrated patient. Normal urine specific gravity in a healthy dog is 1.015 to 1.040, and in a healthy cat it is 1.015 to 1.050. When fluid therapy has been administered, the urine specific gravity should normalize once rehydration has occurred.

Fluid Therapy for Specific States

Systemic Disease

In addition to dehydration, a number of systemic diseases adversely affect the body's natural ability to stay in equilibrium. In these situations, fluids are used to maintain hydration status, provide adequate perfusion to all tissues, diurese both endotoxins and exotoxins, restore normal serum osmolality, and help prevent shock secondary to sepsis. Many of these diseases also adversely affect electrolyte and protein levels. Careful monitoring of these parameters helps to determine the appropriate fluid therapy.

Supportive Care

Fluid therapy can also be used to help support the cardiovascular system when procedures are performed that may decrease the circulating blood volume and pressure. Anesthetic agents, in general, decrease cardiovascular output, and in many surgical procedures a certain amount of blood volume is lost. Cardiovascular support from fluid therapy can reduce the morbidity rate of anesthesia in the very young, very old, or critically ill patient.

Diuresis

Fluid therapy can be used to increase urine production, assisting the body in eliminating substances that can be excreted by the kidneys. Instances in which diuresis are warranted include renal failure, liver failure, diabetes, electrolyte imbalances, and poisonings. Fluid rates for diuresis can be adjusted from 1.5 maintenance to 3 times maintenance, depending on the age of the animal, the nature of the disease, and health of the kidneys and heart. Depending on the laboratory values, the fluids to use for diuresis usually are the isotonic to hypotonic crystalloid and dextrose solutions (Table 4-4).

Hypoproteinemia

If TP levels are below 3.5 g/dl, then the use of colloids may help maintain normal oncotic pressure. If albumin levels are below 2.0 g/dl, then it would be best to use plasma to bring the albumin level back up to this point. Plasma used to treat hypoproteinemia may either be frozen or fresh-frozen plasma. Plasma is usually administered at a dose of 5 ml/kg.

Once albumin volume has been improved, a colloid can be administered. The type of colloid used depends on whether ongoing losses of albumin are caused by capillary leakage. If albumin is low because of lack of production, then the dextrans may be used at a rate no greater than 40 ml/kg/day. Hetastarch can be administered in volumes of up to 30 ml/kg/day.

TABLE 4-4

Selection of Fluids for Certain Diseases

Condition	SERUM					Fluid of Choice
	Na⁺	Cl	K⁺	HCO₃	Volume	
Diarrhea	D	D	D	D	D	Lactated Ringer's + KCl, Normosol-R
Pyloric obstruction	D	D	D	I	D	0.9% NaCl
Dehydration	I	I	N	N/D	D	Lactated Ringer's 0.9% NaCl, 5% dextrose Normosol-R
Congestive heart failure	N/D	N/D	N	N	I	0.45% NaCl + 2.5% dextrose 5% dextrose
End-stage liver disease	N/I	N/I	D	D	I	0.45% NaCl + 2.5% dextrose + KCl
Acute renal failure						
Oliguria	I	I	I	D	I	0.9% NaCl
Polyuria	D	D	N/D	D	D	Lactated Ringer's + KCl, Normosol-R
Chronic renal failure	N/D	N/D	N	D	N/D	Lactated Ringer's solution, 0.9% NaCl
Adrenocortical insufficiency	D	D	I	N/D	D	0.9% NaCl
Diabetic ketoacidosis	D	D	N/D	D	D	0.9% NaCl (±KCl)

D, Decreased; *I*, increased; *N*, normal.

Febrile States

Fever increases an animal's metabolic rate. An increase in temperature of 1.8° F (1° C) will increase the metabolic rate by 13.8%. It is difficult to quantify precisely what this means in regard to H_2O consumption, but generally, maintenance fluid rates should be increased by 10% for each 1.8° F rise in body temperature.

Hypothermia

Patients, especially small animals, suffering from hypothermia will benefit from a rewarming process before fluid administration, because hypothermia causes vasoconstriction. Applying a Bair Hugger (forced warm air blanket), hot water bottles, or blankets will assist in safely increasing the animal's temperature. Catheter placement and fluid resuscitation can be difficult on a severely hypothermic patient because of the vasoconstriction. Without proper rewarming, smaller patients such as cats, rabbits, and ferrets can develop pulmonary edema from aggressive fluid therapy.

Anesthesia

Fluid deficits should be replaced before anesthesia or surgery whenever possible. Anesthetized patients undergo an obligatory H_2O loss of about 1.5 to 3.0 ml/kg/hr. This H_2O should be replaced in addition to H_2O lost from surgical wounds. General supportive fluid therapy for anesthetized patients is 20 ml/kg in the first hour, then 3 to 5 ml/kg each additional hour for dogs, and 3 to 5 ml/kg/hr for cats. The anesthetized patient must be monitored closely and treated with additional fluid therapies, including colloids, to decrease the chance of fluid overload during long procedures.

TABLE 4-5

Routes of Fluid Administration for Dogs and Cats

Routes	Indications and Advantages	Technique	Complications and Contraindications
Oral	For anorexic patients with short-term illnesses More appropriate for small animals (<20 kg) Very appropriate for neonates	Via a stomach tube, pharyngostomy tube, small dosing syringe, or small baby bottle and nipple, depending on animal's size and underlying illness Warm fluid to body temperature	Should not be used in cases of aspiration pneumonia Is not useful for hypovolemic shock Should not be used in vomiting animals Should avoid administering air Should not be used for acute or extensive fluid losses
Subcutaneous	For correcting mild to moderate dehydration For maintenance in patients not severely ill Not appropriate for animals weighing >10 kg	Use isotonic fluid Best to administer through gravity flow through an 18- to 20-gauge needle for adult-sized cat (use smaller needle for pediatric patients) Should not deposit more than 10-12 ml/kg per injection site Fluids should be deposited dorsally along area bordered by scapulae anteriorly and iliac crests posteriorly The average 5 to 6 kg cat can receive 150-200 ml once or twice daily	Avoid using hypertonic, hypotonic, or fluids containing dextrose Should not deposit fluids under infected or devitalized skin Is not useful for hypovolemic shock Should not use irritating solutions Safe for certain owners to be trained to do at home Should avoid hypothermic patients because of vasoconstriction

Routes

Once the patient has been assessed and the fluid type chosen, the administration of fluid therapy begins. Choices for therapy routes include oral, subcutaneous, IV (peripheral or central veins), intraosseous (intramedullary), and intraperitoneal. Oral fluid administration may be the easiest route, but it is contraindicated in life-threatening fluid imbalances. Subcutaneous fluid administration may be appropriate for cases of mild to moderate dehydration. Fluids should be warmed to body temperature and must be isotonic (osmotic pressure equal to that of ECF). However, severe fluid deficits that warrant rapid replacement are best addressed via the IV or interosseous routes. Intraperitoneal fluid administration generally is not recommended because of complications of peritonitis and intraabdominal abscessation (Table 4-5).

Fluid Dosing and Rates

The fluid dosing regimens presented in this section are guidelines. Careful monitoring is essential in determining what is needed to correctly treat the patient's condition.

Shock Doses

Isotonic Crystalloids
Initial rapid infusion

Dogs: 20 to 40 ml/kg is given intravenously for the first 15 minutes, then the patient is reassessed. Shock dose may be continued at 70 to 90 ml/kg over 1 hour, reassessing the patient every 15 minutes.

Cats: 10 to 20 ml/kg is given intravenously for the first 15 minutes, then the patient is reassessed. Shock dose may be continued at 35 to 50 ml/kg over 1 hour.

Hypertonic Crystalloids

7.5% sodium chloride
4 ml/kg over 2 minutes
Response should be seen within 1 to 2 minutes
Duration of response 1 to 2 hours

Colloids

Dogs: 10 to 20 ml/kg
Cats: 10 to 15 ml/kg

In cases of poor perfusion, dextan or hetastarch may be given at these rates as a rapid IV bolus. The technician should be cautious when bolusing fluids to cats. Rapid infusion has been associated with vomiting, hypotension, prolonged bleeding, and collapse. Life-threatening reactions are less frequent with hetastarch. If the patient's underlying disorder is trauma (without an ongoing disease), then a single colloid bolus should be sufficient to bring blood pressure up rapidly while preserving the interstitium of the brain and lungs.

Replacement Doses

Replacement doses are used to correct dehydration and replace fluid loses. One first needs to calculate the volume deficit needed for replacement. Dehydration usually can be corrected in the first 24 hours of therapy. It is generally recommended to correct dehydration by deficit replacement of 75% to 80% on the first day and the remaining 25% on the second day. Another method is called *front-end loading,* in which enough fluids are administered during the first 4 to 8 hours to correct dehydration. The first approach may be more advantageous physiologically, because it allows more time for adequate equilibration of H_2O and electrolytes between body compartments.

The volume needed to correct dehydration is calculated as follows:

% dehydration × body weight (kg)
= liters of fluid to be replaced

% dehydration × body weight (lb) × 500
= milliliters of fluids to be replaced

Maintenance Doses

Maintenance volume is the amount of fluid and electrolytes needed on a daily basis to keep the volume of TBW and electrolyte content normal in a well-hydrated patient. This volume consists of two subcomponents:

1. Insensible losses: Not readily measurable losses from respiratory evaporation, passage of normal feces, and sweat (which is negligible in dogs and cats). This loss can be estimated at 22 ml/kg/day (10 ml/lb/day). These losses can increase during febrile states, panting, and high environmental temperatures.
2. Sensible losses: Readily measurable losses such as urine production. Urine production is approximately 22 to 44 ml/kg/day (10 to 20 ml/lb/day) in normal animals (Table 4-6).

Crystalloids

Dogs: 66 ml/kg/day
Cats: 50 to 60 ml/kg/day

These volumes are based on patients with normal urine output. The normal animal loses approximately 65 to 75 mEq/L sodium and 15 to 20 mEq/L of potassium in the urine on a daily basis. Using these values, maintenance fluids should nearly equal the expected losses (see Table 4-6).

Colloids. A constant rate infusion of large molecular colloids (hetastarch or pentastarch) may be necessary in cases of sepsis or systemic inflammatory response syndrome. After an initial IV bolus, the daily recommended dose is divided over a 24-hour period and administered with crystalloids.

Dogs: 20 ml/kg/day
Cats: 10 to 15 ml/kg/day

Delivery Systems

Intravenous Lines

Many brands of IV fluid lines exist. The major manufacturers are Baxter Travenol, McGaw, Abbott, and Arrow. It is important to remember that the brand of infusion set must be compatible with the infusion pumps that are in the hospital.

TABLE 4-6

Daily Water Requirements for Dogs

Body Weight (kg)	Total Water/Day (ml)	Milliliters per kg (ml/kg)
1	140	140
2	232	116
3	312	104
4	385	96
5	453	91
6	518	86
7	580	83
8	639	80
9	696	77
10	752	75
11	806	73
12	859	71
13	911	70
14	961	68
15	1011	67
16	1060	66
17	1108	65
18	1155	64
19	1201	63
20	1247	62
25	1468	59
30	1677	56
35	1876	54
40	2068	52
45	2254	50
50	2434	49
60	2781	46
70	3112	44
80	3431	43
90	3739	41
100	4038	40

From Ross L: Fluid therapy for acute and chronic renal failure, *Vet Clin North Am* 19:343, 1989.

Extension sets and t-sets should be matched to infusion sets (most brands are compatible with others). Low-volume extension sets are also available for the smaller patient.

Manufacturers will custom make IV sets, extension sets, and t-sets that will be compatible with a number of different infusion pumps. The advantage to a custom set is that its length can be changed in accordance with the hospital's needs; Aseptic technique is maintained when dealing with IV lines. Injection ports are cleaned with alcohol before use, and the fluid lines are changed whenever disconnected or soiled, as well as after 24 hours of use.

The label on the administration set typically identifies the number of drops per milliliter that the set provides. Typically, administration sets can be found that deliver 10, 15, and 60 drops per milliliter. The drops normally are observed passing through a small drip chamber. With this information, drops per minute can be calculated (important when calculating fluid drip rates for gravity feed systems).

Buretrols are fluid chambers that hold 150 ml of fluid. The markers on the buretrol divide the chamber by milliliters, allowing for very accurate measurement of fluid administration in smaller animals. Buretrols can also be used for mixing different concentrations of solutions or drug therapies that must be given over a period of time. For small patients, fewer drops per milliliter allows for a more accurate fluid dose. Buretrol systems, with their attached burettes, offer accurate control of fluid doses in the exceptionally small patient. Medications to be infused can be added directly to the burette (Fig. 4-1).

Fluid Rate Administration

Although administering fluids by gravity flow is a common practice, it can be difficult to maintain regulated flow rates. Using a fluid pump can eliminate many of these complications.

In a gravity feed system, fluids are kept in an elevated position above the patient, and gravity forces the fluids into the body. The drip rate is adjusted manually using the regulator on the fluid line. A timing measure should be affixed to the line so that dosing accuracy can be ascertained. Gravity feed systems depend on patient positioning; thus they must be monitored very closely. Dial-a-Flows are devices attached to the fluid lines and can be adjusted depending on what rate is needed.

Suggested Readings

Aldrich J: *Where did all my fluids flow?* Proceedings of the 10th Annual Meeting of the IVECCS, San Antonio, TX, 2004, pp 257-261.

Antinoff N: *Avian medicine: the basics.* Proceedings of the 10th Annual Meeting of the IVECCS, San Antonio, TX, 2004, pp 207-213.

Antifnoff N: Emergency care of reptiles. Proceedings of the 10th Annual Meeting of the IVECCS, San Antonio, TX, 2004, pp 224-228.

Armstrong SR et al: Perioperative hypothermia, *J Vet Emerg Crit Care* 15:32-37, 2005.

DiBartola S: Introduction to fluid therapy. In DiBartola S: *Fluid therapy in small animal practice*, ed 2, Philadelphia, 2000, Saunders, pp 265-279.

Hohenhaus AE, Rentko V: Blood trans. and blood substitutes. In DiBartola S: *Fluid therapy in small animal practice*, ed 2, Philadelphia, 2000, Saunders, pp 461-462.

Litchtenberger M: *Critical care for rabbits and ferrets.* Proceedings of the 10th Annual Meeting of the IVECCS, San Antonio, TX, 2004, pp 241-245.

Pascoe PJ: Periop mgt of fluid therapy. In DiBartola S: *Fluid therapy in small animal practice*, ed 2, Philadelphia, 2000, Saunders, pp 319-326.

Schertel ER, Tobias TA: Hypertonic fluid therapy. In DiBartola S: *Fluid therapy in small animal practice*, ed 2, Philadelphia, 2000, Saunders, pp 496-504.

Silverstein D: Shock fluid therapy: past, present and future strategies. Proceedings of the 10th Annual Meeting of the IVECCS, San Antonio, TX, 2004, pp 262-270.

CHAPTER 5

Small Animal Transfusion Medicine

DONNA A. OAKLEY

As a result of the increased specialization in veterinary medicine, the demand for blood products has risen dramatically. These specialties (i.e., emergency medicine, critical care, oncology) have created a need for knowledge and expertise in veterinary transfusion medicine. The importance of transfusion education for veterinarians, veterinary technicians, and students continues to unfold. Education is clearly the link to ensuring the overall quality of all aspects of blood banking and transfusion services.

A safe and adequate supply of blood components for transfusion is indispensable. The American Association of Blood Banks has established acceptable standards for the collection, processing, storage, distribution, and administration of human blood and blood components. Each blood bank and transfusion service strictly follows these standards, as well as certain legal requirements of local, state, and federal governments (most importantly, those of the Food and Drug Administration). Strict compliance with these standards reflects a commitment to providing quality products and appropriate care for patients receiving transfusion support. Although government organizations play less of a role in ensuring quality practices in veterinary medicine, the industry is striving to adhere to similar standards. To that end, the Association of Veterinary Hematology and Transfusion Medicine is helping to establish standards in veterinary transfusion medicine and blood banking that guarantee safety and efficacy.

Whole Blood and Components

With the availability of variable speed, temperature-controlled centrifuges and the advent of plastic storage bags with integral tubing for collection, processing, and administration, specific blood component therapy is possible. The goal in veterinary transfusion medicine is to limit whole blood (WB) transfusion and to use component therapy whenever possible. WB can be stored or processed into one or more of the following components: red blood cells (RBCs), platelets, plasma, and cryoprecipitate (CRYO). Blood components permit specific replacement therapy for specific disorders, reduce the number of transfusion reactions as a result of diminished exposure to foreign material, and decrease the amount of time needed to transfuse. Most importantly, appropriate therapeutic use of blood components increases the number of patients who benefit from this limited resource.

Blood is made up of two portions: (1) a cellular portion and (2) the plasma, which acts as a carrier medium for the cells, proteins, gases, nutrients, vitamins, and waste products. Each component of blood has a specific role or function in the body. Certain disease states require replacement of one or any combination of these components. The component or components chosen will depend on the crisis at hand.

Whole Blood

Initial collection yields fresh whole blood (FWB) and is defined as such for up to 8 hours after collection. FWB provides RBCs, white blood cells (WBCs), platelets, plasma proteins, and coagulation factors. Certain components in blood are more fragile than others and will become less effective with time and ambient temperature change. To achieve full benefit of all components when needed, FWB should be administered immediately after collection.

FWB is used in actively bleeding, anemic animals with thrombocytopenia or thrombopathia, anemia with coagulopathies, and massive hemorrhage. Massive hemorrhage is defined as a loss approaching or exceeding one total blood volume within a 24-hour period. In cases of severe hemorrhage, administration of all components may be necessary to support the patient.

After collection, WB must be processed into components or (at the least) refrigerated at 1° to 6° C within 8 hours. After 24-hour storage of WB, platelet function is lost and the concentration of labile coagulation factors decreases (factor V and factor VIII). The product is then defined as *stored WB* and provides RBCs, the more stable coagulation factors, and other plasma proteins (i.e., albumin, globulins). The length of time a unit of WB can be stored under refrigeration depends on the anticoagulant-preservative solution used in collection. With the advantages

in the use of blood components so well documented in both human and veterinary medicine, as well as the improved availability of these products as a result of commercial blood banks, the use of WB is no longer considered the treatment of choice. However, stored WB can be used in patients that require oxygen-carrying support and intravascular volume expansion.

The use of WB, fresh or stored, is not recommended in severe chronic anemia. Chronically anemic patients may have a reduced red cell mass but have compensated over time by increasing their plasma volume to meet their total blood volume. Administration of WB may expose these patients to the risk of volume overload, especially in patients with preexisting cardiac disease or renal compromise.

Packed Red Blood Cells

Packed red blood cells (PRBCs) can be harvested from a unit of WB after centrifugation at 4° C, and stored at 1° to 6° C for approximately 1 month (definitive storage time is determined by the anticoagulant-preservative solution used in collection). In patients who require oxygen-carrying support, PRBCs are the component of choice for increasing red cell mass. Decreased red cell mass may be caused by decreased bone marrow production, increased destruction of RBCs, or surgical or traumatic bleeding. Although it seems logical that blood loss should be replaced with WB, replacing blood volume with PRBCs and crystalloid or colloid solutions is often adequate therapy for the majority of acutely bleeding patients.

Transfusion of PRBCs is not recommended in patients who are well compensated for their anemia (e.g., chronic renal failure). The decision to perform red cell transfusion should never be based solely on hematocrit (HTC) or hemoglobin levels. Patients should be properly evaluated and PRBC administration based primarily on clinical status (e.g., respiratory compromise, tachycardia, poor pulse quality, lethargy).

Plasma Components

Fresh Frozen Plasma. In addition to water and electrolytes, plasma contains albumin, globulins, and coagulation factors. Plasma is primarily used for its coagulation factor value; it does not contain functional platelets. Most coagulation proteins are stable at 1° to 6° C, with the exception of factors V and VIII. To maintain adequate levels of all factors, plasma must be harvested from a unit of WB and frozen at −18° C or colder within 8 hours from the time of initial collection. This product is then labeled as *fresh frozen plasma* (FFP) and will retain its coagulation factor efficacy for 12 months provided it is maintained at the appropriate temperature. FFP can be used to treat most coagulation factor deficiencies (e.g., disseminated intravascular coagulation, liver disease, anticoagulant rodenticide toxicity, hereditary coagulopathies) and potentially other conditions (e.g., acute pancreatitis). FFP is not recommended for use as a blood volume expander or for protein replacement in animals with chronic hypoproteinemia.

Frozen and Liquid Plasma. Plasma may be separated from a unit of WB anytime during storage (through its expiration date). When stored at −18° C or colder after harvesting, the component is called *FP* and may be kept for up to 5 years from the date of initial WB collection. If not frozen, then it is called *liquid plasma* (LP) and has a shelf life not exceeding 5 days after the expiration date of the WB from which it was harvested. Additionally, if FFP is not used within 12 months, then it can be relabeled as *frozen plasma* (FP) and stored for an additional 4 years.

FP and LP may have varying levels of the more stable coagulation factors, as well as albumin; however, FP and LP do not contain functional platelets or the labile coagulation factors V and VIII. FP and LP can be used to treat stable clotting factor deficiencies and certain cases of acute hypoproteinemia (i.e., parvoviral enteritis). If animals are severely or chronically protein deficient, then plasma must be administered in large volumes to have a measurable effect in managing the acute effects of hypoproteinemia (i.e., pulmonary edema, pleural effusion). In this case, synthetic colloid solutions should be considered because they are readily available and more effective in increasing oncotic pressure. As with FFP, FP and LP are not recommended for use as a blood volume expander.

Cryoprecipitate. CRYO is the cold-insoluble portion of plasma that precipitates after FFP has been slowly thawed at 1° to 6° C (i.e., refrigerator). The precipitated material contains concentrated amounts of von Willebrand's factor, factor VIII, fibrinogen, and fibronectin. After production, CRYO can be frozen at −18° C or colder and has a shelf life of 1 year from the original date of WB collection. CRYO can be used in patients with possible or diagnosed von Willebrand's disease, hemophilia A, or fibrinogen deficiency. Each unit of CRYO contains approximately 25 to 50 ml of LP.

Platelets. Platelet-rich plasma (PRP) is harvested from a unit of FWB that is less than 8 hours old and has not been cooled below 20° C. Refrigerated platelets do not maintain function or viability as well as platelets stored at room temperature. The PRP may be administered after centrifugation, or the platelets may be further concentrated by additional centrifugation and removal of most of the supernatant plasma. Under optimal conditions, platelets prepared from a single unit of FWB administered to a 30 kg dog would be expected to result in an increase in the patient's platelet count of 10,000/µl.

The major indication for platelet transfusion is to stop severe, uncontrolled, or life-threatening bleeding in patients with decreased platelet number, function, or both. In situations of platelet destruction, such as idiopathic thrombocytopenia purpura, the survival of transfused platelets is a matter of minutes rather than days; however, platelet transfusion may still be warranted if the patient is acutely bleeding into a vital structure (i.e., brain, myocardium, lung). Patients experiencing massive hemorrhage may also require platelet support to compensate for excessive consumption during hemostasis and the dilution factor associated with volume replacement therapy.

In veterinary medicine, platelet preparation is difficult in regard to the volume needed to measurably increase platelet numbers in larger breed dogs. In some patients, however, cessation of bleeding after platelet transfusion has been achieved without a measurable increase in platelet number. Because of the impracticality associated with production of this component in the required volume necessary for significant effect, as well as the specific storage requirements and short shelf life, veterinary medicine routinely treats patients with thrombocytopenia and thrombopathia (with active bleeding) with FWB through which the patient will receive both platelets and oxygen-carrying support (Table 5-1).

Blood Sources

Historically, veterinarians have relied on donor dogs living within the hospital facility as a source of blood for transfusion purposes. Blood was collected for immediate use, and little emphasis was placed on quality control. However, these few in-house donors failed to meet the growing need for transfusion. During the past few years, several commercial animal blood banks and community-based blood donor programs have been established to help meet blood transfusion needs. These facilities supply safe and high-quality blood products that are processed according to the standards set forth by the American Association of Blood Banks. Blood banking staff also share expertise in transfusion medicine through newsletters and individual case consultation requests. Purchasing products from these blood banks and maintaining an inventory within the hospital may be much more time efficient and cost-effective than maintaining in-house donors and likely provides more specific products to treat specific disorders.

Large blood banks obtain their supplies from closed donor colonies or a volunteer donor programs. Each approach has advantages and disadvantages. Animals rescued from terminal situations (i.e., retired racing dogs, dogs given or claimed by the Society for the Prevention of Cruelty to Animals) may support closed donor colonies. These animals are given a second chance at life and are adopted into homes after a predetermined stay at the blood bank facility. An unknown medical history is the biggest disadvantage in securing donors from these sources.

Other blood banks have opted to establish volunteer donor programs to meet the transfusion needs of the profession. Recruitment of donors is accomplished through employee personal pets, healthy client-owned animals, breeders, and organized dog clubs. Client education as to the importance of blood product availability and the need for blood donors is instrumental in establishing a donor pool. Informed and educated pet owners are valuable assets to this type of program. Most are willing to volunteer their pets for periodic blood donation (i.e., 3 to 4 times a year) once they understand the need for blood products and the elements of the donation process. Comparable to those who volunteer to help human blood donor programs, these pet owners are motivated by altruism. Nevertheless, potential donors may carry illnesses that could possibly affect the safety of the donation

process, the safety and quality of the blood products, or both, thereby further compromising patients. For this reason, it is important to verify donor health status through an extensive medical history, physical examination, and appropriate laboratory testing, all of which are performed on the day of the donation.

Canine donors must meet specific requirements before being accepted into the program. Donors must be a minimum of 1 year of age and weigh at least 25 kg to allow for the collection of a full unit (i.e., 450 ml +/– 10%). They should be healthy, have a current vaccination status for distemper, hepatitis, parainfluenza, parvovirus, and rabies and not be on medication at the time of donation (excluding heartworm and ectoparasite preventative). Because canine donors are not sedated for blood collection, good temperament is required for successful donation. On an annual basis, a complete blood count, serum biochemistry profile, and testing for geographically specific infectious agents (e.g., *Ehrlichia canis, Babesia canis*) should be performed. The HCT or hemoglobin concentration should be ≥40% or ≥13.5 g/dl, respectively, before each donation. Although each donor should be evaluated as an individual, most dogs are retired from the blood donor program by the age of 7 years (Table 5-2).

Blood types are genetic markers on the surface of RBCs, are specific to each species, and are antigenic. A set of blood types of two or more alleles makes up a blood group system. More than 12 blood group systems have been described in dogs. The current nomenclature is listed as dog erythrocyte antigen (DEA) followed by a number. RBCs from a dog can either be positive or negative for any blood group system other than the DEA 1 system. For example, a dog's red cells can be DEA 3 positive or DEA 3 negative. The DEA 1 system, however, has at least two subtypes: (1) DEA 1.1 (also known as *A1*) and (2) DEA 1.2 (also known as *A2*). Thus a dog's red cells can be DEA 1.1 positive or negative, and DEA 1.1 negative cells can be DEA 1.2 positive or negative. Very limited surveys on the frequency of canine blood types have been reported (Table 5-3). Some blood types are rare (e.g., DEA 3), whereas others are more common (DEA 4).

Clinically, the most severe antigen-antibody reaction is observed with the DEA 1.1 antigen. *Significant* naturally occurring alloantibodies are not seen in the dog; therefore antigen-antibody reactions are not likely to occur on initial transfusion. However, dogs that are DEA 1.1 negative can develop alloantibodies

TABLE 5-1

Transfusion Therapy

Component	Contents	Indications	Shelf Life	Preparation	Comments
Fresh whole blood (FWB)	Red blood cells (RBCs), plasma proteins, all coagulation factors, white blood cells (WBCs), platelets (approx. hematocrit [HCT] 40%)	Acute active hemorrhage, hypovolemic shock, thrombocytopenia or thrombopathia with active bleeding	Less than 8 hours after initial collection	Use immediately after collection (temperatures below 20° C compromise platelet viability)	Restores blood volume and oxygen-carrying capacity; may help control some microvascular bleeding in patients with thrombocytopenia/thrombopathia
Stored whole blood (WB)	RBC, plasma proteins (approx. HCT 40%)	Anemia with hypoproteinemia, hypovolemic shock	Greater than 8 hours old and up to 30 days (dependent on anticoagulant-preservative solution used); refrigerate at 1-6° C	Allow to come to room temperature (temperatures exceeding 37° C will result in hemolysis and bacterial proliferation)	Restores blood volume and oxygen-carrying capacity; WBC and platelets not viable; factors V & VIII diminished; not recommended for chronic anemia
Packed red blood cells (PRBC)	RBC (approx. HCT 80%), reduced plasma	Increase red cell mass in symptomatic anemia	Dependent on anticoagulant-preservative solution used; refrigerate at 1-6° C	Allow to come to room temperature (temperatures exceeding 37° C will result in hemolysis and bacterial proliferation); may reconstitute with 0.9% sodium chloride before administration	Same oxygen-carrying capacity as WB but less volume

Product	Composition	Indication	Storage	Handling	Notes
PRBC, adenine-saline added	RBC (approx. HCT 60%), reduced plasma, 100 ml additive solution	Increase red cell mass in symptomatic anemia	28-30 days; refrigerate at 1-6° C	Allow to come to room temperature (temperatures exceeding 37° C will result in hemolysis and bacterial proliferation)	Additive solution extends shelf life of PRBC by improving storage environment; reduces viscosity for infusion
Platelet-rich plasma (PRP)/platelet concentrate	Platelets, few RBCs and WBCs, some plasma	Life-threatening bleeding caused by thrombocytopenia or thrombopathia	5 days at 22° C; intermittent agitation required	Should administer immediately after collection and preparation	Should not refrigerate
Fresh frozen plasma (FFP)	Plasma, albumin, all coagulation factors	Treatment of coagulation disorders/factor deficiencies, liver disease, disseminated intravascular coagulation, anticoagulant rodenticide toxicity	12 months frozen at −18° C or colder	Thaw in 37° C warm-water bath (temperatures exceeding 37° C will result in protein denaturation and bacterial proliferation)	Frozen within 8 hours after collection; no platelets; can be relabeled as *frozen plasma* (FP) after 1 year for additional 4 years; must be administered within 4 hours after thawing
FP	Plasma, albumin, stable coagulation factors	Treatment of stable coagulation factor deficiencies	5 years frozen at −18° C or colder	Thaw in 37° C warm-water bath (temperatures exceeding 37° C will result in protein denaturation and bacterial proliferation)	Frozen after more than 8 hours after collection; no platelets; can be used to treat some cases of acute hypoproteinemia; must be administered within 4 hours after thawing
Cryoprecipitate (CRYO)	Factor VIII, von Willebrand's factor, fibrinogen, fibronectin	Hemophilia A von Willebrand's disease, hypofibrinogenemia	12 months frozen at −18° C or colder	Thaw in 37° C warm-water bath (temperatures exceeding 37° C will result in protein denaturation and bacterial proliferation)	Must be administered within 4 hours after thawing

TABLE 5-2

Canine Infectious Disease Screening

Disease	Disease Agent	Screening
Babesiosis	B. canis, B. gibsoni	Recommended
Leishmaniasis	L. donovani	Recommended
Ehrlichiosis	E. canis	Recommended
	E. ewingii, E. chaffeenis	Conditional
Brucellosis	B. canis	Recommended
Anaplasmosis	A. phagocytophilum	Conditional
	A. platys	
Neorickettsiosis	N. risticii	Conditional
	N. helminthica	
Trypanosomiasis	T. cruzi	Conditional
Bartonellosis	B. vinsonii	Conditional
Lyme	B. burgdorferi	Not recommended
Rocky Mountain spotted fever	R. rickettsii	Not recommended

From Wardrop et al: Canine and feline blood donor screening for infectious disease, *J Vet Intern Med* 19:135-142, 2005.

to DEA 1.1 from a mismatched first transfusion. These anti-DEA 1.1 antibodies can develop within as few as 9 days from initial transfusion and can potentially destroy the donor's RBCs, ultimately minimizing the benefits of the transfusion. However, a previously sensitized DEA 1.1 negative dog can experience an acute hemolytic transfusion reaction after transfusion of DEA 1.1 positive blood. Transfusion reactions may also occur after a previously transfused (and now sensitized) dog receives blood that is mismatched for any red cell antigen other than DEA 1.1. These reactions may occur as early as 4 days after sensitization. For example, a previously sensitized DEA 4 negative dog experienced an acute hemolytic transfusion reaction while receiving DEA 4 positive blood. Despite the variety of identified and unidentified blood types and the limited availability of compatibility testing in clinical practice, transfusion reactions are rarely reported.

Because of the strong antigenicity of DEA 1.1, typing of donors for DEA 1.1 is strongly recommended. A simple in-practice blood-typing kit is commercially available to classify dogs as DEA 1.1 negative or positive. Blood from a DEA 1.1 negative donor can be given to DEA 1.1 negative and DEA 1.1 positive patients. Dogs positive for the DEA 1.1 antigen can be accepted into the donor pool, as long as recipients are typed before administration, with DEA 1.1 positive blood being given only to patients positive for DEA 1.1 (see Table 5-3).

The approach to the feline donor is much more complicated than with its canine counterpart. At present, few commercial feline blood banks exist. In addition, volunteer programs for cats hold many

TABLE 5-3

Blood Type Frequencies in Dogs

Blood Types	% Positive	% Negative
DEA 1		
1.1 (A1)	33-45	55-67
1.2 (A2)	7-20	35-60*
DEA 3	5-10	90-95
DEA 4	87-98	2-13
DEA 5	12-22	78-88
DEA 7	8-45	55-92

*DEA 1.1– and DEA 1.2–negative dogs.

TABLE 5-4

Feline Infectious Disease Screen

Disease	Disease Agent	Screening
Feline leukemia virus	Feline leukemia virus	Recommended
Feline immunodeficiency virus	Feline immunodeficiency virus	Recommended
Hemoplasmosis	*M. haemofelis* *M. haemominutum*	Recommended
Bartonellosis	*B. henselae* *B. clarridgeiae, B. cholerae*	Recommended Conditional
Cytauxzoonosis	*C. felis*	Conditional
Ehrilichiosis	*E. canis*-like	Conditional
Anaplasmosis	*A. phagocytophilum*	Conditional
Neorickettsiosis	*N. risticii*	Conditional
Feline infectious peritonitis	Feline enteric coronavirus	Not recommended
Toxoplasmosis	*T. gondii*	Not recommended

risks. Although dogs will donate blood voluntarily, the majority of cats must be sedated for blood donation purposes. The legal ramifications associated with sedating personal pets for blood donation is far too great. Another concern is that cats can harbor infectious agents more readily than dogs. For this reason, only 100% indoor cats should be used.

Feline blood donors should be young, good-natured adults. They should be large and lean, weighing at least 5 kg to allow for collection of a 40- to 50-ml unit of blood. Good health can be verified through a medical history, physical examination, and routine laboratory testing. Donors should have current vaccination status for rhinotracheitis, calicivirus, panleukopenia, and rabies. Annual laboratory screening includes complete blood count, serum biochemistry profile, feline leukemia virus, feline immunodeficiency virus, *Mycoplasma haemofelis*, and *M. haemominutum*. Before each donation, donor HCT (≥35%) or hemoglobin (≥11 g/dl) is checked (Table 5-4).

One blood group system, the AB system, has been recognized in the cat. It contains three blood types: (1) A, (2) B, and (3) the extremely rare AB. Nearly all domestic short hair and domestic long hair cats have type A blood, the most common. Many purebred cats (and some domestic short hair cats) have been identified with type B blood. The proportion of type A and B varies not only among the different breeds but

also geographically. The rare type AB blood has both the A and B antigen on the red cell surface.

Cats differ from dogs in that they have significant naturally occurring alloantibodies against the other blood group. Cats with type B blood have very strong naturally occurring anti-A alloantibodies, whereas type A cats have relatively weak anti-B alloantibodies. These alloantibodies can cause two serious problems:

1. Transfusion reactions—Cats with rare type B blood can experience potentially fatal reactions if they are given a transfusion of type A blood. Type A cats receiving type B blood may not exhibit clinical signs associated with an acute adverse reaction; however, the half-life of the type B cells will be short and the transfusion ineffective.
2. Neonatal isoerythrolysis—If a queen with type B blood is bred to a tom with type A blood and produces kittens with type A blood, then the antibodies in the colostrum of the queen will destroy type A RBCs in the kittens.

When administering type B blood to a type A cat, an obvious clinical reaction may not occur; however, the transfused red cells have a half-life of approximately 2 days. Ultimately, this has no positive effect on the patient. In administering type A blood to a type B cat, the red cell survival can be minutes to hours with severe clinical (sometimes fatal) signs. Administration of a small amount of blood to test for incompatibility is not an acceptable procedure. Life-threatening acute hemolytic transfusion reactions can be observed with administration of as little as 1 ml of AB-incompatible blood. These reactions can be avoided by typing donors and patients. Blood-typing cards similar to those used in dogs are also commercially available.

Because of the presence of naturally occurring alloantibodies, no universal blood type exists in the cat. All feline blood donors and recipients must be blood typed, and only type-specific blood should be administered. If blood-typing cards are not available, then a blood crossmatch (BCM) should be performed to ensure blood compatibility. The extremely rare blood type AB cat lacks anti-A and anti-B alloantibodies and can be safely transfused with type A PRBCs if type AB blood is not available.

Blood Collection

Quality should be the primary goal in the collection, processing, storage, and administration of all blood products. At each step, it is critical that practices must prevent or delay adverse changes to blood constituents, as well as minimize bacterial contamination and proliferation.

Anticoagulant-Preservative Solutions

Several anticoagulants, anticoagulant-preservatives, and additive solutions are available for blood collection for transfusion purposes. The primary goal of preservative solutions is to maintain red cell viability during storage and to lengthen the survival of red cells posttransfusion. According to American Association of Blood Banks standards, 75% of transfused RBCs must survive for 24 hours after infusion for the transfusion to be considered acceptable and successful. The longer cells are stored, the more viability decreases. Predetermined storage times are based on studies that have investigated adverse biochemical changes that take place during red cell storage. These alterations, referred to as the *storage lesion*, include such things as a decrease in pH and 2,3-diphosphoglycerate (2,3-diphosphoglycerate loss occurs only in dogs), an increase in the percentage of hemolysis, and an increase in ammonia level within the blood

product. All of these changes ultimately lead to a loss of red cell function and decreased viability. Storage time will vary with the anticoagulant-preservative solution used:

1. Citrate-phosphate-dextrose-adenine-1:
   - RBC 2,3-diphosphoglycerate and adenosine triphosphate better maintained
   - Good anticoagulant-preservative solution; WB may be stored for 30 days, PRBCs may be stored for 21 days
   - Used at ratio of 1 ml citrate-phosphate-dextrose-adenine-1 to 7 to 9 ml WB
2. Citrate-phosphate-dextrose:
   - PRBCs may be stored for 21 days
   - Used at ratio of 1 ml citrate-phosphate-dextrose to 7 to 9 ml WB
3. Acid-citrate-dextrose:
   - PRBCs may be stored for 21 days
   - Used at ratio of 1 ml acid-citrate-dextrose to 7 to 9 ml WB
4. Heparin:
   - Not recommended for transfusion purposes
5. Additive solutions (e.g., Adsol, Fenwal Laboratories, Baxter Healthcare Corp, Deerfield, IL; Nutricel, Miles, Pharmaceutical Division, West Haven, CT; Optisol, Terumo Medical Corporation, Somerset, NJ):
   - Protein-free solution added to red cells after plasma removal from unit of WB
   - Canine PRBCs may be stored for approximately 30 days

Blood Collection Systems

WB is most often collected into commercially available plastic bags (Baxter Healthcare Corp, Fenwal Division; Miles, Inc., Cutter Biological Division, Elkhart, IN; Terumo Medical Corp, Somerset, NJ). These sterile bags are considered "closed" collection systems in that they allow for collection, processing, and storage of blood and blood components without exposure to the environment, diminishing the risk of bacterial contamination to the product. These systems are available in a variety of configurations that will determine blood component preparation and storage. They all meet human blood banking standards and have been tested successfully in veterinary medicine.

A single blood collection bag is used for the collection of WB when it is to be administered as WB. This system consists of a main collection bag containing anticoagulant-preservative solution and integral tubing with a 16-gauge needle attached. A single blood collection bag is not recommended for component preparation because the bag must be entered to harvest components, risking environmental exposure and potential bacterial contamination. If the bag is entered, then the definition of this system then becomes "open," and the product must be used within 24 hours. Other collection systems consist of a primary collection bag containing anticoagulant-preservative solution and one, two, or three satellite bags intended for component preparation. One of the satellite bags may contain 100 ml of an additive solution used for red cell reconstitution after plasma removal. Additive solutions (i.e., saline, dextrose, adenine) extend PRBC storage time.

Vacuum glass bottles containing acid-citrate-dextrose anticoagulant-preservative solution have always been a popular collection system used for canine blood donation. Although blood collection is more rapid with this system, many limitations and disadvantages exist. For example, a vacuum glass bottle is considered an open collection system, the glass activates platelets and certain clotting factors, the foam created during collection will disrupt the red cell surface and cause hemolysis, and component preparation is not possible. Therefore vacuum glass bottles are not recommended. Vacuum chambers that allow for more rapid collection into blood collection bags are available.

In the dog, blood may be collected using the human blood collection bags; however, the size of these systems prohibits their use in cats. Currently, smaller closed collection systems are not commercially available. In addition, blood component preparation is difficult because of the small volume of blood with which to work. Recommendations have been made to use the 450 ml citrate-phosphate-dextrose-adenine-1 blood collection system used in humans and dogs. The majority of anticoagulant is expressed from the main collection pack into a satellite container via integral tubing. The remainder of the anticoagulant solution in the collection tubing will be appropriate for 1 U of WB (e.g., 40 to 50 ml). Using this approach to blood collection maintains a closed system. Because of the size of both the collection bag and its attached needle (16 gauge), the author does not recommend this method.

Because of the lack of commercially prepared closed blood collection systems for cats, the difficulty in preparing blood components from small WB

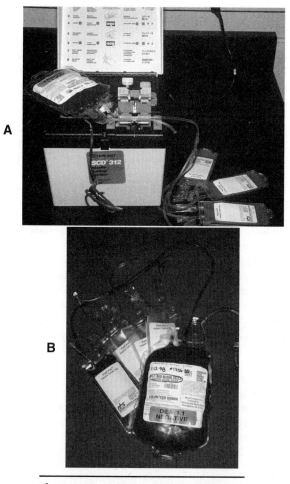

Fig. 5-1 **A,** Tubing welder. **B,** Finished product.

units, and limited storage time allowed for blood collected with an open system, cats in need of transfusion support have most often received FWB. By modifying current blood collection protocols, the Penn Animal Blood Bank has developed a closed collection system for small blood volumes (20 to 50 ml) by using commercially available blood collection products. All connections are established and sterility is maintained by using a tube-welding instrument (Terumo Sterile Tubing Welder 312) (Fig. 5-1). This newly developed system may serve as a prototype for a commercially manufactured closed collection system for cats that will allow for collection, processing, and storage of feline blood components.

Blood Collection Techniques

Plastic bag collection systems can be placed within a vacuum chamber and blood withdrawal facilitated by establishing negative pressure. The blood collection bag is hung from a hook on the chamber lid. The collection line with attached needle is brought through a notch between the cylinder and lid, and a hemostat is clamped on the line distal to the needle. A vacuum source is connected via tubing to an inlet in the chamber. The chamber is placed on a scale, the scale is turned to zero, and the suction is adjusted to less than 3 inches of mercury. The needle is inserted into the jugular vein, the hemostat is removed, and blood flows into the collection line to the bag as the scale measures the grams of blood collected (i.e., 1 ml of WB weighs approximately 1.06 g). When the desired amount is collected (i.e., 405 to 495 ml), the hemostat is clamped on the line, the needle is removed, and pressure is applied to the collection site. Successful collection depends on many factors (e.g., animal restraint, venipuncture technique, vacuum pressure). After collection, the WB unit can be used immediately, stored as WB, or processed into components and stored according to established blood banking protocols (Fig. 5-2).

Alternatively, blood can be collected using separate, single syringes. A butterfly catheter attached to a three-way stopcock and sterile 10- to 60-ml syringes containing anticoagulant may be used. During collection, the syringes should be gently inverted to allow for mixing of blood and anticoagulant, preventing clot formation. Blood collection using this technique is effective but considered an open system. After collection, blood can be transferred from the syringes into an empty sterile bag or transfer pack, making delivery more efficient. Products collected via syringe are not suitable for storage.

Avoidance of hypotension is a concern during blood collection. Careful monitoring of the donor is essential, because hypotension can be encountered despite all precautions, particularly in the feline donor. Some institutions routinely administer intravenous or subcutaneous 0.9% sodium chloride at a dose of two to three times the volume of blood drawn to feline blood donors immediately after donation. Others only treat the donors if symptoms of hypotension occur. To avoid hypotension, the target unit collection time is usually 4 to 10 minutes.

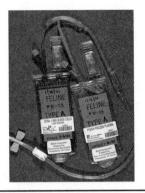

Fig. 5-2 Feline blood collection system.

Processing and Storage

The centrifuge rotor size, speed, and duration of spin are the critical variables in preparing components by centrifugation. Each individual centrifuge must be calibrated for optimal speed and specific time of spin for each component. The technician can harvest PRBCs from WB (fresh or stored) by centrifuging the unit at $5000 \times g$ at 4° C for 5 minutes. If a refrigerated centrifuge is not available, then the RBCs may be allowed to separate from refrigerated WB by sedimentation over a period of time. Unfortunately, the process of natural sedimentation decreases the volume of plasma that can be removed and increases the chance of red cell contamination to the final product. After separation has occurred, plasma is removed (ideally with a plasma extractor), leaving enough plasma in the unit to maintain a HCT that does not exceed 80%. Removal of more plasma than recommended will provide insufficient preservative solution to support storage. Ideally, PRBCs should be reconstituted with a nutrient solution before storage to maintain the cells in a healthier environment. The use of additive solutions allows for increased plasma yield and extended storage time. In addition, reconstitution of the cells will reduce viscosity of the PRBCs during administration. If a nutrient solution is not used at the time of processing, then PRBCs can be reconstituted with approximately 100 ml of 0.9% sodium chloride before administration to reduce viscosity. Only isotonic saline should be used to dilute blood components, because other intravenous solutions may cause red cell damage (e.g., dextrose 5% in water) or initiate blood coagulation (e.g., lactated Ringer's solution). The technician should remember that PRBCs can be refrigerated at 1° to 6° C, with storage time defined by the anticoagulant-preservative or additive solution used in collection and processing. If the red cells were separated in a system that was open at any time, then the product must be used within 24 hours.

Fresh plasma will provide plasma proteins and coagulation factors; it does not contain viable platelets. The same value is retained for up to 1 year if fresh plasma is frozen at –18° C or less within 8 hours from the time of collection. If plasma is harvested from a unit of WB more than 8 hours after collection but before the unit's expiration date, then the product is labeled as *FP* and has a shelf life of 5 years from the date of initial WB collection. FFP has a shelf life of 1 year from the original date of collection; however, if it is not used within this time, then it can be relabeled as *FP* and stored for an additional 4 years.

CRYO is harvested from a unit of FFP that has been allowed to thaw slowly at 1° to 6° C for approximately 12 to 18 hours. The slurried plasma is centrifuged at 5000 × g at 4° C for 6 minutes. The supernatant plasma is expressed using a plasma extractor, leaving behind a white foamy precipitate (mostly adhered to the bag) in 25 to 50 ml of LP. Units of CRYO can be pooled before storage or administration. If pooled before freezing, then the process should happen immediately after preparation and then frozen. If thawed and then pooled, the product must be administered within 4 hours.

PRP is harvested from FWB that has been centrifuged at 1000 × g at 20° to 24° C for 4 minutes, a much slower speed and warmer temperature than used for routine plasma harvesting. The WB should not be cooled below 20° C before the PRP is removed, and the separation must occur within 8 hours from the time of collection. After centrifugation, the bag is allowed to sit undisturbed for 30 minutes and the PRP is removed. Platelets can be further concentrated by additional centrifugation of the PRP at 5000 × g at 20° to 24° C for 6 minutes. After centrifugation, the platelet-poor plasma should be expressed into an attached satellite bag and the platelet concentrate allowed to rest undisturbed for approximately 1 hour to ensure even resuspension of the platelets. Refrigerated platelets do not maintain function or viability as well as platelets stored at room temperature; therefore this component should be prepared and administered as quickly as possible after collection.

The shelf life of blood components is determined by the type of system used for blood collection; the anticoagulant-preservative solution used; the time between collection, processing, and storage; and the temperature and conditions under which products are stored. It is critical that appropriate temperatures are consistently maintained to secure the quality of both red cell and plasma products. Refrigerators and freezers for blood component storage should be dedicated for this purpose, and evaluation of their temperatures should be performed daily. Commercially available blood refrigerators and freezers are built to continuously monitor and record temperature, with audible alarm systems that activate before blood products reach unacceptable temperatures (Fig. 5-3).

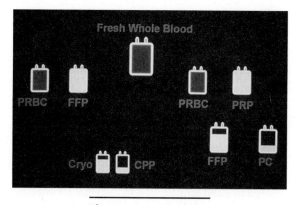

Fig. 5-3 Component chart.

Blood Administration

Blood Compatibility

Pretransfusion testing is necessary to ensure the best possible results of a blood transfusion. Compatibility testing includes testing of the donor, selection of appropriate donor units based on the patient's blood type, and BCM. Although pretransfusion testing will help to determine incompatibility between the donor and recipient, normal survival of transfused cells in the patient's circulation cannot be guaranteed. Blood samples for initial testing should be collected from all patients before infusion of any donor blood products.

Blood Types. Ideally, all canine blood donors and all recipients should be blood typed for DEA 1.1 before a transfusion. The erythrocyte antigen DEA 1.1 is very antigenic and responsible for most blood incompatibilities in dogs. A blood-typing kit is commercially available to classify dogs as DEA 1.1 positive or negative. The assay is based on the agglutination reaction that occurs when erythrocytes that contain DEA 1.1 antigen on their surface membranes interact with a murine monoclonal antibody specific to DEA 1.1. DEA 1.1 negative blood can be given to DEA 1.1 negative and DEA 1.1 positive patients. DEA 1.1 positive blood can only be given to patients positive for DEA 1.1. In an emergency situation, or with specific medical conditions that preclude conclusive typing (e.g., autoagglutination in a patient with immune-mediated hemolytic anemia), DEA 1.1 negative blood should be used to avoid sensitization to the DEA 1.1 antigen.

Blood-typing cards similar to those used in dogs are available for cats. This blood-typing test card is used to classify cats as type A, B, or AB. The assay is based on the agglutination reaction that occurs when erythrocytes interact with a murine monoclonal antibody specific for the A antigen—an anti-B solution (wheat germ lectin, *Triticum vulgaris*, or both), which at a specific concentration causes agglutination of only type B cells. RBCs from type A cats will agglutinate with anti-A monoclonal antibody (labeled *A* on the card), and RBCs from type B cats will agglutinate with anti-B solution (labeled *B* on the card). RBCs from type AB cats will agglutinate with both anti-A and anti-B reagents.

Samples need to be evaluated for autoagglutination. If macroscopic autoagglutination exists, then washing RBCs three times with phosphate-buffered saline (see BCM procedure following) may eliminate the problem, otherwise blood typing cannot be performed. The RapidVet-H (canine DEA 1.1 and feline) blood-typing test cards are manufactured by DMS Laboratories (2 Darts Mill Road, Flemington, NJ 08822; [800] 567-4367).

Blood Crossmatch. A BCM is performed to detect serologic incompatibility by identifying antibodies in donor or recipient plasma against recipient or donor RBCs. A BCM is divided into two parts: (1) the major crossmatch consists of mixing the patient's plasma with the donor's RBCs; (2) the minor crossmatch consists of mixing the donor's plasma with the patient's RBCs. Of the two tests, the major BCM is much more important in determining survival of the transfused RBCs.

Dogs lack significant naturally occurring alloantibodies; therefore they may be safely transfused without a BCM before the first transfusion. However, all dogs that have received RBC transfusions more than 4 days previously must be crossmatched before receiving any additional RBC transfusions. Because

---

BOX 5-1   ⚛

Procedure for Blood Crossmatch

1. Collect blood into an (EDTA) tube from the recipient and possible donor or donors.
2. Centrifuge (1000 × g for 5 minutes) to separate plasma from red blood cells (RBCs), remove plasma from each sample with a pipette, and transfer the plasma to clean, labeled glass or plastic tubes. Note any hemolysis.
3. Wash RBCs three times with phosphate-buffered saline.
   a. Add 4 to 5 ml of phosphate-buffered saline.
   b. Mix well.
   c. Centrifuge 1 to 2 minutes.
   d. Remove saline, leaving a pellet of RBCs at bottom of tube.
4. Resuspend with phosphate-buffered saline to make a 3% to 5% RBC suspension.
5. Prepare (for each donor) three tubes labeled *major*, *minor*, and *recipient control*. Add to each tube 2 drops (50 µl) of plasma and 1 drop (25 µl) of RBC suspension as follows:
   a. Major—recipient plasma + donor RBCs
   b. Minor—donor plasma + recipient RBCs recipient—control recipient plasma + recipient RBCs
6. Mix gently and incubate for 15 to 20 minutes at 37° C in a warm-water bath.
7. Centrifuge for 15 seconds at 1000 × g.
8. Examine supernatant for hemolysis.
9. During the gentle resuspension of the pellet of RBCs (by tapping the tube), examine for macroscopic agglutination and classify as *1+* (fine), *2+* (small), *3+* (large), or *4+* (one large agglutinate).

---

cats have naturally occurring alloantibodies and may experience a severe reaction to their first transfusion, a BCM should be performed before any blood transfusion if blood typing is not available. A BCM is typically not necessary for a first transfusion if the blood types of the feline recipient and donor are known. As with dogs, feline patients that have received RBC transfusions more than 4 to 7 days previously should be crossmatched before receiving any additional RBC transfusions (Box 5-1).

An autocontrol with recipient RBCs and plasma is included, because some recipients may have autoagglutination interfering with the BCM. If the

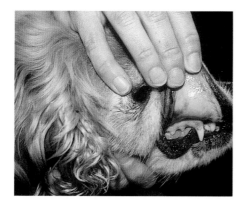

Color Plate 1

Icterus mucous membrane color in a cocker spaniel with liver disease.

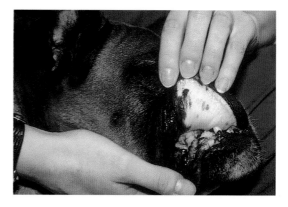

Color Plate 2

Pale mucous membrane color in a boxer with a packed cell volume of 13%.

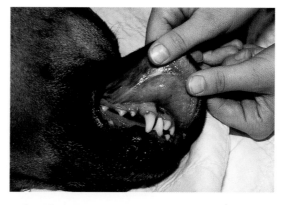

Color Plate 3

Brick red mucous membranes in a mongrel with septic shock.

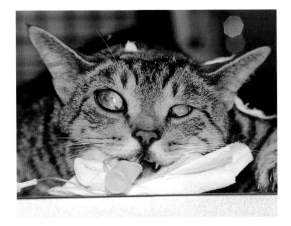

Color Plate 4

A cat with buthalmia (enlargement and distention of the globe) in the right eye caused by glaucoma.

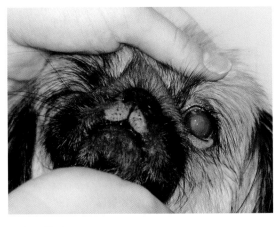

Color Plate 5

A Pekinese with conjunctival hyperemia, with mucopurulent discharge in the left eye caused by a corneal ulcer.

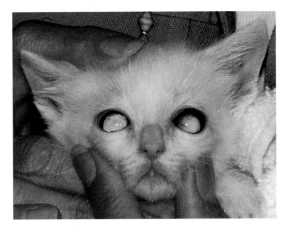

Color Plate 6

A kitten with congenital cataracts in both eyes.

patient control is positive (i.e., agglutination is present), then one cannot draw conclusions about blood compatibility between patient and donors. Any hemolysis, agglutination, or both in the major or minor BCM (but not the control) indicate an incompatibility and the need to choose a new donor. The minor BCM should be compatible in dogs but is of lesser importance in that canine donor plasma should not contain significant antibodies. Feline patients must be given type-specific plasma products because of the presence of naturally occurring alloantibodies.

A compatible BCM does not prevent sensitization or delayed transfusion reactions; it simply indicates that at the present time no antibodies against the RBCs are detected.

Component Preparation

Allowing it to sit at room temperature for approximately 30 minutes may gently warm refrigerated blood. Properly administered cold blood will not increase the chance of a transfusion reaction; however, large amounts of cold blood given at a rapid rate can induce hypothermia and cardiac arrhythmias. Routine warming of red cell products is not recommended except in neonates, hypothermic patients, and those receiving massive transfusions. Several types of blood warmers are commercially available. In an emergency situation, the tubing of the administration set can be placed in a warmwater bath, not to exceed 37° C, so warming can occur as blood passes through the tubing. The entire unit should not be immersed in the bath. Frozen products should also be thawed in a 37° C warmwater bath. Once thawed, products should remain at 37° C for no longer than 15 minutes to minimize the degradation of certain coagulation factors. No blood product should be exposed to temperatures exceeding 42° C to avoid damage to RBCs and denaturation of blood proteins. Once refrigerated or frozen products are brought to room temperature, they should not be rechilled. Warming red cell products or thawing plasma products in a microwave oven is not recommended.

Administration Volume

The aim of transfusion in the patient with anemia is not to return the packed cell volume to normal values but to correct the clinical signs. The volume of blood administered depends on the onset and degree of anemia, clinical status of the patient, and body weight. The following doses are used to determine the required blood component volume:

- 10 to 20 ml/kg = milliliters of WB needed
- 6 to 10 ml/kg = milliliters of PRBCs needed
- 6 to 10 ml/kg = milliliters of plasma needed

Clinical evaluation of the patient after the transfusion will determine whether further blood product support is necessary.

Administration Routes

Blood and blood components can be administered via the intravenous or intraosseous route. Intravenous is obviously the most effective route because the infused RBCs or plasma products are immediately available to the general circulation. The intraosseous route is used in puppies or kittens when vascular access is difficult or unsuccessful. When delivering blood products intraosseously, infused cells and proteins are available to the general circulation within minutes. The most common sites for intraosseous catheter placement are the trochanteric fossa of the femur, the wing of the ilium, and the shaft of the humerus. Care should be taken in the placement of these catheters because of the increased risk of osteomyelitis.

Administration Rates

Administration rates are variable. For example, a patient with massive hemorrhage may require a more rapid transfusion than a normovolemic patient with a chronic anemia. Blood should not be administered at a rate exceeding 22 ml/kg/hr; however, rate is less critical in a hypovolemic animal than a normovolemic animal where circulatory overload is a potential problem. Cardiovascularly compromised animals cannot tolerate infusion rates that exceed 4 ml/kg/hr.

It is recommended that blood components always be infused slowly (e.g., 1 ml/kg) for the first 10 to 15 minutes while the technician closely observes the animal for signs of an acute transfusion reaction. The blood product should then be infused as quickly as will be tolerated, but infusion should not take longer than 4 hours. Before infusion, baseline values of attitude, rectal temperature, pulse rate and quality, respiratory rate and character, mucous membrane color, capillary refill time, HCT, total plasma protein, and plasma and urine color should be monitored. The majority of these parameters should be checked every 30 minutes during transfusion and evaluated routinely after the transfusion to ensure the desired effect has been achieved.

Transfusion Reactions

Animals should be carefully monitored for any adverse reactions during and for several weeks after transfusion. Transfusion reactions can be classified as immune mediated or nonimmune mediated in origin.

Immune-mediated transfusion reactions can be hemolytic in origin, with either an acute (because of preexisting alloantibodies or prior sensitization) or delayed (can be exhibited >4 days posttransfusion) presentation. Hemolytic transfusion reactions are the most serious but are less common. In acute situations, intravascular hemolysis is caused by preexisting antibodies, as seen in the mismatched transfusion of feline type A blood to a cat with type B blood or in a previously sensitized DEA 1.1 negative dog receiving DEA 1.1 positive blood. Clinical signs include, but are not limited to, fever, tachycardia, weakness, muscle tremors, vomiting, collapse, hemoglobinemia, and hemoglobinuria.

Nonhemolytic transfusion reactions are a result of antibodies to WBCs, platelets, or plasma proteins. These reactions are most often transient in nature and do not cause life-threatening situations. Clinical signs include urticaria, pruritus, and pyrexia. Vomiting can be noted with any type of transfusion reaction; therefore patients receiving blood products should not be fed during or just before transfusion.

A variety of factors is associated with nonimmune-mediated transfusion reactions. Any type of trauma to the RBCs will potentially cause hemolysis: (1) overheating RBC products (also will cause protein denaturation and may increase bacterial growth during infusion), (2) freezing RBC products, (3) mixing RBC products with nonisotonic solutions causing cellular damage, (4) warming and then rechilling blood products, and (5) collecting or infusing blood through small needles or catheters.

Bacterial pyrogens and sepsis can be a complication of improperly collected and stored blood. Dark-brown to black supernatant plasma in stored blood indicates digested hemoglobin from bacterial growth. Any blood with discolored supernatant should be immediately discarded. Patients experiencing this complication will most often mount a febrile response 15 to 20 minutes from start of infusion.

Citrate intoxication may occur when citrate/blood volume ratio is disproportionate or in massively transfused patients, particularly in patients with liver dysfunction. Common clinical signs include involuntary muscle tremors, cardiac arrhythmias, and decreased cardiac output. This compromised state can be confirmed by obtaining ionized serum calcium. If citrate toxicity is in question, then blood administration should be discontinued and calcium gluconate administered.

The appropriate volume of blood must be administered to each patient. Specific component therapy should be used to treat each disorder, and the patient's cardiovascular status should always be assessed before determining the required volume and administration rate. Because blood is a colloid solution, vascular overload is a potential complication. Clinical signs include coughing (as a result of pulmonary edema), dyspnea, cyanosis, tachycardia, and vomiting. If volume overload is of concern, then blood administration should at the very least be temporarily discontinued and supportive care instituted.

All blood products should be filtered to help prevent thromboembolic complications. Standard blood infusion sets have in-line filters with a pore size of approximately 170 to 260 mcm. A filter of this size will trap cells, cellular debris, and coagulated protein. Trapped debris combined with room temperature conditions may promote proliferation of any bacteria that may be present; therefore blood infusion sets may be used for several units of blood products or for a maximum time of 4 hours. Microaggregate filter systems with a pore size of 20 to 40 mcm may be used for low-volume transfusion (i.e., <50 ml WB, <25 ml PRBC or plasma).

Conclusion

Many positive changes have taken place in veterinary transfusion medicine in the last 2 decades that have ultimately improved the quality of medicine practiced. Inevitably, this evolution will continue as it has in human medicine. The Association of Veterinary Hematology and Transfusion Medicine will help to develop standards in veterinary blood banking and investigate some exciting future trends in blood banking and transfusion medicine.

Suggested Readings

Brecher ME, ed: *Technical Manual (15th ed)*, Bethesda, American Association of Blood Banks, 1999.

Cotter SM, ed: *Advances in Science and Comparative Medicine: Comparative Transfusion Medicine*, San Diego, 1991, Academic Press.

Day M, Mackin A, Littlewood J, eds: *Manual of Canine and Feline Haematology and Transfusion Medicine*, United Kingdom, 2000, British Small Animal Veterinary Association.

Feldman BF, Sink CA, Burton DL, editors: *Practical Transfusion Medicine for the Small Animal Practitioner*, Jackson, 2004, Teton New Media.

Giger U: Blood typing and cross matching to ensure compatible transfusions. In Bonagura JD: *Kirk's Current Veterinary Therapy XIII*, Philadelphia, 2000, Saunders, pp 396-399.

Giger U, Gelens J, Callan MB, et al: An acute hemolytic transfusion reaction caused by dog erythrocyte antigen 1.1 incompatibility in a previously sensitized dog, *J Am Vet Med Assoc* 206:1358-1362, 1995.

Harmening DM, ed: *Modern Blood Banking & Transfusion Medicine (5th ed)*, Philadelphia, 2005, FA Davis Company.

Hohenhaus AE, ed: *Problems in Veterinary Medicine: Transfusion Medicine*, Hagerstown, 1992, Lippincott.

Kristensen AT, Feldman BF, editors: *The Veterinary Clinics of North America, Small Animal Practice: Canine and Feline Transfusion Medicine*, Philadelphia, 1995, Saunders.

Messick MB, ed: *The Veterinary Clinics of North America, Small Animal Practice: Hematology*, Philadelphia, 2003, Saunders.

Silverstein DC, Hopper K, eds: *Small Animal Critical Care Medicine*, St Louis, Elsevier, in press.

Willard MD, Tvedten H, eds: *Small Animal Clinical Diagnosis by Laboratory Methods (4th ed)*, St Louis, 2004, Elsevier.

6

Nutritional Support for the Critically Ill Patient

Daniel L. Chan

Critically ill animals undergo several metabolic alterations that put them at high risk for the development of malnutrition and its subsequent complications. During periods of nutrient deprivation, a healthy animal primarily will lose fat. However, sick or traumatized patients will catabolize lean muscle rather than fat when they are not provided with sufficient calories and nutrients. This loss of lean tissue reduces the animal's strength, immune function, wound healing, and overall survival. Inadequate calorie intake is commonly the result of a loss of appetite, an inability to eat or tolerate feedings, vomiting, or dehydration that accompanies many diseases processes. Because malnutrition can occur quickly in these animals, the technical staff plays a vital role in identifying animals at risk for malnutrition, as well as in providing nutritional support. In those patients requiring nutritional support, it is important to first identify the most appropriate route for nutrition—either enteral (using the gastrointestinal tract) or parenteral (IV) nutrition if oral intake is not adequate. The goals of nutritional support are to treat malnutrition when present and, just as important, to prevent malnutrition in patients at risk. Whenever possible, the enteral route should be used because it is the safest, most convenient, and most physiologically sound method of nutritional support. However, when patients are unable to tolerate enteral feeding or unable to use nutrients administered enterally, parenteral nutrition (PN) should be considered. Ensuring the successful nutritional management of critically ill patients involves selecting the right patient, making an appropriate nutritional assessment, and implementing a feasible nutritional plan.

Nutritional Assessment

As with any medical intervention, risks of complications are always possible. Minimizing such risks depends on patient selection and patient assessment. The first step in formulating a nutritional strategy involves making a systematic evaluation of the patient, referred to as a *nutritional assessment*. Nutritional assessment identifies malnourished patients who require immediate nutritional support and also identifies patients at risk for developing malnutrition in which nutritional support will help to prevent malnutrition.

Indicators of overt malnutrition include recent weight loss of at least 10% of body weight, poor haircoat quality, muscle wasting, and signs of poor wound healing. However, these abnormalities are not specific to malnutrition and are not present early in the process. In addition, fluid shifts may mask weight loss in critically ill patients. Factors that predispose a patient to malnutrition include anorexia lasting longer than 3 days, serious underlying disease (e.g., trauma, sepsis, peritonitis, pancreatitis, gastrointestinal surgery), and large protein losses (e.g., protracted vomiting, diarrhea, draining wounds). Nutritional assessment also identifies factors that can affect the nutritional plan, such as cardiovascular instability, electrolyte abnormalities, hyperglycemia, and hypertriglyceridemia, as well as concurrent conditions such as renal or hepatic disease that will influence the nutritional plan. Appropriate laboratory analysis should be performed in all patients to assess these parameters. Before implementation of any nutritional plan, the patient must be cardiovascularly stable, with major electrolyte, fluid, and acid-base abnormalities corrected.

An important aspect of nutritional assessment involves determination of a body condition score (BCS). Various systems have been proposed, and each of these systems seeks to qualitatively assess whether an animal is emaciated, thin, in ideal body condition, overweight, or obese. These systems incorporate both a visual and a tactile assessment of the animal's body, paying careful attention to abdomen, ribs, pelvic bony prominences, and tailhead. The most commonly used systems use either five or nine categories. Neither system is superior; the most important point is that a practice should adopt one of these systems and use it consistently. The entire staff should use BCS in every assessment of both healthy and hospitalized patients. By consistently using the BCS, one can effectively communicate the progression of an animal's body condition during the course of a disease and recovery. Many pet food companies will provide BCS charts that can be used to train both staff and clients. To communicate which BCS system it is being used, the BCS should

reflect the scale being used. For example, a dog that is in ideal body condition should be listed as 3/5 or 5/9, depending on the system being used. This will eliminate any confusion.

Goals of Nutritional Support

Even in patients with severe malnutrition, the immediate goals of therapy should focus on resuscitation, stabilization, and identification of the primary disease process. As steps are made to address the primary problems, formulation of a nutritional plan should strive to prevent (or correct) overt nutritional deficiencies and imbalances. By providing adequate energy substrates, protein, essential fatty acids, and micronutrients, the staff ensures that the animal's body will support wound healing, immune function, and tissue repair. A major goal of nutritional support is to minimize metabolic derangements and catabolism of lean body tissue. During hospitalization, restoration of previous healthy body weight is *not* a priority, because weight restoration will only occur when the animal is recovering from a state of critical illness. The goal of nutritional support during hospitalization is to prevent further losses to lean tissue and provide energy and nutrients required for healing. With these principles in mind, it is prudent to provide nutritional support in a conservative and gradual manner with frequent reassessment.

Nutritional Plan

Proper diagnosis and treatment of the underlying disease is the key to the success of nutritional support. Based on the nutritional assessment, a plan is formulated to meet the patient's energy and other nutritional requirements and, at the same time, address any concurrent condition or conditions requiring adjustments to the nutritional plan. The anticipated duration of nutritional support, which will largely depend on clinical familiarity with the specific disease process and sound clinical judgment, should be estimated and factored into the plan. For each patient, the best route of nutrition should be determined—enteral nutrition versus PN. This decision should be based on the underlying disease and the patient's clinical signs. Whenever possible, the enteral route should be considered first. If enteral feedings are not tolerated or the gastrointestinal tract must be bypassed, then PN should be considered.

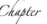

Nutritional support should be introduced gradually and reach target levels in 48 to 72 hours.

Calculating Nutritional Requirements

The patient's resting energy requirement (RER) is the number of calories required for maintaining homeostasis while the animal rests quietly. The RER is calculated using the following formula:

$$RER = 70 \times (\text{body weight in kilograms})^{0.75}$$

For animals weighing between 2 and 30 kg, the following linear formula gives a good approximation of energy needs:

$$RER = (30 \times \text{body weight in kilograms}) + 70$$

Traditionally, the RER was then multiplied by an illness factor between 1.0 and 1.5 to account for increases in metabolism associated with different conditions and injuries. Recently, less emphasis has been placed on these subjective illness factors, and current recommendations are to use more conservative energy estimates to avoid overfeeding. Overfeeding can result in metabolic and gastrointestinal complications, hepatic dysfunction, increased carbon dioxide production, and weaken respiratory muscles. Of the metabolic complications, the development of hyperglycemia is most common (and possibly the most detrimental).

Currently, the RER is used as an initial estimate of a critically ill patient's energy requirements. It should be emphasized that these general guidelines should be used as starting points, and animals receiving nutritional support should be closely monitored for tolerance of nutritional interventions. Continual decline in body weight or body condition should prompt the clinician to reassess and perhaps modify the nutritional plan (e.g., increasing the number of calories provided by 25%).

Role of the Veterinary Technician

The technical staff is absolutely crucial in providing nutritional support. Because technical staff spend the most contact time with patients, they are best suited in identifying patients in need of nutritional support, using the nutritional plan, and assisting in placement of feeding tubes, placement of catheters for PN, and monitoring the patient for complications. In most practices, the technical staff should be empowered to assist clinicians in formulating the nutritional plan for a patient and help assess the response to treatment. The next few sections are devoted to the role of technical staff in the provision of the different types of nutritional support.

Enteral Nutrition

As previously mentioned, the enteral route of nutritional support is usually preferable. Enteral nutrition is safer and less expensive than PN, and it helps to maintain intestinal structure and function. Enteral nutrition includes all forms of oral feeding (e.g., hand feeding, syringe feeding) and tube feedings (e.g., nasoesophageal [NE], esophagostomy [E], gastrostomy [G], jejunostomy [J] feeding tubes). Even with the use of feeding tubes, patients can easily be discharged for home care with good owner compliance. Most feeding tube complications include tube occlusion and localized irritation at the tube exit site. More serious complications include infection at the exit site or, rarely, complete tube dislodgment and peritonitis if the tube was a G or J tube. Staff can avoid feeding tube complications by using the appropriate tube, making proper food selections, and preparing and carefully monitoring clients (encouraging pet owners to follow home care guidelines and watch for potential problems).

Assisted feedings (either by hand or by syringe) are usually ineffective in providing adequate amounts of calories. Nevertheless, these techniques are important in two ways. First, assisted feeding can aid in assessing whether the patient's gastrointestinal tract can tolerate feedings. Should the patient vomit after assisted feeding, consideration should be given for PN. Second, assisted feeding can help determine when a patient's appetite is improving. Appetite stimulants such as cyproheptadine are usually not very effective when given to completely anorexic patients; however, they can stimulate animals to eat more consistently when beginning to eat with assisted feeding.

The important point to remember with syringe feeding is that it should never be a stressful event. If the animal resists or objects to syringe feeding, then placement of a feeding tube should be considered. Should a patient begin to associate eating with a stressful situation, the animal may develop a food aversion that further complicates nutritional support (this is especially true in cats). Another important point is that syringe feeding should never be done to a patient that is dyspneic or with compromised ability to protect its airways (e.g., patients with laryngeal paralysis), because the risk for aspiration or decompensation is too great.

If a feeding tube is required for nutritional support, the next step is selecting the type of feeding tube to be used (Table 6-1). Feeding tubes commonly used in dogs and cats include NE, E, G, and J tubes. The veterinary technician can play a major role in the placement of such tubes, because placement techniques often require more than one person. Moreover, the staff can be extremely helpful in setting up and preparing the tubes and patients for these procedures. Once the desired feeding tube is placed, radiography should be used to confirm satisfactory tube placement.

NE tubes are very easy to place and require very little sedation. Application of local anesthetics to nasal mucosa and proper lubrication of the tube can improve the animal's tolerance for such a tube placement. However, NE tubes have disadvantages. First, only liquid diets can be used, and these diets are usually only 1 kcal/ml; therefore administering an adequate amount of calories to the patient is difficult. Secondly, this tube usually requires placement of an Elizabethan collar to prevent removal by the animal; therefore placement is not well tolerated. Feeding via NE tubes should be limited for very short-term use or in particularly unstable animals who cannot tolerate anesthesia. In some animals, bolus feedings of liquid diets through NE tubes elicit nausea and vomiting. A useful strategy in such cases is to attempt NE feedings via a slow continuous infusion with a syringe or infusion pump. The technician should start with 1 to 2 ml/hour infusions and increase gradually until the caloric goals are met.

E tubes are much more versatile and can be used for effective nutritional support. Placement requires a brief period of anesthesia; the technique is easily

TABLE 6-1 📖

Feeding Tube Selection

Feeding Tube	Duration	Advantages	Disadvantages
Nasoesophageal (NE tube)	Short term (<5 days)	Inexpensive Easy to place No anesthesia required	Requires liquid diet Some animals will not eat with NE tube in place
Esophagostomy (E tube)	Long term	Inexpensive Easy to place Can use calorically dense diets	Requires anesthesia Cellulitis can occur if tube is remove early
Gastrostomy (G tube)* Percutaneous endoscopically guided (PEG) Surgically placed	 Long term Long term	Easy to place Can use calorically dense diets Can use calorically dense diets	Requires anesthesia Requires endoscope Requires anesthesia and laparotomy
Jejunostomy (J tube)	Long term	Bypasses stomach and pancreas Can be used in patients with pancreatitis	Requires anesthesia and laparotomy For all in-hospital use Requires continuous rate infusion Requires liquid diet Peritonitis can occur if tube is removed

*For all the G tubes, peritonitis is a possible complication if the tube leaks or is removed early.

mastered and allows feeding for prolonged periods of time. The technique for placement is detailed in Box 6-1, and a step-by-step procedure is also described. Both the tube and the feedings are well tolerated by patients, and most clients can become adept at this feeding method. Flushing of the tube with water after each use will prevent clogging. Oral liquid medications can also be administered via the E tube; however, crushed and dissolved medications should not be administered via the E tube because of the high likelihood of clogging of the tube. Feedings should be done using gently warmed foods and done over a 10- to 15-minute period.

Surgically placed G tubes and percutaneous endoscopically placed gastrostomy (PEG) tubes require more involved procedures using anesthesia and special equipment. These types of tubes are more appropriate for long-term nutritional support. Cases in which G or PEG tubes may be indicated include severe esophageal dysfunction (e.g., megaesophagus, severe esophagitis, esophageal stricture, esophageal or pharyngeal neoplasia) or protracted debilitating diseases (e.g., end-stage chronic renal failure). Special kits for these tubes are available; more commonly, Pezzer mushroom tip catheters can be modified for use. A step-by-step description is listed in Box 6-2. These larger tubes allow for feeding of "blenderized" diets that could not be administered via NE or E tubes. The exit site for the G or PEG tube should be frequently assessed (for signs of infection) and appropriately managed. Feeding through a G or PEG tube should never cause the patient discomfort. Should discomfort occur, the tube should be immediately investigated. With patients in whom the G or PEG tube is to be used for more than a couple of months, these tubes could be replaced by more cosmetic (and often costly) low-profile feeding tubes. The only advantage of these tubes is that they are largely inconspicuous and may be less easily dislodged.

In cases in which the patient undergoes abdominal surgery and reason exists to bypass the upper GI tract (i.e., severe pancreatitis, pancreatic abscesses or masses, pancreatic or duodenal resections), the surgeon may place a J tube. This will allow jejunal feedings while the upper GI tract heals. Although previous recommendations included using enteral products designed for humans, the use of veterinary liquid diets such as CliniCare are usually well tolerated. It is vital that patients with J tubes be carefully monitored, because leakage or displacement usually results in peritonitis. Care must also be used in properly labeling J tubes, because critically ill patients typically have other concurrent IV and urinary catheters that can be confused, resulting in serious consequences. Feeding through J tubes should be administered as continuous infusions via pumps rather than bolus feeding, which may be associated with nausea or pain.

Based on the type of feeding tube chosen and the disease process being treated, an appropriate diet should be selected. Diet selection will also depend on the animal's clinical parameters and laboratory results (Box 6-3). The amount of food is then calculated, and a specific feeding plan is devised. Generally, NE, E, and G tube feedings are administered every 4 to 6 hours, and feeding tubes should be flushed with 5 to 10 ml of water after each feeding to minimize clogging of the tube. By the time of discharge, however, the number of feedings should be reduced to three to four times per day to facilitate owner compliance.

For E and G tubes, a volume of 5 to 10 ml/kg per individual feeding is generally well tolerated (may vary with the individual patient). In patients who are generally healthy but cannot consume food orally (e.g., jaw fracture), larger volumes of food per feeding (15 to 20 ml/kg) may be tolerated. Because enteral diets are mainly composed of water (most canned food is >75% water), the amount of fluids administered parenterally should be adjusted accordingly to avoid volume overload. Prevention of premature removal of tubes can be accomplished using an Elizabethan collar and wrapping the tube securely. Care should be taken to avoid wrapping the tube too tightly (doing so could lead to patient discomfort and possibly compromise ventilation).

Parenteral Nutrition

PN is more expensive than enteral nutrition and is only for in-hospital use. Indications for PN include vomiting, acute pancreatitis, severe malabsorptive disorders, and severe ileus. Although PN terminology can be confusing, two major types exist: (1) total parenteral nutrition (TPN) is typically delivered via a central venous (jugular) catheter and provides all of the patient's energy requirements; (2) partial parenteral nutrition (PPN) only provides a portion of the animal's energy requirements (40% to 70%). However, because of the lower osmolarity of the PPN solution, it can usually be administered through a

BOX 6-1

Esophagostomy Tube Placement

1. Proper placement of an esophagostomy (E) tube requires the distal tip to be placed in the distal esophagus at the level no further than the ninth intercostal space. This may require premeasuring the tube. Rather than cutting the distal tip and creating a sharp edge, the exit side hole should be elongated using a small blade.

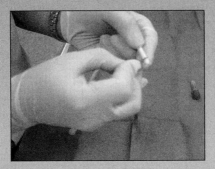

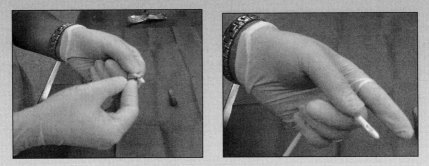

2. The patient should be anesthetized and preferably intubated. While in right lateral recumbency, the left side of the neck should be clipped and a routine surgical scrub performed.

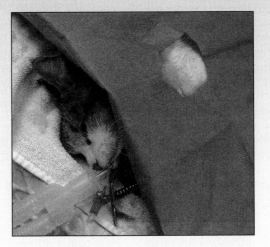

3. A curved Rochester-Carmalt forceps is placed into the mouth and down the esophagus to the midcervical region. The jugular vein should be identified and avoided.

BOX 6-1

Esophagostomy Tube Placement—cont'd

4. The tip of the Rochester-Carmalt is then pushed dorsally, pushing the esophagus toward the skin.

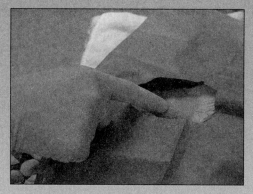

5. The tip of the Rochester-Carmalt is palpated over the skin to confirm its location, and a stab incision is made through the skin and into the esophagus. The mucosa of the esophagus is relatively more difficult to incise than the skin.

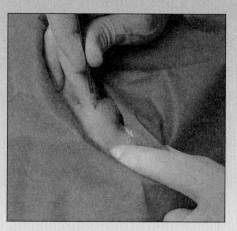

6. The tip of the instrument is then forced through the incision, which can be slightly enlarged with the blade to allow opening of the tips of the Rochester-Carmalt and placement of the E tube within the tips.

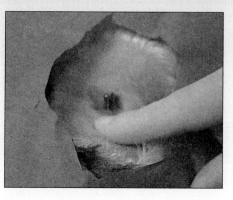

Continued.

BoX 6-1

Esophagostomy Tube Placement—cont'd

7. The Rochester-Carmalt is then clamped closed and pulled from the oral cavity.

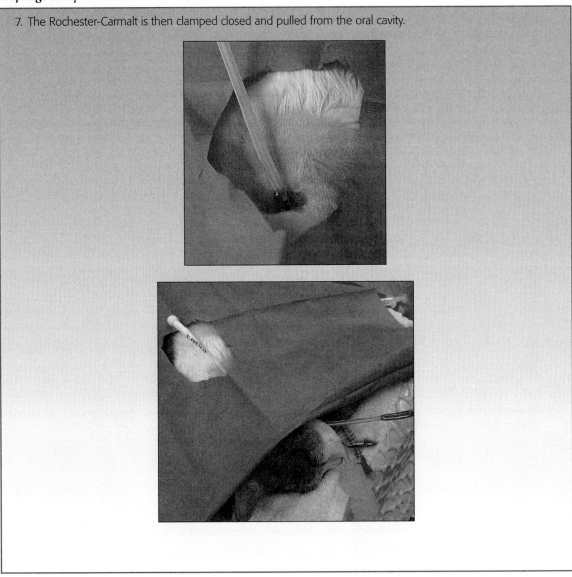

large peripheral vein (e.g., lateral saphenous in dogs, femoral in cats). Because PPN only provides a portion of the patient's requirements, it is only intended for short-term use in a nondebilitated patient with average nutritional requirements. Regardless of the exact form of PN, IV nutrition requires a dedicated catheter that is placed using aseptic technique. Once PN is initiated, the catheter should no longer be used for administration of IV medications or collection of blood (it should only be used to administer PN). Long catheters composed of silicone, polyurethane, or polytetrafluoroethylene are recommended for

BOX 6-1

Esophagostomy Tube Placement—cont'd

8. The tips of the Rochester-Carmalt should be disengaged and the tip of the E tube curled back into the mouth and fed into the esophagus. As the curled tube is pushed into the esophagus, the proximal end is gently pulled simultaneously. This will result in a subtle "flip" as the tube is redirected within the esophagus. The tube should easily slide back and forth a few millimeters, confirming that the tube has straightened.

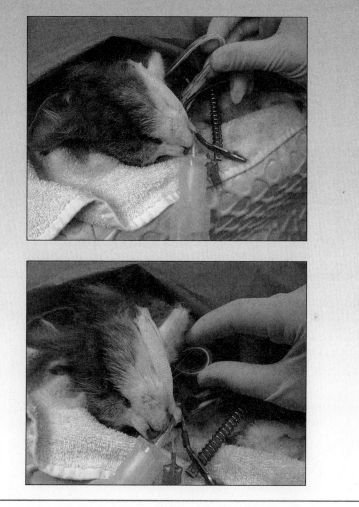

Continued.

use with PN to reduce the risk of thrombophlebitis. Multilumen catheters are often recommended for PN because they can remain in place for longer periods of time (as compared with normal jugular catheters) and provide other ports for blood sampling and administration of additional fluids and IV medications. Most PN solutions are composed of a carbohydrate source (dextrose or glycerol), a protein source (amino acids), and a fat source (lipids). Vitamins and trace metals can also be added.

Because of the high osmolarity of the TPN solution (usually 1100 to 1500 mOsm/L), it must

BOX 6-1

Esophagostomy Tube Placement—cont'd

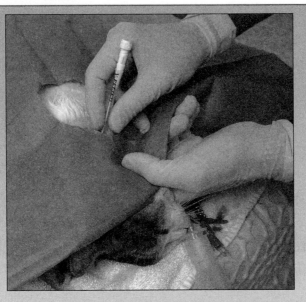

9. The clinician should visually inspect the oropharynx to confirm that the tube is no longer present within the oropharynx.
10. The incision site should be briefly rescrubbed before a purse-string suture is placed, followed by a "Chinese finger trap" (further securing the tube in place).

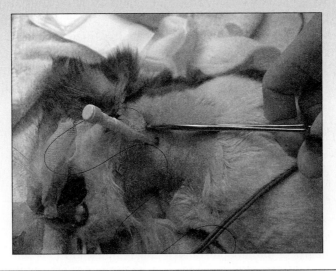

BOX 6-1

Esophagostomy Tube Placement—cont'd

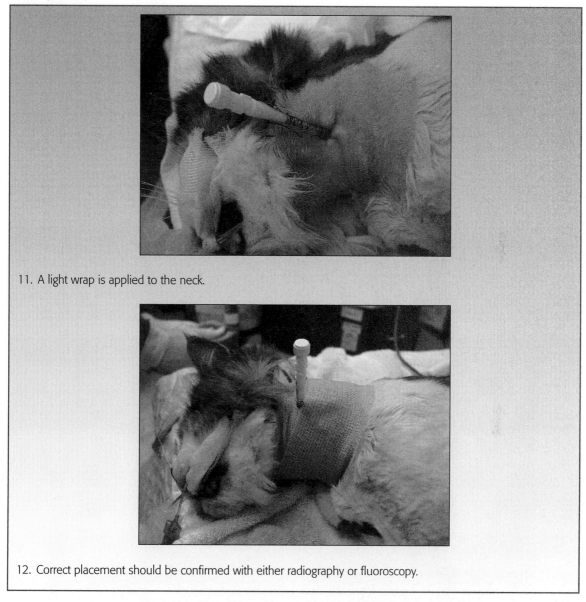

11. A light wrap is applied to the neck.

12. Correct placement should be confirmed with either radiography or fluoroscopy.

be administered through a central venous (jugular) catheter. PPN is formulated so that it can be administered through a peripheral catheter; however, because it is more dilute (usually <750 mOsm/L), PPN can only provide a portion of the patient's energy requirements. Formulation of TPN and PPN solutions require special equipment and training; therefore it is best obtained from a local human hospital or human home healthcare companies. Usually an order provides 3 to 5 day's

BOX 6-2

Percutaneous Endoscopic Gastrostomy Tube Placement

1. The first step in placement of a percutaneous endoscopically placed gastrostomy (PEG) tube is preparation. Although a variety of ready-made PEG tube kits exist, one can also modify simple mushroom tip catheters and produce acceptable feeding tubes. The depicted setup is what one usually needs: an appropriate-sized mushroom tip tube, some large-gauge hypodermic catheters (16 gauge, 1.5- to 2.0-inches long), sharp micropipette tips, a blade, scissors, forceps, and strong nylon suture.

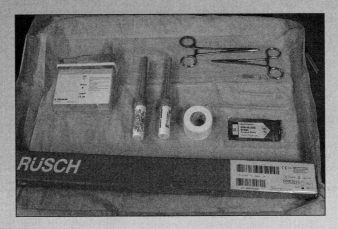

2. First, the flared, open end of the catheter should be cut off and discarded; then another two pieces of tubing (2 to 3 cm each) should be cut off for use as internal and external flanges.

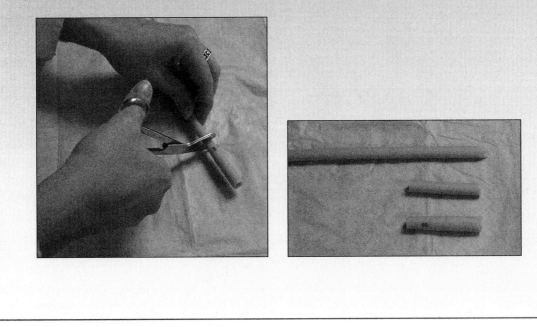

BOX 6-2

Percutaneous Endoscopic Gastrostomy Tube Placement—cont'd

3. The end of the catheter opposite of the mushroom tip is trimmed to facilitate its introduction into the larger opening of a disposable plastic micropipette tip.

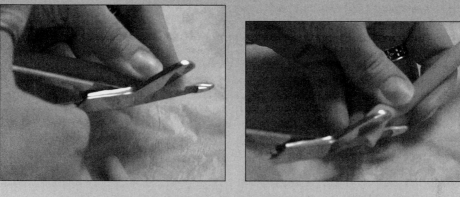

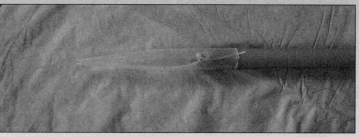

4. A stab incision is made through the center of each flange, allowing each flange to be inserted through the catheter.

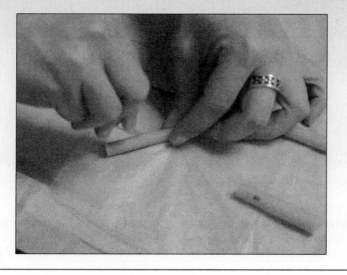

Continued.

BOX 6-2

Percutaneous Endoscopic Gastrostomy Tube Placement—cont'd

5. The clinician should insert a closed hemostat through the incision on the flange, then open and grasp the trimmed end of the catheter with the hemostat. Now he or she should slide the flange down until it rests against the mushroom tip. The other flange will be used as an external flange that will lie against the abdominal wall.

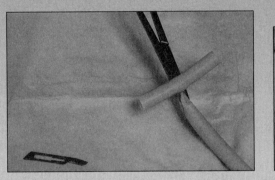 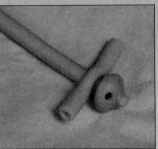

6. The animal is anesthetized and placed in right lateral recumbency so that the stomach tube can be placed through the greater curvature of the stomach and the left body wall. The animal is clipped, and surgical preparation is applied caudal to the left costal arch. The endoscope is introduced into stomach, and the stomach is inflated until the abdomen is distended (but not drum tight). The left body wall is transilluminated with the endoscope to ensure that the spleen is not positioned between the stomach and body wall. An appropriate site for insertion of the tube is determined by endoscopically monitoring digital palpation of the gastric wall.

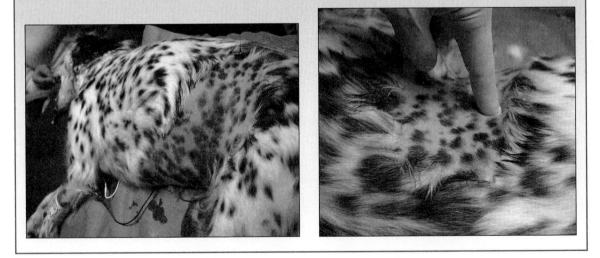

worth of PN for a patient and should be stored in the refrigerator. Each bag of PN holds 1 day's worth of solution and should be administered via constant rate infusion over 24 hours. Cyclical PN (i.e., providing PN during certain hours of the day and discontinuing it at night) is discouraged, because it increases the likelihood of catheter contamination. If the practice cannot provide 24-hour care, then consideration should be made to refer the case to another facility.

BOX 6-2

Percutaneous Endoscopic Gastrostomy Tube Placement—cont'd

7. A small skin incision is made with a blade and an IV catheter (16 to 14 gauge, 1.5- to 2-inches long) is stabbed through the body wall into the lumen of the stomach and visualized with the endoscope.

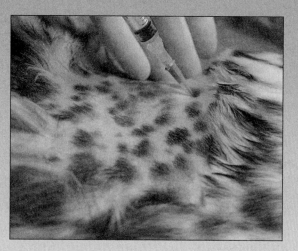

8. Via the endoscope, the IV catheter can be seen entering the stomach. The stylet is removed, and nylon is threaded through the catheter into lumen of stomach.

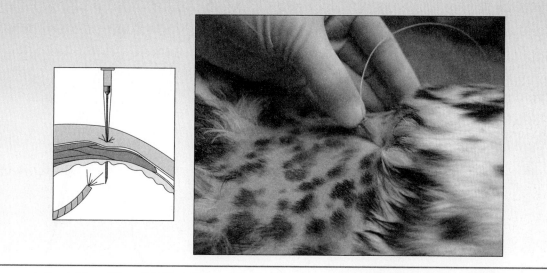

Figure on bottom left from Ettinger S, Feldman E, editors: *Textbook of veterinary internal medicine*, ed 6, St Louis, 2005, Saunders.

Continued.

Percutaneous Endoscopic Gastrostomy Tube Placement—cont'd

9. The suture material that was fed through IV catheter is grasped with the endoscopic biopsy forceps, and the endoscope and forceps are carefully withdrawn through the esophagus and out of the mouth.

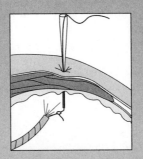

10. The suture now needs to be secured to the feeding tube. The micropipette is placed through the suture, the suture is threaded through a hypodermic needle on the trimmed end of the feeding tube, and a knot is tied. The clinician then slides the micropipette tip and pushes the trimmed catheter tip into the micropipette.

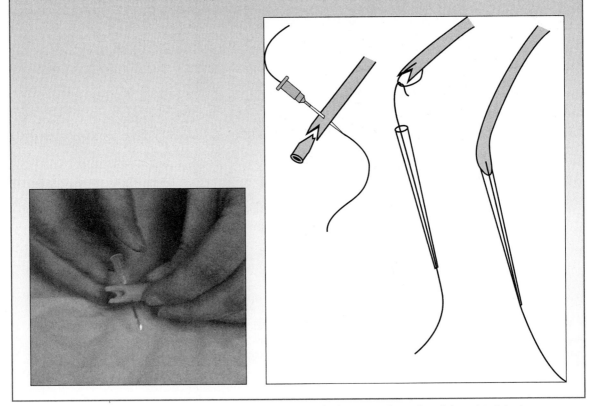

Top and bottom right figures from Ettinger S, Feldman E, editors: *Textbook of veterinary internal medicine*, ed 6, St Louis, 2005, Saunders.

Percutaneous Endoscopic Gastrostomy Tube Placement—cont'd

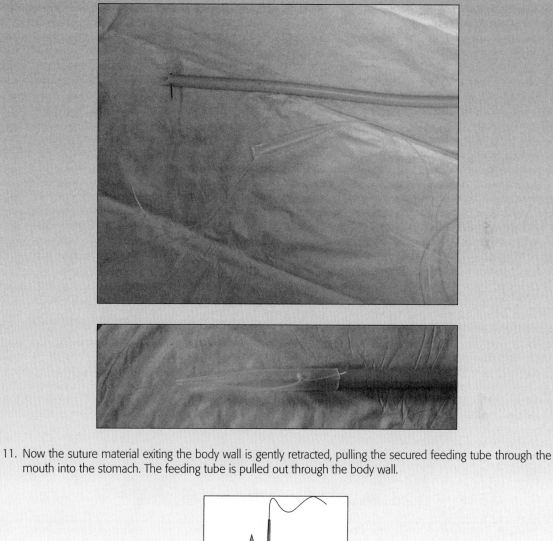

11. Now the suture material exiting the body wall is gently retracted, pulling the secured feeding tube through the mouth into the stomach. The feeding tube is pulled out through the body wall.

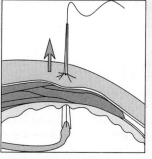

Bottom figure from Ettinger S, Feldman E, editors: *Textbook of veterinary internal medicine*, ed 6, St Louis, 2005, Saunders.

Continued.

BOX 6-2

Percutaneous Endoscopic Gastrostomy Tube Placement—cont'd

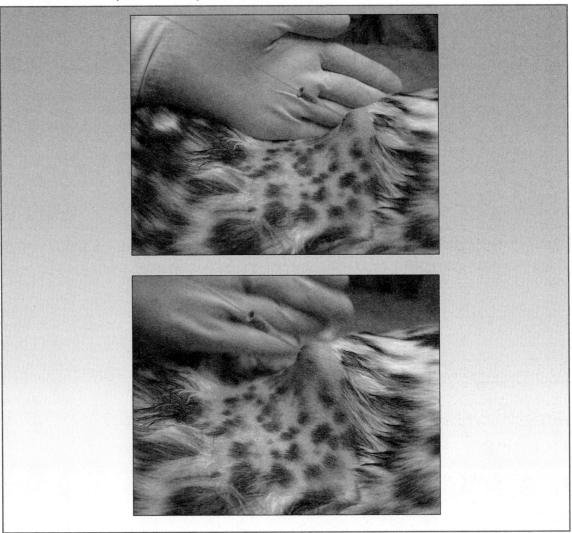

After 24 hours, a new bag of PN must be used (first allowing it to warm to room temperature), with fresh setups and IV lines. Bags, lines, and catheters should always be handled aseptically. Once a patient is started on PN, the system should be maintained as a closed system (no medications are to be injected either into the bag or line, and the lines should not be disconnected during walks or diagnostic procedures). The technician should simply disengage the line from the infusion pump and carry the bag and line with the patient while adjusting the drip flow regulator to a slow drip. Dong this will prevent the catheter from becoming occluded and avoid backflow of blood into the line. Should the line or bag ever be compromised (e.g., chewed lines, dislodged catheters, disconnected inadvertently), the entire setup (including the bag) should be discarded and a new setup and bag hung.

BOX 6-2

Percutaneous Endoscopic Gastrostomy Tube Placement—cont'd

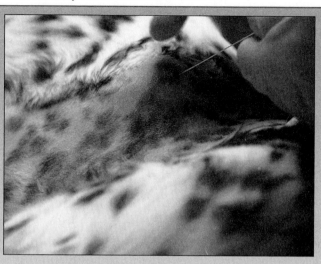

12. The exit site will need to be slightly enlarged with a blade. The clinician should be especially careful not to cut the suture while enlarging the incision. Using the IV catheter that was used to introduce the suture into the stomach may aid in protecting the suture from being cut.

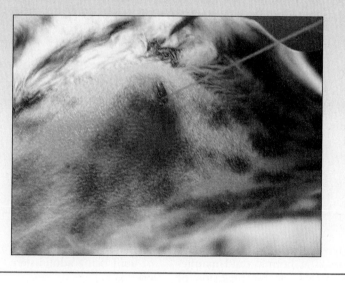

Continued.

An alternative, specially formulated TPN (commercial ready-to-use preparations of glucose and amino acids) is available for peripheral use; however, these formulations provide approximately less than 50% of required calories (when administered at maintenance fluid rate), and they should only be used for short-term or in conjunction with enteral nutrition. One such product is ProcalAmine (Mc-Graw), which is a 3% amino acid solution and 3% glycerol (carbohydrate source). This product, which

BOX 6-2

Percutaneous Endoscopic Gastrostomy Tube Placement—cont'd

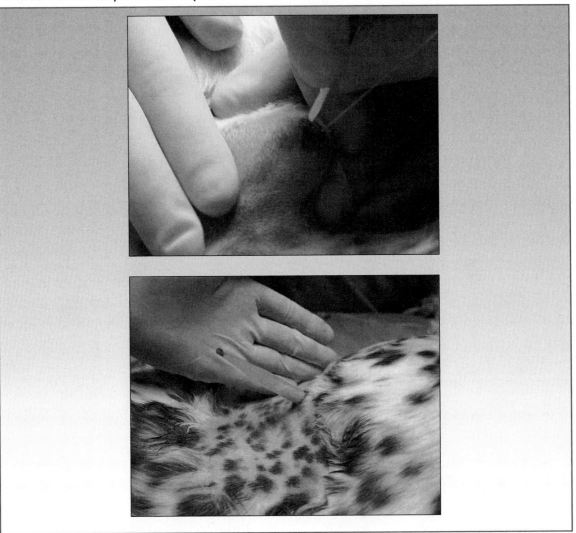

contains approximately 24 mEq/L of potassium chloride, is administered at normal fluid maintenance rates (limited because of the inclusion of maintenance potassium concentrations), either via a central or peripheral IV catheter and provides 245 kcal/L of solution administered. As with enteral nutrition, PN should be instituted gradually over 48 to 72 hours. With both TPN and PPN, the animal's catheter and lines must be handled with aseptic technique to avoid complications. It is important to adjust other IV fluids accordingly for the amount of fluid being administered to avoid fluid volume overload.

Monitoring and Reassessment

Body weight should be monitored daily when providing enteral nutrition or PN. However, the team should take into account fluid shifts in evaluating changes in body weight. For this reason, assessment

BOX 6-2

Percutaneous Endoscopic Gastrostomy Tube Placement—cont'd

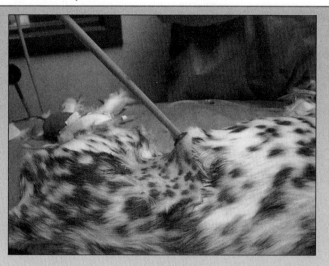

13. The feeding tube is pulled until the mushroom tip rests against the gastric mucosa and can be visualized with the endoscope.

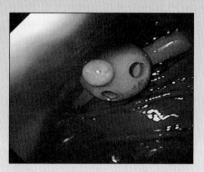

14. To place the outer flange, a closed forceps are placed through the side of the flange. The forceps are then used to grasp the trimmed end of the feeding tube and the flange is slid down the feeding tube to anchor at the skin surface.

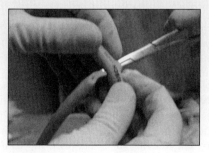

Continued.

Percutaneous Endoscopic Gastrostomy Tube Placement—cont'd

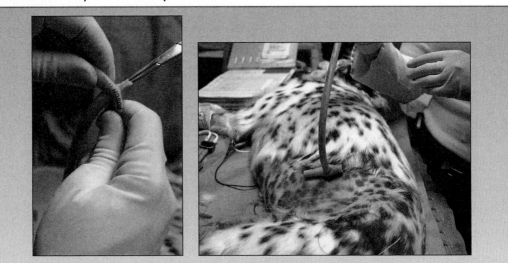

15. The exit incision should be cleaned aseptically again. A Christmas tree adapter is placed on the end of the feeding tube. Additional anchoring suture may be placed to decreased tension at the body wall exit site.

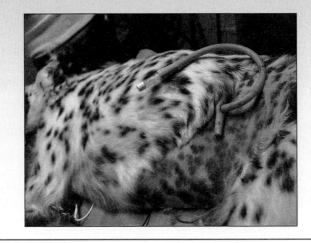

of BCS is important as well. The use of the RER as the patient's caloric requirement is merely a starting point. The number of calories provided may need to be increased to keep up with the patient's changing needs (typically by 25% if well tolerated). In patients unable to tolerate the prescribed amounts, the clinician should consider reducing amounts of enteral feedings and supplementing the nutritional plan with PPN.

Possible complications of enteral nutrition include mechanical complications such as clogging of the tube or early tube removal. Metabolic complications include electrolyte disturbances, hyperglycemia, volume overload, and gastrointestinal signs (e.g., vomiting, diarrhea, cramping, bloating). In critically ill patients receiving enteral nutritional support, the team must also be vigilant for the development of aspiration pneumonia. Monitoring

BOX 6-3

Worksheet for Calculating Enteral Nutrition

1. Resting energy requirement (RER):
   RER = 70 × (current body weight in kilograms)$^{0.75}$
   or, for animals weighing between 2 and 35 kg:
   RER = (30 × current body weight in kilograms) + 70 = _____ kcal required/day
2. Product selected _____
   Contains _____ kcal/ml
3. Total volume to be administered per day:
   $\frac{kcal\ required/day}{kcal/ml\ in\ diet}$ = ___ ml/day
4. Administration schedule:
   One half of total requirement on day 1 = ___ ml/day
   Total requirement on day 2 = ___ ml/day
5. Feedings per day:
   Divide total daily volume into 4 to 6 feedings (depending on duration of anorexia, patient tolerance) = ___ feedings/day
6. Calculate volume per feeding
   $\frac{Total\ ml/day}{Number\ of\ feedings/day}$ = ___ ml/feeding (day 1)
   = ___ ml/feeding (day 2)
*Be sure to adjust the animal's IV fluids accordingly.

Diet Options
Esophagostomy (E) and gastrostomy (G) tubes
Eukanuba Maximum Calorie (canned)
- Supplies 2.1 kcal/ml straight from can but needs to be diluted for tubes

- 1 can + 50 ml water = 1.6 kcal/ml
- 1 can + 25 ml water = 1.8 kcal/ml (for larger tubes)

Hill's a/d (canned)

- Supplies 1.3 kcal/ml straight from can but needs to be diluted for tubes
- 1 can + 50 ml water = 1.0 kcal/ml
- 1 can + 25 ml water = 1.1 kcal/ml (for larger tubes)

Royal Canin low-fat canine diet (canned)

- When a low fat enteral diet is required
- 1 can blenderized with 360 ml water, then strained = 0.8 kcal/ml

Nasoesophageal (NE) and jejunostomy (J) tubes
Veterinary liquid diets

- CliniCare canine/feline liquid diet (1.0 kcal/ml)
- CliniCare RF feline liquid diet (reduced protein formula —1.0 kcal/ml)
- Human enteral products

Note: Most human liquid diets provide 1.0 kcal/ml but do not meet canine or feline requirements (and must be supplemented).

---

parameters for patients receiving enteral nutrition include body weight, serum electrolytes, tube patency, appearance of tube exit site, gastrointestinal signs (e.g., vomiting, regurgitation, diarrhea), and signs of volume overload or aspiration pneumonia.

Possible complications with PN include sepsis, mechanical complications of the catheter and lines, thrombophlebitis, and metabolic disturbances such as hyperglycemia, electrolyte shifts, hyperammonemia, and hypertriglyceridemia. Avoiding serious consequences of complications associated with PN requires early identification of problems and prompt action. Frequent monitoring of vital signs, catheter exit sites, and routine biochemistry panels may alert the staff to developing problems (Box 6-4). If the therapist believes the patient may have a catheter infection, then PN should be discontinued and discarded and the catheter removed and cultured. The development of persistent hyperglycemia during nutritional support may require an adjustment to the nutritional plan (e.g., decreasing dextrose content in PN) or administration of regular insulin and, therefore, will necessitate more vigilant monitoring.

With continual reassessment, the team can determine when to transition the patient from assisted feeding to voluntary consumption of food. The discontinuation of nutritional support should only begin when the patient can consume approximately its RER without much coaxing. In patients receiving TPN, transitioning to enteral nutrition should occur over the course of at least 12 to 24 hours, depending on patient tolerance of enteral nutrition.

BOX 6-4

Monitoring Parameters of Patients on Parenteral Nutritional Support

The monitoring required will depend on the individual patient. However, at least the following should be measured daily:

- Heart/respiratory rate
- Catheter site
- Attitude
- Body weight
- Temperature
- Glucose, total solids (should check hematocrit tubes for lipemia)
- Electrolytes, especially potassium (should be monitored at least every other day)

Summary

Although critically ill patients are often not regarded as in urgent need of nutritional support (given their more pressing problems), the severity of their injuries, altered metabolic condition, and necessity of frequent fasting place these patients at high risk of becoming malnourished during hospitalization. Proper identification of these patients and careful planning and execution of a nutrition plan can be key factors to successful recovery. Therefore the inclusion of the technical staff in the formulation and administration of nutritional support to critically ill patients is absolutely essential.

Suggested Readings

Buffington T, Holloway C, Abood A: Clinical dietetics. In Buffington T, Holloway C, Abood S: *Manual of veterinary dietetics*, St Louis, 2004, Saunders, pp 49-141.

Chan DL: Nutritional requirements of the critically ill patient, *Clin Tech Small Anim Pract* 19:1-5, 2004.

Chan DL: Parenteral nutritional support. In Ettinger S, Feldman, editors: *Textbook of veterinary internal medicine*, ed 6, St Louis, 2005, Elsevier, pp 591-596.

Chan DL et al: Retrospective evaluation of partial parenteral nutrition in dogs and cats, *J Vet Intern Med* 16:440-445, 2002.

Freeman LM, Chan DL: Parenteral and enteral nutrition, *Compend Stand Care Emerg Crit Care* 3:1-7, 2001.

Lippert AC, Fulton RB, Parr AM: A retrospective study of the use of total parenteral nutrition in dogs and cats, *J Vet Intern Med* 7:52-64, 1993.

Marks SL: Nasoesophageal, esophagostomy, and gastrostomy tube placement techniques. In Ettinger S, Feldman E, editors: *Textbook of veterinary internal medicine*, ed 6, St Louis, 2005, Elsevier, pp 329-335.

Michel KE: Interventional nutrition for the critical care patient: optimal diets, *Clin Tech Small Animal Pract* 13:204-210, 1998.

Michel KE, Higgins C: Nutrient-drug interactions in nutritional support, *J Vet Emerg Crit Care* 12:163-168, 2002.

Remillard RL, Armstrong PJ, Davenport DJ: Assisted feeding in hospitalized patients: enteral and parenteral nutrition. In Hand MS et al, editors: *Small animal clinical nutrition*, ed 3, Philadelphia, 2000, WB Saunders, pp 351-399.

Reuter JD et al: Use of total parenteral nutrition in dogs: 209 cases (1988-1995), *J Vet Emerg Crit Care* 8:201-213, 1998.

Waddell LS, Michel KE: Critical care nutrition: routes of feeding, *Clin Tech Small Animal Pract* 13:197-203, 1998.

Zsombor-Murray E, Freeman LM: Peripheral parenteral nutrition, *Compend Contin Educ Pract Vet* 21:512-523, 1999.

Products Listed

NE tube: Feeding tube, Professional Medical Product Inc, Greenwood, SC

E tube: (Silicone esophagostomy catheters)—Global Veterinary Products, Daphne, AL

G tubes: Pezzer mushroom tip catheters, Rusch, High Wycombe, UK

Low-profile G tube: Corflo-Cubby low-profile gastrostomy device, VIASYS Healthcare Medsystems, Wheeling, IL

J tube: Enteral feeding tube, VIASYS Healthcare Medsystems, Wheeling, IL

CliniCare canine and feline liquid diet, Abbott Animal Health, Abbott Park, IL

CliniCare feline RF liquid diet, Abbott Animal Health, Abbott Park, IL

ProcalAmine, McGraw Inc, Irvine, CA

CHAPTER 7

Oxygen Therapy Techniques

ANDREA M. BATTAGLIA, DON SHAWVER

Respiratory care for humans has been established as a necessary part of the medical profession since the early 1960s. Specific treatment protocols and the use of modern technology have made the respiratory care technician an important part of the life-support team.

Veterinary respiratory care offers new challenges because of anatomic species differences. As veterinary medicine continues to advance, treatment options and therapies must meet the demands placed on the industry by pet owners. The technician must be creative in devising methods that meet the animal's respiratory needs and comfort. One must first have the necessary tools to deal with various clinical situations. The following equipment should be available:

- Regulator (50 psi) with flow gauge
- Pressure-compensated flowmeter
- Oral suction
- E-size oxygen cylinder
- Oxygen connecting tubing (¼ inch)
- Suction catheter
- Nasal catheters (varying sizes)
- Elizabethan collar
- Endotracheal tube

It is important to first determine if the animal needs oxygen therapy. Hypoxemia is defined as a partial pressure of oxygen in the arterial blood of less than 80 mm Hg. A partial pressure of oxygen in arterial blood (Pao_2) of less than 60 mm Hg is considered severe hypoxemia, and immediate intervention is necessary. Cyanosis is a blue discoloration of the mucous membranes that occurs because deoxygenated hemoglobin is present. This indicates severe hypoxemia (Pao_2 <50 mm Hg).

By observing the animal's respiratory pattern and effort, one can assess the animal's degree of hypoxia. Nasal flaring, use of abdominal muscles, panting, and irregular chest wall movement can indicate some degree of hypoxia. Cyanosis is a late indicator of respiratory failure.

Chest wall auscultation can support information obtained by observation. The chest can be palpated and examined for swelling, contusions, punctures, or distortion of any kind. Listening for bubbling, gurgling, wheezing, or any other unusual sounds associated with breathing also assists in locating the primary problem.

Ausculting and differentiating different types of lung sounds can assist in identifying the problem. Immediate treatment, including surgery to remove an obstruction, may be necessary; however, oxygen support may be sufficient for stabilization.

These determinations must be made swiftly and accurately. At the first sign of hypoxemia, oxygen should be administered.

Monitoring Devices

Oxygen-monitoring devices are available at a variety of prices and with various functions. Pulse oximetry is a commonly used monitoring system in veterinary medicine. Many types of oxygen-monitoring devices are available, and the best are monitors that are durable and have different sensors. Importantly, the user must understand the limits of this device and how to position the sensor most effectively. Pulse oximetry will determine how well the hemoglobin is saturated by a percentage. It does not determine how well the animal is ventilating (Fig. 7-1).

Blood gas analysis is the most valuable tool in assessing the animal's ability to oxygenate and ventilate. Many systems are now available that require a small amount of blood to obtain this information.

In addition to oxygen saturation and blood gas analysis, fractional inspired oxygen (Fio_2) must be factored into evaluating whether the animal is able to oxygenate normally. The Pao_2:Fio_2 ratio is a quick way to determine if the animal has the ability to oxygenate normally. The Pao_2 measurement is divided by the Fio_2 decimal value for an assessment of the oxygenation ability. A Pao_2:Fio_2 ratio of 300 to 500 is consistent with mild disease, a ratio of 200 to 300 is associated with moderate disease, and a ratio of less than 200 is associated with severe pathologic conditions.

The Fio_2 is measured as a percentage and is multiplied by five to determine the approximate expected Pao_2 (this is known as the *five times percent inspired oxygen rule*). In a normal, healthy animal, the Pao_2 is approximately 100 mm Hg. It will increase to approximately 500 mm Hg on 100% oxygen. In an animal with lung disease, the Pao_2 will not increase the expected five times.

When oxygen is administered, one should evaluate the effect of the intervention. The best means is arterial blood gas measurement; however, if this means is not available, then pulse oximetry should be used. This analysis should be made 15 to 20 minutes after the initial intervention or change in parameters to allow physiologic compensation to take place.

Visual assessments are made continually to evaluate change in behavior and breathing patterns. Oxygen therapy may not be enough support for animals

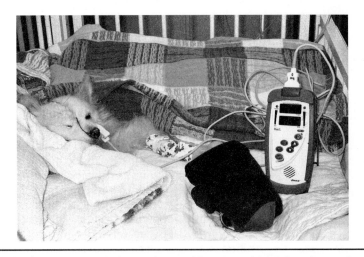

Fig. 7-1 Pulse oximeter monitoring a patient receiving oxygen therapy through a nasal cannula.

that are not ventilating properly, and assisted ventilation may need to be initiated before the animal dies from exhaustion.

Administration of Oxygen Therapy

Each animal in respiratory distress presents a unique set of circumstances. First, the animal's condition must be assessed to determine whether respiratory compromise is present and what intervention is needed. Once the animal's condition has been evaluated, oxygen can be administered. The technician must consider the anatomic characteristics of each species and the level of support the animal needs. If the animal is breathing spontaneously and visual signs indicate that hypoxia may be present, then oxygen therapy is started. A noninvasive method is used while other tests are being performed to determine whether or not long-term therapy will be necessary for treating the condition. Oxygen has a relaxing effect on many animals. Oxygen in high concentrations can have a euphoric effect. When determining any therapy protocol, the technician should remember, above all, to do no harm.

Blow by Oxygen Therapy. The easiest method for most species is to attach an oxygen tube to the gas source, turn the flow to 6 L/min, and hold the open end of the tube approximately 6 inches from the animal's mouth and nose. The flow should not be pointed directly into the nares, because the flow can irritate the delicate nasal passage (Fig. 7-2).

Using this method allows the animal to use less effort to reach the necessary oxygen levels. It is not necessary to add humidification to this method of oxygen delivery, because the overall fractional oxygen concentration being delivered in the lung is probably less than 35% (because it is mixing with ambient air). If one finds that the animal is overly anxious and continues to move its head, then it may be necessary to administer a sedative or use a different administration technique.

Sedated or mildly sedated animals with respiratory distress should be monitored very closely for potential apnea, which necessitates supported ventilation. A manual resuscitator should be available.

Bag Method. Animals, especially cats, with respiratory compromise must be handled cautiously. A fractious cat with respiratory compromise is a good

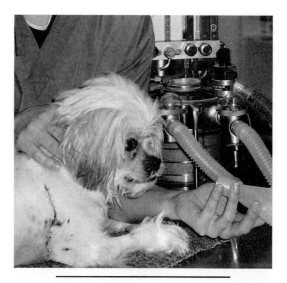

Fig. 7-2 Administering blow by oxygen.

candidate for the bag method. The cat is left in its carrier or box, and a clear plastic bag is wrapped around the box. The oxygen line can be inserted through a hole in the bag, and high-flow oxygen can be administered. This allows the animal to be treated without the stress of being handled. It is a temporary solution until further evaluation is completed and a decision can be made regarding the treatment plan. This method is not to be used for more than 30 minutes, because of the lack of proper ventilation and potential for carbon dioxide buildup within the container.

Nasal Catheters and Prongs. Use of a nasal catheter also is a satisfactory method of administering supportive oxygen to the compromised animal. The nasal cannula can be fashioned from a red rubber feeding tube, or a premade cannula can be purchased from various sources. Premade cannulas usually are available in more appropriate lengths and materials, such as silicone, which is less irritating to the nasal mucosa and to which dried mucus does not adhere. Humidification is recommended. Most dogs and cats best tolerate 3- to 8-French catheters. Larger and smaller catheters are available from various sources for use in other species (Technical Tip Box 7-1).

Nasal prongs also can be used to administer oxygen in some species. The determining factor in this instance is the distance between the right and

BOX 7-1

Technical Tip: Nasal Catheterization

Patient with a Nasal Cannula

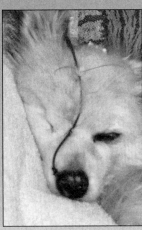

Catheter length is determined by measuring the distance from the tip of the nares to the second upper premolar or the medial canthus. Mark this distance on the catheter.

A suture should be placed close to the external nares, with long ends for tying the catheter in place.

Desensitize the nasal passages with a local anesthetic. Proparacaine solution or 2% lidocaine can be used. Instill 1-2 drops. Wait 30-60 seconds, and repeat if necessary.

Tip the head slightly upward and gently press the tip of the nose upward with the thumb.

Advance the lubricated catheter (surgical lube or lidocaine gel) into the ventral meatus in a ventromedial direction (not necessary in the cat) up to the mark indicated. Be gentle and do not force it.

Suture the catheter in place using two additional points. The most common sites are the bridge of the nose and between the eyes. Suturing to the side of the face is another option. Secure to the oxygen tubing.

Place tape around neck and anchor the tube. Attach a disposable humidifier to the flowmeter.

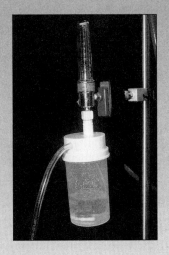

Flow Rates

These rates provide tracheal oxygen of approximately 40%-50% (50-100 mL/kg/min). Oxygen should be administered immediately but gradually. A sudden burst of oxygen can be very uncomfortable for the animal.

- Cats and small dogs <10 kg: 0.5-1.0 L/min
- Dogs 10-20 kg: 1.0-2.0 L/min
- Dogs 20-50 kg: 2-4 L/min
- Dogs >50 kg: 5 L/min

left nostril. This device is one of the most common oxygen administration devices in human oxygen therapy. The nasal prongs are placed at the nares so that each prong is aligned with the opening of one nostril. These devices can slip out of place easily because only the tips of the prongs are in the nares. The technician should be sure to secure both prongs with a suture or surgical staples, taking care not to obstruct the lumen. Oxygen flow rates of 3 to 6 L/min are common, with percentages of oxygen delivered similar to those delivered by nasal catheters. Although the prongs are not placed as far into the nasal cavity as the nasal catheter, the use of topical anesthetic at least initially to reduce mucosal irritation, particularly if flows higher than 3 L/min are used, is advisable. Nasal prongs are available in newborn, pediatric, and adult sizes; the space between the prongs depends on the size selected. The technician should check these devices frequently to ensure proper position is maintained (Fig. 7-3).

Tracheal Oxygen Therapies. Nasal tracheal catheters are used in many veterinary emergency training programs as a way to administer oxygen at percentages greater than 50%, especially for laryngeal paralysis or collapsing trachea. These devices are placed the same way as the nasal catheter, except that the nasal tracheal catheter is advanced to the epiglottis and then slid into the trachea. These catheters are not tolerated well because they can cause the animal to cough frequently, which can dislodge the cannula from the trachea. A topical anesthetic is applied to the laryngotracheal area before insertion to minimize coughing, and a mild tranquilizer can be used to keep the animal sedated. These factors can be risky in animals with severe trauma or disease because they can cause hypoventilation. Because the catheter is left in the trachea, the epiglottis is propped open and the animal can aspirate vomitus or saliva.

A better approach might be transtracheal oxygen. The same catheter used for tracheal and nasal oxygen delivery can be used for transtracheal oxygen. In human medicine, cannulas designed for this purpose are available. Silicone catheters are best for this purpose because silicone is softer, less irritating, and less damaging to the tracheal mucosa. These devices are placed surgically using a scalpel or large-bore needle. The area between the fourth and

fifth cartilaginous ring is prepared and anesthetized locally, and a puncture slightly larger than the catheter is made in this space. The catheter is advanced into the trachea so that its tip is directly above the carina. The catheter position can be verified by oral observation: a laryngoscope is used to lift the epiglottis and observe the catheter position. The proximal end of the catheter is connected to the oxygen source tube and the flow is turned on to approximately 3 L/min. The flow rate is determined by the animal's minute ventilation. If the animal's breathing is deep and rapid, higher flow rates may be necessary.

Oxygen Collars. An oxygen collar is less restrictive than an oxygen mask and less invasive than a cannula. This is a very effective oxygen delivery method, and high levels can be reached very quickly using low flows. It is a technique used for animals with head trauma. One can make an oxygen collar from an Elizabethan collar (Fig. 7-4). An oxygen tube is taped at the base of the collar, with the tip approximately 2 inches from the end of the collar. Clear cellophane wrap is placed across the front of the collar, covering two thirds of the front and taped securely to the sides. The opening acts as a vent, which reduces the confining effect and releases the excess oxygen and exhaled carbon dioxide. This vent size can be increased or decreased depending on the desired oxygen percentage that should be monitored with an oxygen analyzer. Oxygen is heavier than air

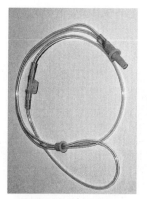

Fig. 7-3 Nasal prongs.

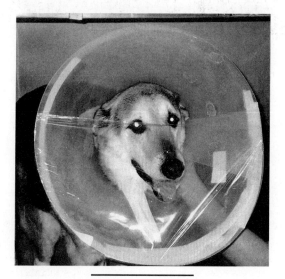

Fig. 7-4 Oxygen collar.

and will remain in the lower two thirds of the collar, which acts as an oxygen reservoir. Flow must meet the animal's ventilatory demand. Monitoring the oxygen saturation in the blood by using a pulse oximeter is a good way to determine effectiveness. It is also important to monitor the buildup of heat and humidity inside the collar. Oxygen is very drying to the mucous membranes. Lubricating the eyes periodically with ophthalmic ointment is recommended with this method of oxygen administration.

Oxygen Cages and Cribs

Oxygen cages and cribs are environmental control devices. They consist of a box, connecting tubes to an oxygen source, filters, and a circulating fan to move the air. Some may have climate controls for temperature and humidification. Because of their size, these devices are not the best choice when

oxygen control and accurate delivery are critical. It takes time for the oxygen concentration to stabilize in this system. Flows as high as 15 L/min are needed to maintain 40% oxygen. These units also develop dead spaces, areas that are not saturated with the proper percentage of oxygen. The cage must be opened frequently to evaluate the animal, and the gas concentration decreases every time the door is opened. This creates an unstable environment for the animal and can be fatal when oxygen concentration control is critical. Animals that are in need of high flows of oxygen immediately but are too fractious to handle can be placed in an oxygen cage, initially. An oxygen tank with a flowmeter is used to infuse high oxygen flows directly into the unit until it reaches the desired percentage (Fig. 7-5).

Oxygen concentration should be monitored with an oxygen analyzer to ensure that proper levels are maintained in the cage (Fig. 7-6). Pulse oximetry and

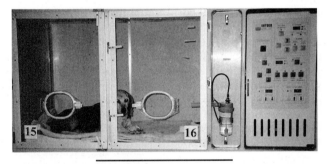

Fig. 7-5 Oxygen therapy cage.

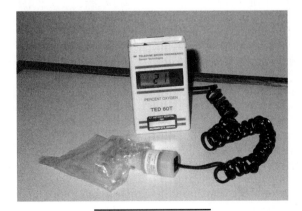

Fig. 7-6 Oxygen analyzer.

visual assessments should be used to ensure that adequate levels of gas are being delivered to meet the animal's physiologic demand.

Humidification systems also must be checked frequently for bacterial growth. Some older oxygen cages were equipped with pass over humidifiers in which air flowed over a pan of water and humidity was derived from surface evaporation. These systems were difficult to clean, and water was often not replaced frequently enough, leading to the growth of bacteria, particularly *Pseudomonas aeruginosa*.

Oxygen can be administered to animals with respiratory compromise in many ways, and some ways work better than others. To determine whether a particular method meets the animal's physiologic demand, the technician must monitor the animal's physiologic response. Devices such as pulse oximeters, oxygen analyzers, and blood gas measuring devices are invaluable in monitoring the animal with respiratory compromise.

Hyperbaric Oxygen

Hyperbaric oxygen therapy is a medical treatment administering 100% oxygen to the entire body greater than normal atmospheric pressures. The increased pressure, combined with an increase of oxygen to 100%, dissolves oxygen in the blood and in all body tissues and fluids up to 20 times normal concentration.

Hyperbaric chambers where developed in the 1920s. Research using animals to test the devices began as early as the 1800s, and many successful treatment protocols for animals are now available.

Hyperbaric chambers have been used successfully to treat nonhealing wounds, birth asphyxia, bone and joint infection secondary to bacterial septicemia in foals, carbon monoxide poisoning, and crush injuries. A few veterinary facilities have hyperbaric chambers on site.

Conclusion

Effective oxygen therapy depends on the technician's understanding of respiratory care devices and their function. In addition, knowledge of the respiratory physiology of different species is needed to understand what is normal. Monitoring specific oxygen parameters is very helpful in determining the extent of respiratory compromise and the extent to which compensation and correction are taking place. Careful observation also is important in determining how well the animal is tolerating the therapy.

As previously mentioned, oxygen can be administered to an animal in many ways, and some ways are more effective than others. Understanding the available methods enables the team to choose the appropriate therapy. Some animals tolerate one type of delivery system better than another. Oxygen therapy should calm the animal and improve its condition. If it causes the animal to struggle and become anxious, then another delivery system should be used. As new and improved methods are developed for using oxygen therapy to treat critically ill and injured small animal patients, the percentage of successful treatments will increase.

Suggested Readings

Bain FT, Slovis NM: *They shoot horses don't they?* The American Association for Hyperbaric Awareness, 2006 (online). Available at www.aaha-us.com

Bistner SI, Ford DB: *Handbook of veterinary procedures and emergency treatment*, ed 6, Philadelphia, 1995, WB Saunders.

Clare M, Hopper K: Mechanical ventilation: indications, goals and prognosis, *Compendium* 27(3):195-207, March 2005.

Crowe DT: Seminar notes. Case-based discussion at the 5th Annual Emergency Medical Conference, Kansas State University, March 1, 1997, Kansas State University Student Chapter of the Veterinary Emergency and Critical Care Society.

McPherson SP, Spearman CB: *Respiratory therapy equipment*, ed 3, St Louis, 1995, Mosby.

Shawver DM: *Clinical notes on airway management, Cambridge University, England*, Bloomington, Ind, 1995, Cook Veterinary Products.

Spearman D, Sheldon RL, Egan DF: *Egan's fundamentals of respiratory therapy*, ed 4, St Louis, 1982, Mosby.

Whelan HT: *The healing powers of hyperbaric oxygen treatment*. HealthLink Medical College of Wisconsin, 2001 (online). Available at www.healthlink.mcw.edu

White GC: *Equipment theory for respiratory care*, ed 3, Albany, NY, 1998, Delmar.

Wingfield WE, Raffe M: *The veterinary ICU book*, Jackson, Wyo, 2002, Teton New Media, pp 289-290.

8

Mechanical Ventilation

ANDREA M. BATTAGLIA, DON SHAWVER

Normal ventilation is the inspiration and expiration of air to and from the lungs. The respiratory cycle has four stages: (1) inspiratory flow, (2) inspiratory pause, (3) expiratory flow, and (4) expiratory pause. Gas exchange does not occur during the pause phase. Downward movement of the diaphragm creates negative pressure, allowing air to enter the lungs. Ventilators alter these cycles to provide more efficient patterns of breathing in animals with ventilatory compromise.

Mechanical ventilation is the act of assisting or controlling the patient's breathing by the use of a machine-driven or hand-operated device. Positive pressure in the lungs drives mechanical ventilation. Reversing the normal respiratory pattern stresses all body systems. The technician responsible for administering mechanical ventilation must understand the system being used and monitor the patient frequently at specific intervals.

When to Mechanically Ventilate

Trauma and various disease processes can impair an animal's ability to breathe properly. The animal in respiratory distress must be assessed quickly and treated immediately. Oxygen therapy is started immediately, and the patient's response is assessed. Visual assessment includes observing the animal's ventilatory pattern, respiratory rate, and posture. Lung auscultation also is important (Table 8-1). If the patient does not have the muscular ability and control to breathe effectively and efficiently, then administering oxygen alone will not be effective. The animal must be able to move the oxygen from the lungs to the tissues to maintain stable oxygen saturation. Cyanosis is not a good indication of when to begin mechanical ventilation; it is a late sign of hypoxemia.

Once the physical assessments are complete, response to oxygen therapy can be evaluated. The patient's respiratory effort and anxiety should decrease if the treatment is effective. Pulse oximetry can be used to determine oxygen saturation but should not be used exclusively. Normal readings are approximately 95% to 98%, depending on

TABLE 8-1

Interpreting Chest Sounds

Sound	Possible Cause
Wheezes	Obstruction
Crackles	Fluid in airspace
Gurgles or bubbles	Heavy secretions in upper airway
Rhonchi, harsh or coarse sounds	Irritated bronchial mucosa
Quiet or diminished lung sounds	Collapsed air sacs, pneumothorax
Drum sound (tympanic resonance) to tapping	Possible pneumothorax or air trapping

respiratory rate and oxygen flow rate. Even low flows will result in blood gases above 100 mm Hg and oxygen saturations of 100% if the pulmonary system is working correctly. Arterial blood gas is the best indicator of oxygen therapy effectiveness. (Blood gas analysis is discussed in detail in Chapter 2.)

Normal values are as follows:

- pH—7.35 to 7.45
- Partial pressure of carbon dioxide in arterial blood ($Paco_2$)—35 to 45 mm Hg
- Partial pressure of oxygen in arterial blood (Pao_2)—94 to 100 mm Hg
- Bicarbonate (HCO_3)—22 to 26 mEq/L
- Base excess—2 to 2

If improvements are noted and the blood gas results are normal, then mechanical ventilation may not be needed immediately. In this case the animal remains on oxygen therapy, and the causes of its respiratory distress are analyzed.

If no improvements are noted or the patient's condition begins to decline, then ventilation must be considered. When hypoxia increases, the work of breathing increases. Total body and system fatigue can occur, which leads to death rapidly.

Once it is determined that assisted ventilation is necessary, a protocol for the animal is developed. The type of sedation and type of airway access is determined initially. Protocols can be established so that if immediate ventilation is required, then time is not wasted.

Airway

The ventilator is only as good as the link to the patient. The endotracheal tube is used most often; however, for patients with upper airway trauma or those under mild sedation, a tracheostomy tube may be necessary.

The tube should be made of a material such as silicone that has very little erosive effect on the tracheal wall and minimal impedance of capillary blood flow when used correctly. The tube is cuffed to allow the ventilator to cycle effectively. The cuffed tube will also aid in preventing stomach content aspiration into the trachea. High-volume, low-pressure cuffs are more desirable for the long term.

Silicone cuffs are a porous material, and air can leak over a longer period of time. To correct this effect, distilled water can be inserted into the cuff in place of air. A minimal leak technique for cuff inflation will reduce the likelihood of tracheal trauma. Once the tube is placed and secured, it is connected to the functioning ventilator. The cuff is inflated slowly until air stops leaking. The cuff is then deflated until a slight hissing sound is heard. If the inspiratory phase does not terminate, then the leak is too large. In this case the technician should reinflate the tube and repeat the withdrawal procedure.

Cuffs are deflated and the tubes are rotated periodically to prevent pressure necrosis of the trachea. Cuff pressure can be measured with a Posey cuff manometer (Box 8-1).

Types of Ventilation

A complete understanding of ventilator terminology and types of ventilators enables the technician to care for patients receiving mechanical ventilation.

- *Controlled ventilation* is the total control of all ventilatory activity (used for apnea).
- *Assisted ventilation* is the intermittent control of ventilation (used for periodic episodes of suppressed respiratory effort).
- *Positive end expiratory pressure* is the elevated pressure maintained in the lung during mechanical ventilation, which increases the functional residual capacity. It prevents exhalation of the entire tidal volume to prevent atelectasis and improve gas exchange. Spring valves or other devices are

BOX 8-1

Technical Tip: Airway Care

Suctioning

The airway must be suctioned to remove secretions.
Tools needed for suctioning include the following:

- Suction kit
- Sterile gloves and catheter
- Suction unit
- Saline
- Sterile endotracheal tube

Suctioning the airway regularly may be necessary and should be anticipated.

Technical tip:

1. Connect the manual resuscitator to the airway and hyperventilate the patient with 10 breaths. Oxygen is being suctioned, as well as the mucus and debris.
2. Infusing a small amount of saline may be necessary to facilitate breaking down thick mucous secretion.
3. Sterile technique is a very important aspect of good airway management. Lubricate the sterile catheter with saline and insert it into the airway with a sterile gloved hand. A red rubber catheter can be used as a suction catheter if a regular manufactured catheter is not readily available. A small thumb port can be cut just below the suction adapter at the proximal end of the catheter to allow for intermittent control over the suction. Hold the distal tip of the suction catheter and the distal suction tip with the sterile gloved hand (hold the proximal end of the catheter in the sterile gloved left hand). This method allows easy control of the amount of suction and control of insertion depth.
4. Advance the tube rapidly to just beyond the distal end of the endotracheal tube with a back-and-forth rotation of the tip between the thumb and index fingers. Once the tip is advanced just beyond the end of the endotracheal tube, place the left thumb over the port, which will activate the suction through the catheter. With the continued back-and-forth rotation, withdraw the catheter from the airway. Suctioning can be very uncomfortable for the patient and may be met with resistance.
5. Reconnect breathing system on the original settings.

6. Observe secretions and note the amount, consistency, and color.

Caution: Reduction of oxygen levels, trauma to the tracheal mucosa, and introduction of infection can occur during suction. All staff should understand the importance of suctioning and sterile technique.

7. Rinse and lubricate the tip in a small cup of sterile distilled water or a small pan of sterile distilled water. Dip the tip of the catheter in the distilled water while applying suction to clear tenacious mucus from the suction catheter.

Suction time will vary depending on the size of the patient. Larger patients may tolerate 5 seconds of suction from start to tip withdrawal. Smaller patients may only tolerate 2 seconds or less. Suctioning a tracheostomy tube will require less time than an endotracheal tube because suction catheter insertion depth is less.

Humidification

The patient's normal humidification system is bypassed during mechanical ventilation. It is important to humidify the air to maintain a healthy airway. Cold aerosol mists and warm-water vapors usually are ancillary ventilator components. Nebulizers and artificial noses are connected to the breathing circuit to provide continual humidification.

Changing the Airway Tube

The airway tube is changed only when necessary.

- Suction the internal lumen and upper airway. Suction the patient's mouth, including the area around the cuff, to remove debris.
- Hyperventilate or increase oxygen to 100% for 10 breaths.
- Suction the upper airway above the cuff.
- Deflate the cuff and immediately but gently remove the tube. Replace it if hypoxia or apnea is apparent.
- Reconnect the ventilator if mechanical ventilation is to be continued.

Note: Airway exchange catheters are available and allow oxygen therapy to continue during the tube exchange.

used to add expiratory resistance to continuous airflow (can reduce cardiac output).

- *Continuous positive airway pressure* is the maintaining of an end expiratory pressure above ambient pressure during spontaneous breathing (also increases functional residual capacity and diffusion).

- *Continuous positive-pressure ventilation* involves applying positive pressure with every breath. This is necessary for animals that cannot breathe spontaneously.

- *Intermittent positive-pressure ventilation* involves applying positive-pressure breaths intermittently during spontaneous breathing (necessary for animals that have a depressed respiratory drive or periods of apnea and is used often for administering gas anesthesia).

- *Dead space ventilation* is the portion of the tidal volume that does not take part in gas exchange between the alveolar sac and the pulmonary blood stream. Approximately one third of the tidal volume is dead space, about 2 ml/kg. This factor cannot be easily measured.

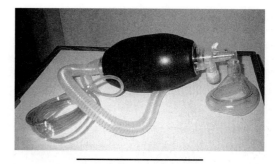

Fig. 8-1 Manual resuscitator.

Most Common Types of Ventilators

Manual Ventilator

Manual ventilators are manual compression bags that can be connected quickly and easily to an endotracheal tube. Reservoir tubes or bags can be connected to the compressible bag to assist in short-term ventilation or cardiopulmonary resuscitation. Portability and availability are the main advantages of manual ventilators.

However, manual ventilators have some limitations. Because of the manual operation, time use is limited. In addition, volume delivery and inspired oxygen cannot be controlled. These devices are best suited for short-term use. The Ambu-Bag is one type of manual resuscitation device (Fig. 8-1).

Pressure-Cycled Ventilator

Pressure-cycled ventilators terminate inspiration based on a preset pressure. To control the percentage of oxygen to be delivered, a blender must be connected to the ventilator. Without a blender, the inspired oxygen levels can reach 90% continually. For long-term ventilation, the technician must be

able to control the oxygen concentration to avoid the negative effects of oxygen toxicity. High flows of 100% oxygen over a period of time can lead to alveolar injury, decreased pulmonary function, and eventually, death. Animals should not receive 100% oxygen for more than 12 to 24 hours and should be maintain at levels below 50% during long-term therapy.

Pressure-cycled ventilators are pressure limited. A control regulates the amount of pressure delivered to the patient's lungs and ventilator system. Tidal volume is the result of the flow of gas from the ventilator to the patient's lungs over a period of time. The resistance and compliance of the ventilatory circuitry and the patient's physiologic condition create pressure readings on the ventilator's manometer. When a patient needs a specific tidal volume to maintain a stable pH, this pressure limit can create a problem. Lungs can become less compliant and demand an increase in pressure to reach the desired tidal volume. The pressure-cycled ventilator may not be able to meet this demand because of premature inspiratory termination.

The advantage of these machines is that they are less expensive than others and more readily available. The disadvantage is that it is impossible to ensure adequate tidal volume. Tidal volumes can be monitored with a spirometer.

The Bird Mark 7, Puritan Bennett PR II, and Puritan Bennett PR I are types of pressure-cycled ventilators (Figs. 8-2 and 8-3).

Volume-Cycled Ventilators

The volume-cycled ventilator terminates inspiration when a predetermined volume is reached. The desired volume is delivered even if resistance in the system occurs.

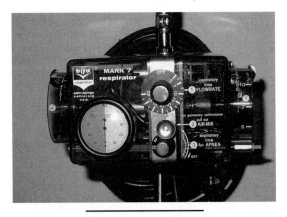

Fig. 8-2 Bird Mark 7 IPPB.

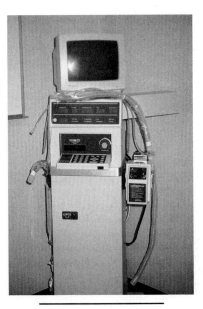

Fig. 8-4 STAR model 300A.

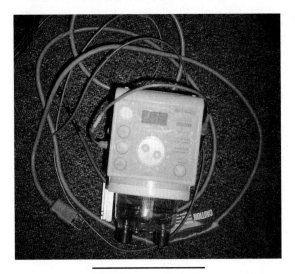

Fig. 8-3 Oxygen blender.

Time-Cycled Ventilators

The time-cycled ventilator terminates the inspiratory phase after a set period of time. These ventilators are commonly used as anesthetic delivery devices. The Bird Mark 11 and the Hallowell Ventilator are examples of time-cycled ventilators.

High-Frequency Jet Ventilators

High-frequency jet ventilators are highly specialized machines. They deliver the gases at a rapid rate so that small volumes are stacked, forcing the gases to permeate the alveolar capillary membranes. These ventilators are used primarily in cases of shock lung syndrome or fibrosis (Fig. 8-5). The Sechrist IV-100B, Life Pulse Jet Ventilator, and Healthdyne Impulse Jet Ventilator are examples of high-frequency jet ventilators.

Parameters critical to the support of the patient must be monitored and maintained at all times. The type of ventilator chosen must be able to deliver adequate volumes in a given period of time at an oxygen saturation that meets the patient's physiologic demands.

The care and monitoring of the patient on the ventilator are important factors in successful treatment (Box 8-2).

Disadvantages include the high cost and low availability of these machines. The ability to control the inspired oxygen percentage (Fio$_2$) and tidal volume, and the availability of positive end expiratory pressure, continuous positive airway pressure, and alarm systems are the benefits of the volume-cycled ventilator.

The Puritan Bennett MA1, MA11, Servo 300/400 (blender separate), and STAR ventilator are types of volume-cycled ventilators (Fig. 8-4).

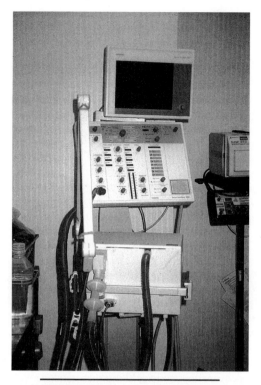

Fig. 8-5 STAR jet ventilator model 3010.

Troubleshooting

Understanding the mechanics of the specific ventilator used enables the technician to support the patient and solve problems as they arise. If the machine cycling begins to fail, then gas and electrical sources should be checked first. Tanks should be filled, and all electrical connections confirmed.

Most of these devices are pressure or volume limited, so leaks are the most common cause of malfunction. The leaks may be around hose connections or the cuff of the endotracheal tube. Feeling around all connections and listening for air escaping will assist in determining if leaks are present.

Excess humidification in the system can cause problems. Water pooling in any of the hoses can increase pressure within the system.

The airway must be evaluated continually. Excess secretions, mucous plugs, or an improperly sized endotracheal tube can cause malfunctions.

True mechanical failure can occur, so a backup system must be available.

Weaning off the Ventilator

When the patient is ready to be weaned and the acid-base status has been stabilized, the Fio_2 is decreased in 10% decrements. The patient's responses are observed and blood gases checked every 20 minutes. This process is continued until the percentage of atmospheric air (21%) is reached.

The mandatory ventilation rate is decreased every 2 to 4 minutes by a couple of breaths. Observing for spontaneous breaths, inspiratory effort, and frequency is important.

Once the patient can breathe spontaneously with adequate effort, extubation can occur. Blood gas is checked after extubation, and oxygen therapy may be necessary for minimal support if the patient is mildly hypoxic (see Box 8-2).

Complications of Mechanical Ventilation

The decision to ventilate mechanically is not made lightly. Mechanical ventilation is a serious commitment made by the veterinary care facility and the owners. The procedure is time-consuming, expensive, and carries a risk of complications.

Upper airway trauma can result if the type of tube used is wrong for the patient or if the cuff is inflated improperly. Pulmonary barotrauma and pneumothorax can result from high ventilatory pressures.

Inadequate ventilation is the result of misplaced endotracheal tubes or improper use of the machine's functions. Nosocomial infections can result from improper aseptic techniques.

Knowledge of respiratory physiologic conditions, mechanical ventilation, patient monitoring, and overall patient care enables the veterinary technician to minimize complications and administer mechanical ventilation successfully.

Record Keeping

One person should be assigned to each patient receiving ventilation (to keep forms and observations consistent throughout the shift). Records must be accurate and detailed, especially with regard to change of ventilator settings and assessments made during treatment. Shift changes must

BOX 8-2

Technical Tip: Care of the Patient Receiving Mechanical Ventilation

Mechanical ventilation is stressful for the patient, but the technician can alleviate some of the stress by using continuous monitoring equipment to optimize treatment. Many available monitors incorporate many features in one system, and some units can be upgraded.

Continuous Monitoring Equipment
- Electrocardiogram
- Pulse oximeter
- Carbon dioxide analyzer
- Thermometer (temperature probes)
- IV fluid pumps
- Blood gas analyzer
- Suction
- Stethoscope
- Doppler for blood pressure monitoring
- Supplies
- Suction catheters
- Endotracheal tubes (multiple sizes)
- Manual resuscitator
- Warming units
- Syringe for cuff inflation
- Items for padding
- Towels
- Blankets
- Support wedges
- Absorbent pads
- Possible indwelling tubes to maintain
- Endotracheal tubes or tracheostomy tube
- IV catheters
- Jugular catheter
- Peripheral catheter
- Arterial catheter
- Urinary catheter with closed system
- Nasogastric feeding tube or stomach tube

Treatment List
- Perform airway tube maintenance as needed.
- Lubricate the eyes every 4 hours with sterile ophthalmic ointment.
- Wipe and moisturize the nose as needed.
- Apply olive oil to the tongue as needed (for moistening).
- Rinse the mouth clean of excess secretions as needed. Suction to collect the solution.
- Use a mouth gag to prevent clamping down on the endotracheal tube and tongue. This is not necessary if a tracheostomy tube is in place.
- Change the patient's position every 2 hours. Animals should not be placed in a complete lateral position.
- Perform physical therapy every 2 hours. Massage the patient's legs. (This step must be performed very carefully. Depending on the type of sedation or depth of anesthesia, massage may be too stimulating.)
- Perform catheter care every 24 hours or as necessary.
- Check the settings on the ventilator and vital parameters every hour and adjust them as needed.

overlap at least 30 minutes so that the next technician has enough time to review updates and patient status.

Conclusion

The method of respiratory support provided by veterinary professionals is very different from the patient's natural respiration. One accomplishes lung ventilation by creating a negative pressure in the chest and allowing air to flow into the lungs. Respiration takes place as an exchange between carbon dioxide and oxygen at the tissue level. When applying mechanical devices to the lung, we create an abnormal situation that can have side effects and complicate the course of treatment. Pulmonary barotrauma, impeded venous return, renal shutdown, tracheal malaise, and pneumothorax are some of the potential complications. Pet owners must understand the cost and risks of mechanical ventilation before treatment can begin.

Anesthesia can cause other complications, such as suppressed respiratory function and central nervous system depression. By being aware of these complications and the factors that create them, veterinary professionals can take steps to minimize or eliminate them.

To maximize the patient's chances of survival and recovery, the critical care team must be trained to operate each machine being used, as well as have a firm understanding of blood gas analysis and respiratory therapy.

Suggested Readings

Martz KV, Joiner JW, Sheperd RM: *Management of the patient-ventilator system*, ed 2, St Louis, 1984, Mosby.

McPherson SP, Spearman CB: *Respiratory therapy equipment*, ed 3, St Louis, 1985, Mosby.

West JB: *Respiratory physiology*, ed 3, Baltimore, 1985, Williams & Wilkins.

White GC: *Equipment theory for respiratory care*, Albany, NY, 1995, Delmar.

CHAPTER 9

Pain Assessment and Treatment

Nancy Shaffran

Philosophers and scientists have long debated the issues of animal pain. Until recently, practical pain treatment in veterinary patients has not been adequately addressed. This oversight may have resulted from the following beliefs:

- Animals do not experience pain.
- Pain may be experienced but not in a way that is detrimental to an animal's well-being or that warrants treatment.
- Signs of pain are too subjective to be assessed.
- Pain is good because it limits activity.
- Analgesia is bad because of adverse side effects or because it interferes with the ability to accurately monitor patients.

The veterinary community has recognized that animals experience pain and that pain must be managed for optimum health. The emerging specialty of veterinary critical care has brought greater attention to pain management. Critically ill patients present unique challenges in pain recognition and treatment option selection, and their analgesic needs are likely to be greater than the needs of more stable patients. Choosing the correct analgesic therapy requires an understanding of the pharmacokinetics of a wide range of drugs, as well as the levels or type of pain associated with various conditions. Failure to adequately manage pain in a critically ill patient lessens the chance of recovery and can result in shock and even death.

Critically ill and injured patients are subjected to numerous painful treatments and diagnostic procedures. The commitment to treat critically ill animals must include alleviating or minimizing their pain throughout treatment.

Patients who are critically ill are the most likely ones to be in pain and in need of treatment; however, because of their fragile condition, these animals may be less able to express their needs than the average, healthy animal. It has been suggested that these animals inspire less affection and greater detachment from caregivers than do healthier animals with "personality," which is thought to diminish the attention paid to their pain needs. However, one might argue that to some caregivers, critically ill patients inspire greater compassion in response to an increased perception of helplessness.

The ambiguity in pain management rests largely in the subjective nature of pain assessment. Veterinary pain assessment is based solely on the ability to recognize often subtle, varying signs and symptoms of non-verbal patients. The study of pain in nonverbal patients (i.e., human neonates, infants, animals) is fairly recent. The first human work examining pain manifestations in preverbal children was conducted in 1986. This research showed that healthy full-term newborns display painful distress in response to tissue damage. Crying, body movements, avoidant behaviors, and facial expressions were described as manifestations of pain in neonatal patients. Despite these acknowledgments, neonates were not routinely treated for pain for nearly 10 more years. The inability to distinguish pain from other stress, the extreme subjectivity of assessment, and persistent argument about the existence of neonatal pain confounded clinicians' efforts. Even now, human neonatal pain assessment and management remains an area of research, growth, and ethical debate.

In veterinary medicine, the issue is further confounded by several factors. First, a natural variation exists in the experience and display of pain between species, breeds, and individual animals. Veterinary technicians are expected to recognize pain in cats, dogs, and other small companion animals. There may appear to be very little similarity between a cat who sleeps curled in the back of its cage, avoiding movement or contact, and a crying, restless dog. However, both animals may be exhibiting signs of pain. Even within species, breed variations are strong. It has become customary to discriminate between perceived stoic and weak animals. Animals that do not display overt signs of pain are praised for their fortitude. Patients that show excessive signs of pain are assumed to be weak. Collies and borzois, for example, are stereotyped as fragile and without strong will to survive grave illness. Conversely, Labradors seem to be oblivious to pain and able to survive where other dogs might not. Although some may argue the specifics, most veterinary professionals probably have preconceived ideas about breed predisposition and ability to handle pain, stress, and illness. Some actual differences may exist in breed pain threshold and response; however, it is dangerous to make general assumptions about pain rather than to consider each patient individually.

Second, veterinary technicians often make assumptions about which procedures are most painful.

For example, most would agree that a thoracotomy is a painful procedure, whereas an ovariohysterectomy is considered by many to be mildly to moderately painful. An examination of how these conclusions were reached is useful. No valid reason exists to make generalizations about procedures other than to assume that invasive surgical or nonsurgical procedures are likely to cause some degree of pain. Each patient must be evaluated. Ultimately, pain treatment often is determined arbitrarily, based on a combination of limited information, subjective assessment, and personal beliefs. One can best approach a scientific and humane course of pain assessment and treatment by studying the physiology of pain, how it is manifested in nonverbal patients, and when and how pain should be treated.

Physiology of Pain

Pain has a physiologic explanation. Pain receptors, called *nociceptors*, in the nervous system are stimulated by noxious events. The stimulus may be chemical, mechanical, or thermal. For example, chemical injury often is caused by substances such as prostaglandins and histamines produced in response to inflammation. Once a painful stimulus reaches a nociceptor cell, the information is transmitted to the brain via the spinal cord and the pain response begins. This includes the release of endogenous opioid endorphins, which function as natural analgesia. Often, in both chronic and acute situations, the level of pain exceeds the body's ability to provide relief. Chronic pain is prolonged and persistent; the body becomes habituated to nervous system responses and no longer provides adequate endogenous pain control. Acute pain is of severe, sudden onset that overwhelms endogenous analgesic mechanisms. Regardless of whether pain is acute or chronic in nature, untreated pain can result in long-term changes in the nervous system that lead to persistent pain nonresponsive pain states. Acute pain is the predominant concern among critically ill patients.

Assessment and Recognition

What Does Pain Look Like?

In an effort to form a consensus on what animal pain looks like, several hundred veterinary personnel from four leading veterinary institutions were surveyed. The survey was a simple form asking the participant to list all criteria he or she used to determine whether a patient was experiencing pain. The results were tabulated and categorized by frequency of response and subcategorized by professional group (i.e., technician, clinician). The top responses, in order of frequency, were vocalization, increased heart rate, increased respiratory rate, restlessness, increased body temperature, increased blood pressure (BP), abnormal posturing, inappetence, aggression, unwillingness to move, frequent changes in position, facial expression, trembling, depression, and insomnia. Also mentioned but less statistically significant were anxiety; nausea; pupillary enlargement; licking, chewing, or staring at site; poor mucous membrane color; salivation; decreased carbon dioxide; and head pressing.

More than 50% of all participants cited "known painful condition or procedure" as a reason to treat for pain. Listed criteria other than physical manifestations were the presence of one or more of the preceding signs without other attributable cause, intuition, and responsiveness to pain medication.

These findings are similar to those found in human neonates and infants, although more attention has been paid to their facial expressions and measured hormonal responses. Increased heart rate and respiratory rate, vocalization, and increased body movements are listed among the top pain manifestations in both human and veterinary patients. Several things become clear from this study. Various types of veterinary personnel have similar criteria for evaluating pain in their patients. This means that agreement exists regarding what pain looks like, although it is not necessarily scientifically conclusive. It is also clear that the list of manifestations is extensive and at times contradictory (e.g., unwillingness to move, frequent position changes). The following signs and symptoms, in the absence of any other reasonable explanation, are reasons to suspect that the animal is in pain and consider treatment. The reader should note that although the following are the most commonly described signs, they are by no means the only indicators of pain in veterinary patients.

- Increased heart rate
- Increased respiratory rate
- Increased BP
- Increased temperature
- Vocalization
- Inability to rest or sleep
- Trembling
- Inappetence

When and How Should Pain Be Treated?

Scientific data support beneficial aspects of pain: it limits further aggravating activity, causes homeostatic regulating hormone release, and motivates the patient to seek medical attention. It has also been demonstrated that severe acute pain can have the following deleterious physiologic effects:

- Neuroendocrine responses (e.g., excessive release of pituitary, adrenal, and pancreatic hormones), possibly resulting in nutritional, growth, development, and healing disturbances, as well as immunosuppression
- Cardiovascular compromise (increased arterial BP, heart rate, and intracranial pressure and decreased perfusion)
- Respiratory rate increases accompanied by decreased partial pressure of oxygen or dyspnea
- Coagulopathies (e.g., thrombotic events, increased platelet reactivity, disseminated intravascular coagulation)
- Complications associated with long-term recumbency caused by pain or depression
- Poor nutritional intake and hypoproteinemia, resulting in slow healing

Much less is known about the psychologic effects of pain on animals, but it appears that these manifestations are numerous and detrimental and may include inappetence, insomnia, and depression. It is probably safe to assume that any behavioral change not attributable to another known cause is likely to be an indication of pain in patients with a sight of past or present tissue injury.

Pain should always be treated to inhibit its deleterious effects. Although rarely as serious as the effects of painfulness, analgesia is not benign and carries some degree of risk and potential complications. Fear of side effects from analgesic drugs precludes their use in many cases. The most common arguments for withholding analgesia are as follows:

- Pain medication may cause cardiovascular compromise in fragile patients.
- Sedation may inhibit movement and lead to respiratory complications.
- Anesthetics and analgesics may mask signs of progress or regression, complicating evaluation

of patient status. Cardiovascular monitoring may be obscured by sedation.

- Pain is self-protective (i.e., animals limit their own activity to minimize pain, and eliminating pain allows the patient to do further damage).
- Pain control measures may result in longer hospital stays and higher costs.

Because the best interest of the patient is to alleviate animal pain, these concerns must be addressed without withholding analgesia. The expected changes in heart rate, respiration, BP, and mentation that accompany analgesic use must be understood. Baseline assessments should be made before treatment. After treatment, follow-up assessments should be made at regular intervals. More frequent cardiovascular monitoring may be needed in patients treated for severe pain. Pain treatment may result in diminished activity and a slower return to normal body functions (e.g., eating, drinking, walking), but these effects may be less detrimental than the recovery delays associated with persistent pain.

Pain Relief

Nonpharmacologic Interventions

Before pain medication is administered, every effort should be made to provide nonpharmacologic comfort to the patient. Differentiating between physical pain and other types of stress is the first step in assessment. Stressors such as boredom, thirst, anxiety, and the need to urinate or defecate can mimic the signs of pain. All these stressors must be addressed before one can determine whether the patient needs medication. In some cases, these efforts may obviate further treatment. Even when pain medication is administered, these comfort needs must be addressed continually.

Providing comfort includes attention to physical surroundings and perceived psychologic needs. It should not be assumed that the patient will automatically assume a comfortable position. The patient may need to be placed in a position that reduces pressure on painful areas, facilitates adequate ventilation, and promotes sleep. Bedding, padding, and pillows can be used to provide additional support. Reducing light and sound can also encourage rest or sleep.

Assessing the patient's emotional needs may be more difficult because of the great variation in individual response to pain and stress. The critical care technician must become adept at recognizing the unique needs of each patient. Gentle stroking and calming speech can be potent means of easing stress. When distraction is more effective, the animal can be placed in an active area with many visual and auditory stimuli. In some cases, owner visits are very comforting to the patient. In others, the patient becomes too agitated by the visit or the apparent benefits are negated by the response to owner's leaving.

Patient comfort can also be improved by reducing painful events. Because many nursing interventions entail painful procedures (e.g., injections, venipuncture, catheter placement, suturing), increasing technical proficiency can prevent pain. Organizing treatments efficiently to reduce the total number of disturbances is another nonmedical pain reduction intervention.

Once the patient's physical and emotional needs have been addressed, the patient's comfort is reassessed. The following questions should be asked:

- Is the patient at an acceptable comfort level?
- Is it possible that the clinical signs are manifestations of pain?
- Are there any contraindications to giving pain medications?
- Can the patient be supported through any adverse effects of drug administration?
- What is the appropriate (safe and effective) medication for the patient?

It is common practice in human and veterinary medicine for technicians to assess pain status and administer appropriately ordered analgesia by continually asking themselves these questions.

Analgesic Drugs

The options for analgesia are increasing as more is understood about pain processing. Choosing the correct analgesic therapy involves understanding the pharmacokinetics of a wide range of drugs and the levels or type of pain associated with various conditions (Technical Tip Box 9-1).

Great individual variation in human responsiveness to drugs has been recognized recently. In other words, the same drug can produce vastly different results in different patients. These differences are partly a result of individual genetic differences, as well as a result of the nonphysiologic factors that influence any pain state: anxiety, fear, sense of control, ethnocultural background, and meaning of the

BOX 9-1

Technical Tip: Epidural Anesthesia and Analgesia

Increasing the percentage of inspired oxygen with a face mask or endotracheal tube helps prevent the sedated or anesthetized patient from becoming hypoxic. IV fluids should be administered (crystalloids, 10 ml/kg/hr) to help prevent hypotension that may result from autonomic blockade. The animal should be placed on a padded surface, and its temperature should be measured and corrected if necessary. The monitoring should include respiratory frequency and adequacy, heart rate, pulse quality, and blood pressure (BP).

The animal is placed on the surface in sternal recumbency (or lateral if a more ipsilateral effect is desired) with the legs bent forward (to expose the lumbosacral junction). For ipsilateral anesthesia or analgesia, the patient must be left for the duration of onset in an unchanged position.

Items needed:
- Clippers
- Sedatives, if animal is not anesthetized
- Antiseptic solutions for surgical preparation
- Sterile gloves
- Sterile drapes
- Sterile saline solution (0.9%)
- Local anesthetic (2% lidocaine) for infiltration at the puncture site if the patient is not anesthetized
- New vial of the preservative-free drug(s) to be administered
- Three sterile syringes (one for infiltration of anesthesia, one for sterile saline, one for drugs to administer epidurally) and suitable sterile needles
- Spinal needle (18- to 22-gauge Tuohy, Crawford, or Quincke)
- Epidural catheter tray

Procedure:
Clip area generously; surgically prepare and drape the animal.

Place the thumb and middle of the finger of one hand on the iliac crests. With the index finger, palpate the dorsal processes of the lumbar and sacral vertebrae in a cranial and caudal direction. The dorsal process of the seventh lumbar vertebrae is identified, and the three fingers should form a triangle with its base between thumb and middle finger. Just caudal to this is the lumbosacral junction, which generally is perceivable as the deepest depression between the midline bone structures. In obese dogs, it can be helpful to mark (with an indelible marker) iliac crests, seventh lumbar, and first sacral dorsal spinal processes before the surgical preparation is done.

Surgically prepare the area.

Infiltrate the puncture site with 1 to 2 ml of 2% lidocaine solution.

Insert the needle caudal to the spinal process of the seventh lumbar vertebra (where the index finger is) and, strictly on midline, advance it until a distinct popping sensation is felt. This resistance results from penetration of the interarcuate ligament (ligamentum flavum), which the needle should penetrate perpendicularly (which causes less damage). The positioning in the epidural space can be identified in two ways:

1. Loss of resistance test—A test injection of 2 to 3 ml with air or 0.9% sterile saline should be feasible with no resistance.
2. Hanging drop test—A few drops of sterile saline are placed in the hub of the needle. If the positioning is correct, then the saline should be drawn into the epidural space. This method is not always a reliable indicator and is not applicable with an animal in lateral recumbency.

Allow 30 to 60 seconds to observe the needle for outflow of cerebrospinal fluid (CSF) or blood. The presence of CSF indicates a puncture of the subarachnoid space. Under these circumstances, the injections could still be made, but with a 50% dose reduction. Presence of blood flow from the needle indicates the puncture of a vessel or hematoma. Epidural injection should not be made.

If the needle has been positioned correctly, the injection can be made slowly (over 60 to 90 seconds). This should avoid stinging (bupivacaine) or patchy anesthesia or analgesia.

If a sacrococcygeal or intercoccygeal injection is planned (i.e., in cats), the procedure is analogous. The sacrococcygeal junction can be identified easily by slightly moving the tail up and down. (Draping of the tail is necessary.)

If epidural analgesia is necessary for continued pain control, insert the catheter through the needle (directed cranially). This can be secured to the animal and left in place for intermittent injections or a slow continual drip of the chosen drug.

pain state to the patient. This phenomenon appears to hold true for animals as well. Individual personality, breed traits, and the psychologic states of fear and anxiety all seem to play a role in the animal's perception of pain and response to treatment. This is one reason protocols for treating pain in veterinary patients have been difficult to develop. Ultimately, pain relief is the only true measure of successful treatment. The following information is meant as a guide to forming an initial treatment plan.

Drug Options

Nonsteroidal Antiinflammatory Drugs. Nonsteroidal antiinflammatory drugs (NSAIDs) are among the most widely used analgesics in the treatment of chronic pain. More recently, NSAIDs have been shown to be extremely effective in treating acute pain, especially when used preemptively (i.e., before tissue injury). Most surgical patients will require more than just NSAIDs to manage their perioperative pain, but many patients can be weaned to NSAIDs alone as the pain diminishes. NSAIDs are convenient to administer, inexpensive, and provide long-lasting pain relief.

NSAIDs have been referred to as *antiprostaglandins*. Actually, NSAIDs do not directly inhibit prostaglandins but rather inhibit cyclooxygenase (COX), which synthesizes prostaglandin. Two types of COX exist: type 1 (COX-1) and type 2 (COX-2). NSAIDs have an effect on both types of COX. COX-2 gives rise to the group of prostaglandins that mediate the inflammatory response associated with pain; therefore COX-2 inhibition reduces inflammation, the desired effect of treatment with NSAIDs. However, COX-1 gives rise to the group of prostaglandins that maintain platelet function and gastrointestinal mucosal integrity; therefore the main disadvantage of extended NSAID administration is COX-1 inhibition resulting in mucosal sloughing, GI ulceration, and bleeding. Non–COX-specific NSAIDs commonly used in the past include aspirin, phenylbutazone, and flunixin meglumide and have produced both pain relief and expected unwanted side effects. Ideally, NSAID therapy should be directed at selectively inhibiting COX-2 while sparing COX 1, thereby reducing inflammation while eliminating many negative effects. The newer NSAIDS are COX-2 selective but have varying inhibition of COX-2 versus COX-1. Recently the COX-2 enzyme has been shown to have very important effects in restoration of GI and renal health in the face of ulceration and hypotension, respectively. This new finding has cast doubt on the optimum ratio of COX-1 versus COX-2 inhibition. To date, real-world data are the most reliable predictors of safety in this important class of drugs.

Opioids. Opioids are the most commonly used analgesics in hospitalized critically ill or injured patients because of their efficacy, rapid onset of action, and safety. The efficacy of various opioids is determined by the specific receptors in the brain and spinal cord they affect. The receptors are classified as μ, κ, and Σ; μ and κ receptors are responsible for sedation, analgesia, and respiratory depression. κ Receptors are responsible for analgesia and sedation. Σ Receptors are less clinically relevant and are thought to be responsible for the adverse effects of opioid administration (e.g., dysphoria, excitement, restlessness, anxiety). Opioid drugs are classified as *agonists* (meaning that they stimulate the opioid receptors) or antagonists (meaning that they block particular opioid receptors). In addition, mixed agonist and antagonist opioids stimulate some receptors while blocking others (and partial agonists with lesser effects). In general, pure agonists are the most potent opioids but also have the most severe adverse side effects. Side effects include vomiting, constipation, excitement, bradycardia, and panting. In humans the most severe side effect is respiratory depression, but this effect is rarely observed in veterinary patients. Pure antagonists reverse the narcotic properties of agonists. The availability of opioid antagonists makes opioid use safe because the drug effects can be removed rapidly. Mixed agonist and antagonist and partial agonist opioids can provide reasonably good analgesia without many of the deleterious side effects of pure agonists. Opioids are metabolized by the liver and excreted via the kidneys; they should be used with some caution in patients with renal or hepatic disease.

Pure Agonists

Pure agonists are the most potent opioid drugs. They provide excellent analgesia but can have adverse effects including mild respiratory and CNS depression, GI motility changes, bradycardia, and hypotension. Regimented treatment, or dosing at regular intervals, is helpful in maintaining an analgesic plane. Otherwise, a roller coaster effect occurs, leaving the patient in varying degrees of pain between treatments.

Administration by constant rate infusion (CRI) or epidural injection minimizes this variability in treatment. The type of opioid is chosen based on the degree of analgesia needed and the specific needs or limitations of the individual patient. The most commonly used pure agonists in the United States are morphine, hydromorphone, oxymorphone and fentanyl.

Morphine Sulfate

Morphine is the gold standard for pure opioid agonists. All other drugs in this class are compared with morphine in terms of efficacy, duration of action, and cost. Morphine is commonly used to provide maximal analgesia and sedation. Its relatively low cost and similar efficacy makes it preferential over other opioids in some cases. However, it has additional side effects (particularly systemic hypotension and vomiting) that make it less desirable in many instances. Cats are particularly sensitive to morphine; therefore lower doses are used in the cat. The typical dose for dogs is 0.5 to 2.2 mg/kg subcutaneously (SC), intramuscularly (IM) and 0.1 to 0.5 mg/kg IV, slowly. Cats typically receive 0.1 to 0.5 mg/kg SC, IM.

Oxymorphone

Oxymorphone has potency approximately 10 times greater than that of morphine and moderate duration (4 to 6 hours). Oxymorphone may cause less respiratory depression and gastrointestinal stimulation than morphine. Some patients experience dysphoria, which may include vocalization, panting, and sensory hypersensitivity. The cost of oxymorphone also may be prohibitive. The typical dose is 0.05 to 0.1 mg/kg IV or IM.

Hydromorphone

Hydromorphone shares similar characteristics with oxymorphone but has been more widely available in recent years. The cost is less than oxymorphone. Typical doses are 0.1 to 0.2 mg/kg SC, IM in the dog and 0.05 to 0.1 mg/kg SC, IM in the cat.

Fentanyl Citrate

Fentanyl is an extremely potent synthetic opioid with rapid onset but short duration of action when administered IV or IM. It is efficiently used as a transdermal patch for long-term (3 days) analgesia.

BOX 9-2

Technical Tip: Procedure for Applying Fentanyl Patch

- Clip the area over the scapula, lower back, or flank larger than the surface area of the patch to be applied. This should be a close clip to remove all hair, but extra care should be taken to avoid creating a clipper-related rash or other damage to the skin.
- Gently wipe the site with dry gauze; no alcohol, water, or scrubbing maneuver should be used.
- Remove the plastic backing from patch and affix it to the skin.
- Place the hand firmly over the patch and hold it in place for 2-3 minutes.
- Date the patch using an indelible marker.

Removal and Disposal of Patch
- Patches can be easily removed with the use of spray adhesive remover (such as that used by athletes to remove skin tape) or Avon Skin-So-Soft. Spray the product on a corner of the patch and gently pull it up; then spray it under the patch and slowly remove the patch (using additional remover as needed).
- Patches are disposed as biohazardous waste.
- For patients discharged with a patch, the animal can be returned to the hospital for patch removal or the owner can remove and return the patch to the veterinary hospital.
- For proper disposal in biohazardous waste, encourage owners to return patches by imposing a $10.00 refundable deposit at the time of discharge.

Fentanyl is contained in an adhesive patch of varying concentration to deliver 25, 75, or 100 μg/hr. Once applied to shaved, cleaned skin, the drug is absorbed continuously (Technical Tip Box 9-2).

Onset of action is from 12 to 24 hours, so supplemental analgesia is recommended during the initial treatment period. Concurrent use of mixed agonist and antagonist opioids reverses the effects of the fentanyl patch and should be avoided.

Mixed Agonist and Antagonist Opioids

Mixed agonist and antagonist opioids provide analgesia at some opioid receptors while inhibiting or decreasing stimulation at the μ receptors. Their action results in diminished analgesia and decreased side effects. These drugs partially reverse pure agonists by blocking action at the μ receptors.

Butorphanol Tartrate

Butorphanol is a κ agonist and a μ antagonist. The overall effectiveness of butorphanol as an analgesic is questionable because of its mild effects and short duration of action. Although the analgesic effects are thought to last only 45 minutes to 1 hour, butorphanol does appear to provide reasonable sedation for about 2 hours. It is expensive compared with morphine but has significantly lower associated incidence of vomiting and dysphoria. Butorphanol is used in patients experiencing mild to moderate pain. It is available in oral and injectable forms. The typical dose is 0.2 to 0.8 mg/kg SC, IM or 0.1 to 0.4 mg/kg IV in the dog and 0.1 to 0.4 mg/kg SC, IM or 0.5 to 0.2 mg/kg IV in the cat.

Buprenorphine

Buprenorphine is a partial μ agonist that is 30 times more potent than morphine and of longer duration because of its slow dissociation from receptors. Its best use is in dogs with moderate pain and in cats with moderate-to-severe pain. Recent work has been done to demonstrate that buprenorphine is readily absorbed across mucous membranes in the feline. This allows for transmucosal administration in the cat, providing analgesia for up to 8 hours from a single dose.

The typical dose is 0.01 to 0.03 mg/kg SC, IM, IV in the dog or cat. Cats can also receive the same dose via the buccal mucosa.

Antagonists

Opioid agonist analgesia, sedation, and side effects can be reversed rapidly with antagonists such as naloxone hydrochloride. Antagonists work by blocking opioid action at the μ receptors. Onset of reversal occurs within 1 to 2 minutes of IV administration and can last for 1 to 4 hours. Treatment can be repeated when reversing narcotics with a longer duration. The typical dose is 2 µg/kg IV.

Anatomic Aspects

Three different layers of protective and supportive sheets known as *meninges* (singular, *meninx*) surround the spinal cord. Firmly adhered to the cord,

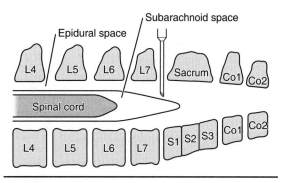

Fig. 9-1 Spinal column of the dog at the lumbosacral junction.

the pia mater is the deepest, most vascular layer. It is highly cellular and has attachments to the most external meninx, the dura mater, along the lateral margin of the spinal cord (denticulate ligaments). These ligaments suspend the spinal cord within the cavity formed by the dura mater.

The intermediate meninx is the arachnoid membrane, another mainly cellular layer that is connected to the pia mater by numerous membranous bridges, the arachnoid trabeculae. The space between the arachnoid and the pia mater contains cerebrospinal fluid (CSF). CSF pressure holds the arachnoid against the dura mater. Only a very thin layer of fluid separates the two. This fluid film allows sliding of the arachnoid with respect to the dura mater. The depth of the subarachnoid space varies, because the arachnoid contacts the dura mater, whereas the pia mater follows every irregularity of the spinal cord's surface.

The most superficial of the three layers, the dura mater, is a tough, fibrous sheath that encloses the spinal cord and the nerves that originate in the spinal cord. Around these nerve roots the dura mater forms protective cuffs (the dural sheaths that accompany the nerves traversing the vertebral canal).

The epidural space is located between the dura mater and the bony walls of the vertebral canal. This space contains loose connective tissue, blood vessels, and adipose tissue. In larger dogs, the spinal cord terminates approximately at the caudal margin of the sixth (or the cranial margin of the seventh) lumbar vertebra (Fig. 9-1). In smaller dogs and in cats, the spinal cord extends further caudad, about the length of one vertebral body (L7-S1, the lumbosacral junction); therefore in these animals it seems to be safer to administer epidural injections at the sacrococcygeal junction or first intercoccygeal space. The cavity formed by the dura mater (dural sac) generally extends about two vertebral bodies more caudal than the spinal cord.

Consequently, in larger dogs (more than 15 kg of body weight), the dural sac (but not the spinal cord) is accessible at the level of the lumbosacral junction. In smaller dogs and in cats, the spinal cord probably is present at the lumbosacral junction.

Definitions and Clinical Implications

The epidural space occupies the large volume between the walls of the vertebral canal and the dura mater. The amount of fat in the epidural space is not necessarily correlated to the amount of body fat. In patients who have lost a lot of weight within a short period of time, a considerable amount of fat may still be found in the epidural space. The more fat in the epidural space, the more cranial the effects of epidurally administered drugs extend.

Old age also can influence the volume of injection necessary to produce a clinical effect. Calcified and fibrous tissue can occlude the intervertebral foramina (where the spinal nerves exit the vertebral canal) and decrease the amount of injectate that leaks from the epidural space, thereby increasing the cephalad distance over which a given volume will travel in the epidural space.

On the bottom of the vertebral canal are large venous plexi. In a patient with reduced venous return, these plexi are engorged, which increases the probability of injecting into the vascular bed. This can lead to increased and potentially toxic plasma levels of the injected substances.

Spinal or intrathecal injection aims for the space filled with CSF that lies between the arachnoid and the pia mater. When drugs are injected into the spinal column, they can be administered inadvertently into this space. This is more likely in cats because of the more caudal spread of the subarachnoid space in this species. Most drugs that clinicians administer epidurally can be injected safely into this subarachnoid space. However, injection volumes have to be much lower (50% to 60%) to obtain the same spatial distribution because the subarachnoid space is much smaller; therefore injected substances are likely to be carried further cephalad with CSF flow.

In the literature about epidural techniques, the terms *epidural anesthesia* and *epidural analgesia* often are used interchangeably. For didactic reasons, the term *epidural anesthesia* should be for injection of local anesthetics into the epidural space and *epidural analgesia* used for administration of drugs that produce analgesia (e.g., opioids, α-2 agonists, ketamine).

Injection Volumes

Because of variations in age, nutritional status, and desired segment of anesthesia or analgesia, no golden rule exists for determining epidural injection volume. However, most authors consider volumes of 1 ml/4.5 to 5 kg body weight (0.22 to 0.24 ml/kg) for anesthesia or analgesia of segments caudal to the umbilicus and 1 ml/3.5 to 3.8 kg (0.26 to 0.28 ml/kg) for the segments as cranial as the tenth to thirteenth thoracic vertebra (T10-T13) to be effective.

Calculating injection volumes based on body weight presents several problems. If the patient is obese, then the calculated volume could be too large for the size of the vertebral canal, because the large amount of adipose tissue in the epidural space could cause a given volume to spread further forward than expected.

The volume of the epidural space also varies among individuals. Some authors consider injection volumes to be safe up to approximately 6 ml for animals up to 35 kg. As in cats, the spinal cord is likely to extend to the lumbosacral junction or even further. Therefore epidural administration could be performed more safely at the sacrococcygeal junction or the first intercoccygeal space with injection volumes of 0.3 to 0.9 ml total (although it has been done at the lumbosacral junction with volumes of 0.2 ml/kg).

For animals with an increase in intraabdominal pressure (e.g., ascites, pregnancy), the calculated volume should be reduced by approximately 25%. If the calculated dose of a drug gives a smaller volume, then it should be made up to the calculated volume with 0.9% sterile saline solution.

Local Anesthetics

Local anesthetics are the substances most commonly injected into the epidural space and produce reliable, dose-dependent epidural anesthesia. These anesthetics stabilize the axonal membrane of a nerve by blocking the influx of sodium and, in this way, interrupting the passage of nerve impulses. It is unclear where exactly this local anesthetic block has its effect after epidural administration. Three possibilities are considered: (1) a paravertebral block after foraminal leakage, (2) a block of the intradural spinal nerve roots (this seems to be the most prominent mechanism), and (3) a spinal cord block. However, local anesthetics do not act on specific receptors, and their effects on different types of nerves are dose dependent. The smaller the diameter of a nerve fiber, the lower the local anesthetic dose needed to produce a block of conduction. Therefore sympathetic nerves are the first, sensory nerves intermediate, and motor nerve fibers the last to be blocked with increasing concentrations of local anesthetics.

Local anesthetics administered epidurally may enter the CSF, the epidural venous blood, and the lymph. A variety of local anesthetics have been used for epidural anesthesia, and the selection is based on the patient's size and the extent, onset, and duration of the desired anesthesia.

A 2% solution of lidocaine, procaine, or Carbocaine produces anesthesia after 10 to 15 minutes for 60 to 90 minutes. The addition of 1:200,000 epinephrine or adrenaline to the local anesthetic may prolong the duration of action. Bupivacaine as a 0.75% solution has a slower onset (20 to 30 minutes) but a longer duration of action (about 4 hours). Etidocaine in a 1% solution has been shown to produce surgical anesthesia for 4 to 6 hours. Ropivacaine (0.75%) has a time of onset similar to that of bupivacaine, and the duration of motor blockade has been found to be about 1 hour and 40 minutes.

Epidural application of local anesthetics produces some loss of motor function. The extent and duration are dose (concentration and volume) dependent. However, at the suggested doses, a nearly constant motor blockade exists for the hind limbs.

Epidural anesthesia as far cranial as the first thoracic segments (T4-T5) has been reported not to affect cardiovascular or respiratory function in healthy, awake dogs. However, in anesthetized, aged, or sick dogs, hypotension can occur. Therefore under these circumstances, IV fluids should be administered and vasopressors held on hand.

In general, the side effects that can be associated with epidural or subarachnoid administration of local anesthetics include hypoventilation (caused by respiratory muscle paralysis), sympathetic blockade-related hypotension, hypoglycemia, and Horner's syndrome, and toxic plasma levels can cause muscle twitches, coma, convulsion, and circulatory depression (i.e., after inadvertent IV injection). The initial sign of hypoventilation usually is the change from thoracic to abdominal breathing as the intercostal muscles become paralyzed.

Opioids

Since the discovery of opioid receptors in the spinal cord (μ, κ, Δ, Σ), several opioids have been used for epidural or intrathecal administration. However, it is still unclear whether they act directly on the opioid receptors of the spinal cord or after systemic absorption and redistribution.

Because opeoids alleviate somatic and visceral pain (antinociceptive action) but do not block impulses of sensory, motor, or sympathetic function, their effect is called *selective spinal analgesia*. This and the prolonged duration of analgesic effects compared with other drugs and compared with other methods of administration are the major advantages of epidurally administered opioids. Furthermore, epidural administration of opioids produces a lower level of sedation than does IM administration.

The analgesic efficacy of opioids increases if they are given preemptively. Therefore preoperative epidural administration is recommended. In addition, epidurally administered opioids reduce the need for inhalant anesthetics.

For a better understanding of the different times of onset and duration of action of the single opioids, it is important to understand that their lipid solubility affects the spread of the administered solution in the epidural and subarachnoid space. The less lipid soluble an opioid, the longer it is present in an unbound form in the spinal canal and consequently the more time is available for cephalad distribution. This explains why low-efficacy (low-lipid solubility) opioids, such as morphine, must be injected very slowly into the spinal canal (over 1 to 2 minutes). Moreover, low-lipid solubility opioids have been found to produce a greater magnitude of tolerance. On the other hand, low-lipid solubility opioids have a longer duration of action.

The most important side effect of epidural opioids is respiratory depression, which can be biphasic or delayed (for up to 12 hours). This may be even more marked for the less lipid-soluble opioids such as morphine. Animals that have been given epidural or intrathecal morphine should be held in a controlled environment (e.g., intensive care unit, dyspnea watch) and observed for at least 24 hours. Centrally mediated increases in vagal tone are responsible for the bradycardia sometimes associated with systemic

TABLE 9-1

Epidural Opioids: Doses and Time Factors in Dogs

Opioid	Dose (mg/kg)	Onset (min)	Duration (hr)
Morphine sulfate PF	0.05-0.15	30-60	10-24
Meperidine hydrochloride	0.5-1.5	10-30	5-20
Oxymorphone hydrochloride	0.05-0.15	20-40	7-10
Fentanyl citrate	0.001-0.01	15-20	4-6

PF, Preservative free.

absorption of epidural opioids. Urinary retention has been found to be present in 15% to 100% of people who received epidural morphine. Although the incidence in animals has not been studied so far, the bladder should be emptied before recovery from general anesthesia. Delayed gastrointestinal motility and nausea seem to be related to epidural morphine in people as well, but it is not clear whether these side effects also occur in animals. Pruritus has been reported as a side effect in dogs and in humans (Table 9-1).

The opioids shown are ordered with increasing lipid solubility. The lower end of the dose ranges is more applicable to larger breed dogs, and the higher doses are for smaller dogs. Because cats occasionally have adverse reactions to higher opioid doses, the lower doses should be applied to cats. In cats, morphine has been given successfully to produce epidural analgesia at 0.1 mg/kg.

Other Drugs

α_2-Adrenergic agonists act primarily by stimulating α_2 adrenoceptors, inhibiting neurotransmitter release. In the human spinal cord, a high density of α_2 adrenoceptors is found. This primary site of activity may be augmented by a secondary local anesthetic-like effect, blocking axonal conduction.

Xylazine given epidurally or intrathecally is an effective analgesic in cattle, horses, and sheep. At a dose of 0.2 to 0.25 mg/kg given epidurally to dogs, xylazine has analgesic effects but only minimal cardiovascular side effects.

Medetomidine has been given to dogs epidurally at a dose of 0.005 to 0.015 mg/kg. It can provide analgesia similar to that of epidural oxymorphone,

but bradycardia and second-degree atrioventricular block are common side effects. Enhanced analgesia has been found when medetomidine is given with an opioid.

Contraindications

Absolute contraindications for epidural or subarachnoid injection are infection at or near the injection site, hypovolemia, bleeding disorders and anticoagulation, central or peripheral nervous diseases, anatomic abnormalities of the spinal column, and spinal trauma. Bacteremia, sepsis, and neurologic disorders are relative contraindications (see Technical Tip Box 9-2).

Local and Regional Anesthetics. Recently a great deal of research has involved local and regional nerve-blocking techniques. Applying analgesia directly to the affected nerve endings can provide excellent pain control while reducing or eliminating the need for systemic drugs. Local anesthetics work by disrupting neural information transmission by axons at the treatment site. Blocking neuronal activity also results in an expected loss of sensation and sometimes affects motor function. This loss of motor control is not seen with systemic analgesia. Local anesthesia should be used with caution in patients who are at risk for self-injury, such as those who have undergone orthopedic surgery.

Lidocaine, the most widely used local anesthetic, takes effect in 3 to 5 minutes and is effective for 60 to 90 minutes. The duration of lidocaine can be extended by combination with a 1:200,000 dilution of epinephrine, which causes local vasoconstriction. Epinephrine should *never* be used in circumferential limb block such as feline declaw. Bupivacaine takes longer to take effect (15 to 20 minutes), but its anesthetic and analgesic effects last 3 to 6 hours. Bupivacaine is not effective as a topical analgesic, but it is an excellent choice for local infiltration.

Drugs similar to lidocaine and bupivacaine are relatively safe when correctly administered. Most cases of toxicity in small animals occur as a result of accidental overdose or inadvertent IV administration. Signs of toxicity include seizures, coma, neurotoxicity, and cardiovascular collapse. Local anesthetics can directly damage tissues and cause allergic reactions or methemoglobinemia.

Topical Analgesia

Applying topical analgesia to the surface skin or mucosa can reduce pain associated with minor procedures such as wound suturing, venipuncture, arterial puncture, or nasal cannulization. Solutions of lidocaine, bupivacaine, tetracaine, and epinephrine can be used alone or in various combinations to desensitize the application site. Gauze pads soaked with solutions can be applied directly to the site. Alternatively, several commercially prepared topical anesthetic creams and jellies can be applied as a thick paste. Regardless of application method, 20 to 30 minutes of direct contact time is needed to ensure effective analgesia.

Local Infiltration

Injecting lidocaine or bupivacaine into local tissue can reduce pain associated with various painful procedures. This technique is useful for arterial catheter placement, thoracocentesis, abdominocentesis, and bone marrow sampling. The entry area is infiltrated with small amounts of anesthetic. Pain reduction is expected at 5 to 10 minutes after injection.

Dental Nerve Blocks

The entire muzzle can be anesthetized by blocking the infraorbital and mandibular foramen. This relatively simple technique is quite effective for dental extractions, oral mass removal, fracture repair, mandibulectomy, maxilectomy, and nasal biopsy.

Joint Space

Effective analgesia before and during orthopedic surgery has been achieved by injecting local anesthetics directly into the joint space. Intraarticular morphine has also been shown to reduce joint pain. It has been suggested that applying a tourniquet above the joint for 10 minutes after injection greatly enhances drug efficacy.

Peritoneal Space

Patients with abdominal pain, generally from abdominal surgery or acute pancreatitis, may benefit by local anesthetic infusion. The anesthetic must be delivered in fairly large volumes of saline to provide maximum interperitoneal surface contact. Risks of the increase in abdominal pressure must be weighed against the benefit of analgesia.

Pleural Space

Interpleural bupivacaine infusion after thoracotomy surgery may have some analgesic benefit. Bupivacaine (1.5 to 2 mg/kg) is injected via an indwelling chest tube into the pleural space. Analgesia is thought to occur by direct blocking of the intercostal nerves. For maximum coverage, the patient should be positioned with the affected side down for 10 minutes after the injection to allow the analgesic to follow gravity and travel to the pain site. Drug absorption through the pleural tissue should be considered.

Alpha₂ Agonists

Alpha$_2$ (α_2) agonists inhibit release of the excitatory neurotransmitter norepinephrine to produce analgesia and sedation. α_2 Agonists are short-duration analgesics and can be rapidly reversed with α_2-antagonists. This characteristic makes these drugs suitable for procedures requiring short-term restraint and analgesia. α_2 Agonists may bind to the same receptors as opioids and act synergistically with them. Opioid doses can be significantly reduced if given concurrently with an α_2 agonist. α_2 Agonists can have profound effects on the cardiovascular and nervous systems, but the clinician can minimize these adverse events by using low doses. Bradycardia and vomiting are the most common side effects with α_2 agonists.

Medetomidine is a dose-dependent sedative analgesic commonly used as a preanesthetic agent in healthy animals. Onset of effect takes 5 to 15 minutes depending on route of administration (IV or IM), and sedation can last up to 90 minutes. Medetomidine administration results in physiologically normal peripheral vasoconstriction, temporary decreased heart rate, and a transient increase in BP. All cardiovascular parameters smoothly return to presedation levels upon reversal with atipamezole. Xylazine has a short duration of analgesia (30 minutes), and its central nervous system effects can be reversed with yohimbine or atipamezole. Both drugs can cause vomiting and cardiovascular suppression.

Constant Rate Infusion

Analgesia can be safely and efficaciously administered by CRI. Many agents can be delivered by this method, but the most commonly used agents are local anesthetic (lidocaine), opioids (morphine or fentanyl), and N-methyl-D-aspartate antagonists (NMDA) (ketamine). Regardless of the drug, a loading dose is typically given immediately before beginning a CRI. These drugs can be used as single agents or in combination with one another.

Morphine

The main advantage of giving morphine as a CRI is the avoidance of peaks and valleys typically seen with opioid bolus dosing. A lower dose of morphine can be used in a CRI than in bolus dosing, which can reduce the unwanted side effects of morphine such as dysphoria or panting. Morphine CRI is useful to manage any severe pain and can be safely combined with ketamine, lidocaine, or both.

The CRI dose for morphine is as follows:

Dogs: 0.2 to 0.5 mg/kg SLOW IV loading bolus followed by 0.1 to 0.3 mg/kg/hr CRI
Cats: 0.05 to 0.1 mg/kg IV loading bolus followed by 0.025 to 0.2 mg/kg/hr CRI

Fentanyl

Fentanyl is a full opioid agonist with similar properties to morphine. The main advantage of fentanyl over morphine is a rapid onset of action and short half-life, which allows for rapid cessation of unwanted side effects. The major disadvantage is that fentanyl is considerably more expensive.

The CRI dose for fentanyl is as follows:

Dog: 2 to 5 μg/kg IV loading dose followed by 5 to 20 μg/kg/hr CRI intraoperatively
Cats: 1 to 2 μg/kg IV loading dose followed by 5 to 20 μg/kg/hr CRI

Lidocaine

Lidocaine is a local anesthetic that provides excellent systemic analgesia when delivered intravenously. Because it is safe for use in patients with GI disturbances, lidocaine is a good choice for analgesia in patients with gastric dilation volvulus or other similar disorders. Lidocaine seems to also provide benefit for patients undergoing procedures with excessive nerve trauma such as complicated back surgeries or limb amputations. IV lidocaine is extremely short acting and can be discontinued without residual effect almost immediately. Lidocaine CRI should be discontinued if the patient shows signs of toxicity including muscle tremors, seizures, nausea, or vomiting.

The CRI dose for lidocaine is as follows:

Dog: 2 mg/kg IV followed by 20 to 50 μg/kg/min

Lidocaine CRI doses are reported for cats, but typically lidocaine is not recommended for use in cats because of the potential for severe cardiotoxic effects.

Ketamine

Ketamine is a dissociative anesthetic and an NMDA antagonist. Stimulation of NMDA receptors in the spinal cord results in firing of neurons that transmit pain signals. Prolonged bombardment of these receptors such as occurs with intense surgical pain or long-term chronic pain results in amplification of the signals. This means the spinal neurons are now more easily excited by less stimulation, a condition called *hyperalgesia*. A second phase called *allodynia* follows, in which even nonpainful stimuli are perceived as painful by the spinal cord neurons. This phenomenon, collectively called *windup*, will be most evident in the postoperative period once the patient has regained consciousness. However, as an NMDA receptor antagonist, ketamine given as an intraoperative CRI binds at these CNS receptors and prevents windup. Because of its mechanism of action, ketamine is best used to manage neuropathic types of pain, particularly when the pain has been long standing and the patient has not responded well to other analgesics. Ketamine should be always be given in combination with an opioid, and both can be delivered in the same infusion.

The CRI dose for ketamine is as follows:

Dog and cat: 0.5 mg/kg IV loading bolus, followed by 10 μg/kg/min CRI during surgery and 2 μg/kg/min for 24 hours after surgery

Adjunctive and Adjuvant Analgesics. In addition to the classic analgesic agents, medications with other indications can be used to help manage pain. These drugs are referred to as *adjunctive analgesics* and come from many separate classes of pharmacological compounds. *Adjuvant analgesics* are agents that can enhance analgesic drugs when coadministered but have few or no analgesic properties when given alone. The following are examples of adjunctive and adjuvant analgesics:

- Tranquilizers (phenothiazines, benzodiazepines) alter an animal's response to pain, can relax muscles, and are used in combination with true analgesics. These drugs also reduce anxiety and fear, which exacerbate pain.
- Dissociative anesthetics (ketamine) can enhance analgesia by blocking sensitization of neurons in the spinal cord (i.e., block NMDA receptors, act as NMDA antagonists) and are especially useful for managing chronic pain.
- Corticosteroids (prednisolone) have powerful antiinflammatory and immunosuppressive effects, "dampening the fires" of acute inflammation.

Epidural Anesthesia and Analgesia

Lumbosacral epidural administration of local anesthetics and analgesics is a valuable way to produce segmental anesthesia or analgesia in dogs and cats. It is an easy, safe, and effective way to alleviate pain, especially after procedures involving body parts caudal to the ribs, and should be considered an adjunct or alternative to other drug administration methods.

Monitoring Drug Effects

Perhaps the most confounding aspect of pain management is assessing pain and pain relief after treatment. The abatement or cessation of clinical signs associated with pain is the best indicator of successful treatment. Careful monitoring of cardiovascular status and mentation are vital to achieving good pain management without detrimental side effects. Effective treatment may result in cardiovascular or respiratory depression, diminished movement, inability to eat or drink, urinary and fecal incontinence, and hypothermia. Supportive care is integral to pain management. The complications and side effects of treatment are monitored and corrected aggressively. Temperature, heart rate, pulses, respiratory rate and effort, mucous membrane color, and capillary refill time should be measured frequently. Treatment may include fluid volume and hydration support, nutritional supplementation, urinary catheterization, external warming, and even oxygen augmentation. Veterinary critical care professionals must eliminate pain and stress wherever possible and treat the adverse consequences as needed.

Pain Management Checklist

Veterinary technicians play a vital role in pain management. The technician is most likely to first detect signs of pain and request pain treatment. Critical care technicians can improve pain management practice in the following ways:

- Establish pain alleviation as a standard of care.
- Recognize the signs of pain.
- Respect owners' observations and assessment of pain in their pets.
- Understand and overcome the barriers to assessment and treatment.
- Be aware of known painful procedures and surgeries, and encourage preemptive and immediate postprocedure treatment.
- Reduce incidence of painful procedures by combining treatments efficiently.
- Use techniques to minimize pain (e.g., use electrocardiogram snaps instead of alligator clips; use indwelling catheters to obtain blood samples).
- Minimize pain associated with critical care techniques by improving technical skill and helping to develop new technologies that minimize pain.
- Differentiate pain from other distress such as confinement, boredom, separation from owners, insomnia, fear, and need to urinate or defecate.

- Understand the treatment options and encourage appropriate types of therapy.
- Monitor the effects of various drugs in a coherent manner to evaluate treatment efficacy.
- Educate other animal caregivers about pain management issues.

Suggested Readings

Bradley R et al: Epidural analgesia in the dog, *Vet Surg* 9:153, 1980.

Branson KR et al: Duration of analgesia induced by epidurally administered morphine and medetomidine in dogs, *J Vet Pharmacol Ther* 16:369, 1993.

Bromage P et al: Rostral spread of epidural morphine, *Anesthesiology* 56:431, 1982.

Broome ME, Tanzillo H: Differentiating between pain and agitation in premature neonates, *J Perinat Neonatal Nurs* 4(1):53, 1990.

Craig KKD et al: Pain in the preterm neonate: behavioral and physiological indices, *Pain* 52:287, 1993.

Day T et al: Comparison of intra-articular and epidural morphine for analgesia following stifle arthrotomy in dogs, *Vet Surg* 24:522, 1995.

Dodman N, Clark G, Court M: Epidural opioid administration for postoperative pain relief in the dog. In Short C, Pozrak A, editors: *Animal pain*, New York, 1992, Churchill Livingstone.

Durant P, Yaksh T: Epidural injections of bupivacaine, morphine, fentanyl, lofentanyl, and DADL in chronically implanted rats: a pharmacologic and pathologic study, *Anesthesiology* 64:43, 1986.

Fletcher T: Spinal cord and meninges. In Evans H, Christensen G, editors: *Miller's anatomy of the dog*, Philadelphia, 1979, WB Saunders.

Golder F et al: The effect of epidural morphine on the minimum alveolar concentration of isoflurane in cats, *J Vet Anaesth* 25, 1998.

Greene S, Keegan R, Weil A: Cardiovascular effects after epidural injection of xylazine in isoflurane-anesthetized dogs, *Vet Surg* 24:283, 1995.

Heath RB: Lumbosacral epidural management, *Vet Clin North Am Small Anim Pract* 22:417, 1992.

Hellyer PW: Management of acute and surgical pain, *Semi Vet Surg Small Anim* 12:2, 1997.

Hendrix P et al: Epidural administration of bupivacaine, morphine, or their combination for postoperative analgesia in dogs, *J Am Vet Med Assoc* 209:598, 1996.

Keegan RD, Greene SA, Weil AB: Cardiovascular effects of epidurally administered morphine and a xylazine-morphine combination in isoflurane-anesthetized dogs, *Am J Vet Res* 56:496, 1995.

Klide AM: Anatomy of the spinal cord and how the spinal cord is affected by local anesthetics and other drugs, *Vet Clin North Am Small Anim Pract* 22:413, 1992.

Maierl J, Reindl S, Knospe C: Observations on epidural anesthesia in cats from the anatomical viewpoint, *Tierarztl Prax* 25:267, 1997.

Mathews KA: *Veterinary emergency and critical care manual*, Eden Mills, Ontario, 1996, Lifelearn.

McMurphy RM: Postoperative epidural analgesia, *Vet Clin North Am Small Anim Pract* 23:703, 1993.

Nolte J, Watney C, Hall L: Cardiovascular effects of epidural blocks in dogs, *J Small Anim Pract* 24:17, 1983.

Otto K et al: Effects of epidural xylazine on EEG responses to surgical stimulation during isoflurane anaesthesia in dogs, *J Vet Anaesth* 24:33, 1997.

Papich MG: Principles of analgesic drug therapy, *Semin Vet Med Surg (Small Anim)* 12:2, 1997.

Pascoe PJ: Local and regional anesthesia and analgesia, *Semin Vet Med Surg (Small Anim)* 12:2, 1997.

Pascoe PJ: Advantages and guidelines for using epidural drugs for analgesia, *Vet Clin North Am Small Anim Pract* 22:421, 1992.

Popilskis S, Kohn D, Laurent L: Efficacy of epidural morphine versus intravenous morphine for post-thoracotomy pain in dogs, *J Vet Anaesth* 20:21, 1993.

Pybus D, Torda T: Dose-effect relationships of extradural morphine, *Br J Anaesth* 54:1259, 1982.

Rollin BE: *The unheeded cry*, New York, Oxford University Press, 1989.

Sackman JE: Pain management. In McCurnin DM, editor: *Clinical textbook for veterinary technicians*, Philadelphia, 1994, WB Saunders.

Short CE, Van Poznak A: *Animal pain*, New York, 1992, Churchill Livingstone.

Skarda R: Local and regional anesthetic and analgesic techniques: dogs. In Thurmon J, Tranquilli W, Benson G, editors: *Lumb & Jones' veterinary anesthesia*, ed 3, Baltimore, 1996, Williams & Wilkins.

Stevens BJ, Johnson CC, Grunau RV: Issues of assessment of pain and discomfort in neonates, *J Obstet Gynecol Neonatal Nurs* 24(9):849-855, 1995.

Tyler DC, Krane EJ: Pediatric pain, *Adv Pain Res Ther* 432, 1990.

Valverde A et al: Use of epidural morphine in the dog for pain relief, *Vet Comp Othop Traumatol* 2:55, 1989.

Vesal N, Cribb PH, Frketic M: Postoperative analgesic and cardiopulmonary effects in dogs of oxymorphone administered epidurally and intramuscularly, and medetomidine administered epidurally: a comparative clinical study, *Vet Surg* 25:361, 1996.

Yaksh T, Sosnowski M: Spinal opioid analgesia: characterization of acute tolerance in an animal model. In Estefanous F, editor: *Opioids in anesthesia II*. Stoneham, MA, 1991, Butterworth-Heinemann.

CHAPTER 10

Anesthesia in the Critically Ill or Injured Animal

Jennifer J. Devey, Dennis T. Crowe, Jr.

Introduction

Anesthesia is defined as the loss of sensation. The goal of general anesthesia is to provide a state of reversible unconsciousness, with adequate analgesia and muscle relaxation, in such a way that it does not jeopardize the patient's health. Delivering safe anesthesia to a critically ill small animal patient is one of the most important, and often one of the most challenging and stressful tasks, for a technician. In many emergency situations, under direct supervision of the attending veterinarian, the technician must be both the anesthetist and the circulating nurse in the operating room. The practice, although often necessary, is not recommended, because critically ill or unstable patients demand the undivided attention of an anesthetist.

The old adage of no safe anesthesia (just safe anesthetists) holds true, especially for anesthesia of the critically ill or injured patient. It would be ideal to be able to stabilize all patients before anesthetizing them; however, some patients cannot be stabilized without surgery. The patient who cannot breathe because of a diaphragmatic hernia, the patient who was hit by a car and has a severe hemoabdomen that is continuing to bleed, and the patient with septic peritonitis are all examples of animals that require surgery even though they are high risk. The technician must be familiar not only with anesthetic agents and their use but also with invasive and noninvasive means of monitoring of critical patients. These patients may have little in the way of reserves, and the anesthetist must understand not only respiratory and cardiovascular physiology but also the pathophysiology of the disease process. Only in this manner can anesthesia be provided safely and the patient be supported effectively.

Some of these patients may need anesthesia as they arrive in the emergency department; some of them may need surgery within the first few minutes or a few hours after arrival. This chapter attempts to provide an overview of anesthesia for this group of critically ill or injured patients. The focus will be on balanced anesthesia, which involves the administration of multiple drugs to the patient, each given for a specific purpose. It is assumed that the reader has a basic understanding of anesthetic equipment, anesthetic drugs, and basic monitoring (the reader is referred to general anesthesia texts for these specifics).

Goals for Success

Maintaining the *ABCs* of airway, breathing, and circulation is as important in the anesthetized patient as in the awake patient. The goals are to establish and maintain a patent airway, ensure breathing is as normal as possible, and ensure adequate circulation. Young, healthy patients undergoing elective surgery usually can cope with the adverse effects of general anesthesia; however, this may not be so for the critical patient. Five physiologic goals of general anesthesia exist regarding the cardiopulmonary system: the veterinary technician should (1) ensure adequate hemoglobin levels, (2) ensure adequate preload (venous volume returning to heart), (3) ensure adequate cardiac contractility, (4) ensure adequate delivery of oxygen (O_2) to the cells, and (5) ensure adequate elimination of cellular waste products (primarily carbon dioxide [CO_2]).

The patient must be intubated and maintained on 100% O_2. Hypoventilation is extremely common, and assisted ventilation always is indicated (either using mechanical ventilation or by hand bagging the patient) and may make the difference between adequate and inadequate O_2 delivery to the alveoli and removal of CO_2. High CO_2 levels cause acidosis, which in turn leads to vasodilation, poor cardiac function, and dysfunction of metabolic enzyme systems. Sufficient hemoglobin must be available to carry the O_2. It is recommended to keep the packed cell volume (PCV) between 25% and 30%. Cardiac output (or the blood that is carrying the O_2 to the peripheral tissues) depends on adequate preload and an effective pump (heart muscle). Decreased preload can result from inadequate circulating volume, vasodilation, or a combination of the two problems. Tachycardia should be avoided because it shortens diastole so that the heart does not have time to fill properly, which may decrease cardiac output, increase the myocardial O_2 demands, and negatively impact coronary circulation. Irregular

rhythms, which may indicate poor coordination of the heart muscle as it contracts, frequently require treatment.

Critically ill or injured patients will respond to analgesics, sedatives, and anesthetics differently than healthy animals for a variety of reasons (e.g., decreased volume of distribution; decreased plasma protein levels; acidosis leading to higher concentrations of the active form of the drug; decreased metabolism secondary to decreased hepatic function, and hypothermia). For these reasons, doses of most anxiolytics, analgesics, and anesthetics should be reduced to 25% to 50% of normal and titrated to effect. Ideally all drugs should be given via the IV or the epidural route, because absorption from the oral and subcutaneous (SC) routes is unpredictable. If needed, then intramuscular (IM) injections should be given in the epaxial muscles (the muscles dorsal and lateral to the vertebra in the region of the thoracolumbar spine), because the blood flow is more sustained to these muscles even during lower flow states. The intraosseous route of drug administration can be effective in very small patients, birds, and exotic animals.

Principles of General Anesthesia

1. A safe general anesthetic agent does not exist (only safe anesthetists).
2. The veterinary professional must be prepared with equipment, basic medications, O_2, emergency drugs, knowledge, skills, and support.
3. Each patient handles drugs differently (i.e., uptake, distribution, effect, metabolism).
4. Drugs, doses, and techniques should be chosen based on the patient's age, condition, and surgery needed.
5. Monitoring is essential to prevent complications (i.e., observe, record, report, act).
6. Practice (including drills) is vital to success and efficiency (i.e., rapid setup, monitoring, emergency contingency plans).
7. Preemptive sedation and analgesia should be used when possible.
8. Patients with airway or respiratory compromise should be preoxygenated, and induction should be performed rapidly.
9. All patients under general anesthesia will hypoventilate and need ventilatory support.

10. Equipment maintenance and an understanding of how it works are as vital as monitoring.
11. The anesthesia does not end when the surgery ends. Preoperative support must continue through the postoperative period.
12. All patients need physiologic support to prevent secondary decompensation of various body systems (including the pulmonary, cardiovascular, renal, and gastrointestinal systems).

Preanesthetic Examination, Evaluation, and Readiness

Physical Examination and Preanesthetic Diagnostic Tests

All patients must have a complete physical examination. The technician and the veterinarian need a baseline of physical parameters from which to work. Only in this manner can early changes in the patient's status be noted. The focus on the physical examination will vary somewhat depending on patient's reason for presentation, and close communication must occur between the veterinarian and the technician in regard to the underlying disease, injury, and anesthetic concerns.

The patient's respiratory rate and effort should be noted, and tracheal and bilateral thoracic auscultation should be performed (this will help localize the source of any airway or respiratory disease or problem that may be encountered during intubation or anesthesia). The presence of respiratory distress, stridor (indicating at least a 75% decrease in airway diameter), or very loud airway sounds, wheezing, crackles, areas of dullness, and SC emphysema indicate ventilatory compromise, which may be worsened under anesthesia. Guttural or sonorous noises indicate pharyngeal disease. High-pitched or stridorous sounds indicate laryngeal or tracheal disease. Lung sounds should be compared on both sides of the thorax. Heart tones should be ausculted and pulses palpated for both strength and presence of any deficits. Jugular veins should be clipped and evaluated for distention. A flat jugular vein that does not distend with digital pressure at the thoracic inlet is consistent with hypovolemia. The jugular that is distended with the patient standing or sitting may indicate a pneumothorax, pericardial effusion, or other causes of right-ventricular heart failure. The presence of abdominal distention should be noted.

Distended superficial epigastric veins suggest high intraabdominal pressure. When this patient is placed in dorsal recumbency, additional pressure may be placed on the vena cava, thus compromising venous return to the heart and potentially leading to cardiovascular collapse. Mucous membranes should be evaluated for color, capillary refill time, and presence of petechiation.

An accurate weight (in kilograms for drug doses) should be recorded whenever possible to ensure accurate drug doses are administered; however, in some patients an approximation of the weight may be all that is possible, because moving the patient to the weigh scale may compromise care. Vital signs including a blood pressure (BP) should be taken before administration of any drugs. If the veterinary team suspects that the animal has cardiac injury or disease, then a lead II electrocardiogram (ECG) should be run (and possibly an echocardiogram, if available). Thoracic radiographs are indicated in patients with a history of trauma, those with cardiorespiratory disease, and those going to surgery for possible neoplasia. Laboratory tests will vary; however, PCV, total solids, electrolytes (sodium, chloride, potassium), blood gas, glucose, blood urea nitrogen, creatinine, albumin, liver enzymes, coagulation tests (prothrombin time and activated partial thromboplastin time or activated clotting time), and platelet count should be evaluated in most critical patients. A buccal mucosal bleeding time should be evaluated in breeds with a high risk for von Willebrand's disease. A urinalysis, complete blood count with manual differential, and complete chemistry panel should be evaluated if time permits.

Vascular Access

One or two peripheral large bore catheters should be placed in all patients going to surgery. If the diameter of the T-port tubing is narrower than the catheter, then it should be removed because it may interfere with rapid fluid infusion. Ideally a jugular catheter should be placed in any patient that is hemodynamically unstable or has underlying heart disease to monitor central venous pressure (CVP). Maintaining adequate preload while avoiding fluid overload is paramount to the survival of these patients. An indwelling arterial catheter for direct BP monitoring and arterial blood gas determination is ideal in any critical patient.

Preanesthetic Stabilization

Every attempt should be made to stabilize the patient; however, as stated previously, in some situations anesthetizing the patient may play a role in patient stabilization. Patients who need O_2 should be provided with it; those with severe pulmonary edema may need diuretics. Bilateral thoracentesis usually is necessary in patients with air or fluid in the pleural space. A chest tube is indicated in all patients with a pneumothorax when a thoracotomy is not being performed. BP should be normal if possible (unless hypotensive resuscitation is being performed). Venous volume should be adequate. Potentially life-threatening arrhythmias should be controlled. Body temperature should be normal. Rectal temperature measurement should be avoided in patients with compromised respiration, because a vagally mediated hypotensive episode may be stimulated. All potentially life-threatening laboratory abnormalities should have been corrected, or should be in the process of being corrected. For example, the patient with signs of a coagulopathy should be receiving a fresh frozen plasma transfusion. The transfusion can be continued intraoperatively if the patient is not stable enough to wait for surgery until the transfusion is completed.

Setting Up for Anesthesia

The anesthetic machine should be ready to be used at a moment's notice, because emergency or critical patients may require anesthesia as part of their resuscitation. The veterinary technician should check O_2 tanks for adequate levels of O_2. The canister for CO_2 absorption and hoses should be in good working order. The vaporizer should be full of inhalant anesthetic. A variety of sizes of clear endotracheal tubes and a laryngoscope must be available. Clear endotracheal tubes are preferred over red ones because they allow for visualization of any secretions (e.g., blood, mucus, vomitus) that may cause an airway obstruction. In addition, clear tubes are less prone to cracking, easier to clean, and are more flexible. If the red tubes are placed incorrectly, then they easily may cause deviation of the trachea. Cuffed tubes should be placed, because ventilation cannot be effectively provided without a good seal (and ventilation is essential in these patients). To help prevent iatrogenic injury to the trachea, high-volume, low-pressure cuffs should be used. Red tubes have cuffs that are higher pressure than clear tubes.

Monitoring equipment should be available and in good working order. Basic equipment should include an esophageal stethoscope, a BP device (preferably a Doppler ultrasonic blood flow detector so that flow and BP can be monitored), an ECG with continuous readout, a pulse oximeter, a capnometer, and a thermometer. If the patient has a chest tube, then a large syringe should be available for aspiration.

Each patient must have an anesthetic plan. Planning helps the technician anticipate and prevent possible complications. Planning should include consideration of patient positioning. For instance, patients with head trauma should not be positioned with the head lower than the heart, and patients with a diaphragmatic hernia should be positioned with the thorax higher than the abdomen. Standard drugs to be given in case of emergency should be written down, with the drug dose in milligrams, as well as the volume needed for the particular patient. During an emergency, no time is available to perform these calculations. Consideration should be given to the types of fluids that will need to be administered intraoperatively. Because many of these patients require delivery of fluid volumes at precise rates, fluid pumps should be available. If the veterinary technician suspects that the patient may need a certain drug, such as a dopamine infusion, then it is much better to set up the infusion in advance. Syringes, needles, and all medications should be present. A flow sheet should be used for recording all drugs administered, as well as the patient's vital signs (Technical Tip Box 10-1).

Setting Up for Surgery

The operating room should be kept in a constant state of readiness. Surgical packs, gowns, and gloves should be laid out. A warm-air or warm-water circulating blanket (or other safe, active-warming device) should be on the surgical table. The ground plate for the electrocautery should be in place and the electrocautery unit plugged in. A suction canister should be in place, with a spare available. Portable suction units should be plugged into the electrical supply.

Time under anesthesia must be minimized. Clipping and surgical preparing should be done as much as possible before induction of anesthesia. Some patients with a severe hemoabdomen may be close to exsanguination, which means preparation may be limited to clipping the area of the incision followed by a quick wipe with the surgical scrub before

BOX 10-1

Technical Tip: Setting Up for Anesthesia

Preparing the Anesthetic Machine
Ensure sufficient oxygen (O_2) for 6 hours
Ensure vaporizer full of inhalant
Ensure carbon dioxide (CO_2) absorption granules do not need to be changed
Check all hoses for cleanliness and cracks
Ensure three sizes of rebreathing bag present
Check machine for leaks
Ensure anesthetic ventilator (if available) ready to be turned on

Items Needed for Induction
Anesthetic plan
    Premedication drug
    Induction protocol
    Emergency drug doses and volume calculated
    Type of IV fluid and rate
    Patient positioning
Clear, cuffed endotracheal tubes with ties and cuff-inflating syringe
Laryngoscope and blade

Monitoring Equipment
Esophageal stethoscope
Blood pressure (BP) monitor (Doppler, oscillometric)
Capnometer
Electrocardiogram (ECG) with printer
Pulse oximeter
Thermometer

Miscellaneous Supplies
Warming blanket
Fluid and syringe pumps
Emergency crash cart

Airway
Laryngoscope and two to four Miller blades
Stylets (flexible) and lubricating jelly
Clear low-pressure high-volume cuffed tubes (3 to 12 mm)
IV line for securing tubes and syringe for inflating cuffs

Suction
Ear syringe
Hand-held and automated suction devices
Tracheal suction catheter
Yankauer or dental suction tip for pharyngeal suctioning
Additional tubing and canisters for floor or wall or machine suction device

Ventilation
Ambu-Bag with reservoir and positive end expiratory pressure valve (variable 2 to 20 cm)
Infant Ambu-Bag with reservoir and positive end expiratory pressure valve
O_2 Tubing to connect to the O_2 supply source
Backup O_2 supply source such as an E tank connected to regulator and flowmeter
Syringe (60 ml) attached to a stopcock and attached to an extension set for thoracentesis

Vascular Access
Hypodermic needles (18, 20, and 22 gauge)
Syringes (3, 6, 12, 35, and 60 ml)
Catheters (14, 16, 18, 20, 22, and 24 gauge)
Guidewire central catheters (4 and 5 French)

Drugs
Syringes (1 and 6 ml) with needles attached for each of the following drugs:

Epinephrine
Norepinephrine
Dobutamine
Dopamine
Isoproterenol
Calcium gluconate
Lidocaine
Atropine
Sodium bicarbonate
Glucose
Diphenhydramine
Methylprednisolone sodium succinate

draping. Surgeons should be gowned and gloved and instrument packs opened before induction (which should be performed in the operating room). This will allow the surgeon to enter the abdomen immediately and gain control of the hemorrhage.

Need for Balanced Anesthesia

Balanced anesthesia involves the delivery of specific drugs for analgesia or amelioration of pain, sedation, amnesia, and muscle relaxation. Because critically ill or injured patients often need to be taken to surgery in the face of an unstable respiratory or cardiovascular system, the use of balanced anesthetic techniques becomes vital. To provide balanced anesthesia the technician must be familiar with many different drugs and their effects in the patient with altered metabolism or organ function. The critically ill animal may have no reserves left, so it is essential the patient receive only enough drug to achieve the analgesia and anesthesia necessary to complete the surgery.

The following are principles of safe anesthesia in the critical patient:

1. Medication should always be titrated to effect.
2. Preemptive analgesia should be used to prevent windup and to decrease the dose of induction drugs.
3. Local anesthesia should be used when appropriate.

Analgesics, Local Anesthetics, and Preanesthetic Agents

Analgesia

One of the main goals of anesthesia is to eliminate pain. Pain has detrimental effects on cardiopulmonary function, metabolism, endocrine status, and immune function. This can lead to serious physiologic effects (e.g., ventricular premature contractions [VPCs], hypoxia, muscle weakness, delayed tissue healing), affect the patient's well-being, and even lead to death.

Analgesia is vital in the surgical patient because every surgical procedure causes pain. No situation exists in which analgesics cannot be administered. As stated previously, the windup phenomenon should be avoided as much as possible by providing preemptive analgesia. Windup, or a resetting of the pain threshold that makes the patient more sensitive to pain, occurs when pain is induced before adequate analgesia is provided. This may not be completely avoidable in patients who arrive at the clinic in pain because of underlying injury or disease. Doses usually need to be adjusted and titrated to effect, because the effective dose in critically ill patients may be only 25% to 50% of normal.

Opioids are the most common analgesics used because of their effectiveness and safety. These include drugs such as buprenorphine, butorphanol, fentanyl, morphine, and oxymorphone. All opioids cause varying degrees of sedation, respiratory depression, bradycardia, and hypotension. These effects are dose related and can be avoided to a large extent by using lower doses than would be used in the healthy, active patient. If significant bradycardia develops (i.e., it is causing hypotension), then administration of an anticholinergic such as atropine or glycopyrrolate will counteract this effect and should be given. Because bradycardia is seen infrequently, routine premedication is not recommended (because the ensuing tachycardia can be detrimental).

Whenever opioids are administered, the respiratory rate and depth should be monitored. Opioids cause respiratory depression; however, at low doses this problem rarely is a clinically significant issue. Ideally, critical patients under general anesthesia should be ventilated, in which case the respiratory depression will not be a problem. Opioids decrease intracranial pressure, but the concurrent respiratory depression may lead to hypercarbia, cerebral vasodilation, and secondary hypertension. If opioids are to be used when a change in intracranial pressure is a concern, then positive pressure ventilation should be provided. The respiratory depression seen with oxymorphone and fentanyl can be reversed with butorphanol, without decreasing the analgesic qualities of the opioids. Opioids and inhalant anesthetics routinely are used together; however, their effects are synergistic, and the combination may lead to significant decreases in heart rate and BP. The doses of the opioid and the inhalant anesthetic must be decreased to avoid these complications. The liver metabolizes opioids, and a decrease in liver function may prolong their effect.

The choice of opioid used depends on availability and familiarity with the drug. Buprenorphine probably is the only opioid not frequently indicated in the critical patient, because its longer onset of action makes it more difficult to titrate. Morphine is a short-acting opioid that has excellent analgesic qualities. It may cause emesis and vasodilation secondary to histamine release when given via IV. These side effects are not seen commonly with the low doses used in critical patients and often can be avoided by administering the drug slowly. Morphine is very effective when delivered as a constant rate infusion (CRI). Butorphanol is a short-acting analgesic that is useful because it has very minimal sedative and respiratory-depressant effects in addition to its mild analgesic properties. Oxymorphone is an intermediate-acting opioid that can be used effectively in the critical patient. Hydromorphone is similar in duration to oxymorphone but typically requires a higher dose to achieve a similar analgesic effect. Fentanyl is a very potent short-acting opioid that is most useful when administered as a CRI, although it can be given by bolus injection.

In general, nonsteroidal antiinflammatory drugs are contraindicated in patients with hypotension or decreased tissue perfusion, those with gastrointestinal or renal disease or dysfunction, and those with thrombocytopenia or platelet dysfunction. Therefore these medications should not be administered to the critical patient.

Local or Regional Anesthesia

Infiltration of nerve endings using local anesthesia is a very effective way of providing analgesia and is recommended highly. Because the systemic effects of drugs used to produce local or regional anesthesia are minimal, this is a safe technique to use in the compromised patient. Local or regional anesthesia can be used in combination with sedation, systemic analgesia, and anxiolysis (i.e., relief of anxiety). In the severely debilitated patient, local anesthetics in combination with systemic analgesics and sedation may be sufficient to perform the necessary surgery.

Lidocaine and bupivacaine typically are used for local, regional, or epidural anesthesia. Lidocaine can be placed directly onto the wound surface and into the skin edges to help decrease the pain associated with débridement, flushing, and suturing. Infiltration of surgical incisions with bupivacaine or lidocaine as a line block (preoperatively or postoperatively) helps to decrease the pain associated with the incision. These medications can be infused as regional blocks, as intraarticular injections, or intrapleurally.

Local anesthetics are very acidic drugs and can cause irritation when injected locally. This effect can be lessened by warming the solution to body temperature or by adding sodium bicarbonate into the syringe with the local anesthetic (10% sodium bicarbonate by volume). If a large volume of local anesthetic is required, then it can be diluted by 50% with any fluid that has an acidic or neutral pH. By combining lidocaine and bupivacaine, the clinician helps the patient to benefit from the rapid onset of action of the lidocaine and the long duration of effect of the bupivacaine.

Epidural Analgesia and Anesthesia

Epidurally administered analgesic and anesthetic agents are effective in controlling pain. When given preoperatively, a significant decrease occurs in the amount of analgesic agents required postoperatively. Epidural anesthesia significantly lowers the requirement and may even eliminate the need for inhalant anesthesia in unstable patients.

Local anesthetics such as lidocaine and bupivacaine in combination with morphine, oxymorphone, or hydromorphone typically are used for delivering epidural anesthesia. Oxymorphone is thought to bind to receptors near the site of injection better than morphine because of its lipophilic nature; therefore oxymorphone is more likely to have an effect at the site of injection than morphine. Bupivacaine and morphine in combination are more effective than morphine alone, and bupivacaine alone has been shown to be more effective than morphine alone. Onset of action is approximately 30 to 60 minutes, and duration of effect is from 6 to 24 hours.

Placement of an epidural catheter permits supplemental dosing intraoperatively and postoperatively for anesthesia and analgesia of the thorax, abdomen, or pelvic limbs. It is easier to administer high epidural analgesia more accurately if a catheter is placed.

Potential complications of epidural anesthesia include hypotension from sympathetic blockade, respiratory depression, motor paralysis, hypothermia, urinary retention, and infections. The higher the epidural is, the greater the likelihood of respiratory depression and hypotension.

Premedication

Premedication involves administration of some combination of tranquilizers, sedatives, hypnotics, analgesics, and anticholinergic drugs. It decreases the doses needed for induction and maintenance anesthesia and helps ensure a smoother recovery.

Many of these drugs may not be indicated in or tolerated by the critical patient; however, opioids can be used safely even in fragile patients.

Anticholinergic drugs include atropine and glycopyrrolate; these drugs are effective at reversing bradycardia secondary to increased vagal tone, decreasing airway secretions, and causing airway dilation; however, the resulting increase in heart rate increases the myocardial O_2 demands. The increased myocardial O_2 demands may cause myocardial hypoxia and malignant arrhythmias, and anticholinergic drugs should not be given routinely to critical patients. Exceptions include those animals with high resting vagal tone when it is anticipated that surgical manipulation will lead to increased vagal tone, as well as those with significant bradycardia, significant liquid airway secretions, or increased salivation (cats being more predisposed than dogs to this side effect). If in doubt, then it is always better to administer the anticholinergic once the effects of the other administered drugs are known.

Phenothiazines, administered as a sole agent, generally are not indicated in critically ill or injured patients because of their vasodilatory and hypotensive side effects. These side effects can be a significant problem when normal or high doses are administered, and even low doses can cause a significant problem if the patient is not hemodynamically stable. However, very low doses may have several beneficial effects. The vasodilatory effects improve microcirculatory flow or perfusion. When used in combination with opioids, the effects of both drugs are synergistic. Some of the clinical signs exhibited by the ill or injured patient may be interpreted as pain; however, they may be caused in part by anxiety. Acepromazine is an excellent anxiolytic and may help reduce stress (and its detrimental effects on patient metabolism). A dose of 0.01 to 0.025 mg/kg can be used safely in many patients to help decrease anxiety, increase the effectiveness of the opioid, and help decrease the dose of induction and maintenance agents. This dose also has been shown to reduce the chance of arrhythmias while minimally affecting BP. Phenothiazines have no effect on cerebral blood flow in the face of normal systemic BP, but the vasodilatory effects can be detrimental to cerebral blood flow if the patient becomes hypotensive.

Some of the side effects of acepromazine reported in the literature are rarely a clinical problem, especially at low doses; however, because many of the critical patients may be unstable and may lack the ability to deal with side effects of drugs, the anesthetist should be aware of potential complications. Acepromazine can cause red blood cell sequestration in the spleen, a decrease in plasma protein levels, platelet dysfunction. In addition, although the position is controversial, some researchers believe that phenothiazines may lower the seizure threshold and ideally should not be used in patients with a history of seizures. Phenothiazines are metabolized in the liver.

Anesthetic Agents

General Concerns

General anesthesia can be provided with injectable drugs, with a combination of injectable drugs and an inhalant, or by administration of inhalational agents alone.

Critical patients should be anesthetized using drugs that allow rapid airway control and rapid institution of positive pressure ventilatory support. Mask or tank inductions should not be performed. The only exception may be the extremely fractious cat that has been injured but cannot be approached to give an IM injection or intraoral ketamine. After they have been premedicated, critical patients should be preoxygenated for 5 minutes.

Neuroleptanalgesia

Neuroleptanalgesia implies a tranquil, dissociative, analgesic state produced by the synergism between an opioid and a tranquilizer. The combination of the two drugs allows lower doses of each drug to be administered. Neuroleptanalgesia may provide anesthesia in the severely debilitated patient. In less debilitated patients, doses of inhalants can be reduced significantly. Awake intubation, or insertion of an orotracheal tube in the patient that is not unconscious, often can be performed with these combinations.

Etomidate

Etomidate is an imidazole derivative that is classified as a *nonbarbiturate, nonnarcotic, sedative-hypnotic agent*. It has poor analgesic qualities, and opioids or other means of providing analgesia should be administered if etomidate is being used. It causes mild respiratory depression but minimal change in cardiopulmonary function even in hypovolemic dogs. It does have mild negative inotropic effects, but they are not significant, making it a very useful drug in patients with severe cardiovascular instability. Vomiting, excitement, tremors, and apnea may be seen on induction. The neurologic signs are thought to be the result of disinhibition of subcortical neural activity and are not seizures. Etomidate decreases cerebral blood flow and metabolic O_2 requirements similar to barbiturates and can be used in patients with intracranial disease. Etomidate causes cortisol suppression for up to 6 hours after a single injection. This is of unknown significance but may be a concern in the critically ill or injured patient. Even though etomidate is metabolized in the liver, liver disease does not seem to affect its metabolism.

Ketamine and Benzodiazepine Combinations

Ketamine in combination with benzodiazepine such as diazepam or midazolam makes an excellent combination for induction of anesthesia in critical patients. Midazolam is a water-soluble benzodiazepine with similar effects to diazepam but a longer half-life. Midazolam and diazepam can be used in titrated doses under anesthesia to help maintain anesthesia when injectable drugs are being used or to decrease the amount of inhalant required.

Ketamine is a dissociative anesthetic that has good musculoskeletal analgesic properties, weak visceral analgesic qualities, and poor muscle relaxant properties. It exerts a positive inotropic effect on the myocardium and increases cardiac output, BP, pulmonary artery pressure, and CVP. For these reasons it may be contraindicated in patients with elevated left atrial pressures or pulmonary hypertension. It should be avoided in cats with hypertrophic cardiomyopathy. Because it increases myocardial O_2 demands, ketamine should be used with caution in patients with significant myocardial dysfunction. The cardiovascular effects can be prevented or diminished by concurrently administering a sedative such as a benzodiazepine or acepromazine. Ketamine may cause seizures, an increase in cerebral metabolic rate, an increase in intracranial pressure, and a decrease in cerebral perfusion pressure. Therefore ketamine should be used with caution in patients with intracranial disease or head trauma. Nystagmus is common, so it is a poor choice for patients requiring ocular surgery. Ketamine increases airway secretions, and anticholinergic drugs may be indicated, especially in the cat. It is important for the veterinary technician to remember that anticholinergic drugs should not be used prophylactically because of the potential detrimental side effects.

Benzodiazepines are metabolized in the liver and should be used with caution in severe liver disease. Ketamine is metabolized in the liver in the dog; however, in the cat it is excreted primarily unchanged in the urine.

Medetomidine

α2 Agonists such as xylazine and medetomidine usually are contraindicated in critical patients, because they cause a decrease in heart rate of up to 50% of baseline. These drugs also can cause atrioventricular block and VPCs. Medetomidine has a diuretic effect lasting up to 4 hours, which may be detrimental in the dehydrated or hypovolemic patient.

Propofol

Propofol is an alkylphenol classified as *nonbarbiturate, nonnarcotic, sedative-hypnotic* that has poor analgesic qualities. Its advantages lie in rapid induction and recovery with no cumulative effects even after multiple doses. Disadvantages include a high rate of apnea (seen on induction) and systemic hypotension. The hypotension is secondary to a decrease in myocardial contractility, as well as both vasodilation and venodilation. This effect, which is similar to that seen with thiopental, is of greater significance in hypovolemic patients. VPCs may be seen, and it also causes hypothermia. Tremors and opisthotonus, which may be seen, are thought to be the result of disinhibition of neural activity and are not seizures. Premedicating the patient with an anxiolytic can prevent these effects. Propofol is a good choice in patients with intracranial disease as long as they are not hypotensive, because it decreases cerebral metabolic O_2 requirements. This drug is metabolized extensively in the liver, but its effects do not appear to be prolonged in patients with significant liver dysfunction.

Barbiturates

Both thiobarbiturates (e.g., thiopental) and oxybarbiturates (e.g., pentobarbital) can be used for providing general anesthesia; however, because they have significant respiratory-depressant qualities and negative inotropic properties that can cause significant hypotension, they must be used with caution. The negative effects are intensified in the presence of shock, acidosis, hypothermia, and hypoproteinemia. Because of severe depressant effects, barbiturates should not be used for induction without premedication. They have no analgesic qualities and must be used in combination with opioids. Advantages of barbiturates include rapid induction, which allows for rapid intubation and control of ventilation; they also decrease cerebral metabolic O_2 consumption and can be used safely in patients with intracranial disease. Lack of body fat and liver dysfunction significantly prolong recovery from thiobarbiturates.

Inhalants

Inhalant anesthetics most commonly used include isoflurane and sevoflurane. Both inhalants cause significant dose-dependent decreases in BP and cardiac output, which could be life threatening in the critical patient. This is related to a combination of negative inotropic effects and vasodilatory properties because of the calcium channel–blocking effects. Injectable anesthesia has been recommended when hypotension develops. Although it causes similar cardiovascular effects to isoflurane, sevoflurane sensitizes the myocardium less to the arrhythmogenic effects of catecholamines and recovery is more rapid. Unlike sevoflurane, isoflurane is an airway irritant and has the potential to cause airway spasm. Both inhalants cause dose-related respiratory depression (centrally and as a result of direct effects on the diaphragm). Neither inhalant has any analgesic qualities, but they do provide some muscle relaxation.

Neuromuscular Blocking Agents

General

Neuromuscular blocking agents are very useful in the critically ill or injured patient; they help gain airway control without inducing gagging, coughing, or laryngospasm. These agents do not affect the cardiovascular system, thus the patient remains more stable under anesthesia. Good muscle relaxation is provided, which increases chest compliance and allows for more effective ventilation with lower peak inspiratory pressures (PIPs). The muscle relaxation is useful during reduction of a luxation and when treating fractures. Neuromuscular blockers do not cause any central nervous system depression.

The patient is paralyzed but aware and must receive both analgesics and sedatives or dissociative agents; however, because movement is eliminated, amounts of other drugs are decreased. Because the animal is paralyzed, positive pressure ventilatory support is required.

Depolarizing Muscle-Blocking Agents

Two classes of neuromuscular blockers exist: (1) depolarizing and (2) nondepolarizing. Depolarizing agents act like acetylcholine at the neuromuscular junction, causing the muscle to contract, and their effect is longer than acetylcholine, which leads to persistent contraction (muscle paralysis). Depolarizing agents are broken down by plasma cholinesterase. No antagonists are available for these drugs.

Succinylcholine is the most commonly used drug in this class. It has a rapid onset of action (within 30 to 60 seconds) and rapid recovery (within 5 to 20 minutes). Muscle fasciculations may be seen as the membranes depolarize, which can cause a transient increase in potassium levels of 0.5 to 1 mEq/L. Because of its rapid onset of action, succinylcholine it is an effective drug to use if rapid airway control is required. It should be used with caution in patients with renal disease, severe liver dysfunction, myopathy, penetrating eye injury, or chronic debilitating disease. Succinylcholine is not recommended in patients in whom increased intraabdominal or increased intrathoracic pressures are undesirable (e.g., tension pneumothorax, gastric dilation volvulus). Hypokalemia, hypothermia and exposure to organophosphates will prolong the effects of succinylcholine. Succinylcholine may cause malignant hyperthermia.

Nondepolarizing Neuromuscular Blocking Agents

Nondepolarizing neuromuscular blocking agents bind to acetylcholine receptor sites at the muscle end plate, thus preventing acetylcholine from binding with the receptor sites. This prevents muscle contraction and causes a flaccid paralysis. Nondepolarizing drugs are not metabolized by cholinesterase, but anticholinesterase drugs such as edrophonium or neostigmine can antagonize them. An anticholinergic usually is administered concurrently with the reversal drug, because they may cause parasympathetic side effects such as bradycardia, salivation, miosis, and increased gastrointestinal motility. Reversal will be effective only if at least some muscle function has returned.

Atracurium is the most common nondepolarizing neuromuscular blocker used in veterinary medicine and has a slightly longer onset of action than succinylcholine. Atracurium may not be the best first choice if rapid airway control is being attempted using just the neuromuscular blocker (because a period of time will occur when the patient cannot breathe properly but is not paralyzed sufficiently to be able to intubate). A patient should never be allowed to struggle to breathe. Atracurium is degraded by Hoffman elimination, which is spontaneous degradation that is not dependent on hepatic metabolism or renal excretion; however, atracurium's effects will be prolonged by acidosis and hypothermia.

Atracurium has an onset of action of as short as 1 minute to as long as 5 minutes and duration of effect of 20 to 45 minutes. A loading dose can be followed by repeat IV doses (using 40% of the initial dose) or a CRI. At high levels, atracurium may cause histamine release.

Monitoring with Neuromuscular Blocking Agents

Peripheral nerve stimulators using a train of four should be used to monitor neuromuscular blockade if available. The stimulator can be attached to the facial or ulnar nerve. If a peripheral nerve stimulator is not available, then it will be impossible to assess the depth of the block until muscle function starts to return. The patient must be artificially ventilated until good ventilatory function returns, and the patient should never be extubated until it is able to sit up. It is more difficult to monitor patients under anesthesia with neuromuscular blockade, because the normal neuromuscular reflexes are abolished. Lacrimation, salivation, slight muscle movement of the limbs or face, curling of the tip of the tongue, increased resistance to ventilation, and increased BP may be indicators that the patient is aware of its surroundings or is in pain. One of the best guides to general anesthetic depth when a neuromuscular blocker is not being used is jaw tone; it should always be present to some extent (Table 10-1).

Intubation

General

All critical patients should be preoxygenated before induction by placing a mask over the patients face or simply by placing a tube from an O_2 source in front of the patient's face (i.e., blow-by). The tube should be placed into the patient's mouth if it is gasping or panting. High flow rates should be used.

All patients should be intubated with the largest endotracheal tube that fits comfortably in the trachea. The anesthetist should feel comfortable intubating a patient in lateral, dorsal, and sternal recumbency. Intubating the patient in dorsal recumbency allows insertion of a tube ½ mm to 1 mm larger than would be placed with the patient in sternal recumbency, and it allows the patient to be intubated unassisted. To avoid aspiration, the patient should not be intubated in dorsal recumbency if the stomach is distended.

In very unstable patients awake, intubation may be indicated (done by administering an opioid and a benzodiazepine to provide mild sedation and anxiolysis). A neuromuscular blocking agent also may be required to allow the animal to tolerate the endotracheal tube. The patient is sedated only, so a general anesthetic agent, which may decompensate the patient, is avoided.

Resistance to ventilation is determined primarily by the diameter of the endotracheal tube (the larger the tube, the less the resistance). Cuffed endotracheal rubes should be placed in all patients because ventilation cannot be provided effectively without a good seal. The cuff should be inflated to provide a seal at 15 to 20 cm water. If the team is concerned about tracheal disease, then the cuff should be inflated to provide a seal at 10 to 12 cm water. The cuff should not be overinflated, because this may lead to mucosal injury and ischemia (and in the cat can lead to tracheal disruption by tearing the dorsal tracheal muscle). Whenever the patient is turned, the endotracheal tube should be disconnected from the anesthetic machine to avoid applying torque to the tube, which may cause trauma to the trachea.

A laryngoscope should be used in all patients, and topical lidocaine (0.2 ml of 2% lidocaine per 5 kg body weight) should be used on the arytenoid cartilages if laryngospasm, gagging, or coughing on induction needs to be avoided. If topical lidocaine

TABLE 10-1

Anesthetic Drugs

Drug	Doses IV (unless otherwise indicated)
Premed and Postoperative Analgesia	
Atropine	0.02-0.04 mg/kg
Glycopyrrolate	0.01-0.02 mg/kg
Acepromazine	0.005-0.2 mg/kg (max 3 mg)
Ketamine	3.0-8.0 mg/kg
Oxymorphone	0.04-0.3 mg/kg
Fentanyl	5.0-10.0 mg/kg
Fentanyl patch	One-half, covered 25 µg/hr patch if <2.5 kg
	25 µg/hr 5-10 kg
	50 µg/hr 10-20 kg
	75 µg/hr 20-30 kg
	100 µg/hr > 30 kg
Morphine	0.5-2.2 mg/kg; 0.05-1.0 mg/kg/hr constant rate infusion (CRI)
Butorphanol	0.2-0.4 mg/kg
Buprenorphine	5.0-20.0 µg/kg
Induction	
Thiopental	6.0-10.0 mg/kg 2% solution
Ketamine	5.0-10.0 mg/kg
Etomidate	0.5-2.0 mg/kg
Propofol	3.0-6.0 mg/kg
With diazepam use	0.2-0.5 mg/kg
Propofol with diazepam	1.0-3.0 mg/kg
Oxymorphone with diazepam	0.2 mg/kg
Fentanyl with diazepam	20 µg/kg
Etomidate with diazepam	0.25-0.4 mg/kg
Maintenance	
Oxymorphone	0.05-0.1 mg/kg q20min
Fentanyl	0.5-1.0 µg/kg/min
Propofol	0.1-0.6 mg/kg/min
Diazepam	0.2-0.5 mg/kg/hr
Midazolam	0.5-1.5 µg/kg/min
Pentobarbital	0.05-2.6 mg/kg
Ketamine with diazepam	1.25-2.5 mg/kg
Diazepam	0.05-0.2 mg/kg

TABLE 10-1

Anesthetic Drugs—cont'd

Drug	Doses IV (unless otherwise indicated)
Neuromuscular Blockers	
Atracurium	mg/kg load; 0.1 mg/kg redose; 2.0-8.0 µg/kg/min
Pancuronium	0.04-0.11 mg/kg; 0.04 mg/kg/hr
Succinylcholine	0.22-0.44 mg/kg; 0.2 mg/kg/hr
Reversal	
Naloxone	0.01-0.02 mg/kg 50% IV, 50% intramuscular (IM); 0.02-0.04 mg/kg IM
Nalbuphine	0.03-0.1 mg/kg IV
Buprenorphine	10-20 µg/kg IV 20 min pre reversal
Atropine w/edrophonium	0.01-0.02 mg/kg followed by 0.5 mg/kg IV
Atropine w/neostigmine	0.04 mg/kg followed by 0.06 mg/kg IV
Local Anesthesia	
Epidural	If spinal or CSF decrease dose by 75%; 0.3 ml/kg volume; 1 ml/15 kg will block to T5; max volume 6 ml
Oxymorphone	0.1 mg/kg
Morphine	0.1 mg/kg
Buprenorphine	0.03 mg/kg
Bupivacaine	2 mg/kg 0.5% solution (1 ml/4.5 kg)
Lidocaine	2-4 mg/kg 2% solution (1 ml/4.5 kg)
Intercostal	
Bupivacaine	2 mg/kg 0.5% solution; 0.5 ml/nerve
Intrapleural	
Bupivacaine	1.5-2.0 mg/kg diluted to 1 ml/kg q6h
Local	
Lidocaine	0.5-2.0% max 6 mg/kg with bicarbonate 1 ml per 10 ml lidocaine

Opioids	Mu (µ)	Kappa (κ)	Sigma (σ)
Analgesia	+	+	−
Respiration	Depression	Depression	Stimulation
Behavior	Euphoria	Sedation	Dysphoria
Dependency	+	−	−

Pain Management	Duration	Receptors	Potency
Morphine	4-6 hr	µ, κ, σ Agonist	
Fentanyl	30-45 min	µ, κ, σ Agonist	100 × Morphine
Oxymorphone	1-6 hr	µ, κ, σ Agonist	10 × Morphine
Buprenorphine	10-12 hr	Slow µ dissociation	30 × Morphine
Butorphanol	3-4 hr	Weak µ, strong κ	3-5 × Morphine

is used, then the anesthetist should wait at least 10 seconds before intubating. Nontraumatic intubation is most important, because stimulation of the larynx can invoke a vagally mediated bradycardia and potentially an arrest in the hypoxemic patient. In the severely hypotensive patient, the head should not be raised during intubation (because this may decrease cerebral blood flow to the point of causing cardiorespiratory arrest). In this situation, the patient should be intubated in dorsal or lateral recumbency. If a stylet is used, then care should be taken to ensure the tip does not protrude past the end of the endotracheal tube (it can cause damage to the trachea).

Lidocaine can be given via IV as part of an induction protocol to help decrease arrhythmias and decrease the gag or cough response to intubation. Giving lidocaine also allows for a decrease in the doses of other induction agents, and it is particularly useful in patients with preexisting VPCs or in patients with possible elevated intracranial pressure.

Once the patient is intubated and the tube is secured, the lungs should be ausculted bilaterally. Doing this allows the anesthetist to confirm that the tube is in the trachea (not the esophagus) and that the tip of the tube has not been inserted into a mainstem bronchus.

Intubating a Patient with a Possible Airway Disruption

Intubating a patient with a possible airway disruption is more complex than regular intubation. Cervical bite wounds may create a tear in the cervical trachea, and the tip of the tube must project past the suspected area of injury. Cats that have a possible trachealis dorsalis muscle tear secondary to an anesthetic complication may have a tear that starts at the mid- or distal cervical region and ends at the bronchial bifurcation. In these patients the tube should be passed more distally than it normally would (generally to the level of the bronchial bifurcation). Artificial ventilation of this patient should be avoided until the tear is located and it is confirmed that the tube projects past the injury. If the patient must be ventilated, then it should be closely monitored for signs of a developing tension pneumomediastinum. Clinical signs include loss of Doppler blood flow sounds, hypotension, increasing difficulty in ventilation, and worsening SC emphysema.

Intubating a Patient with Upper Airway Swelling or Obstruction

If the team is concerned that the airway will be too edematous or disrupted to intubate the animal orotracheally, an awake tracheostomy should be performed under local anesthesia (and sedation, if required) before induction. If considerable edema exists, as in the case of the bulldog with possible laryngeal paralysis, then a single dose of dexamethasone sodium phosphate (0.5 mg/kg IV) may help alleviate some of the swelling.

Maintaining a Patient under General Anesthesia

Critical patients should be maintained on 100% O_2 and controlled ventilation. Metabolic O_2 requirements are approximately 5 ml/kg/min (O_2 flows should not be less than this). With semiclosed anesthesia, O_2 flow rates of 100 to 300 ml/kg/min are indicated. Low-flow anesthesia is ideal for the critical patient, because less moisture is lost from the airways and, because O_2 flow rates are low, less heat loss occurs. During low-flow anesthesia, the O_2 flow rates are, by definition, slightly greater than metabolic O_2 requirements. Because critical patients may have a higher demand for O_2, low-flow anesthesia should not be less than 10 ml/kg/min. Many anesthetic machines have small leaks that lead to losses of 100 to 200 ml/min, and flow rates should rarely decrease below this level. During low-flow anesthesia, the canister that traps CO_2 should be checked more frequently (this method relies more on removal of CO_2 by the canister than by flow). Monitoring end-tidal carbon dioxide ($ETCO_2$) levels via capnography is very important during low-flow anesthesia.

Critically ill or injured patients under anesthesia often need modifications in their anesthetic protocols and fluids rates because they are not stable. Many of these patients will develop severe hypotension with normal inspired concentrations of inhalant anesthesia. Therefore injectable drugs often are needed intraoperatively. When patients appear to be responding to surgical stimulation, they may be perceiving pain and analgesics should be used judiciously throughout the surgical procedure. This will allow the anesthetist to significantly lower the amount of other anesthetic agents being used. Most opioids will need to be redosed every 15 to 20 minutes. If benzodiazepines are being used to create neuroleptanalgesia, then it may be necessary to redose these drugs every 15 to 20 minutes as well. In most cases subsequent doses of all drugs should be given at increasing intervals and lower amounts, because hypothermia and acidosis prolong their effects.

Controlled Ventilation

All anesthetic agents are ventilatory depressants, so ventilatory support is essential in the critical patient. In general, tidal volumes should be set at 12 to 15 ml/kg (lean body weight), at a rate of 12 to 20 breaths/min. PIPs should be kept below 15 cm of water whenever possible. The veterinary technician should remember that tidal volumes as high as 20 ml/kg and PIPs as high as 25 cm of water may be needed. Tidal volumes are adjusted based on observation of chest movement during ventilation, lung auscultation, capnometry (and blood gases if available), and BP. To avoid complications, the lowest volumes and pressures the patient will tolerate should be used.

Ventilator parameters must be adjusted according to the patient's condition. For example, patients with less complaint lungs or masses pushing on the diaphragm may require higher tidal volumes and PIPs than patients with compliant chest walls. In addition, the tubing from the anesthetic machine to the patient will absorb some of the pressure from the ventilator. If a lot of tubing is used or the tubing is compliant, then higher than expected tidal volumes and pressures may need to be used in smaller patients. The tubing becomes less of a factor in larger patients. If higher-frequency ventilation is being used, then tidal volumes can be decreased. Overventilation can lead to a decrease in preload and a secondary decrease in cardiac output and BP. Increased tidal volumes or inspiratory pressures may be needed in patients with a large amount of dead space (i.e., large amount of anesthetic tubing compared with the tidal volume), restrictive pulmonary disease, or impaired diaphragmatic movement (e.g., gastric dilation volvulus, obesity). Increases may also be required in patients restrained in dorsal recumbency with limbs stretched, because chest wall movement will be restricted in this position.

Manual ventilation is provided by hand bagging the patient. Respiratory and ventilatory parameters should be monitored. Mechanical ventilation is recommended to provide consistent, continuous ventilatory support in all critical patients. Mechanical ventilation frees up the technician so that he or she can do a better job of monitoring the patient. Many economical ventilators are available that are simple to use and will help save lives of the critical patient under anesthesia.

An Ambu-Bag with a reservoir and 100% O_2 should be used to ventilate all patients during transport from the preparation area to the operating room or to radiology.

Monitoring

Close monitoring of the critically ill or injured anesthetized patient is mandatory. Most parameters should be recorded every 5 minutes in the unstable patient (to a maximum of every 15 minutes in the stable patient). All vital signs, ventilatory parameters, drugs administered, fluids, and surgical interventions should be noted on an anesthesia flow sheet (Box 10-2).

Hands-On Physical Parameter Monitoring—The Essentials

The anesthetist should not rely solely on monitoring equipment but should check the patient physically at regular intervals using eyes, ears, and hands to confirm that the machine readouts are accurate. A machine cannot pick up changes such as cyanosis and pallor.

The seriously ill or injured patient who is undergoing surgery is at risk for serious complications such as airway compromise, respiratory depression, hypercarbia, hypoxemia, arrhythmias, coagulopathy, metabolic acidosis, and even cardiac arrest. Absolute numbers are vitally important, but often the trend of change is an early indicator of whether or not the patient is beginning to decompensate. This section discusses monitoring of the patient under anesthesia.

The respiratory rate should be measured. If necessary, then the lungs should be ausculted using an esophageal stethoscope (if drapes prevent direct auscultation). The earliest way to detect pulmonary edema is with an esophageal stethoscope. With interstitial pulmonary edema, the breath sounds change (normally from a very quiet exhalation sound to that of breath sounds getting louder on exhalation). As alveolar edema becomes evident, crackles become audible—first just on exhalation; later crackles

BOX 10-2   ⓐ

Recommended Monitoring Check List for Anesthesia of the Critical Patient

Continuous monitoring by devices (able to see numeric values and waveforms):

- Electrocardiogram (ECG), end-tidal capnography, pulse oximetry
- Doppler blood flow (qualitative evaluation by listening to generated sounds)
- Respiratory rate and effort (by impedance), arterial and central venous pressure (CVP) (if available)

Monitoring as often as required and recorded every 5 minutes:

- Respiratory rate, heart rate, blood pressure (BP), oxygen (O_2) saturation, end-tidal carbon dioxide ($ETCO_2$)
- Pulse strength, mucous membrane color, eye position, muscle tone by estimating tone in muscles of mandible (jaw tone test)*

Monitoring as often as required and recorded every 15 minutes:

- Temperature
- Fluids infused (type, rate, and running total of each), estimated blood loss (based on sponges and blood in suction reservoir)
- Urine output if catheter present
- Lung sounds and heart tones*
- Stage of operation, manipulations done*

Monitoring if intraoperative concerns present or surgery longer than 2 to 3 hours:

- Packed cell volume (PCV), total solids, venous blood gas, arterial blood gas, glucose, electrolytes, albumin, coagulation parameters

*Monitored but generally recorded only if findings deviate from those expected or if abnormality develops intraoperatively.

will be heard on both inhalation and exhalation. An esophageal stethoscope can be used to assess lung sounds and heart tones. Abnormalities such as crackles (which are consistent with pulmonary edema) and dullness (consistent with obstruction or atelectasis) can be ausculted. Chest excursion should be assessed with both spontaneous respiration and assisted ventilation (both by hand bagging and mechanical ventilation).

Jaw tone should be assessed along with eye position; however, neither assessment provides a very accurate measurement of depth (which depends on the drugs being administered to the patient). Extreme laxity of the jaw and extreme ventral strabismus suggests a depth of anesthesia that may be excessive.

Electronic Monitoring of Ventilation and Oxygenation

More sophisticated methods of assessing ventilatory function include the following:

- Pulse oximetry readings should indicate an oxygen saturation (SpO_2) above 98%. The most accurate location for placement of the O_2 sensor is on the tongue. A good pulse signal (either indicated by waveform or signal intensity light) is necessary to get valid SpO_2 readings. Tongue clips in smaller animals often will apply sufficient pressure to interfere with circulation and cause inaccurate readings. This can be corrected by moving the clip at regular intervals to a slightly different location on the tongue; O_2 saturation reaches 100% at an arterial pressure (PaO_2) of about 95 mm Hg. The PaO_2 should be 4.5 to 5.0 times the fraction of inspired oxygen (FiO_2); therefore with an FiO_2 of 1 (100% O_2, which is the concentration given during anesthesia), the PaO_2 should be 450 to 500 mm Hg. The SpO_2 will read 100% from a PaO_2 of 500 mm Hg to below about 95 mm Hg. This makes SpO_2 a very inaccurate means of monitoring oxygenation in the patient that is receiving 100% O_2. If the team is concerned about pulmonary function, then arterial blood gases should be assessed. Pulse oximetry is a very important tool, however, when the patient is not on supplemental O_2 (i.e., is breathing room air) or is receiving low levels of O_2 supplementation (i.e., nasal, nasopharyngeal, nasotracheal) during recovery.
- Capnometry should be assessed in all patients. Waveform analysis (capnography) is preferred to Capnometry, which only gives a number corresponding to $ETCO_2$. Waveform analysis allows the anesthetist to detect changes in ventilatory mechanics. For example, a steep slope means a clear airway, whereas a slow rise in the slope indicates an obstructive airway problem. The $ETCO_2$ corresponds to air exhaled from the alveoli and,

assuming no ventilation perfusion mismatch, corresponds to pulmonary arterial blood carbon dioxide tensions ($Paco_2$); it is the only way of assessing adequacy of ventilation noninvasively. $ETCO_2$ levels will generally be about 3 to 5 mm Hg lower than $Paco_2$ because of dead space ventilation. The $ETCO_2$ should remain between 25 to 35 mm Hg.

- The PIP must be monitored whenever the patient is being ventilated. Peak airway pressure should be no higher than 15 to 20 cm of water whenever possible. Higher pressures may lead to barotrauma with subsequent air trapping in the alveoli, pneumothorax, or pneumomediastinum. Periodic sighing every 2 to 5 minutes with pressures from 20 to 30 cm of water also is recommended to prevent atelectasis in patients who are not being mechanically ventilated.

Monitoring Cardiovascular Parameters

Heart rate should be measured by esophageal auscultation or listening to a Doppler blood flow detector. Low heart rates can be associated with a low cardiac output and hypotension. High heart rates can lead to inadequate cardiac filling and low cardiac output with subsequent hypotension. High heart rates also lead to increased myocardial O_2 demands and may lead to arrhythmias.

To adequately assess cardiovascular status, the veterinary technician must have a means of measuring BP, either directly or indirectly. To ensure adequate renal and splanchnic perfusion, systolic BP should be maintained above 100 mm Hg and mean arterial pressure should be kept above 60 mm Hg.

When monitoring cardiovascular parameters, the following should also be kept in mind:

- A Doppler ultrasonic blood flow detector is recommended, because it allows accurate determination of BP (systolic and diastolic in many patients), as well as flow based on the strength of the sound. Arrhythmias also are audible using a Doppler. It is important to note the heart rate whenever a BP measurement is taken.
- An oscillometric BP monitor detects pulse waves under a cuff that is placed around the limb (or tail). Systolic, diastolic, and mean arterial pressures along with the heart rate are displayed on the screen. It is simpler to use and is much less labor intensive than the Doppler method, but its major disadvantage is that flow cannot be evaluated. If the heart rate does not match the patient's actual rate, then the BP measurement likely is inaccurate. If the patient is small, significant arrhythmias are seen, or the signal is weak, then readings may be inaccurate. Oscillometric BP monitors also are very sensitive to motion artifact.
- CVP correlates with right atrial pressure, which correlates with the volume reaching the right atrium during diastole (preload). Ideally, CPV should be 4 to 8 cm of water. CVP will be falsely elevated in any condition that increases intrathoracic pressure (e.g., positive pressure ventilation, pneumothorax). If a jugular catheter is not present, then jugular distention and filling should be evaluated.
- If an indwelling urinary catheter is in place, then the patient should be producing a minimum of 1 ml/kg body weight of urine per hour. If a catheter is not present and abdominal surgery is being performed, then the surgeon should be asked to monitor the urinary bladder for signs of urine production. This helps confirm adequate BP and circulating blood volume.
- An ECG allows monitoring of electrical rhythm only; therefore it is a vital tool for detecting arrhythmias but may not correlate with cardiac function. Changes in the ST segment and T wave configuration can be used to determine the possible myocardial hypoxia. The anesthetist must be able to identify sinus tachycardia, sinus bradycardia, atrioventricular block (first, second, and third degree), VPCs, atrial fibrillation, and ventricular fibrillation. Arrhythmias noted on the ECG can be confirmed by auscultation with an esophageal auscultation. Electrical equipment, such as electrocautery, can interfere with the ECG.
- Mucous membrane color and capillary refill time should be monitored. Lingual pulse strength and rhythm should be compared with BP measurements and the ECG.

Temperature

Temperature is best monitored by direct thermometry with a thermistor that attaches to physiologic recorders so that every few seconds the temperature is recorded and displayed. The thermistor is placed down the esophagus, rectum, or ear canal, or it is taped to the patient's toe web space (to allow core or peripheral temperature monitoring, respectively). Indoor-outdoor temperature probe devices can also be used to monitor temperature. Although these devices are much less expensive than thermistors, they but do not provide as accurate information and data cannot be recorded. However, indoor-outdoor temperature probes do allow simpler and more accurate temperature monitoring than simple rectal thermometers.

Teamwork in Anesthesia

The circulating veterinary technician, the anesthetist, the surgeon, and the surgical assistant must work together to treat the critically ill or injured patient. Constant communication must occur among team members. For example, if the anesthetist notices that the lingual pulses do not feel very strong, then the surgeon should be asked to inspect internal BP (i.e., aortic pulsation). If the surgeon feels that the tissues are starting to look pale, then he or she should ask the anesthetist to check vitals signs and perhaps a PCV.

Supportive Measures Needed during Anesthesia

Temperature Conservation and Preventing Hypothermia

Hypothermia can cause prolonged coagulation times and peripheral vasoconstriction leading to increased peripheral tissue acidosis secondary to anaerobic metabolism. Ventricular fibrillation and asystole may develop, starting at 28° C. Hypothermia should be avoided in a critical patient unless it is undergoing surgery that would benefit from induced hypothermia. Anesthetic requirements will decrease as the patient's temperature decreases.

The use of plastic wrap, bubble wrap, infrared heating lamp, warm irrigation fluids, warm IV fluids, hot-water circulating blankets, and warm-air circulating blankets can be used to reduce hypothermia. The patient should not be placed on a cold surface. Using warm water to perform the surgical scrub and avoiding overwetting the patient may help. Low-flow anesthesia will help slow the development of hypothermia, and the use of a heating circuit in the patient's anesthetic tubing is an excellent way to decrease heat loss during anesthesia. Care always

should be taken with any item used to supply supplemental heat to ensure it does not cause burns. All warm water bottles and warm-water circulating blankets should be covered in a towel before placement next to the patient.

Fluid Support

Fluid therapy is much more important for the critically ill or injured patient under anesthesia than for the healthy patient, but the endpoints are the same. The goal of fluid therapy is to maintain an adequate circulating blood volume, adequate hemoglobin levels, and adequate clotting factors. Crystalloids are redistributed primarily to the interstitium; if increased intravascular volume is required, then a combination of colloids, both synthetic and biologic, and crystalloids are indicated. The PCV ideally should be maintained at a minimum of between 25% and 30%. Albumin levels should be maintained above 2.0 g/dl using plasma. If albumin levels are low and the patient is not hemodynamically stable, then synthetic colloids, such as hetastarch, Dextran 70, or human albumin should be infused.

Based on normal fluid requirements and evaporative fluid losses under anesthesia (with major body cavities opened), a maintenance rate of 10 ml/kg/hr of a balanced electrolyte solution should be administered. If major body cavities are not open, then the rate generally can be decreased by 50% (based on studies in dogs). The authors are not aware of any cat studies, but it seems logical that the rate requirements might be slightly less. If the patient has significant heart or liver disease, then it may be important to use a half-strength sodium solution to avoid sodium (and thus fluid) overload.

If the patient is hypoglycemic, glucose should be supplemented in the fluids, and dextrose supplementation should be considered in any patient when it is anticipated the patient might become hypoglycemic during the procedure. This includes patients with liver disease, endotoxemia, and all pediatric patients. If the patient is significantly hypokalemic, then potassium should be supplemented to help with muscle strength, cardiac function, and to avoid prolonging the effects of drugs such as neuromuscular blockers. If potassium is being supplemented, then the potassium level must not be allowed to rise above normal, and intraoperative monitoring of serum potassium levels may be indicated.

Special Considerations

Sight Hounds

Sight hounds tend to have prolonged recovery for several reasons; they have less body fat than many breeds, and drugs that are redistributed such as thiobarbiturates will have a prolonged effect. They have decreased hepatic microsomal enzyme activity, which will prolong the effects of any drugs metabolized in the liver. Sight hounds also tend to have decreased plasma protein levels, which increase the concentration of the active form of some anesthetics. Although it is always safer to use drugs that require minimal hepatic metabolism, in general, similar drugs can be used in sight hounds as in other breeds. Neuroleptanalgesia combinations of opioids and diazepam can be used (as well as ketamine and diazepam) and inhalants such as isoflurane and sevoflurane. The difference is that the dose should be reduced. Propofol causes similar effects in sight hounds as it does in other breeds. Although the recovery period is longer for sight hounds receiving propofol than it is for other breeds, it appears to be a safe anesthetic agent to use.

Cesarean Section

The important factors in choosing an anesthetic protocol relate as much to familiarity with the technique as the drugs that are used. Hypothermia, hypoxia, and hypotension should be avoided as for any patient. Barbiturates should be avoided in cesarean section, because they readily cross the placenta. Epidural anesthesia is considered the most beneficial method, but postoperative paralysis may be undesirable. The combination of propofol and isoflurane has been shown to be as acceptable (in terms of survival of the offspring) as an epidural. Because of the lack of analgesic effects of these drugs, analgesics should be administered once the puppies or kittens have been delivered. Neuromuscular blocking agents, in general, will not cross the placental barrier because of their large size. To avoid overdosing the dam, she should be dosed according her lean body weight, minus the offspring.

Anesthetic Emergencies and Complications

Any complications that can arise during general anesthesia of the healthy patient can occur in the critical patient under anesthesia (Table 10-2). Of course the best treatment is prevention. The following section focuses on complications specific to critically ill or injured patients and problems that may pose more of a risk to these patients in the intraoperative or perioperative period. Hypoventilation and severe hypotension probably are the two most important complications. If these problems are left unresolved, then they can lead to respiratory and cardiac arrest. If even moderate hypotension is allowed to persist for short periods of time, then significant postoperative morbidity can occur.

Anesthetic drugs, central nervous system disease, airway obstruction, space-occupying intrathoracic masses, pneumothorax (either from the injury or secondary to volutrauma or barotrauma), severe abdominal distention (e.g., gastric dilation volvulus, severe ascites), musculoskeletal disease, obesity, and body position can all cause hypoventilation. If a ventilator is being used, then the cause may be inappropriate ventilator settings, air leak in the system (endotracheal tube cuff, anesthetic hoses), lack of O_2 in tank, airway obstruction, or resistance to lung expansion.

An increase in the respiratory rate or ventilatory effort is not always the result of the patient becoming more aware; therefore deepening the level of anesthesia may be disastrous for the patient. Pain or hypercarbia secondary to hypotension with inadequate pulmonary circulation, airway obstruction, or pulmonary or pleural space disease are the most common causes. Other causes of increased ventilatory rate or effort include hypoxia, opioid pant, hyperthermia, and pressure buildup in the rebreathing bag.

Pneumothorax may occur secondary to volutrauma or barotrauma from artificial ventilation. Clinical signs include hypotension, bradycardia, tachycardia, greater resistance to ventilation, cyanosis, a thoracic cage that does not deflate on expiration, loss of lung sounds on auscultation, SC emphysema, distended jugular veins, increased CVP, and decreased Doppler flow sounds. If the clinician suspects that the patient has pneumothorax, then a thoracentesis should be performed immediately.

Hypotension generally is caused by hypovolemia or anesthetic drugs (leading to bradycardia or vasodilation). The hypovolemia may be an actual volume deficit as occurs with severe blood loss. It can be the result of a relative blood loss that occurs when a patient with a large abdominal mass or a gravid uterus is placed in dorsal recumbency. The

Text continued on p. 163.

TABLE 10-2

Anesthetic Complications

Cause	Diagnostic Test	Treatment
Anaphylaxis*		
Drug induced	Clinical signs (hypotension, facial edema)	Discontinue drug Treat for allergic reaction
Perivascular injection		
Perivascular administration of drug	Clinical sign (perivascular swelling)	Dilute with saline 5-10 × volume (+/− sodium bicarbonate)
Regurgitation/vomiting		
Decreased lower esophageal sphincter (LES) tone Drug-induced	Clinical sign	Suction +/− Nasal irrigation +/− Lavage esophagus +/− Nasogastric tube placement Extubate with cuff partially inflated
Air embolism*		
Vessel or vascular sinus open to air Pneumocystogram	Severe bradycardia progressing to asystole	Position patient so that air floats to apex of heart and aspirate Consider hyperbaric oxygen (O_2)
Malignant hyperthermia*		
Succinylcholine Inhalant anesthetics	Rectal temperature Electrolytes, blood gas	Provide 100% O_2 Discontinue anesthetic Active cooling Dantrolene 3 mg/kg via IV administration
Cyanosis		
Lack of O_2 supply	Check O_2 tanks and flowmeter	Provide 100% O_2
Airway obstruction	Check endotracheal tube Auscult lungs†	Unkink, suction or replace as indicated
Pulmonary failure	Auscult lungs† Arterial blood gas	Increase peak inspiratory pressure (PIP), respiratory rate, positive end expiratory pressure
Inadequate pulmonary circulation secondary to hypotension, pneumothorax, or pericardial tamponade	Auscult lungs† Check blood pressure (BP) Check for jugular distention Check end-tidal carbon dioxide (ETCO$_2$)	Correct underlying cause
Lack of thoracic expansion		
Hypoventilation	See causes of hypoventilation	Correct underlying cause
Barotrauma and pneumothorax	Auscult lungs Check for jugular distention Perform thoracentesis	Perform thoracentesis

*Rare complication; †using esophageal stethoscope.

TABLE 10-2

Anesthetic Complications—cont'd

Cause	Diagnostic Test	Treatment
Hypoventilation		
Anesthetic drugs	Check drug doses	Decrease drugs Discontinue inhalant temporarily Positive pressure ventilation
Airway obstruction Pneumothorax	Check endotracheal tube and hoses Auscult lungs Check for jugular distention Perform thoracentesis	Unkink, suction or replace as indicated Perform thoracentesis
Body position		Loosen limb restraints Alter position if possible
Ventilator problems (inappropriate settings, air leak, lack of O_2)	Check ventilator settings Check for air leak in cuff, hoses	Correct underlying problem
Need for increased PIP		
Airway obstruction	Check endotracheal tube and hoses	Unkink, suction, or replace as indicated
Underlying pulmonary disease (space-occupying mass, fibrosis)	Arterial blood gas	Consider increasing PIP, respiratory rate, or allowing permissive hypercapnia
Barotrauma and pneumothorax	Auscult lungs Check jugular distention Perform thoracentesis	Perform thoracentesis
Decreased oxygen saturation measured by pulse oximetry (SpO_2)		
Insufficient O_2	Check O_2 supply and flowmeter	Provide 100% O_2
Esophageal or bronchial intubation	Visualization, auscult lungs Check $ETCO_2$	Reposition tube
Obstructed endotracheal tube	Check tube	Replace tube
Poor perfusion	Check BP	Correct hypotension
Sensor malfunction	Check tongue clip Arterial blood gas	Reapply clip, moisten tongue Change sensor
Bronchospasm	Tachypnea Auscultation Response to treatment	Treat with bronchodilator
Aspiration pneumonia	Check oral cavity, pharynx, and endotracheal tube	Suction airway
Severe anemia	Check mucous membranes and packed cell volume (PCV)	Blood transfusion

Continued.

TABLE 10-2

Anesthetic Complications—cont'd

Cause	Diagnostic Test	Treatment
Decreased ETCO$_2$		
Hyperventilation	Check ventilation Auscult lungs Check thoracic expansion Check pain	Correct underlying problem
Esophageal or bronchial intubation	Visualization, auscultation	Reposition tube
Obstructed endotracheal tube	Check tube	Replace tube
Poor pulmonary circulation	Check for lung overinflation Check BP	Decrease ventilation Correct hypotension
Pulmonary or pleural space disease	Arterial blood gas	Ventilate based on blood gas
Ventilation perfusion mismatch		Treat underlying problem
Increased ETCO$_2$		
Hypoventilation	Check ventilation Auscult lungs Check thoracic expansion	Correct underlying problem
Carbon dioxide (CO$_2$) absorber not working	Check CO$_2$ absorber	Change absorber
Increased dead space	Tachypnea Check inspired CO$_2$ level Check anesthesia circuit	Increase or institute ventilation Consider neuromuscular blocker Correct underlying problem
Lung disease	History Auscult lungs Blood gas	Alter ventilation parameters Treat underlying disease
Moisture in sensor	Check sensor and tubing	Replace
Hypertension		
Underlying disease	Systolic >180 mm Hg	Increase dose of inhalant
Drug induced	Diastolic >120 mm Hg	Consider nitroprusside
Hypotension		
Hypovolemia	Check BP Check lingual pulses	Colloid and crystalloid administration
Too deep a plane of anesthesia	Check vaporizer settings	Adjust settings
Inadequate preload from pressure on vena cava	Check underlying disease	Increase fluids Correct underlying disease
Bradycardia	Check heart rate	Increase fluids Correct underlying disease
Poor cardiac contractility	Check heart rhythm	Dobutamine infusion Antiarrhythmic drugs
Refractory vasodilation	Rule out other causes	Dopamine at vasopressor doses
Peripheral vasoconstriction, hypothermia	Check temperature	Warm patient

TABLE 10-2

Anesthetic Complications—cont'd

Cause	Diagnostic Test	Treatment
Severe hypotension (arrest pending)		
Severe hypovolemia	Check BP	Discontinue anesthetic agents
Cardiac failure	Check heart rate and	Fluid resuscitation
Extreme depth of anesthesia	electrocardiogram (ECG)	Surgeon to place pressure on cranial
	Check ETCO$_2$	abdominal aorta if abdomen open
		Positive inotropic and vasopressor
		support
Bradycardia		
Too deep a plane of anesthesia	Check anesthetic depth	Decrease or discontinue drugs
		Atropine
Opioids		Atropine 0.04 mg/kg IV*
Severe hypotension	Check BP	Discontinue anesthetic agents
	Check heart rate and ECG	Fluid resuscitation
	Check ETCO$_2$	Surgeon to place pressure on cranial
		abdominal aorta if abdomen open
		Positive inotropic and vasopressor
		support
Surgical manipulation of vagus nerve or organs innervated by vagus nerve	Check with surgeon	Decrease surgical stimulation
Tachycardia		
Pain	Check level of anesthesia/analgesia	Administer analgesics
Hypoxia	Check for airway obstruction	Unkink, suction, or replace as indicated
	Check for tension pneumothorax or mediastinum from barotrauma	Thoracentesis
Supraventricular tachycardia		
Idiopathic	Check ECG	Treat underlying problem
Heart disease		Diltiazem
Pulmonary disease		Avoid beta blockers
Pain		

*High-end doses of atropine (0.05-0.2 mg/kg IV) should be used because lower doses may lead to a second-degree atrioventricular block and worsening of the problem. If the patient does not respond, the clinician should consider doses up to 0.5 mg/kg IV or epinephrine to effect (beginning at 0.001 mg/kg/min).

Continued.

TABLE 10-2

Anesthetic Complications—cont'd

Cause	Diagnostic Test	Treatment
Multifocal ventricular premature contractions (VPCs), ventricular tachycardia		
Myocardial hypoxia (traumatic myocarditis)	Check ECG Check BP Check central venous pressure (CVP) Check electrolytes	Ensure O$_2$ being provided Ensure appropriate analgesia Ensure adequate volume Lidocaine 2 mg/kg followed by constant rate infusion (CRI) at 25-75 μg/kg/min If unresponsive, consider procainamide 6-8 mg/kg over 5 min followed by CRI at 15-40 μg/kg/min or magnesium sulfate at 1 mEq/kg over 30 min
Splenic disease	Check ECG Check BP Check electrolytes	As in previous section
Acidosis	Check ETCO$_2$ Check blood gas Check BP Check CVP Check electrolytes	Improve perfusion Antiarrhythmic drugs as in previous section
Sinus arrest, severe or second-degree atrioventricular block		
	Check ECG	Atropine 0.05-0.2 mg/kg IV*
High CVP		
Hypervolemia	Check CVP	Diuretics Decrease or stop fluids
Pneumothorax, pneumomediastinum	Auscult lungs Check jugular distention Perform thoracentesis	Thoracentesis
Pericardial tamponade	Auscult heart Check ECG	Pericardiocentesis
Low CVP		
Hypovolemia	Recheck CVP Check BP	Increase fluid administration
Pallor		
Anemia	Check PCV	Blood transfusion
Hypotension	Check BP	Blood transfusion
Hypothermia and vasoconstriction	Check temperature Check ECG	Warm patient Correct arrhythmias

*High-end doses of atropine (0.05-0.2 mg/kg IV) should be used because lower doses may lead to a second-degree atrioventricular block and worsening of the problem. If the patient does not respond, the clinician should consider doses up to 0.5 mg/kg IV or epinephrine to effect (beginning at 0.001 mg/kg/min).

pressure on the vena cava in these patients can cause partial occlusion of the vessel. In a small percentage of patients, cardiac arrhythmias may be the cause. Primary signs of hypotension include an increasing heart rate (assuming the baroreceptor reflex has not been overridden), vasoconstriction, poor pulses, decreasing $ETCO_2$, and signs of deepening anesthesia.

Anesthetic drugs, hypoxemia, hypotension, hypothermia, acidosis, anemia, hyperthermia, toxemia, and cardiac trauma usually cause cardiac arrhythmias that appear when patients are under anesthesia. They must be identified rapidly and treated accordingly.

Postoperative Analgesia and Ventilatory and Cardiopulmonary Support

Critically ill or injured patients should be kept on O_2 until they are extubated. The patient should be monitored during trials on room air via pulse oximetry or arterial blood gases for signs of hypoxemia and hypercarbia. If hypoxia is present, the patient may need to be placed on supplemental O_2 and a nasopharyngeal or nasotracheal O_2 tube may be indicated. To place a nasopharyngeal catheter, the tube is premeasured from the naris to the lateral canthus of the eye. (This location allows the patient to tolerate higher concentrations of O_2 than a tube measured to the medial canthus of the eye.) Nasotracheal intubation helps to decrease the work of breathing in patients with upper airway compromise who otherwise would have increased respiratory effort. If the patient is significantly hypercarbic (especially in the face of hypoxemia), then continued ventilatory support may be needed.

The patient should be kept intubated until it is able to maintain a normal $ETCO_2$ level and shows signs of a strong gag response. The cuff should remain inflated until the time of extubation. Regurgitation and aspiration may occur during the recovery period, and it is important that the airway be kept protected. If evidence of regurgitation is seen, the oropharynx should be suctioned (along with the esophagus if a large amount of liquid is present), and the tube should be removed with the cuff partially inflated.

Patients should be aggressively rewarmed if they are hypothermic, being careful to ensure burns do not occur. Vital signs, including BP, should be checked every 5 to 10 minutes until the patient is sternal. The patient should not be left unattended until it is sternal. Fluid support should be continued as required to maintain normal CVP and urine production. Any positive inotrope, vasopressor, or antiarrhythmic drugs should be continued as required to maintain normal BP and cardiac rhythm.

Analgesia is vitally important in the postoperative period, and the patient should be given medication according to need (not a set schedule). Often CRIs are required and doses may need to be reduced. A syringe pump is recommended. Regional and epidural analgesia can be repeated postoperatively as required.

These patients often have received a number of drugs and large amounts of fluids during anesthesia. Significant metabolic abnormalities may have occurred secondary to the underlying disease. Laboratory tests should be checked in the immediate postoperative period, including a minimum of a PCV, total solids, glucose, albumin, electrolytes, and venous or arterial blood gas. Abnormalities should be corrected as indicated.

Suggested Readings

Funkquist PM, Nyman GC, Lofgren AJ et al: Use of propofol-isoflurane as an anesthetic regimen for cesarean section in dogs, *J Am Vet Med Assoc* 211:313-317, 1997.

Hendrix K, Raffe MR, Robinson EP et al: Epidural administration of bupivacaine, morphine or their combination for postoperative analgesia in dogs, *J Am Vet Med Assoc* 209:598-607, 1996.

Ilkiw JE, Pascoe PJ, Haskins SC et al: Cardiovascular and respiratory effects of propofol administration in hypovolemic dogs, *Am J Vet Res* 53:2323, 1992.

Lukasik V: Neuromuscular blocking drugs and the critical care patient, *JVECC* 5:99-113, 1993.

Marshall M: Capnography in dogs, *Compend Contin Educ Pract Vet* 26:761-778, 2004.

Mazzaferro E: Hypotension during anesthesia in dogs and cats; recognition and treatment *Compend Contin Educ Pract Vet* 23:728-736, 2001.

McCrackin MA, Harvey RC, Sackman JE et al: Butorphanol tartrate for partial reversal of oxymorphone-induced postoperative respiratory depression in the dog, *Vet Surg* 23:67-74, 1994.

Miller RD: *Miller's anesthesia*, ed 6, Philadelphia, 2005, Elsevier.

Spoonamore G: Epidural anesthesia: backing up pain relief, *Vet Tech* 25(3):168-175, 2004.

Tefend M: Hemodynamic monitoring of critically ill patients, *Vet Tech* 25(7):468-480, 2004.

11

Isolation Techniques in Clinical Practice

Ed Park

Isolating a small animal patient is sometimes a necessary requirement in emergency and critical-care medicine. Patients are isolated in clinical practice for several reasons, including the following:

- To prevent the spread of infectious diseases
- To protect immunocompromised patients from developing secondary infections that may be nosocomial in origin
- To protect patients who may be sensitive to sensory stimuli (e.g., visual, auditory, olfactory) in association with particular disease states
- To protect other patients in the hospital from a disruptive patient

For veterinary hospitals to provide the best care for patients who need to be isolated, an area must be available to allow them to be physically separated from other patients. However, like other critical patients, they require careful monitoring. Oftentimes the tendency exists for patients who are not in the immediate vicinity (i.e., away from the intensive care unit [ICU]) to be unintentionally ignored for long periods at a time. Whether or not this factor may contribute to the mortality of isolated patients has never been qualified; however, it cannot be emphasized enough that these patients must never be overlooked.

The following text describes five levels of isolation in clinical practice, and each of these levels is explored in this chapter. The reader should note that the classification used in this section does not represent an official classification used by a recognized international medical organization but should serve more as a guideline.

Level V

Level V isolation entails the isolation of a patient who has been diagnosed or is of high clinical suspicion of having a highly infectious disease. Infectious diseases comprise conditions that are caused by an organism that may be easily transmissible from one animal to another. The most common routes of horizontal transmission are fecal-oral, aerosol, bite-salivary, urine, and less commonly, through transfusions or dermal contact. People who are in contact with animals with potentially infectious diseases should ideally wear proper isolation disposable attire consisting of the following:

- Long-sleeve isolation gowns
- Gloves
- Shoe covers
- Mask
- Caps

In addition to isolation attire, personnel who are in contact with animals in isolation should also ideally have limited contact to the other animals in the hospital. If this is not possible, then personnel should make all attempts to try to handle animals with infectious diseases last.

Whenever a patient with a potentially infectious disease is admitted, proper procedure should be used before allowing entrance of a patient into the hospital. Personnel who will be allowed come in contact with these animals should have proper isolation attire *before* handling the patient. In addition, entrance into the isolation facility should be separate from the main entrance to prevent potential contamination of the waiting area and other parts of the hospital. Typically, the isolation area will be outfitted with its own examination and treatment equipment that should never leave the isolation area except for routine maintenance and cleaning. The most important items that all isolation units should have include the following:

- Examination table
- Scales
- Examination equipment (e.g., stethoscopes, thermometers, disposable gloves, hemostats, clippers, ear swabs, blood pressure monitoring devices, pulse oximeters, electrocardiogram machine)
- Treatment equipment (e.g., catheters, T-connectors, bandage material, extension sets, fluid bags, heating units, fluid pumps, syringes, emergency drugs, oxygen therapy, lab materials)

Many hospitals use the practice of using disposable equipment from outside the isolation facility—a technique that is acceptable under the premise that

---

BOX 11-1

Common Infectious Diseases Seen in Clinical Practice

Dogs
- Canine parvovirus
- Canine distemper
- *Bordatella bronchiseptica*
- Canine influenza

Cats
- Feline upper respiratory infection
- Feline infectious peritonitis (FIP)
- Feline panleukopenia (feline distemper)

---

the disposable equipment should not be allowed to reenter the rest of the hospital.

Many infectious diseases warrant the hospitalization of patients in the isolation unit. Although the list in Box 11-1 is by no means complete, it highlights the most common infectious diseases seen in clinical practice.

Canine Parvovirus

Canine parvovirus is an infectious viral disease of dogs that is typically transmitted through fecal-oral contact. On infection of a dog with parvovirus, the virus replicates itself in various lymphoid tissues before systemic dissemination. The virus itself requires actively dividing cells to replicate, because it lacks its own ability to do so. As a result, the cells that are most susceptible to parvovirus are the crypt cells of the gastrointestinal (GI) tract, cells of the bone marrow, and in very young puppies (less than 6 weeks of age), the myocardium (the muscle cells of the heart). Typically, the time from initial infection to the time of active fecal shedding of the virus is anywhere from 5 to 12 days. The clinical course of the disease will last on average, from 1 to 2 weeks. The diagnosis of parvovirus in clinical practice is readily made through the in-house snap test (IDEXX, Westbrook, Maine) that involves taking a sample of the animal's fecal material onto a cotton swab. Keeping in mind that recently vaccinated animals can have weak positive results is important. It is also important to understand that infected dogs that are early in the clinical course of the disease may have false negatives; thus retesting all animals that may have initial negative results is important. The classic clinical signs of parvovirus infection are bloody diarrhea (often foul smelling), vomiting, severe dehydration, lethargy, anorexia, weight loss, and in severe cases, sepsis. Less common clinical findings include signs of congestive heart failure and also an abdominal mass effect as the result of an intussusception. Treatment for parvovirus consists of IV isotonic fluids, systemic antibiotics, GI protectants, antiemetics, plasma transfusions, and introducing enteral nutrition when the puppies are able to tolerate it. The prognosis for parvovirus is guarded to poor, and animals with parvovirus commonly remain in the hospital from 3 to 10 days. The virus is relatively hardy in the environment, and the only effective disinfectant for destroying the virus is bleach.

Canine Distemper

Canine distemper is a multisystemic infectious disease that is rare because of widespread vaccination. The disease is most prevalent in young, unvaccinated dogs, and the clinical signs associated with this disease are variable. Most canine distemper infections are likely subclinical or characterized by mild upper respiratory signs that resolve without treatment. In other dogs, patients have nonneurologic signs with ocular or nasal discharge (or both), dyspnea, coughing, vomiting, and diarrhea. Neurologic signs include seizures (appearance can vary depending on the region of the brain involved), vestibular and cerebellar signs (e.g., ataxia, nystagmus, head tilt), and paresis. Diagnosis of this disease is dependent on a consistent history (i.e., respiratory or GI signs preceding neurologic signs), clinical suspicion, physical examination, and laboratory findings. Immunofluorescence of conjunctival smears of affected animals may detect infection early in the course of the disease. After the early stage, diagnosis may be obtained using viral detection in respiratory epithelium (from transtracheal wash samples) and from immunologic detection of biopsies of skin and footpads. Blood tests (using reverse-transcriptase polymerase chain reaction) and cerebrospinal fluid taps can also aid in the diagnosis of canine distemper. The treatment of canine distemper is typically palliative and unrewarding, because progressive neurologic disease typically results in death or humane euthanasia. The best treatment for this disease is prevention through proper vaccination.

Bordatella Bronchiseptica *Pneumonia*

Bordatella bronchiseptica, the causative agent of kennel cough in dogs, usually results in upper respiratory signs. The cough is usually a loud, hacking, unproductive cough that can be induced in animals with tracheal stimulation. Dogs that have recently come into contact with infected dogs (usually while being boarded, in a common play area, or at a shelter or pet store) are at risk of contracting the disease. Kennel cough is a relatively common disease in clinical practice and is usually treated with Clavamox or another antibiotic that is effective against the gram-positive organism. Technicians that are responsible for triaging incoming patients should remove dogs with a loud hacking cough, unless they are dyspneic, away from other dogs in the waiting room. One of the complications of kennel cough occurs when the organism spreads to the lower respiratory system, resulting in pneumonia. Animals with pneumonia typically will have fevers, crackles on lung auscultation, noticeable dyspnea (e.g., open-mouth breathing, extended neck, elbows adducted, abdominal component to breathing), and a loud hacking cough that may or may not be productive. It should be mentioned that not all dogs with pneumonia are infected with *B. bronchiseptica*; therefore these patients are usually not immediately placed in isolation unless the clinical history is suspicious for the disease. The diagnosis of pneumonia is derived from clinical suspicion and thoracic radiographs. As with any dyspneic patient, radiographs are taken when patients are able to tolerate this procedure. Classically, pneumonia in dogs in characterized by alveolar and interstitial pattern with air bronchograms present; the air bronchograms signify the presence of fluid or cells around airways. If the patient is stable enough to undergo sedation for a transtracheal wash, then the procedure should ideally be performed before starting antibiotic therapy. The sample derived from a transtracheal wash is submitted for both cytology and culture and sensitivity; the culture results of which can confirm the diagnosis of *B. bronchiseptica* pneumonia. Patients with confirmed *Bordatella* pneumonia should be placed in an isolation unit that can provide oxygen therapy if needed. Treatment for *Bordatella* pneumonia consists of antibiotics (initially a broad-spectrum antibiotic is chosen but may be altered based on culture results), IV fluids, saline nebulization, coupage, and oxygen therapy (either through nasal or cage) if necessary.

Prognosis for patients with pneumonia is guarded, and therapy with antibiotics is typically over a long course (typically 4 to 6 weeks). Clinical improvement of pneumonia proceeds radiographic improvement; radiographic improvement may not occur for several weeks after the initiation of therapy.

Canine Influenza

Canine influenza is a newly emerging respiratory infection of dogs and is caused by a virus that is believed to have mutated from the equine influenza virus. The disease was first discovered in racing greyhounds in Florida early in 2004; however, the virus has now been diagnosed in many other states since being first recognized. Canine influenza is typically spread between dogs via respiratory secretions; however, transmission of the virus can also occur through fomite transmission from contaminated objects. The clinical syndrome induced by canine influenza occurs in one of two forms: (1) mild and (2) severe. Clinical infection with the mild form involves a wet or dry cough (the dry cough is similar to that seen in kennel cough). Like other respiratory viral infections, infected dogs are more susceptible to the development of secondary bacterial infections; thus mucopurulent nasal discharge may be a clinical feature of the mild form. Infection with the severe form of canine influenza is characterized by moderate to severe fever, along with signs consistent with pneumonia (e.g., dyspnea, tachypnea, crackles on auscultation). Diagnosis of the disease involves clinical suspicion along with viral antibody testing (antibodies to the virus can be present 7 days after infection). The mild form of canine influenza must be differentiated from kennel cough; the distinction may be difficult to make, however, because considerable overlap of clinical signs exists. Treatment for canine influenza is largely symptomatic and typically consists of IV fluids, oxygen therapy (if needed), coupage and nebulization therapy (in cases of pneumonia), and antibiotics (to treat secondary bacterial infections). Most cases of canine influenza are that of the mild form, and the current mortality rate in dogs is less than 10%.

Feline Upper Respiratory Infection

Upper respiratory infections are common in cats, and the two most prevalent viruses responsible for these infections are feline herpes virus and feline calicivirus. These viruses comprise 90% of feline upper respiratory infections (URIs); less common causes include infections with *Bordatella bronchiseptica*, *Chlamydophila felis*, or mycoplasma. Cats are usually infected after contact with clinically affected cats, fomites, or carrier cats (cats that are not clinically affected but are shedding the virus). After a state of clinical infection, cats may remain carriers for months to years. Clinical signs of feline URI in the acute stage include fever, sneezing, nasal or ocular discharge (serous to mucopurulent in nature), anorexia, and dehydration. Chronic disease is characterized by chronic nasal discharge (usually secondary to damage to the upper respiratory passage) and sneezing. Feline calicivirus can cause oral ulcerations, pneumonia, and joint disease, whereas feline herpes virus can cause corneal disease and miscarriage in pregnant queens. The diagnosis of feline URI is made through history, physical examination, and by ruling out other causes of chronic nasal discharge. Immunologic testing can be performed to identify the infectious organisms from conjunctival, pharyngeal, or tonsillar specimens. Treatment for feline URI is typically supportive, and most cases will resolve without therapy. Supportive care for infected cats includes fluid therapy, nebulization, periodically clearing nasal secretions, and antibiotics (to treat secondary bacterial infections). The prognosis for cats with URI is good; cats with chronic disease may need periodic symptomatic care, and owners should be made aware that infected cats may periodically have bouts of respiratory disease.

Feline Infectious Peritonitis

Feline infectious peritonitis (FIP) is a fatal disease that is caused by a coronavirus that has undergone mutation to a more virulent form in affected cats. Normally, when corona viruses clinically affect cats, the disease produces diarrhea that results from the loss of the normal villous epithelium in the GI tract (the villous epithelium is required for GI nutrient and water absorption). Through mechanisms that are not completely understood, coronaviruses that cause clinical FIP undergo a genetic mutation to a more virulent form. FIP produces two clinical syndromes: (1) the dry form and (2) the wet form. The wet form of FIP is the form that is more clinically prevalent and is called such because of the effusions associated with this syndrome. The effusions may be pleural or abdominal in nature (usually a modified transudate). The fluid removed from cats with FIP usually has a yellow, viscous consistency; on microscopic examination the fluid is characterized by a sterile, pyogranulomatous nature. The dry form of FIP is characterized by neurologic signs (e.g., depression, seizures) and is caused by the inflammation of the brain and its choroid plexus (the structures in the brain that produce cerebrospinal fluid). The diagnosis of FIP is difficult, and the only definitive diagnosis involves histopathologic analysis of postmortem samples. Detecting coronavirus is a cat with possible FIP is not diagnostic for the disease, because non-FIP cats can have coronaviruses in their fecal matter. A cat that is febrile, with a high protein count caused by the hyperglobulinemia, as well as neurologic signs or abdominal and pleural effusions, should be suspected of having FIP. Other tests that can be performed to help increase the clinical suspicion include polymerase chain reaction on effusions, protein electrophoresis, and cerebrospinal fluid analysis. As previously mentioned, the only diagnostic method to confirm the diagnosis of FIP is on postmortem histopathology. Cat owners and shelter personnel should be encouraged to pursue a necropsy of cats with possible FIP to confirm the diagnosis (because the virus tends to be prevalent in catteries and other situations where multiple cats are housed together). The virus itself is very difficult to destroy, and all items that have come into contact with a cat confirmed to be FIP positive should be discarded. Unfortunately, the prognosis for cats with FIP is grave; supportive care consisting of fluids, steroids, and antibiotics is largely palliative.

During the admission of a patient classified under Level V, an alternative entrance from the one normally used for other patients should be used. Typically the alternative entrance is located in close proximity to the isolation unit to minimize the probability of contact of the patient with the rest of the ICU. Another common practice to minimize contact of an infected patient with random personnel in the ICU is to have the personnel responsible for handling Level V patients involved in their admission.

Personnel and materials used in the care of Level V isolated patients should enter and exit the unit in a one-directional pattern. The use of this technique helps to minimize the contamination and spread of infectious organisms within the isolation ward, as well as to the rest of the hospital. An effective technique that has used in practice is that of the *U* pattern, which is shown in Fig. 11-1.

Many variations to the technique are shown here. The main point, however, is the unidirectional movement of personnel and items through the isolation unit. Near the entrance of the unit, isolation attire consisting of disposable gowns, gloves, caps, and booties should be made available to personnel who are to handle isolated patients. Again, personnel who are to handle isolated patients should be restricted to handling only those patients. If this is not possible because of staffing, then isolated patients should be handled last to minimize any potential exposure of other patients to infectious organisms. When personnel are not directly handling isolation patients, monitoring devices should be installed in the isolation unit. The best monitoring devices consist of a camera with sound and zoom capabilities that allow real-time monitoring. It should emphasized that the availability of sound is extremely important, because alarm signals emitted by monitoring devices and fluid pumps will not be audible from a distance. Alternatively, windows can be used to allow monitoring of the isolated patients from outside the isolation ward; however, if this technique is chosen, then sound devices should also be installed to facilitate monitoring.

On average, most patients who are admitted into an isolation ward will stay between 3 to 7 days depending on the clinical course of the disease. Unfortunately, many of these patients do not survive the disease and are either humanely euthanized or succumb to the clinical course of the illness. Discharge of the isolated patient should occur from an exit that is separate from the exit used by other patients. The same port used for entry of the patient is typically used for this process.

Level IV

Level IV isolation involves the isolation of a patient with an infectious disease that requires the direct contact of a susceptible individual with secretions or bodily material to transmit infection. Oftentimes Level IV patients are not placed into an isolation facility (as are those requiring Level V isolation); however, precautions should be undertaken by personnel to prevent the spread of infectious disease. In the ideal situation, isolation gear such as gowns, gloves, caps, and booties should be worn when handling Level IV patients. Usually, however, only disposable gloves are used. Personnel handling Level IV

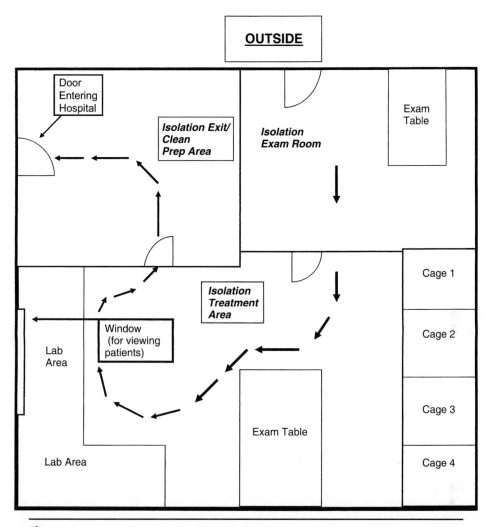

Fig. 11-1 Traffic Flow Diagram. The diagram represents the isolation area within a hospital. Many hospitals will not have the space to accommodate such a large unit but will be able to design a similar setup with the same type of traffic flow pattern. The flow of traffic is very important to eliminate the spread of infectious disease.

- The owner enters the examination room with the pet with the possible contagious disease from the outside entrance.
- The medical staff enters the examination room through the outside entrance with isolation attire including gowns, masks, and gloves. The pet is examined, and it is determined whether isolation will be necessary.
- The pet is moved into the isolation area by the medical staff only. Owners are not allowed to visit inside the isolation area. The medical staff puts shoe covers on before entering the isolation ward area.
- The flow of traffic continues to move in a *U*-shaped pattern, avoiding contamination of the entire area. The pet is not allowed beyond the treatment table.
- Gowns, gloves, masks, and shoe covers are disposed of at the entrance into the clean area. A change of clothes can be stored here. A footbath is placed at the exit door, and the medical staff steps into the footbath before entering the hospital area.
- A window is available to view the isolation patients (for medical observation or owner viewing). It helps control frequent traffic in and out of isolation.
- Isolation is entered only through the outside entrance.
- A videotape and sound monitor are in place to monitor the pet continuously while in the hospital.

patients should avoid handling other patients in the ICU. If this is not possible, then these patients should be handled last.

The following list comprises the most common clinical conditions under the Level IV designation:

Leptospirosis
Feline leukemia virus (FeLV)
Feline immunodeficiency virus (FIV)
Rabies
Toxoplasma gondii
Neospora caninum

Leptospirosis

Leptospira spp. are infectious organisms that are spread via contact of susceptible patients to the urine of infected animals; the organisms can also be spread via contact of susceptible patients to standing water or other aqueous sources. Several major serovars of *Leptospira* exist, not all of which are covered in the vaccine that is administered in clinical practice. The most recent Fort Dodge vaccine covers the following serovars:

- *Leptospira icterohemorragicae*
- *L. pomona*
- *L. hardjo*
- *L. canicola*

However, two other serovars *(Leptospira bratislava and L. autumnalis)* have been identified as causes of clinical disease in domestic species. The two organ systems that are most affected include the renal system and hepatic system. Clinically affected animals typically have signs of acute renal failure including lethargy, anorexia, vomiting, diarrhea, polyuria, and polydipsia. Affected animals may also have signs of hepatic disease such as icterus, lethargy, anorexia, vomiting, and diarrhea. The diagnosis of this disease is based on clinical suspicion, history, clinical signs, blood work, and response to therapy. When clinical suggestion of the disease occurs, blood tests should be submitted to evaluate for serum antibody titers in response to an active infection. It is not uncommon for patients to have a urinary catheter placed (especially when acute renal failure is present), which can help to prevent contaminated urine from spreading within the facility. The mainstay of treatment for Leptospirosis involves IV fluids along with antibiotic therapy; other supportive therapy (e.g., GI protectants) is given according to the clinical presentation of the patient. The prognosis of a patient with leptospirosis is guarded and patients who recover typically need to be placed on antibiotic therapy for at least 4 weeks. Care should be taken when handling patients with leptospirosis because a zoonotic disease may be transmitted to people. Gloves should be worn at all times when handling these patients.

Feline Leukemia Virus

Feline leukemia virus (FeLV) is an infectious disease of domestic and wild Felidae that is caused by a virus of the Retroviridae family. The virus itself is typically spread between cats via salivary contact and nasal secretions; thus mutual grooming and sharing of food or water sources are common methods of infection. Once infection occurs, the virus replicates in the oropharynx before systemic infection; eventually the virus will enter the bone marrow. Cats infected with FeLV can harbor the virus without clinical consequence for long periods. Clinically affected cats succumb to a number of clinical syndromes associated with the virus. The virus is capable of inducing anemia and leukopenia that can potentially make the cat susceptible to secondary infections. In addition to directly affecting blood cell lines, the virus can also predispose affected cats toward the development of lymphoma, a malignant tumor of lymphocytes. A FeLV vaccine is available for owners who wish to vaccinate their cats. Generally speaking, only cats that are at risk of contacting the infectious virus are recommended for vaccination; these cats include outdoor cats and cats exposed to cats that go outdoors. Although the vaccine has been associated with the development of sarcomas at the vaccination sites, it has been shown to prevent infection in approximately 90% of cats.

Feline Immunodeficiency Virus

Feline immunodeficiency virus (FIV) is an infectious disease of cats that is transmitted via bite wounds. A virus of the *Lentivirus* genus causes the disease. FIV is spread primarily through bite wounds, although the virus is present in semen of infected males and can be transmitted through insemination. Queens can also transmit the virus to kittens during pregnancy. The virus replicates in white blood cells (WBCs), specifically lymphocytes and macrophages, during the active phase of initial infection in which a low-grade fever, neutropenia, and reactive lymphandeonopathy can occur.

After the initial infection, the virus enters a variable latent state. Eventually, an immune deficiency state, similar to acquired immunodeficiency syndrome in people, can develop with concurrent infections exacerbating the clinical state of the patient. Clinical signs associated with FIV include fever, generalized lymph node enlargement, anorexia, uveitis, and weight loss; other clinical signs observed can vary depending on concurrent infections. The most common hematologic changes observed in clinically infected cats include neutropenia, thrombocytopenia, and anemia; chemistry panel changes are variable. The most common method of diagnosis is an in-house snap test (which also tests for FeLV). Kittens less than 180 days old should be tested every 60 days until results are negative (because colostrum-derived antibodies can result in a false-positive test). Isolating the virus and also performing polymerase chain reaction to test for the virus can aid in the diagnosis. A recently developed vaccine has been released by Fort Dodge for use in clinical practice. Various therapies including antiviral medications and other immunotherapies have been developed to treat both FeLV and FIV with variable success. The best therapy for FIV is through prevention via having cats housed indoors and FIV-positive cats placed into single-cat households. The virus itself is not easily spread through fomite contact, because the virus dies outside the host within minutes and is easily killed by disinfectants; therefore all items including dishes and boxes should be cleaned regularly with disinfectants and hot water when used by FIV-positive cats.

Rabies

Rabies is an infectious disease that affects all species and is spread by the bite of an animal that is infected with this fatal disease. The most common route of infection occurs via bite wounds from infected raccoons, skunks, foxes, and bats; transmission of the virus from bats, however, has been known to occur in the absence of a bite wound. The virus causes inflammation of the brain and spinal cord (a term that is referred to as *encephalomyelitis*) and must be differentiated from other diseases that cause this type of inflammation. With the widespread use of the rabies vaccine, rabies is fortunately rare; thus any unvaccinated animal that has progressive neurologic disease

(especially with a history of a bite wound) should be suspected of having rabies. An animal infected with rabies can have a variable incubation period (anywhere from 7 days onward) before the onset of clinical signs. The clinical signs of rabies can be variable and include depression, aggression, dysphagia, ataxia, paraparesis, tetraparesis, excessive salivation, and varying cranial nerve deficits. Ultimately, animals that are clinically infected with rabies will succumb within 7 days. Any personnel that come into contact with potentially infected animals should wear gowns, gloves, and masks. Viral shedding from infected animals can last up to 2 weeks before the onset of clinical signs. As a zoonotic disease, full precautions should be made in regard to handling these animals because of the public health considerations of this disease. Although diagnostic testing in the form of blood samples and cerebrospinal fluid samples may help in the diagnosis of this disease, definitive diagnosis can only be made via immunofluorescent antibody testing of brain samples. Although transfer of the virus between patients in a hospital facility is unlikely, many hospitals have gone to the practice of treating potential rabies patients as Level V patients; thus many of these animals are placed into a separate isolation facility. The typical in-hospital quarantine period for rabies observation is 10 days for a potentially infected animal; however, the time period for quarantine may be variable for each individual state.

Toxoplasmosis

Toxoplasma gondii is an infectious protozoa parasite that is a rare cause of clinical disease in an infected animal. The natural host of the parasite is the cat; thus shedding of the organism can occur only through the feces of a feline host. All other animals (including humans) that are infected by this organism cannot shed the organism and are referred to as *aberrant hosts*. In small animal practice, clinical infection from *Toxoplasma* affects multiple organs including the central nervous system (with varying clinical signs depending on the location of the CNS affected), muscles, eyes (particularly in cats), lungs, and liver. It should be noted that not all infected animals come down with clinical disease; clinical disease typically occurs in patients who are immunosuppressed and also in neonate patients. The diagnosis of toxoplasmosis can be difficult; typically, rising IgG antibody titers in two separate blood samples (or an elevated IgM antibody titer in a single sample) aids in the diagnosis. It should be noted that a positive IgG antibody titer does not confirm active infection; this finding only confirms exposure to the parasite. Treatment for infected animal involves administration of clindamycin or trimethoprim-sulfa for at least 1 month. Because of the zoonotic nature of toxoplasmosis, all personnel handling animals with confirmed toxoplasmosis should wear at gloves and other protective clothing. In addition, toxoplasmosis can cause miscarriage when infection occurs during pregnancy; this can also occur in humans. Therefore pregnant women should avoid handling cats that are shedding the organism and should also avoid handling feces of infected cats.

Neosporosis

Neospora caninum is an infectious protozoal parasite whose natural host is the dog. Clinical disease in infected dogs typically occurs in the form of neurologic signs with varying manifestations; neurologic signs associated with neosporosis include hind limb paresis, seizures, neuromuscular weakness, and cerebellar signs (e.g., nystagmus, hyperreflexia, truncal swaying). Infected bitches can also pass the parasite to offspring, and clinical neosporosis in puppies is typified by hind limb extension (because of muscle contraction and inflammation of the nerve roots to the hind limbs). Diagnosis of neosporosis in the live animal can be difficult, but rising antibody titers can be used to aid in the diagnosis. The diagnosis can be confirmed via immunocytochemical staining of tissue biopsies; this technique can also be used to differentiate *Neospora* from *Toxoplasma*. The treatment for neosporosis involves the administration of clindamycin for at least 1 month. The prognosis for clinically affected animals is poor.

All hospital personnel should identify patients with Level IV diseases using labeled signs on their cages. Another approach advocated with Level IV patients is to avoid placing infected animals adjacent to a cage in which an animal of the same species is located. Fomite transmission is not as likely with Level IV diseases as with Level V diseases. Nonetheless, hospital personnel must dispose of materials used in handling Level V patients and, most importantly, must wash the hands. In addition, once Level IV animals are discharged, cages where these animals are kept should be completely disinfected as with Level V diseases. Depending on the disease process, a certain period should be allowed to lapse before placing another patient in the same cage. On discharge, care should be taken to prevent the contact of these patients with other patients in the waiting room and discharge area.

Level III

Level III isolation involves the proper handling of patients who are susceptible to the development of infectious diseases (including nosocomial infections). Patients who fall into the Level III category include immunocompromised patients, patients with critical traumatic injuries, and patients in the postoperative period.

A patient who is immunocompromised implies a patient who is susceptible toward the development of secondary infections as a result of a disorder or dysfunction of the immune system. The most common reason for an immune system disorder is a WBC deficiency, a term that is referred to as *leukopenia*. Less commonly, patients can be immunocompromised as a result of a dysfunction in leukocyte function.

Patients with Leukopenia

The term *leukopenia* is defined as a deficiency in the total WBC count of a patient. WBCs play a critical role in the immune system; patients with leukocyte deficiency are at particular risk for developing infectious diseases, including nosocomial infections (i.e., infections that develop within the hospital facility). This is particularly critical when dealing with diseases in the Level V category. The most common reasons for leukopenia in veterinary patients include the following:

Patients Undergoing Chemotherapy. The term *chemotherapy* comprises the various oncologic treatment modalities used for the treatment of neoplasia. A large majority of these treatments inhibit the normal replication of deoxyribonucleic acid in fast-dividing cells (characteristic of malignant neoplasia). However, malignant neoplasia in cancer patients does not comprise the only population of fast-dividing cells. The other major populations of these cells include crypt cells of the GI epithelium and progenitor cells of the bone marrow. As a result, patients treated with chemotherapy are prone to develop leukopenia and GI signs including vomiting and diarrhea. Therefore caution should be taken when dealing with chemotherapy patients who develop leukopenia, because they will be prone toward the development of secondary infections. Sterile gloves should be worn when handling these patients; personnel handling patients with infectious diseases should avoid contact with immunosuppressed chemotherapy patients.

Special mention should also be made regarding the isolation of chemotherapy patients in the period immediately after therapy. Because chemotherapy patients will urinate radioactive particles for 24 hours after therapy, caution should be used when handling these patients. The cages of these patients should be properly disinfected after hospitalization, and cages should not be used in the immediate period after these patients are discharged.

Patients with Infectious Diseases. Leukopenia can also be observed in patients with overwhelming infections because of the consumption of WBCs in response to an infectious organism. The main WBCs used during an acute infection are neutrophils and macrophages; however, lymphocytes and eosinophils can also become decreased during an active infection. When the use of these white cells exceeds the host's ability to produce new WBCs, leukopenia results; thus the patient is predisposed toward developing other infections. As discussed previously, cats that are infected with FeLV and FIV are prone toward the eventual development of leukopenia. Therefore precautions should be taken toward avoiding contact of these patients with infectious diseases.

Patients with Bone Marrow Disorders. Disorders of the bone marrow such as neoplasia, immune-mediated diseases, infectious diseases, aplasia, and other degenerative disorders can also predispose a patient toward the development of leukopenia. The bone marrow is responsible for the production of WBCs (with the exception of lymphocytes), red blood cells, and platelets. Thus any disorder of the bone marrow can leads to the potential development of leukopenia, anemia, or thrombocytopenia (depending on the cell line that is affected). Therefore patients developing leukopenia secondary to a bone marrow disorder should avoid contact with patients with infectious diseases.

Patients on Immunosuppressive Medications

Patients diagnosed with immune-mediated disorders such as immune-mediated hemolytic anemia or immune-mediated thrombocytopenia are typically placed on a course of immunosuppressive medications for their disease syndromes. In addition, animals diagnosed with severe inflammatory diseases (which can be secondary to an infectious disease) are occasionally placed on immunosuppressive medications. These medications include prednisone, azathioprine, cyclosporine, and other medications. Each of these medications suppresses the host immune system through differing mechanisms. Although immunosuppression is necessary to control the systems of the immune-mediate disease process, use of these medications can predispose patients toward the development of infectious diseases. Thus care should be taken to minimize the exposure of patients taking immunosuppressant drugs to infectious disease.

Patients with Traumatic Open Injuries

Patients who sustain traumatic open wounds are prone toward the development of infections at the sites of injury. All open wounds, at the very minimum, are flushed thoroughly to maintain cleanliness at the wound site. Depending on the preference of the attending clinician, the wound may or may not be flushed with a disinfectant. Common disinfectants used in clinical practice include Nolvasan-based and iodine-based solutions. After disinfectant therapy, all wounds should be thoroughly flushed with a sterile, nondisinfecting solution such as sterile saline. Importantly, disinfecting solutions should not be allowed to remain at the wound site because these solutions may be irritating to the underlying tissues. Commonly, a sterile saline bag is attached with a three-way stopcock attached to an extension set with a syringe for flushing. An 18-gauge needle (or larger) is often attached to the syringe to promote high-flow wound flushing. High-flow flushing promotes the dislodging of particulate matter that may contaminate the wound and is generally more effective than low-flow therapy. After flushing, the wound may or may not be immediately débrided or closed. Closure depends on the type of wound involved and the size of the actual wound. For example, small puncture bite wounds are not routinely closed, because drainage through these wounds is encouraged. However, if the wound is large or has a significant pockets, closure often is performed with Penrose drains to promote drainage from the wound site. Although patients with traumatic open wounds are not isolated into a separate ward, care should be undertaken when handling these patients to minimize the chance of allowing infection to enter the wound site. Strict hygiene involving the washing of hands with a proper disinfectant should be undertaken before handling these patients and their wound sites (Table 11-1).

Postoperative Patients

Surgery is a form of controlled trauma, and care should be taken to minimize the exposure of these patients to infectious diseases, particularly in the immediate postoperative period. This type of care is especially critical with patients who have chest tubes placed postoperatively and with patients who have abdominal drainage (either open or closed) performed. Although most patients are placed on antibiotics postoperatively, precautions should be taken to avoid nosocomial infections from developing at the wound site. Likewise, it should be understood that many of these postoperative patients are in critical condition and thus may be immunosuppressed and susceptible toward the development of other disease processes. Stress should be minimized in postoperative patients to allow them the optimal chance to heal.

A few special precautions are typically made with regard to the admission of Level III patients. Patients who have traumatic open wounds should be triaged to the ICU for immediate evaluation, immediate therapy, or both. Patients who are actively bleeding should be immediately brought back to the ICU for immediate evaluation and intervention if needed. No special precautions are typically made when these patients are discharged.

Level II

Level II isolation involves the isolation of patients who may be sensitive to sensory stimuli as a result of a particular underlying condition. These stimuli include olfactory stimuli, visual stimuli, auditory stimuli, and in some cases, tactile stimuli. In an ideal setting, Level II patients should be kept in a quiet area to minimize their exposure to these stimuli. However, for practical reasons they are kept in the same arena as other patients to facilitate monitoring. No special consideration is given to the actual admission process of a Level II patient; however, special effort should be made to place Level II patients in a cage where the flow of traffic is relatively low.

The following list indicates some of the common conditions seen in clinical practice that would require Level II isolation:

Patients with Seizure Disorders

A seizure is a syndrome that results from excessive electrical activity in the brain (specifically the part of the brain known as the *prosencephalon*). Seizures are classified as *generalized seizures, partial seizures,* or *psychomotor seizures.* The type of seizure disorder present in a patient can vary based on multiple factors (e.g., underlying cause, severity and location of disease in the brain). Generalized seizures are characterized by increased muscle rigidity, paddling in all four limbs, lateral recumbency, loss of bowel or bladder control, and chomping movements of the mouth. A partial seizure has variable clinical signs such as focal twitching, focal muscle contraction, head turning toward one side, and other focal one-sided signs (i.e., signs that affect only one side of the body). Psychomotor seizures can also have variable manifestations such as bouts of altered behavior (e.g., aggression, rage, hysteria), biting motions in the air (fly biting), self-mutilation, and tail chasing; these seizures are characterized more by bizarre behavior changes than with abnormal movements of the body.

Seizures can last from just a few seconds to much longer periods at a time. The term *status epilepticus* is used to refer to patients who experience multiple seizures without an intervening period. This represents a true medical emergency that requires immediate stabilization, because these animals are at serious risk of developing hyperthermia, permanent neurologic damage, cardiac arrhythmias, pulmonary edema, and hypoxemia. After a seizure episode, patients commonly experience a clinical state known as the *postictal period,* a state in which patients are disoriented and may have residual neurologic deficits (e.g., blindness).

The primary differential diagnoses for seizures include the following:

- Idiopathic epilepsy (This is a condition mainly seen in dogs younger than 5 years of age.)
- Metabolic disorders (This includes disorders of hypoglycemia, hypocalcemia, hypertension, and a number of other metabolic abnormalities.)
- Trauma (Trauma to the cranial cavity is the main cause.)

TABLE 11-1

Disinfectants

Classification	Generic Name	Dilution	Contact Time	Activity	Comments
Quaternary Ammonium Compounds	KennelSol; Roccal-D	KennelSol (HC) & Roccal-D 1:256	10 minutes	Effective against both gram +, gram −, and enveloped viruses	Works against Canine Parvovirus Inactivated by soap
Hypochlorites	Household Bleach	1:32	10 minutes	Effective against enveloped and nonenveloped viruses, fungi, bacteria, and algae	Works against Canine Parvovirus High concentrations can be irritating to skin, eyes, and mucous membranes Once diluted, shelf-life is 24 hours
Alcohols	Alcohol	Not diluted	10-30 minutes	Effective against bacteria, fungal spores, and enveloped viruses	Typically used as a topical disinfectant Not effective against nonenveloped viruses
Chlorhexidine	Nolvasan	1 oz./1 gallon	5-10 minutes	Effective against bacteria, fungi, and most viruses	Not as effective as most other disinfectants Not toxic to animals
Iodine	Betadine-5%	Typically not diluted	10-30 minutes	Effective as bactericidal, sporicidal, virucidal, and fungicidal	Typically used as a topical disinfectant This product doesn't have cleaning compounds
Oxiding Agents	Hydrogen Peroxide	Not diluted	10-30 minutes	Effective against anaerobic bacteria	Not virucidal Mostly used for cleaning surgical sites
Phenolic Disinfectants	Pine-sol; Lysol	Not diluted	10-30 minutes	Effective against bacteria and enveloped viruses	Toxic to cats Great deodorizer

Courtesy Melissa Ambeau, LVT.

- Infectious diseases (These include viral [e.g., rabies, West Nile virus], bacterial, protozoal [e.g., *Neospora, Toxoplasma*], and fungal diseases [e.g., cryptococcus, blastomycoses].)
- Inflammatory disease (Inflammatory brain diseases can also result in seizures and include diseases such as granulomatous meningoencephalitis and other causes of encephalitis or meningitis.)
- Neoplasia (This is found particularly in older patients who do not have a previous seizure history.)
- Toxicity (The common toxicities include ethylene glycol, metaldehyde, chocolate, pyrethrins, and others.)

Whenever a patient arrives at the clinic seizing, an effort should be made to safely attempt IV catheterization. If IV catheterization is successful, then an anticonvulsant agent is administered to stop the seizure. The most common anticonvulsant used is diazepam at a dose of 0.5 mg/kg. The use of this agent should be avoided in patients with known hepatic disease, because metabolism of the drug can be prolonged. In this situation, another anticonvulsant agent such as propofol should be used. If IV catheterization is not possible, then the alternative route of administration is to give an anticonvulsant rectally at an increased dose.

Although predicting when a patient will experience a seizure is impossible, various physiologic stimuli including tactile, visual, and auditory signals have been theorized to sometimes trigger a seizure episode. Stress and excitement can also precipitate a seizure in a predisposed animal. Thus although these patients must be closely monitored in the event that a seizure may occur, some effort should be made to minimize the stimulation and traffic that occurs in a patient who has a seizure history.

Patients with Vestibular Disorders

The vestibular system is responsible for maintaining the sense of balance in a normal individual. When disease of the vestibular system occurs, patients will have varying clinical signs such as tilting of the head, resting or positional nystagmus, ataxia, and proprioceptive deficits. Lesions of the vestibular system can be broken down into two main areas: (1) central lesions or (2) peripheral lesions. Peripheral lesions (i.e., lesions typically localized toward either the left or right side of the animal) usually involve a disease process that affects the middle or inner ear. The common diseases that are seen in clinical practice include otitis media (i.e., infection of the middle ear) or otitis interna (i.e., infection of the inner ear), idiopathic vestibular syndrome (otherwise known as *old dog vestibular disease*), and ototoxicity (typically secondary to the administration of an aural medication such as gentamicin in patients without an intact eardrum). Typical clinical signs of peripheral vestibular disease include horizontal nystagmus (with the quick phase in the opposite direction of the affected side), head tilt (toward the affected side), and ataxia with the animals falling toward the affected side. Patients who have significant middle ear disease can also have Horner's syndrome because of damage to the sympathetic nerve inputs that go to the eye. The three clinical signs associated with Horner's syndrome include ptosis (elevation of the third eyelid), miosis (papillary contraction), and enophthalmus (retraction of the globe). In contrast to peripheral vestibular disease, an animal that has central vestibular disease has a disease process affecting the brain (specifically the brainstem where the nucleus of the vestibulocochlear nerve is found). The most common lesions affecting this area are mass lesions (e.g., neoplasia, abscess, granuloma), inflammatory or infectious diseases, degenerative diseases, and vascular diseases (e.g., strokes). Typical clinical signs found with central vestibular disease include a head tilt (typically toward the side of the lesion), vertical nystagmus, ataxia, and general proprioceptive deficits (because of disruption of the upper motor neuron tracts) on the same side of the lesion. Confirmatory diagnosis of a central vestibular lesion typically requires an imaging study of the brain (through either an magnetic resonance imaging or computed tomography scan) and possibly through analysis of cerebrospinal fluid samples.

Many owners will confuse the clinical signs observed in vestibular disease with those of a seizure; vestibular animals commonly thrash and paddle in an attempt to right themselves when they are recumbent. For many owners, managing a vestibular patient at home can be difficult because of their unstable neurologic symptoms. As a result, vestibular patients are commonly hospitalized for supportive care. Keeping vestibular patients in a quiet area is important because they can be easily agitated and will thrash inside their cages. The cages they are kept in should be provided with an abundance of soft padding to prevent these patients from injuring themselves.

Tetanus

Tetanus is a disease that is caused by *Clostridium tetani,* an infectious organism that is abundant in the external environment. The organism infects an animal by gaining access through an open wound. The characteristic clinical effects of this disease are caused by the actions of specific toxins produced by the organism. Specifically, the Clostridia organism produces a toxin called *tetanospasm* that prevents the release of an inhibitory neurotransmitter from interneurons in the spinal cord. The inhibitory neurotransmitters glycine and gamma-aminobutyric acid prevent the uncontrolled firing of lower motor neurons in the spinal cord and brainstem. Thus the common clinical signs observed in patients with generalized tetanus are extensor rigidity of all four limbs and retraction of the lips, eyelids, and ears; these animals also have trismus (i.e., difficulty in opening the jaw). An interesting feature of clinical tetanus is that the limbs that are in close proximity to the entrance wound are the first to be clinically affected. Resolution of the clinical signs of tetanus occurs in the reverse order, with the limbs distal to the point of entry resolving first (then the initially affected limbs resolving). Animals can also have localized tetanus, whereby only one or two limbs may be in extensor rigidity. Compared with horses and humans, dogs and cats tend to be resistant to clinical tetanus; cats are known to be the most resistant species. The time from initial infection to resolution can be variable, with most animals improving after 1 week. Some animals, however, may remain clinical for up to 3 to 4 weeks. Animals that ultimately succumb to tetanus do so as a result of respiratory muscle paralysis; therefore some of these patients require mechanical ventilation for their survival. Patients who are clinically affected with tetanus should be kept in a quiet environment where they can be continually monitored, particularly in regard to their ventilatory nature. These patients should have regular pulse oximetry and blood gases performed; in addition, they should be turned at least once every 4 hours if they are fully recumbent. Minimizing the stress in these patients is important; therefore overstimulation should be minimized.

Pancreatitis

Pancreatitis is defined as inflammation of the pancreas. The pancreas has two limbs (a left and a right) and serves a dual function (an exocrine function and an endocrine function). The endocrine function of the pancreas involves the release of four major hormones involved primarily in glucose homeostasis and digestion; the four hormones are insulin, glucagon, somatostatin, and pancreatic polypeptide D. The exocrine function of the pancreas involves the release of digestive enzymes into the small intestine that aid in the digestion of fats, proteins, and carbohydrates. The pancreas possesses a number of self-protective mechanisms designed to prevent autodigestion by its own enzymes. During pancreatitis, however, premature activation of these enzymes occurs within the parenchyma of the pancreas, resulting in the clinical signs of pancreatitis. The typical dog with pancreatitis has a history of vomiting, lethargy, anorexia, abdominal pain, and sometimes diarrhea. On physical examination, dogs with pancreatitis will typically have clinical dehydration, a painful cranial abdomen, and varying degrees of other clinical signs (e.g., dyspnea, abdominal distension). Cats with pancreatitis will typically have only lethargy and anorexia. The diagnosis of pancreatitis is made through a combination of clinical suspicion, blood work changes, and imaging studies (ultrasound is the best modality for diagnosing pancreatitis). Patients with pancreatitis require supportive care involving IV fluids, GI protectants, pain medications, antibiotics, and in certain cases, other treatments such as transfusion, feeding tube placements, surgery, and parenteral nutrition.

When these patients are hospitalized and still actively vomiting, they are usually kept off of food and water. Care should be taken to avoid olfactory stimulation in these patients, because the smell (and possibly the sight) of food can potentially cause pancreatic enzyme release. Thus ICU personnel should avoid placing food of any kind (including their own personal food) in close proximity to the cages of pancreatitis patients. Although placing these patients out of the ICU into a back area is tempting, this practice should be avoided, because pancreatitis can be a life-threatening condition. Instead these patients should be in an area of the ICU where the flow of traffic is minimized.

Cats

A special mention should be made in regard to the hospitalization of feline patients in the ICU. Although most practices (including referral facilities) keep canine and feline patients together in the same unit, some degree of consideration should be made toward the stress level placed on hospitalized cats. Many of these cats have life-threatening conditions, and the stress of barking or fractious dogs can have deleterious effects (some of which are discussed in the next section). In the ideal situation, a separate feline ward with all the same capabilities of an ICU should be present. In most situations, whether because of staffing or spacing issues, this is not available. Thus an effort should be made to keep cats as separate as possible to help minimize their stress level.

No special considerations are made when Level II patients are discharged from the ICU.

Level I

Level I isolation involves isolation of the disruptive patient; disruptive patients are patients who increase the stress level of other patients in the hospital through their behavior (e.g., excessive barking, aggression toward other animals or personnel, destructive behavior, anxiety). These patients tend to increase the anxiety and stress level in the hospital, thereby placing further compromise on the health of fellow patients. Increasing the stress of a patient will increase circulating cortisol level, which can have various deleterious effects. Cortisol is a hormone that is endogenously released from the adrenal glands; these glands are located at the cranial poles of both kidneys. In times of increased stress, such as

during clinical illness, the release of cortisol is up regulated (assuming an animal is not addisonian) in response to various factors to meet the increased metabolic need.

Cortisol has a myriad of functions used for maintaining normal homeostasis in an individual (e.g., gluconeogenesis, normal GI epithelial turnover). When cortisol is increased in response to stress, however, a number of deleterious effects may occur that include GI ulceration, impaired immune function, and impaired wound healing. Because of these effects, placing patients exhibiting behaviors classified under Level I criteria in areas that will cause the least amount of anxiety to other patients is recommended. Typical areas where this is accomplished include dog runs and cages located in a back area where supervision is routinely performed.

These patients should be routinely admitted and are usually given the opportunity to remain in the main ICU. However, Level I patients are usually isolated from other patients when a prolonged period of disruptive behavior is exhibited. The administration of low-dose sedation is sometimes used to calm patients in the Level I category; although the use of excessive sedation should be avoided, sedation can be beneficial to prevent these animals from self-harm. It should be noted strongly, however, that Level I patients deserve the same care as other patients in the hospital. The tendency is to leave these patients in an isolated area where they unsupervised for hours at a time; this practice should be avoided at all costs. No special consideration is given when these patients are discharged.

II

EMERGENCY CARE
FOR SMALL ANIMALS

This section discusses the importance of an organized work space in the emergency department and the types of emergencies seen in the small animal emergency facility. The technician plays a vital role in stabilizing these animals.

CHAPTER 12

Management of the Patient in Shock

HAROLD DAVIS

The veterinary technician plays an integral role in the management of the emergent or critically ill patient. Many of these patients suffer a disease process associated with inadequate tissue perfusion resulting in poor oxygen delivery. The condition is often assessed as *shock*. Shock has been typically classified into several categories (e.g., cardiogenic, septic, hypovolemic), and the causes of shock are numerous. Regardless of the form of shock, the goal is to optimize oxygen delivery. This discussion provides an overview of the determinants of oxygen delivery, a review of the pathophysiology of hypovolemic shock, and a discussion of the management of shock.

Oxygen Delivery

Oxygen delivery (DO_2) represents the amount or volume of oxygen transported to the tissues each minute. DO_2 is the product of cardiac output and oxygen content (Cao_2). Calculating DO_2 is not possible in most practice situations. However, the concept is important, and several components of DO_2 (Fig. 12-1) can be addressed. Cardiac output is the product of stroke volume and heart rate. To improve or increase cardiac output, the heart rate and stroke volume has to increase. Stroke volume is the amount of blood pumped out of the heart with each beat, and three primary determinants of stoke volume exist. Stroke volume is increased in proportion to (1) the stretch of the walls of the ventricles during diastole (preload), (2) the strength of contraction (contractility), and (3) decreases in the forces that oppose blood flow from the heart (afterload) (i.e., in the absence of valvular stenosis, arterial blood pressure [BP]).

Cao_2 is the amount of oxygen in arterial blood. Oxygen is either dissolved in plasma or bound to hemoglobin (Hb). Cao_2 is defined by the equation in Fig. 12-2.

Hb is the main carrier of oxygen in the blood. Each gram of Hb has the capacity to carry 1.34 ml of oxygen: 20.1 ml of oxygen per deciliter

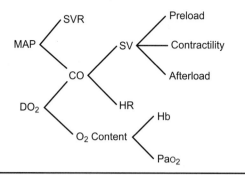

Fig. 12-1 Determinants of DO_2. *CO,* Cardiac output; *Hb,* hemoglobin; *HR,* heart rate; *MAP,* mean arterial pressure; *Pao₂,* partial pressure of oxygen; *SV,* stroke volume; *SVR,* systemic vascular resistance.

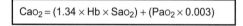

$$Cao_2 = (1.34 \times Hb \times Sao_2) + (Pao_2 \times 0.003)$$

Fig. 12-2 Oxygen content (Cao_2) equation.

Forms of Oxygen in Arterial Blood

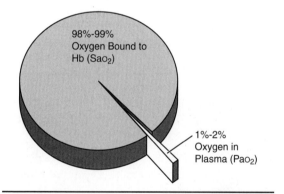

98%-99%
Oxygen Bound to
Hb (Sao_2)

1%-2%
Oxygen in
Plasma (Pao_2)

Fig. 12-3 Percentage of oxygen bound to hemoglobin (Hb) and dissolved in plasma.

of blood when the Hb is 15 g/dl. Only 0.3 ml of oxygen per deciliter blood is dissolved in the plasma when the partial pressure of oxygen in arterial blood (Pao_2) is 100 mm Hg (Fig. 12-3).

Definitions of Shock

Many different categorization schemes have been used to define shock. In some instances, overlap between categories exists. For the purposes of this discussion, shock is categorized into four different forms based on the causative pathophysiologic mechanism. Ultimately, the focus of therapy will be to optimize oxygen delivery. *Cardiogenic* shock is a form of shock that results from heart failure but excludes those factors outside the heart (i.e., cardiac tamponade, caval syndrome). Pump failure may be caused by hypertrophic or dilative cardiomyopathy, valvular insufficiency or stenosis, arrhythmias, or fibrosis. *Distributive* shock is often used to describe shock states associated with flow maldistribution. Initiating causes for this form of shock include sepsis, anaphylaxis, trauma, and neurogenic problems. *Obstructive* shock results from a physical obstruction in the circulatory system. Heartworm disease, pericardial effusion, pulmonary embolism, and gastric torsion can all contribute to impaired blood flow. *Hypovolemic* shock is the result of decreased intravascular volume. The decreased volume may be caused by blood loss, third-space loss, or fluid losses because of excessive vomiting, diarrhea, and diuresis. Hypovolemic shock is the most common form of shock seen in small animals.

Pathophysiology of Hypovolemic Shock

Shock is a complex and dynamic process involving many compensatory mechanisms. An initiating cause results in a decreased intravascular volume. As a result of the decreased intravascular volume, venous return and ventricular filling (i.e., preload) is decreased. With the decreased ventricular filling, decreased stroke volume and cardiac output occur. The end result is inadequate tissue perfusion and oxygen delivery.

Decreased cardiac output and hypotension cause a baroreceptor-mediated sympathoadrenal reflex that activates the patient's compensatory mechanisms to help maintain perfusion. Norepinephrine, epinephrine, and cortisol are released from the adrenal gland. Epinephrine and norepinephrine cause an increase in heart rate and contractility, arteriolar constriction (which increases systemic vascular resistance and redirects blood flow to the heart and brain and away from skin, muscles, kidneys, and gastrointestinal tract). Cortisol enhances the effects of the catecholamines on arterioles. Sodium and water is conserved, because of renin-angiotensin-aldostrone system activation, causing an increased intravascular volume.

Initial Assessment and Recognition

The initial recognition of hypovolemic shock is based on historical and physical findings (Table 12-1). Historically, the owner may be able to provide information that supports a reason for hypovolemia such as trauma, excessive urination, diarrhea, or vomiting. Typically the physical findings are indicative of sympathoadrenal activation (tachycardia and vasoconstriction). In the early stage or compensatory phase of shock, tachycardia, decreased pulse quality, prolonged capillary refill time (CRT), pale mucous membrane color, and cool extremities are seen. This may be called *stage I, compensated shock*. In stage II, *decompensated shock*, the patient is tachycardic, has decreased pulse quality, variable CRT, "muddy" mucous membrane color, decreasing BP, and obtunded mental status. When the patient is suffering from severe systemic hypoperfusion and therapies cease to be effective, the patient is said to be in stage III, irreversible shock. The stages of shock are a continuum. Progression through the stages is based on patient-related factors, as well as the timeliness and effectiveness of therapy.

TABLE 12-1

Nursing Assessment Parameters for Shock

Parameter	Assessment
Level of consciousness	Assess for alertness, obtundation, stupor, coma
Pulse	Assess for rate, rhythm, strength, quality
Respiration	Assess for rate, depth, effort, breath sounds
Cutaneous	Assess temperature (rectal/extremity), mucous membrane color/moistness, capillary refill time (CRT), skin turgor
Urine production	Assess output, specific gravity
Blood pressure (BP)	Assess for changes in values

Therapy

The goal of therapy is to improve oxygen delivery (Box 12-1). The veterinary technician energy should be directed at correcting or improving the components of the oxygen delivery algorithm (see Fig. 12-1).

Oxygen Therapy

Maintaining oxygen saturation is one of the primary goals in maintaining blood oxygenation. If any question exists concerning a patient's blood oxygenation, then supplemental oxygen should be provided until assessment of arterial blood gases or Hb saturation confirms that oxygen supplementation is not necessary. When this equipment is not available, assessment will have to be based on clinical dyspnea or auscultable abnormalities and clinical signs of hypoxia: cyanosis of the mucous membranes or

BOX 12-1

Summary of Therapy to Improve Oxygen Delivery (DO_2)

Correct Primary Problem
- Control fluid loss
- Treat infection

Oxygenation
- Provide supplemental oxygen (mask, nasal or transtracheal catheter, cage)

Fluid Resuscitation
- Crystalloids:
  Dogs 80-90 ml/kg
  Cats 50-55 ml/kg
  7.5% Hypertonic saline 4-6 ml/kg
- Synthetic colloids:
  Dogs 10-40 ml/kg
  Cats 5 ml/kg increments over 15 to 20 minutes
- Plasma 10-40 ml/kg
- Whole blood 10-30 ml/kg
- Red blood cells 5-15 ml/kg

Note: All fluids given to effect. Consider sympathomimetics—dopamine 5-10 µg/kg/min, dobutamine 5-15 µg/kg/min.

TABLE 12-2

Fluid Flow Rates Based on Catheter Gauge and Height of Fluid Bag

Catheter Gauge	HEIGHT, 3 FEET Flow Rate (ml/min)	HEIGHT, 6 FEET Flow Rate (ml/min)
16	88	152
18	75	114
20	45	75

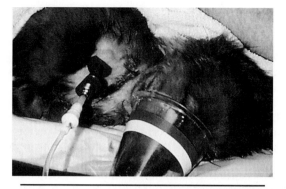

Fig. 12-4 Fluid administration via intraosseous catheter.

dark-colored blood, tachypnea, tachycardia, and anxiety. Individually, the clinical signs do not prove hypoxemia, but together they are suggestive of hypoxemia.

A variety of methods of oxygen therapy exist. The method selected depends on the expected duration of therapy, the demeanor of the patient, and equipment availability. Available methods include the use of face masks, oxygen bags (hoods), oxygen cages, as well as transtracheal and nasal insufflation. The ultimate goal of oxygen therapy is to provide adequate oxygen to the blood, using the lowest possible inspired oxygen concentrations.

Venous Access

Selection of a vein to catheterize depends on several factors such as the size and species of the animal, the skill of the operator placing the catheter, therapeutic goals, and the animal's problem or disease. Any vessel that is visible or palpable should be considered a candidate for percutaneous catheterization. The cephalic and saphenous veins offer easily accessible routes that can be catheterized quickly. The internal diameter and the length of the catheter and height of the fluid bag above the patient primarily determine the maximum fluid flow rate of a catheter (Table 12-2).

A short, large-gauge catheter is needed if fluids are to be rapidly administered. Keeping administration tubing short is also advisable, as well as avoiding excessive use of extension tubing and unnecessary connectors that reduce flow rates.

In the event vascular access cannot be obtained, the establishment of an intraosseous line (Fig. 12-4)

is a reasonable alternative. Fluid or drugs administered by this route are rapidly taken up into the circulatory system.

Fluid Resuscitation

The most effective way to improve oxygen delivery is to increase cardiac output by optimizing preload with the administration of fluid.

Crystalloids. Isotonic crystalloids, which have electrolyte concentrations (i.e., sodium, chloride, potassium, and bicarbonate-like anions) similar to extracellular fluid, are commonly used in the treatment of hypovolemic shock. These fluids freely and rapidly distribute between the intravascular and interstitial compartments. After 30 minutes, 98% of the volume of fluids infused into the intravascular compartment shifts into the interstitial compartment. Examples of commonly used crystalloids include lactated Ringer's, normal saline, Normosol-R (Abbott Laboratories, North Chicago, IL), and Plasmalyte 148 (Baxter Healthcare, Deerfield, IL). A commonly cited fluid dose goal of isotonic crystalloids is 80 to 90 ml/kg/hr for the dog and 50 to 55 ml/kg/hr for the cat (equivalent to one blood volume). Individual animal requirements are variable; therefore it may be necessary to administer 0.5 to 1.5 times the previously mentioned volume to effectively resuscitate the patient. Frequently reassessing the patient's condition (i.e., about every 10 to 15 minutes) is necessary during large or rapid volume fluid administration.

Hypertonic crystalloids such as 7.5% saline have been recommended for use in shock therapy in cases in which it is difficult to administer large volumes of fluids rapidly enough to resuscitate the patient. Hypertonic saline causes fluid shifts from the intracellular space to the extracellular (including intravascular) space, resulting in improved venous return and cardiac output. Hypertonic saline also causes vasodilation and improves tissue perfusion. The recommended dose range is 4 to 6 ml/kg over 5 minutes. Dextran 70 has been added to hypertonic saline to potentiate and sustain vascular volume augmentation. Because of the fluid "steal" that occurs, isotonic crystalloids should be subsequently administered at 40% to 60% of the shock dose of fluids.

Hypotonic fluids such as 5% dextrose in water, half-strength saline, and half-strength lactated Ringer's should not be used to treat hypovolemic shock. These fluids contain too much free water and distribute excessively to the intracellular compartment.

Colloids. Colloids are large molecular weight solutions that do not cross capillary membranes readily. Colloids are better blood volume expanders than are isotonic crystalloids, because 50% to 80% of the infused volume remains in the intravascular space. Colloids should be administered when crystalloids are not effectively improving or maintaining blood volume restoration. Intravascular colloid oncotic pressure (COP) is important in maintaining intravascular volume. Large volumes of crystalloids decrease COP, whereas colloids increase COP. Colloids should be administered when the total protein or albumin are decreased below 4.0 g/dl or 1.5 g/dl, respectively. Colloids include plasma, blood, and the synthetics—dextran 70 (Gentran 70, Baxter Healthcare, Deerfield IL) and hetastarch (Hespan, DuPont, Wilmington, DE). Plasma provides albumin, immunoglobulins, platelets, and clotting factors. The approximate dose of plasma is 10 to 40 ml/kg; however, it should be administered to effect. Large volumes of plasma may be required to affect total protein or albumin concentrations.

Hb must be available in sufficient concentrations to ensure adequate Ca_{O_2}. If Hb decreases from 15 g/dl to 10 g/dl, then Ca_{O_2} is reduced by one third; cardiac output will need to increase to maintain adequate delivery of oxygen (see Fig. 12-1). In the absence of Hb measurements, Hb can be estimated from the microhematocrit (micro-HCT). The Hb is usually about one third of the HCT values. The HCT should be maintained around 30%. Oxygen delivery is limited when the HCT decreases below 20%. Whole blood and packed red blood cells are administered at 10 to 30 ml/kg and 5 to 15 ml/kg, respectively; again, this will need to be administered to effect. These doses will increase the HCT approximately 5% to 15%.

As an alternative to plasma, synthetic colloids may be administered. In cases in which the patient is a cat or thought or known to have closed cavity hemorrhage, head trauma, pulmonary contusions, or cardiogenic shock, fluid therapy should be conservative: the colloid should be administered no faster than 5 ml/kg increments over 15 to 20 minutes. The 5 ml/kg boluses are titrated to effect. It has been reported that rapid administration of colloids may cause nausea in cats. Otherwise, dextran and hetastarch may be given as a bolus of 10 to 40 ml/kg to effect. Because the synthetic colloids only replace intravascular volume, crystalloids still must be given to replace interstitial fluid deficits. Crystalloids are given at 40% to 60% of the dose used if crystalloids had been used alone.

Dextran and hetastarch can interfere with platelet function and can increase coagulation parameters somewhat more than can be attributed to simple hemodilution. Blood products and oxypolygelatins can cause allergic reactions.

Sympathomimetics

Sympathomimetics, such as dopamine (Intropin, DuPont Critical Care) and dobutamine (Dobutrex, Lilly) are indicated when the patient is unresponsive to vigorous fluid therapy and arterial BP, vasomotor tone, and tissue perfusion have not returned to acceptable levels. These drugs support myocardial contractility and BP with minimal vasoconstriction. BP monitoring is recommended. Dopamine, a precursor of norepinephrine has dose-dependent effects. At 0.5 to 3.0 µg/kg/min, dilation of renal, mesenteric, and coronary vascular beds will occur because of the dopaminergic effect. Increase of heart rate or contractility (or both) is seen at a dose range of 3.0 to 7.5 µg/kg/min (a result of beta 1 activity). At doses greater than 7.5 µg/kg/min, alpha receptor stimulation and vasoconstriction occurs. Dobutamine has primarily beta activity. It increases contractility and has minimal effect on heart rate and peripheral vascular resistance except at higher doses. The dose range is 5 to 15 µg/kg/min. Sympathomimetics should not be a substitute for adequate

> Dosage (µg/kg/min) × (kg)(body weight) = Drug (mg) to place in 250 ml/fluids
>
> Administer at 15 ml/hr

Fig. 12-5 Quick formula for calculating µg/kg/min constant rate infusions.

volume restoration. Fluid resuscitation remains the cornerstone of shock therapy.

The technician should be able to calculate constant rate infusions using the formula shown in Fig. 12-5.

Monitoring

Many of the signs associated with shock are related to the compensatory mechanism the body invokes to maintain life. Frequently assessing clinical signs is important because the hemodynamic and metabolic sequelae of shock are continually changing. The monitoring process begins with the physical assessment and is integrated with physiologic monitoring and evaluation of cellular function (acid-base balance and other laboratory values).

Physical Parameters

Respiratory Parameters. When evaluating the patient's respiratory parameters, the veterinary technician should ask the following questions:

- Is the patient able to meet its ventilation and oxygenation requirements?
- Is the rate and tidal volume adequate?
- Is the breathing effort smooth and easy?
- Is the breathing pattern regular?
- Can normal breath sounds be auscultated? (Abnormal breath sounds could be described as crackles, wheezes, squeaks, muffled and quiet.)

Cardiovascular Parameters. Assessment of the cardiovascular system may begin with the heart rate. Tachycardia and bradycardia have several causes. If arrhythmias are auscultated, then an electrocardiogram is indicated. Indicators of peripheral perfusion include mucous membrane color, CRT, urine output, and appendage temperature. Normal mucous membrane color is pink. Pale mucous membranes may indicate anemia and or vasoconstriction. Brick red or hyperemic mucous membranes may indicate vasodilation and is seen in the early phases of septic shock. Normal capillary refill is 1 to 2 seconds. Prolonged CRT is associated with decreased peripheral perfusion. Normal urine production is 1 to 2 ml/kg/hr; it decreases when perfusion is decreased or when mean arterial pressure is less than 60 mm Hg. Appendage temperature decreases as a result of vasoconstriction and poor peripheral perfusion. A full, strong pulse indicates a good pulse pressure and stroke volume, whereas a weak pulse indicates decreased stroke volume.

Physiologic Monitoring Parameters

Oxygen Saturation. Hb saturation measured by pulse oximetry (SpO_2) provides noninvasive and continuous information about the percent of oxygen bound to Hb. Normal SpO_2 is greater than 95%. The patient is seriously hypoxemic when the SpO_2 is less than or equal to 90%. Caution should be exercised when interpreting SpO_2 values with animals breathing 100% oxygen. Animals with a PaO_2 of 500 mm Hg still show a SpO_2 from 98% to 99%.

Arterial Blood Pressure. Arterial BP (measured by indirect and direct methods) is the product of cardiac output, vascular capacity, and blood volume. The three determinants work in concert to maintain BP. Should one of the three become subnormal, the other two determinants should compensate. Normal systolic, diastolic, and mean BP are approximately 100 to 160, 60 to 100, and 80 to 120 mm Hg, respectively. Systolic and mean BPs below 80 mm Hg and 60 mm Hg, respectively, warrant therapy. Causes of hypotension include hypovolemia, peripheral vasodilation, and decreased cardiac output. Hypertension may be caused by chronic renal failure, an adrenal tumor, pheochromocytoma, or any other factor that causes increased cardiac output.

Central Venous Pressure. Central venous pressure (CVP) is the BP in the intrathoracic anterior vena cava compared with a column of water in a plastic manometer or a pressure transducer and oscilloscope. Changes in pressure in the thorax produce fluctuations in the water manometer or wave forms on the oscilloscope. CVP is a measure of the heart's ability to pump fluids returned to it and is also an estimate of the relationship of blood volume to blood volume capacity. CVP should be measured when heart failure is suspected or as an aid in determining the end-point to aggressive fluid therapy. Clinicians generally assume that a reasonable preload has been achieved when the CVP approaches 10 cm of water (7.5 mm Hg). If cardiac output, pulse quality, BP, and perfusion parameters (CRT, mucous membrane color, urine output, and appendage temperature) are acceptable, the clinician can assume that effective blood volume restoration has been accomplished. If not, then the clinician can assume that the heart is unable to handle the venous return.

Laboratory Parameters

Hematocrit and Total Solids. HCT and total solids (TS) can be used to gauge fluid therapy, estimate Hb concentration and, to a certain degree, assess blood loss. The two tests should be interpreted together to minimize errors in interpretation. Increase in both HCT and TS indicate dehydration; decrease in both HCT and TS is suggestive of recent blood loss or clear fluid administration. Increase in TS and normal HCT may indicate anemia with dehydration. Both normal HCT and TS may be normal in peracute blood loss. TS may decrease with reduced albumin levels; albumin is a contributor to oncotic pressure.

Electrolytes. Electrolytes play a major role in the maintenance of interstitial compartmental water balance and cell function. Baseline electrolytes should be obtained and monitoring continued as therapy progresses. Fluid therapy can alter various serum electrolyte concentrations, and may require adjustment of the electrolyte composition in the fluids being administered. Commonly measured electrolytes include serum potassium, sodium, chloride, magnesium, and ionized calcium.

Arterial pH and Blood Gases. Arterial blood gases are an excellent way to assess ventilation and oxygenation. Testing $Paco_2$ reveals how well the patient is ventilating. A $Paco_2$ less than 35 mm Hg or greater than 45 mm Hg indicates hyperventilation or hypoventilation, respectively. Testing Pao_2 reveals how well the patient is oxygenating. A Pao_2 less than 80 is considered hypoxemia, although the patient may not be treated until the Pao_2 approaches 60 mm Hg. The pH combined with bicarbonate or base balance reveals the metabolic status of the patient. Normal pH is 7.35 to 7.45; a pH less than 7.35 is termed *acidemia*, and a pH greater than 7.45 is termed *alkalemic*. A patient has metabolic acidosis if the bicarbonate is less than 18 mmol/L or base deficit is more negative than –4. Alkalosis is identified by bicarbonate greater than 27 mmol/L and a base excess greater than +4.

Jugular venous Po_2 samples below 30 mm Hg or greater than 60 mm Hg may be caused by decreased oxygen delivery to the tissues and reduced oxygen uptake by the tissues, respectively. No correlation exists between venous Po_2 and arterial Po_2.

Colloid Oncotic Pressure. COP can be measured and used to guide fluid therapy. COP is a force created by large plasma proteins that do not move freely across capillaries. The presence of colloids in the vascular space has the effect of pulling water from the interstitium into the vascular space. The goal is to maintain a COP greater than 18 mm Hg.

Lactate. When perfusion decreases and oxygen delivery is reduced, the body shifts from aerobic to anaerobic metabolism, resulting in lactate formation. Elevated blood lactate (lactate >2 mmol/L) has been proposed as a indicator of inadequate tissue oxygenation. Although elevated blood lactate levels often signify generalized tissue hypoxia, a normal value does not rule out regional lactate production.

Summary

Shock is a dynamic and complex syndrome; the focus of therapy and monitoring is oxygen delivery. To improve Cao_2 component of oxygen delivery, the veterinary technician might administer oxygen or Hb in the form of packed red blood cells or whole blood. To improve the cardiac output component, a technician might administer fluids in the form of crystalloids or colloids that, in turn, improve preload. Drug therapy may also be needed to improve contractility, heart rate, and in some cases reduce afterload. By improving cardiac output and systemic vascular resistance the patient's BP is improved. Having a basic understanding of the pathophysiologic and compensatory mechanism of this complex syndrome will aid the veterinary technician in meeting therapeutic and monitoring goals.

Suggested Readings

Chandler CF, Waxman K: Monitoring. In Shoemaker WC et al, editors: *Pocket companion to textbook of critical care*, Philadelphia, 1996, WB Saunders, p 113.

Franklin CM, Darovic GO, Dan BB: Monitoring the patient in shock. In Darovic GO, editor: *Hemodynamic monitoring: invasive and noninvasive clinical application*, Philadelphia, 1995, WB Saunders, p 441.

Fulton RB, Hauptman JG: In vitro and in vivo rates of fluid flow through catheters in peripheral veins of dogs, *J Am Vet Med Assoc* 198(9)1473-1696, 1991.

Kirby RR: *Colloids those magic fluids*. Scientific proceedings of the 23rd annual meeting of the Veterinary Emergency and Critical Care Society, San Antonio, TX, 1997.

Lohrman JM: *Clinical aspects of oxygen delivery and consumption*. Proceedings of the Barbara Clark Mims Associates Presents Pathophysiology of Shock, San Antonio, TX, 1997, pp 24-25.

Marino PL: Hemodynamic drugs. *The ICU Book*, Baltimore, 1998, Williams & Wilkins, p 283.

Rudloff E, Kirby RR: Hypovolemic shock and resuscitation, *Vet Clin North Am Small Anim Pract* 24:1015, 1994.

CHAPTER 13

Cardiopulmonary Cerebrovascular Resuscitation

Harold Davis

Cardiopulmonary arrest (CPA) is the sudden cessation of spontaneous and effective ventilation and systemic perfusion (circulation). CPA may be a result of any disease process carried out to its extreme that disrupts cardiac or pulmonary homeostasis (or both). Potential causes of CPA include hypoxia, metabolic disorders, trauma, vagal stimulation, anesthetic or other drugs, and environmental influences (i.e., hypothermia or hyperthermia). In one study the most frequent conditions leading to cardiac arrest in young dogs (up to 1.5 years) were infections (i.e., gastroenteritis, pneumonia) and trauma. Conditions leading to CPA in older dogs (between 6 and 10 years) were of a more chronic nature, such as primary heart disease, autoimmune disease, and malignancy. In the same study the most common medical condition preceding CPA in cats was trauma, with infectious diseases being the next most frequent condition. In another study, CPA was associated with anesthesia with or without preexisting diseases in 55% of the animals, cardiovascular collapse in 28% of the animals, and chronic disease with an imposed stress in 17% of the animals. More than 40 years have elapsed since the combined techniques of mechanical ventilation, external precordial compression, and defibrillation were introduced in human medicine. Today clinicians know these combined techniques as cardiopulmonary cerebrovascular resuscitation (CPCR) and are fortunate that much of the CPCR research conducted has been carried out in animal subjects. Many of the techniques or procedures used in human medicine are also used in veterinary medicine. The goal of CPCR is to provide adequate ventilatory and circulatory support until spontaneous function returns. CPCR has three phases: (1) basic life support (BLS), (2) advance life support, and (3) prolonged life support. This chapter covers preparation for this ultimate emergency, recognition of CPA, and the three phases of CPCR.

Preparation

Staff

Like many other aspects of emergency care, the team approach to the management of the CPA patient is a must. The ideal number of participants in a resuscitation attempt is three to five; all are required to meet several responsibilities (Table 13-1) of CPCR. Each member of the hospital staff (including reception and kennel help) should be trained to carry out one or more of those responsibilities. The team leader is usually the veterinarian; if the veterinarian is not available, then the person with the most experience in performing CPCR should lead the team. People will be needed to provide ventilation, chest compressions, establish IV lines, administer drugs, attach monitoring equipment, record the resuscitation effort, and monitor the team's effectiveness. Practice drills should be held on a regular basis. The benefits are tremendous when the staff can respond quickly and efficiently. A stuffed animal can be used as the patient during these drills. Each person should understand what his or her responsibilities are during an arrest. After each practice session or true resuscitation, a self-evaluation should be performed.

Facilities

The area in which the resuscitation endeavor takes place should provide enough space for a CPCR team (a minimum of three people) and equipment. An oxygen source should be readily available. Good lighting is required; it facilitates endotracheal intubation and visualization of veins. If open chest massage is attempted, then good lighting will allow visualization of internal structures. If CPCR is to be performed on a table, then the height of the table should be adjustable. If a table is too tall for the person performing chest compressions, then he or she will find it difficult to perform effectively. If the height of the table is not adjustable, then a footstool should be made available or CPCR should be performed on the floor. Grated surgical preparation tables should be avoided if at all possible; they have too much "give," which can be counterproductive when performing chest compressions. If the team has no choice and must use a preparation table, then a board should be place on or below the grate to provide extra support. The table must have a solid surface. If some form of crash cart is not used, then the drugs, electrocardiogram (ECG), suction, and defibrillator should be in close proximity. A shelf and a few drawers may be set aside for the emergency supplies.

Equipment

The use of a crash cart or kit makes the resuscitation endeavor more efficient by having the necessary supplies readily available. The crash cart or kit may be as simple as a fishing tackle box or as elaborate as a mobile tool chest (Fig. 13-1). If a cart is used, then in addition to the standard emergency supplies (Box 13-1), additional equipment may be stored on the cart (e.g., suction machine, ECG, defibrillator). The crash cart or kit should be checked at the beginning of each shift and restocked immediately after each use.

TABLE 13-1

Cardiopulmonary Cerebrovascular Resuscitation Responsibilities and Tasks

Responsibility	Task
Airway management	Establish airway Ventilate
Cardiovascular management	Compress chest
Venous access	Place IV lines Start IV fluids
Monitor effectiveness	Attach ECG Check pulse Check mucous membrane color Check Doppler flow Check end-tidal carbon dioxide ($ETCO_2$)
Drug administration	Administer drugs Document drugs given and response

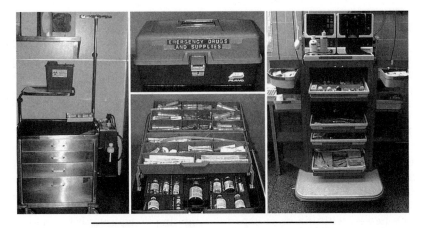

Fig. 13-1 Examples of an emergency kit and crash cart.

Recognition

Veterinary technicians are often in a position to recognize impending problems such as CPA. The technician's efforts should be directed toward identifying those patients who are at risk for developing CPA. The technician should observe for decreasing mentation or lack of response; change in respiratory rate, depth, and pattern; change in pulse rate, rhythm, or quality; abnormal rhythms on ECG; or unexplained changes in anesthetic depth. If the patient's condition begins to deteriorate, then medical and nursing interventions will be required. Preventing an arrest is often easier than treating an arrest. CPCR should be initiated if the patient is apneic, the pulse is absent, or the heart cannot be auscultated. Pupils may become dilated with in 20 to 40 seconds after arrest. Knowledge of recent medications administered should be used when assessing pupils; drugs such as atropine and epinephrine can cause the pupils to dilate. If any questions arise as to whether the patient is in CPA, then CPCR should be initiated until proven otherwise.

Phase One: Basic Life Support

The primary objective of BLS is to temporarily support the patient's oxygenation, ventilation, and circulation. This is accomplished by administering manual artificial ventilation and external chest compressions. Remembering the mnemonic *Airway,* *Breathing, and Circulation* (ABC; Box 13-2) helps to keep the resuscitation team focused on the priorities of BLS. Recent discussions have centered on the idea of reordering the mnemonic from ABC to CAB (Circulation, Airway, and Breathing). The premise is based on human medicine (in which cardiac dysrhythmias secondary to coronary artery disease is the common cause of CPA, and early defibrillation is associated with the best survival rates). In veterinary medicine, respiratory and vagally mediated arrests are common causes of CPA. In addition, CPA in animals is most often a result of conditions that are not primarily cardiac in origin. Given the causes of CPA in the veterinary patient, early ventilation is more appropriate. Therefore it would seem prudent to continue using the ABC mnemonic.

Airway

The first priority for BLS is the establishment of an airway. Usually an endotracheal tube is inserted to ensure a patent airway. On occasion, a tracheostomy tube may be indicated if an upper airway obstruction exists. If tracheostomy tubes are not available and the patient has an upper airway obstruction, then an endotracheal tube may be used like a tracheostomy tube. A variety of different-sized endotracheal and tracheostomy tubes and the associated airway management supplies (e.g., laryngoscopes, stylets, roll gauze, syringes) should be readily available to the team. In addition, suction should be available to remove blood, mucus, pulmonary edema fluid, and vomitus from the oral cavity and trachea. Properly

BOX 13-1

Standard Emergency Supplies

Pharmaceutical Supplies
Atropine
Epinephrine
Vasopressin
Two-percent lidocaine (without epinephrine)
Sodium bicarbonate ($NaHCO_3$)
Calcium chloride or gluconate
Lactated Ringer's (and/or hypertonic saline, dextran 70, or hetastarch)

Airway Access Supplies
Laryngoscope and blades
Endotracheal tubes (variety of sizes)
Lubricating jelly
Roll gauze

Venous Access Supplies
Butterfly catheters (variety of sizes)
IV catheters (variety of sizes)
IV drip sets
Bone marrow needles
Syringes (variety of sizes)
Hypodermic needles (variety of sizes)
Adhesive tape
Tourniquet

Miscellaneous Supplies
Gauze (3 × 3 inch)
Stethoscope
Minor surgery pack
Suture material
Scalpel blade
Surgeon's gloves

BOX 13-2

Mnemonics for Key Steps in Basic Life Support

Airway—Establish airway
Breathing—Once every 3-5 seconds
Circulation—80-120 Compressions/min

should provide moderate hyperventilation to offset any developing metabolic acidosis. Effective ventilation will also help to remove carbon dioxide that is generated with sodium bicarbonate ($NaHCO_3$) administration. Arterial blood gases can be used to determine the effectiveness of the artificial ventilation.

Circulation

The third and final priority of BLS is the initiation of artificial circulation. This can be accomplished through external or internal cardiac compression. The effectiveness of cardiac compression depends on the transmission of force to the heart and intrathoracic vessels.

External Cardiac Compression. External cardiac compression can be carried out with the patient in lateral or dorsal recumbency. With the patient in lateral recumbency, one or both hands are placed on the lateral thoracic wall over the area of the heart (fourth to fifth intercostal space at the costochondral junction). In larger patients (5 kg or greater) the arms should be kept extended and locked. The compressive force is applied by bending at the waist (Fig. 13-2). The person delivering the chest compressions should not compress the chest by bending the elbows; it will be difficult to generate an appropriate force to affect perfusion. In patients less than 5 kg, the thumb and first two index fingers can be used to compress the chest. It has been suggested that the compressions be delivered with enough force to displace the thorax by 25% to 33% of its diameter. The rate of compressions ranges from 80 to 120 per minute. Some researchers suggest placing patients in dorsal recumbency if they weigh more than 15 kg or if they have a barrel chest, providing the patient can be stabilized. Placing the patient in dorsal recumbency and compressing the sternum may aid in increasing intrathoracic pressure and subsequent forward blood flow.

placing the endotracheal tube is imperative. Proper placement is confirmed by visualization; chest auscultation for breath sounds is also helpful.

Breathing

The second priority is to initiate artificial ventilation. The patient is attached to a breathing source that delivers 100% oxygen such as an Ambu-Bag, or anesthetic machine. Initially the patient is given two quick breaths of 1 to 1.5 seconds in duration and then ventilated once every 3 to 5 seconds interspersed between chest compressions. Artificial ventilation

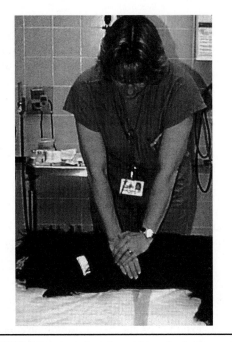

Fig. 13-2 Proper technique for applying chest compressions. Note that the arms are extended and the technician is bending at the waist.

Internal Compression. Internal or direct cardiac compression has been shown to be more effective than external chest compression. The advantages over external compression include greater cardiac output and blood pressure; better cerebral, myocardial, and peripheral tissue perfusion; and higher survival rate with improved neurologic recovery. Other advantages of internal compression include the ability to assess ventricular filling between compressions and to determine what type of cardiac arrest is present in the absence of an ECG monitor. With the chest open, the descending aorta may also be compressed to force blood to the brain and coronary circulation. It has been suggested that a pericardectomy be performed to prevent cardiac tamponade.

Immediate internal compression is indicated if the patient has rib fractures, pleural effusion, pneumothorax, or cardiac tamponade. Otherwise internal cardiac compression should be performed if effective artificial circulation and tissue perfusion are not evident within 5 minutes of cardiac arrest. The thoracotomy is also performed if effective, spontaneous rhythm has not commenced after 10 minutes.

The patient is placed in left lateral recumbency for an emergency thoracotomy. Time is not wasted performing a surgical preparation; however, the coat is clipped in longhaired dogs enough to see the rib spaces. An incision is made at the fourth or fifth intercostal space from just below dorsal epaxial muscles down to 2 cm short of the sternum but not through the pleura. The person ventilating the patient should stop while the chest cavity is entered with a pair of curved Mayo scissors. The scissors are then opened slightly and slid along the cranial edge of the caudal rib to enlarge the opening. A gloved hand is inserted into the chest and the heart compressed between the fingers and the palm of the hand. Small hearts can also be compressed between two fingers. Internal cardiac compression is performed rhythmically. Care should be taken not to puncture the heart with fingertips or twist the heart. Should spontaneous beating return and the patient is stable, the chest cavity is irrigated with sterile saline; a sterile surgical skin preparation is performed, and the chest cavity is closed.

Mechanism of Blood Flow. Two theories explain mechanisms of forward blood flow during CPCR. The classic theory is the cardiac pump theory. The heart is compressed between the two thoracic walls, forcing blood out of the heart and into the arterial circulation. This is equivalent to the systolic phase of a normal heartbeat. Atrioventricular valves prevent retrograde blood flow. Chest relaxation creates subatmospheric intrathoracic pressure, allowing venous return and heart filling, similar to the normal diastolic phase.

The thoracic pump mechanism of blood flow is a newer theory that was recognized a little over 25 years ago. It is hypothesized that chest compressions cause a rise in intrathoracic pressure that is transmitted to the intrathoracic vasculature; intrathoracic structures are compressed. Collapse of venous structures also occurs in the thorax, which prevents retrograde venous blood flow. Intrathoracic pressure falls when chest compressions are relaxed, allowing return of venous blood from the periphery into the thoracic venous system. Determining which mechanism plays the predominant role in blood flow during cardiopulmonary resuscitation (CPR) is difficult; it may depend on several factors. Some of the factors include patient size, chest compliance, the presence or absence of pleural filling defects, and cardiomegaly. Maximizing the affects of both mechanisms is perhaps best.

Assessing Effectiveness. The effectiveness of the team's efforts must be monitored frequently. Improvement in mucous membrane color and the presence of a palpable pulse during CPCR has been used for assessing effectiveness. However, even in the best of circumstances palpation of a pulse can be difficult. The placement of a Doppler flat probe on the cornea is a more reliable method of assessing blood flow through the common carotid artery than the use of the Doppler at peripheral sites. Monitoring peripheral pulses with quantitative Doppler techniques has shown that the pulse generated during compression is, in fact, from venous flow and not arterial flow. If a direct arterial line is in place, then arterial pressure wave forms and pressures can be used to assess effectiveness of therapy. In essence, the clinician will have a compression-to-compression assessment of the technique; the goal is to achieve a diastolic pressure of 40 mm Hg or greater. Some investigators have shown that when aortic diastolic pressure was raised above 40 mm Hg, usually with α-adrenergic drugs or other special maneuvers, dogs could be successfully resuscitated from CPA. End-tidal carbon dioxide ($ETCO_2$) has been suggested as a way to noninvasively assess resuscitation efforts. Studies have shown that $ETCO_2$ varies directly with cardiac output during cardiac arrest. Dramatic decreases in $ETCO_2$ occur during cardiac arrest; with CPCR a dramatic increase is seen and even a more dramatic increase or overshoot when spontaneous circulation returns. In humans the initial $ETCO_2$ measurement obtained at the outset of CPCR is very low (11 to 12 mm Hg), compared with normal $ETCO_2$ of 40 to 45 mm Hg.

If resuscitation efforts are not effective, then the resuscitation techniques must be changed. It may be necessary to increase or decrease the rate, duration, and depth of compression; change the hand or patient's position; change the person performing compressions; or use alternative or augmenting techniques.

Alternate Techniques to Improve Blood Flow. If one technique is not working, then the team should do the following:

- Ventilate with every second or third chest compression. (This has been shown to increase intrathoracic pressure and to improve cerebral [but not myocardial] blood flow.)
- To maximize the thoracic pump mechanism of blood flow in larger breed dogs, compress the chest where it is widest.

- Keep in mind that intermittent abdominal compression, alternating with external chest compression, improves venous return to the chest (This has been reported to improve arterial blood pressure and cerebral and myocardial perfusion.)
- Use abdominal counterpressure (A sandbag or a hand is used to apply steady pressure over the midabdomen; this prevents the posterior displacement of the diaphragm when the chest is compressed. This technique increases intrathoracic pressure and improves cerebral blood flow.)

Phase Two: Advanced Life Support

Once BLS objectives have been achieved, they must be maintained and a shift is made to advanced life support. During advanced life support, drugs and countershock is administered based on ECG and clinical findings. A *D* and *E* can be added to the ABC mnemonic (Box 13-3). The type of cardiac arrest present dictates drug therapy during CPA; therefore ECG monitoring is required.

Drugs

Fluids. CPA is a rapidly vasodilating disease process; therefore crystalloid fluids such as lactated Ringer's are indicated. Dextrose solutions were implicated in increased morbidity and mortality in association with cardiac arrest and should not be used. The initial dose of fluids is 40 ml/kg in the dog and 20 ml/kg in the cat. The fluids should be given rapidly intravenously, in aliquots sufficient to maintain effective circulating volume. When anemia or hypoproteinemia is present whole blood, plasma, hetastarch, or dextran 70 may be indicated.

BOX 13-3 ⦾

Mnemonics for Key Steps in Advanced Life Support

Airway—Establish airway
Breathing—Once every 3-5 seconds
Circulation—80-120 Compressions/min
Drugs—Administer drugs
Electrical—Defibrillate

Atropine. Atropine has predominant parasympatholytic effects. Its use in cardiac arrest is based on its vagolytic action. It plays a central role in the prevention and management of CPA associated with intense vagal stimulation. Atropine is indicated in the treatment of ventricular asystole and slow sinus or idioventricular rhythms. The recommended dose is 0.02 to 0.04 mg/kg.

Epinephrine. Epinephrine possesses both α- and β-adrenergic properties. Epinephrine's strong α-adrenergic properties cause arterial vasoconstriction. Diastolic blood pressure is increased, which results in augmented coronary and cerebral blood flow. Aortic diastolic pressure is the critical determinant of success or failure of resuscitative efforts in animals and humans. The drug also causes constriction of large veins that displace blood out of the venous capacitance vessels. It has been reported that higher doses of epinephrine (0.2 mg/kg) may be more effective than the previously recommended doses (0.02 mg/kg). The higher doses tend to improve cerebral blood flow but also predisposes to ventricular fibrillation. Initial doses of epinephrine should be low and titrated upward until the desired effect is achieved.

Two-Percent Lidocaine. Lidocaine is a class 1 antiarrhythmic agent and is most commonly used to treat ventricular arrhythmias (i.e., premature ventricular contractions, ventricular tachycardia). Lidocaine may be used to supplement treatment of refractory ventricular fibrillation and is used as a background drug to raise the fibrillatory threshold. Studies suggest that lidocaine increases the energy requirements for defibrillation. The dose is 0.5 to 1.0 mg/kg in cats and 1 to 2 mg/kg in dogs.

Magnesium Sulfate or Chloride. Hypomagnesemia has been reported in critically ill dogs and can contribute to the development of lethal ventricular arrhythmias such as ventricular tachycardia and fibrillation. Magnesium has been used to treat such arrhythmias. The exact mechanism of action is not clear. Whether magnesium is effective because it repletes an intracellular or extracellular deficit or because of some intrinsic antiarrhythmic property irrespective of magnesium level is not known. It has been suggested that magnesium therapy be considered for patients suffering refractory ventricular fibrillation. The dose is 30 mg/kg given over 2 minutes.

Sodium Bicarbonate. The use of $NaHCO_3$ has been deemphasized. It was one of the primary drugs used in the treatment of cardiac arrest. The premise for its use was that it corrected metabolic acidosis, which was generated by anaerobic metabolism in hypoxic tissues. It was felt that the metabolic acidosis was associated with decreased cardiac function and lowered ventricular fibrillation threshold. Intracellular pH, not blood pH, determines cardiac viability and the likelihood of resuscitation. Ideally, $NaHCO_3$ administration should be guided by venous blood gas results; however, in the absence of blood gases, $NaHCO_3$ may be given empirically at a conservative dose of 0.5 mEq/kg per 5 minutes of cardiac arrest after the first 5 to 10 minutes, unless the patient is known to have preexisting metabolic acidosis. Moderate hyperventilation helps to offset a developing respiratory acidosis or is necessary as a result of CO_2 development when $NaHCO_3$ is administered.

Vasopressin. Vasopressin is the naturally occurring antidiuretic hormone. In doses higher than required for the antidiuretic hormone effect, vasopressin acts as a direct peripheral smooth muscle vasoconstrictor. Vasopressin is an effective vasoconstrictor and may be used as an alternative to epinephrine in the treatment of cardiac arrest. Vasopressin has been included in the American Heart Association's 2000 CPCR guidelines as a treatment for refractory ventricular fibrillation and pulseless ventricular tachycardia. The guidelines consider its use in asystole and pulseless electrical activity as a *class intermediate*, meaning, not recommended, not forbidden. A single dose is recommended. The half-life of vasopressin in animals with intact circulation is 10 to 20 minutes, which is longer than epinephrine. A suggested dose for vasopressin is 0.8 U/kg given intravenously.

Ten-Percent Calcium. Calcium is not currently recommended in the routine treatment of cardiac arrest. Calcium was used routinely during CPCR to augment cardiac contractility. Excessive intracellular calcium concentrations, however, cause sustained muscular contraction ("stone heart") and myocardial and cerebral vasoconstriction. Calcium has also been implicated in reperfusion injury. Reperfusion injury occurs when ischemic tissue is reperfused or reoxygenated, leading to cellular damage. It remains to be seen whether calcium is beneficial in patients with prolonged arrest. Calcium is indicated when the patient is hyperkalemic, hypocalcemic, or has calcium channel blocker toxicity. The dose of calcium is 0.2 ml/kg of 10% calcium chloride or 0.6 ml/kg 10% calcium gluconate.

Route of Drug Administration. Selecting a site for drug administration during CPCR requires the following considerations:

- Speed with which venous access can be obtained
- Technical abilities of the person attempting venous access
- Difficulties encountered in obtaining venous access
- Rate of drug delivery to the central circulation
- Duration of effective drug levels after injection

Several options (Box 13-4) are available for the delivery of drugs during CPA. Although drug circulation time is dependant on the cardiac output generated during CPCR, it appears that the central or jugular vein is the most desirable, because drugs will be deposited near the heart. Drugs administered at the central venous site have the advantage of providing higher drug concentrations in a shorter period of time. Aside from patient movement during CPCR, placing a jugular catheter in a patient suffering CPA (the jugular vein is usually palpable) is relatively easy. Peripheral venous drug administration tends to deliver the drug to the heart in a lower blood concentration and at a slower rate as compared with the central venous route. Experimental studies in animals demonstrate that drug delivery after peripheral injection is enhanced after the injection with 10 to 30 ml saline flushes and elevation of the extremity. The circulation time was shorter, and the peak concentration was higher. In one study a 0.5 ml/kg flush solution permitted a peripherally administered model drug to reach the central circulation as quickly and in an equivalent concentration as a centrally administered drug during CPCR in a canine cardiac arrest model.

Few studies have examined the intraosseous route for the delivery of drugs during CPCR; however, it remains an option. The intraosseous route has been used in human medicine for treating pediatric CPA. This route requires the placement of an intramedullary cannula inserted into the femur, humerus, and wing of the ilium or tibial crest. "Shock" treatment volumes of fluids and drugs can be injected into the medullary canal and rapid uptake is provided by the abundant endosteum medullary blood supply.

The intratracheal route can be used to administer a limited number of drugs (Box 13-5).

The intratracheal route has been advocated for drug administration when venous access is not accessible, but peak concentrations will be lower than those obtained by other routes. Some studies have indicated that drug uptake from the tracheal surface during resuscitation is sporadic, undependable, and delayed. If this route is to be used, the person administering the drugs should double the IV dose of the drug, then dilute it with 5 to 10 ml of saline (if needed) to provide enough volume, and inject it via a long catheter placed through the endotracheal tube to the carina. Finally, the person ventilating should hyperventilate the patient a few breaths to help disperse the drug.

Several years ago the American Heart Association de-emphasized the use of intracardiac injections. Chest compressions must be stopped while the injection is made. In addition, several potential complications are associated with this procedure: myocardial trauma, lacerated coronary arteries, pericardial effusion, and refractory ventricular fibrillation if the heart muscle is injected with epinephrine. As a result, use of this route is probably best reserved as a last resort after all other methods have failed, if at all.

Regardless of the drug administration route, effective chest compressions must be maintained throughout the CPCR endeavor so that the drug can circulate.

BOX 13-4

Methods of Drug Delivery

- Jugular venous
- Peripheral venous (cephalic)
- Intraosseous
- Intratracheal
- Intracardiac

BOX 13-5

Drugs That Can Be Administered by the Intratracheal Route

Atropine
Lidocaine
Epinephrine

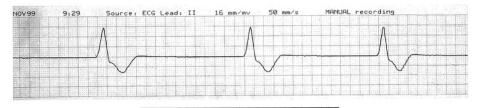

Fig. 13-3 ECG example of pulseless rhythm.

Defibrillation

The purpose of defibrillation is to eliminate the chaotic asynchronous electrical activity of the fibrillating heart. Defibrillation is accomplished by passing an electrical current through the heart, causing the cardiac cells to depolarize and (it is hoped) to repolarize in a uniform manner with resumption of organized and coordinated electrical and contractile activity. Defibrillation stands a better chance of being successful if performed early in the CPCR endeavor. The defibrillator paddles are placed firmly over the heart on each side of the chest after a contact gel has been applied. The person performing the defibrillation should yell "Clear" and make sure that no other personnel is in contact with the patient (or anything associated with the patient) immediately before discharging the defibrillator. An energy level is set, and the defibrillator is discharged. The energy necessary for external defibrillation is at least 3 to 5 J/kg. The internal defibrillation energy level is at least 0.2 to 0.4 J/kg. Excessive energy levels and repeated defibrillation can cause myocardial damage; therefore starting at the lower energy levels and increasing as needed is best.

Cardiac Rhythms

In a study the three types of rhythms noted during CPA were (1) pulseless electrical activity (23.3%), (2) asystole (22.8%), and (3) ventricular fibrillation (19.8%). Additional rhythms that may be encountered during CPCR event include sinus bradycardia (19%), sinus tachycardia, and ventricular tachycardia. Early recognition of the cardiac rhythm will dictate the type of therapy needed. A focused and directed approach is needed to treat CPA. An algorithm or flowchart aids the CPCR team in making therapeutic decisions. An algorithm of the three most common types of rhythms is included in this section. Importantly, if the patient's rhythm changes from one to another, then the CPCR team must do the same with

regard to which algorithm to use. For example, if the patient goes from asystolic rhythm to ventricular fibrillation, then the team must switch from the asystole algorithm to the ventricular fibrillation algorithm.

Pulseless Electrical Activity. The electrical pattern in pulseless rhythms may be near normal in appearance or wide and bizarre QRS complexes (Fig. 13-3). In addition, pulse and heartbeat will not be detectable. Therapy (Box 13-6) should be aimed at determining

---

BOX 13-6

Pulseless Electrical Activity Therapy

Continue Effective Cardiopulmonary Cerebrovascular Resuscitation (CPCR)
- Epinephrine 0.02-0.2 mg/kg

Increase to High Dose if Nonresponsive Search for Treatable Causes
- Hypoxia
- Acidosis
- Hyperkalemia
- Hypovolemia
- Cardiac tamponade
- Tension pneumothorax

Consider the Following:
- Fluid challenge
  Cat: 20 ml/kg bolus
  Dog: 40 ml/kg bolus
- Atropine 0.04 mg/kg (if heart rate is slow)
- Vasopressin 0.8 U/kg
- Sodium bicarbonate ($NaHCO_3$) 0.5 mEq/kg/5 min

Note: If preexisting metabolic acidosis, start at zero time; if no preexisting metabolic acidosis, start at 5 minutes into arrest.

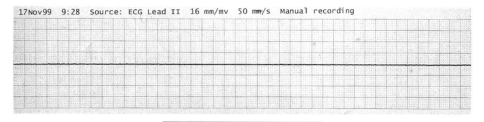

Fig. 13-4 ECG example of asystole.

the underlying cause such as hypoxia, acidosis, hyperkalemia, hypovolemia, cardiac tamponade, and tension pneumothorax. Epinephrine is indicated, and fluid bolus, atropine, and $NaHCO_3$ should be considered.

Asystole. Asystole is characterized by no electrical (a flat line on the ECG) or mechanical activity (Fig. 13-4). End-stage cardiac or pulmonary disease or increased vagal tone may cause this type of arrest. Pulse and heartbeat will not be detectable, and heart movement will not visible (if the heart was viewed). Epinephrine and atropine are the primary drugs (Box 13-7) used to treat this rhythm. Fluid bolus, $NaHCO_3$, pacemaker, and calcium therapy should be considered.

Ventricular Fibrillation. Ventricular fibrillation is characterized by chaotic electrical activity (Fig. 13-5) and no mechanical activity. The ECG display will show no definable pattern, marked irregularity in rhythm; P waves and QRS complexes are unidentifiable. Pulse and heartbeat are undetectable. The heart would look like a quivering bag of worms if viewed. Defibrillation is the treatment of choice (Box 13-8).

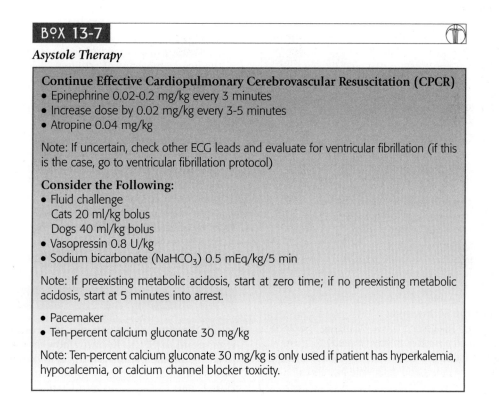

BOX 13-7

Asystole Therapy

Continue Effective Cardiopulmonary Cerebrovascular Resuscitation (CPCR)
- Epinephrine 0.02-0.2 mg/kg every 3 minutes
- Increase dose by 0.02 mg/kg every 3-5 minutes
- Atropine 0.04 mg/kg

Note: If uncertain, check other ECG leads and evaluate for ventricular fibrillation (if this is the case, go to ventricular fibrillation protocol)

Consider the Following:
- Fluid challenge
  Cats 20 ml/kg bolus
  Dogs 40 ml/kg bolus
- Vasopressin 0.8 U/kg
- Sodium bicarbonate ($NaHCO_3$) 0.5 mEq/kg/5 min

Note: If preexisting metabolic acidosis, start at zero time; if no preexisting metabolic acidosis, start at 5 minutes into arrest.

- Pacemaker
- Ten-percent calcium gluconate 30 mg/kg

Note: Ten-percent calcium gluconate 30 mg/kg is only used if patient has hyperkalemia, hypocalcemia, or calcium channel blocker toxicity.

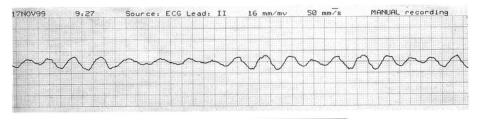

Fig. 13-5 ECG example of ventricular fibrillation.

BOX 13-8

Ventricular Fibrillation Therapy

Continue Effective Cardiopulmonary Cerebrovascular Resuscitation (CPCR)
- Defibrillate
- 3 J/kg external
- 0.2 J/kg internal
- Defibrillate
- 4 J/kg external
- 0.3 J/kg internal
- Defibrillate
- 5 J/kg external
- 0.4 J/kg internal
- Epinephrine 0.02-0.2 mg/kg or vasopressin 0.8 U/kg
- Defibrillate (previous setting)
- Two-percent lidocaine
  Dogs: 2-4 mg/kg
  Cats: 0.2 mg/kg
- Defibrillate (previous setting)
- Search for treatable causes:
  Metabolic disturbances
  Hypothermia
  Hypovolemia
  Epinephrine increase from previous dose

Consider the Following:
- Sodium bicarbonate (NaHCO₃) 0.5 mEq/kg
- Second dose of lidocaine
- Give half of the previous dose
- Defibrillate
- 3-5 J/kg external prn
- 0.2-0.4 J/kg internal prn

Consider the Following:
- Magnesium sulfate or chloride 30 mg/kg if ventricular fibrillation refractory to other therapy
- If ventricular fibrillation persists, repeat epinephrine in increasing doses and defibrillate as needed

---

Phase Three: Prolonged Life Support

Once the heart is beating spontaneously, the patient should be monitored closely. Special attention should be paid to the cardiovascular, pulmonary, and central nervous system. Monitoring as many parameters as possible for each system is helpful. Asking the following questions gives the team a clear overview of the patient's status:

- What is the heart rate and rhythm? (If arrhythmias are present, then antiarrhythmic drugs, correction of electrolyte abnormalities, or oxygen therapy may be indicated.)
- How is the blood pressure, central venous pressure, and pulse pressure? (All are indications of the heart's mechanical activity.)
- How is the patient's mucous membrane color, capillary refill, urine output, and toe web temperature? (These are indications of the peripheral perfusion.)
- What is the patient's respiratory rate and character of breathing?
- Does the patient seem to be taking adequate breaths?
- Can airway sounds be auscultated? (If airway sounds cannot be heard, pleural filling defects must be ruled out.)
- What is the patient's mental status?
- Is the patient's condition improving or deteriorating? (Mannitol, corticosteroids, or diuretics may be indicated.)

Summary

Ideally the team will have an idea of the owner's wishes with regard to CPCR. Knowing how far owners want to go should their animals arrest is important. Do the owners want an emergency thoracotomy performed, closed chest CPCR, or no resuscitation? Many factors come into play when deciding whether CPCR is to be attempted: the patient's current condition, the prognosis for recovery, the age, and the owner's financial limitations. The animals who survive CPCR are often those who were young and healthy before the arrest or those who had a drug reaction. The survival rate or the percentages of patients who suffer cardiac arrest and are discharged from the hospital are not that great.

Two studies report similar findings when compared with humans. The University of California–Davis study reported that 3.8% of dogs and 2.3% of cats were still alive at 1 week. The Colorado State study reported the hospital discharge rate was 4.1% for dogs and 9.6% for cats. Even with the dismal survival rates, if resuscitation is to be undertaken, then it needs to be managed aggressively. The veterinary team needs to have a plan regarding how the CPA will be managed; cases in which resuscitation is successful often is due, at least in part, to a informed, prepared, and efficient CPCR team.

Suggested Readings

Cole SG, Otto CM, Hughes D: Cardiopulmonary cerbral resuscitation in small animals—a clinical practice review (I), *J Vet Emerg Crit Care* 12:261-267, 2002.

Cole SG, Otto CM, Hughes D: Cardiopulmonary cerbral resuscitation in small animals—a clinical practice review (II), *J Vet Emerg Crit Care* 13:20-23, 2003.

Crowe DT: Evaluation of a Doppler flow detector probe on the eye for determining effectiveness of blood flow generation with cardiac massage in dogs, *Proc Int Vet Emerg Crit Care Symp* 3:837, 1992.

D'alecy L et al: Dextrose containing intravenous fluid impairs outcome and increases death after eight minutes of cardiac arrest and resuscitation in dogs, *Surgery* 100:505-511, 1986.

Gaddis GM, Dolister M, Gassis ML: Mock drug delivery to the proximal aorta during cardiopulmonary resuscitation: central vs. peripheral intravenous infusion with varying flush volumes, *Acad Emerg Med* 2(12):1027-1033, 1995.

Gonzalez ER: Pharmacologic controversies in CPR, *Ann Emerg Med* 22(2):317-323, 1993.

Grauer K, Cavallaro D: Sudden cardiac death—the role of electrolytes in cardiac arrest. In *ACLS a comprehensive review,* vol 2, St Louis, 1993, Mosby Lifeline, pp 324-326.

Haskins SC: Internal cardiac compression, *J Am Vet Med Assoc* 200:1945-1946, 1992.

Henik RA: Basic life support and external cardiac compression in dogs and cats, *J Am Vet Med Assoc* 200:1925-1931, 1992.

Jaffe AS: Cardiovascular pharmacology I, *Circulation* 74(suppl IV):IV-70-IV-74, 1986.

Kass PH, Haskins SC: Survival following cardiopulmonary resuscitation in dogs and cats, *J Vet Emerg Crit Care* 2:57-65, 1992.

Kayser SR, Callaham ML: A critical reappraisal of the pharmacologic management of cardiac arrest, *Pharm Ther Forum* 33:6, 1985.

Kern KB, Niemann JT: Perfusion pressure. In Paradise NA, Halperin HR, Nowak RM, editors: *Cardiac arrest the science and practice of resuscitation medicine,* Baltimore,1996, Williams & Wilkins, pp 270-285.

Kerz T, Dick W: Routes for drug administration during cardiopulmonary resuscitation, *Anaesthesist* 45(6):550-565, 1996.

Macintire DK, Drobatz KJ, Haskins SC et al: Cardiopulmonary cerebral resuscitation (CPCR). In *Manual of small animal emergency and critical care medicine,* Baltimore, 2005, Lippincott Williams & Wilkins, pp 16-26.

Marino PL: Cardiac arrest. In *The ICU Book,* Baltimore,1998, Williams & Wilkins, pp 260-277.

Martin LG, Matteson VL, Wingfield WE et al: Abnormalities of serum magnesium in critically ill dogs: incidence and implications, *J Vet Emerg Crit Care* 4:15-20, 1994.

Martin LG, Wingfield WE, Van Pelt DR et al: Magnesium in the 1990s: implications for veterinary critical care, *J Vet Emerg Crit Care* 3:105-114, 1994.

McGeorge F: Diagnosis during cardiac arrest real time monitoring. In Paradise NA, Halperin HR, Nowak RM, editors: *Cardiac arrest the science and practice of resuscitation medicine,* Baltimore, 1996, Williams & Wilkins, pp 562-580.

Rebello CD, Crowe DT: Cardiopulmonary resuscitation: current recommendations, *Vet Clin North Am* 19:1127-1149, 1989.

Rush JE, Wingfield WE: Recognition and frequency of dysrhythmias during cardiopulmonary arrest, *J Am Vet Med Assoc* 200:1932-1937, 1992.

Tomaselli GF: Etiology, electrophysiology, and mechanics of ventricular fibrillation. In Paradise NA, Halperin HR, Nowak RM, editors: *Cardiac arrest the science and practice of resuscitation medicine,* Baltimore, 1996, Williams & Wilkins, pp 301-319.

Waldrop JE, Rozanski EA, Swanke ED et al: Causes of pulmonary arrest, resuscitation management, and functional outcome in dogs and cats surviving cardiopulmonary arrest, *J Vet Emerg Crit Care* 14:22-29, 2004.

Weil MH, Tang W: Wolf Creek Conference IV on cardiopulmonary resuscitation: addressing the scientific basis of reanimation, *New Horiz* 5:97, 1997.

Wingfield WE: Cardiopulmonary arrest and resuscitation in small animals. I. Basic life support, *Emerg Sci Tech Adv Vet Med* 2:21-26, 1996.

Wingfield WE: Controversial issues in cardiopulmonary resuscitation. *Scientific proceedings of the 23rd annual meeting of the Veterinary Emergency and Critical Care Society,* San Antonio, 1997, The Society, pp 63-70.

Wingfield WE, Van Pelt DR: Respiratory and cardiopulmonary arrest in dogs and cats: 265 cases (1986-1991), *J Am Vet Med Assoc* 200:1993-1996, 1992.

Zaritsky AL: Resuscitation pharmacology. In Chernow B, editor: *Essentials of critical care pharmacology,* Baltimore, 1994, Williams & Wilkins, pp 179-192.

CHAPTER 14

Trauma

JENNIFER J. DEVEY, DENNIS T. CROWE, JR.

Introduction

A well-equipped hospital with a well-trained team of doctors, veterinary technicians, and receptionists is essential for treating the seriously injured patient. The team must be prepared to address both the medical needs of the patient and the emotional needs of the owners. Medical skills go hand in hand with caring and compassion. Although the information in this chapter deals primarily with the medical management of trauma, taking care of the distraught owner can be as important as taking care of the medical needs of the animal.

Survival of the injured patient depends on many factors, including the type and severity of the injury and the medical treatment provided. Recognition, assessment, action, and reassessment are the four essential components of effective trauma management. Technicians and doctors must be able to recognize critical injuries quickly, because the outcome of a very severe injury often is determined within the first few minutes. Technicians usually have the first contact with patients in the hospital; therefore they must be able to assess the patient rapidly and determine whether potentially life-threatening problems are present. The veterinary team must be able to act immediately and treat the problems in order of priority. Resuscitation may entail multiple invasive procedures, laboratory tests, advanced diagnostic tests (including contrast radiographic studies and ultrasound), and potentially emergency surgery, often during the first, or so called golden hour after the injury. Therefore the hospital must be equipped and the team trained to deal with all possible emergencies.

Initially it should be assumed always that the patient has a serious injury until proven otherwise. By anticipating the worst, the team is more likely to recognize injuries and their secondary effects. All patients should be evaluated in the same stepwise fashion, starting with the ABCs of *airway, breathing* and *circulation*. A patient with a distal forelimb fracture sustained during a fall also may have pneumothorax, which can be overlooked easily if a complete assessment is not performed.

Once resuscitation has been initiated and after completion, aggressive monitoring is vital. Tracking changes in vital signs and other physiologic parameters allows technicians and doctors to determine if the patient's status is deteriorating. Detailed flow sheets and treatment sheets must be used. Because injured patients are at serious risk for secondary complications such as pneumonia, delayed healing, and the systemic inflammatory response syndrome, intensive monitoring and treatment may help to prevent some of these complications (Box 14-1).

Readiness

Ready Area and Crash Cart

Each hospital should have a ready area, which is where all emergency patients requiring immediate care are brought for examination and treatment. The ready area should also be where in-hospital emergencies are treated. It is usually centrally located, such as a main treatment room, although it can be the surgical preparation area. It should be near the operating room, because seriously injured trauma patients may require surgery as part of their resuscitation. The ready area must have all the necessary equipment for full resuscitation, including open-chest cardiopulmonary resuscitation. Oxygen (O_2), airway and vascular access devices, fluids (e.g., crystalloids, colloids), suction, monitoring equipment, and basic bandaging supplies must be available. A crash cart with multiple drawers should be outfitted with all the necessary supplies. The crash cart should be checked on once or twice daily to ensure all the necessary supplies are present and equipment is in working condition. A piece of tape placed diagonally across the cart can be used as an indicator of whether or not materials have been removed. When the cart is used, the tape is taken down and not replaced until the missing supplies have been replaced. The tape also can be dated and initialed after each check so that other members of the team can be certain that the cart has all the necessary equipment.

Monitoring equipment should be kept on the top of the crash cart and include suction and equipment to continuously monitor electrocardiograms (ECGs), blood pressure (BP), capnography, and pulse oximetry. All equipment should be checked once or twice daily to ensure it is plugged in and in good working condition. Several sizes of BP cuffs should be available (usually 2 to 5 cm widths). Good overhead lighting is essential. Both a wide-beam dish light and a focusing high-intensity cool-beam light should be available. Direct light sources that can be worn, such as a head loupe or inexpensive headlamps or snake lights (available from hardware stores), allow the airway, oral cavity, and wounds to be closely assessed while freeing up both hands.

A limited number of sterile surgical supplies should be kept with the crash cart, including scalpel blades; curved Mayo scissors; curved hemostats; and various sizes of polypropylene suture material (sizes from 2 to 5-0) for vascular suturing, tracheotomy, or resuscitative thoracotomy. Satinsky forceps, although expensive, are invaluable as vascular forceps for controlling hemorrhage from large vessels such as the vena cava or the aorta. Ideally, a pair of Balfour retractors or Finochietto rib retractors also should be available. Laparotomy pads and towels, which can be used to cover and protect open wounds from infection and to apply pressure to bleeding wounds, should be sterilized and available. If a resuscitative thoracotomy is required, then these pads and towels also can be used to pack bleeding areas. Red rubber tubes are effective vascular occlusive devices. When wrapped around a vessel and pulled tightly with hemostats, a red rubber tube acts as an atraumatic Rumel tourniquet.

Suction

Suction equipment should be capable of generating pressures of up to 760 mm Hg. Electronic suction devices are ideal; however, hand-held suction devices (Mityvac, Neward Enterprises, Cucamonga, CA) are an inexpensive but effective alternative. A suction trap placed between the suction tip and the tubing will help prevent clogging of the tubing. Several different types of suction tips should be available. A Yankauer suction tip is useful for oral and pharyngeal secretions. A dental tip can be used to remove vomitus and clots from the rima glottis and trachea. Tracheal whistle-tip catheters can be used for removing frothy secretions, vomit, and blood from the trachea. Suction also can be attached directly to the end of the endotracheal tube if the patient is intubated and fluid or exudate is obstructing the tube. The suction device always should be ready for immediate use. This means that the suction tip should be attached to the tubing and the tubing should be attached to the suction unit. If an electric unit is being used, then the machine should be plugged into an outlet.

Fluids

Trauma patients often need large volumes of IV fluids. Balanced electrolyte solutions that are buffered are the preferred crystalloid solutions (e.g., lactated Ringer's solution, Normosol-R, Plasmalyte-A). Because 70% to 80% of crystalloids infused will have left the intravascular space within 1 hour, many patients require an infusion of colloids to help maintain euvolemia. Both synthetic and biologic colloids should be kept readily available. Synthetic colloids include dextran 70, hetastarch, and pentastarch. Biologic colloids include human albumin, whole blood, and fresh frozen plasma. Blood products should not be administered through the same line as calcium-containing fluids, because the calcium binds with the citrate in the anticoagulant. Because trauma patients are at risk for developing coagulopathies secondary to loss of clotting factors and platelets, fresh whole blood and fresh frozen plasma are indicated frequently in the severely hemorrhaging patient.

Autotransfusion

Autotransfusion equipment should be available. If large volumes of blood are present in the thoracic or abdominal cavity, then the blood can be collected into sterile containers and reinfused as an autotransfusion. When using a suction unit to collect the blood, care should be taken to prevent suctioning air simultaneously. Commercial autotransfusion systems are available, but the cost may be prohibitive for most veterinary hospitals. A simple but effective way to administer autotransfusions is to use a bag designed for delivering liquid enteral nutrition as the transfusion bag. These bags have a large opening at the top with a cap. The cap is removed and the blood is poured into the bag. Blood administration sets can be attached to the food bags and gas sterilized as a unit. A simpler method is to use a sterile 1 L IV fluid bag. The top is cut along approximately 30% of the front panel. In this way the bag can still be hung and blood poured into the bag through this hole. Blood is collected from the patient and placed into the transfusion bag. Ideally, this blood should be administered through a filter; however, in an emergency a filter is not essential. It often is more important that the patient receives the blood rapidly (filters significantly decrease the infusion rate).

Radiology and Ultrasound

A radiograph machine capable of producing high-quality radiographs is a necessary part of evaluating injured patients. A 300 to 500 mA radiograph machine and an automatic processor that can develop films within minutes are needed. The recent availability of digital radiography has significantly enhanced the speed and diagnostic capability of radiographs; however, these systems are still expensive and are only available in larger hospitals. Accurate technique charts should be available for taking the standard lateral and ventrodorsal views (as well as horizontal beam radiographs). Horizontal beam radiography causes much less stress to the patient, especially if the patient is showing any signs of respiratory distress. This type of radiography also provides an effective means of determining the presence of free fluid in the chest or abdominal cavity. The technician should be trained to perform contrast radiographic studies such as IV urography, double-contrast cystography, peritoneography, and barium series. Contrast dyes, tubes, and catheters should be stocked in radiology for these studies. Both positioning charts and protocols for contrast studies should be posted or be readily available.

Injured patients who are nonambulatory or unconscious should be secured to Plexiglas or wood spinal boards and radiographed through the boards. Trauma films or survey radiographs of the animal from nose to tail can be effectively taken through both materials to look for obvious injuries. A variety of positioning devices should be available to help decrease the exposure of the staff to radiation. This includes things such as V trays, foam pads, sand bags, and cushions filled with beads.

Ultrasound is one of the diagnostic tests of choice for rapid evaluation of the internally hemorrhaging trauma patient. Free fluid can be rapidly visualized in the abdominal or thoracic cavities, as well as in the pericardial sac. Depending on the skill of the ultrasonographer it also can be used to determine injuries to liver, spleen, kidneys, and bladder. An ultrasound survey examination can be completed within 5 to 10 minutes.

Laboratory

Laboratory equipment ideally includes a centrifuge for spinning packed cell volumes (PCVs) and for separating serum; a refractometer for blood, urine, and fluid analysis; and capabilities for analyzing blood gases, basic chemistries, complete blood cell counts, and coagulation parameters. Point-of-care devices are fairly inexpensive and allow for rapid (i.e., 1 to 2 minutes) assessment of blood gases, acid-base status, electrolytes, glucose, lactate, and coagulation parameters using very small volumes of whole blood (0.05 ml). A good microscope is essential for performing manual differentials and evaluating urine and fluid cytology.

Surgery

Many seriously injured trauma patients require surgery as part of their resuscitation. Because time is of the essence for many of these patients, the anesthesia machine must be set up and the operating room must be kept ready. A major surgical pack and gowns should be laid out and ready to be opened at a moment's notice. The suction unit must be functional and ready to receive suction tubing from the surgeon. Electrocautery should be plugged in, and the ground plate should be in place. The use of a surgical headlight will greatly enhance visualization of bleeding and traumatized tissues and vessels; it should be a standard part of the operating room equipment. Trauma surgical packs should contain the basic equipment for an exploratory laparotomy

or thoracotomy. In addition, towels and laparotomy pads (for packing large bleeding wounds) and red rubber tubes for use as vascular occlusion devices should be sterilized and ready for use. Many trauma patients are hypothermic or develop hypothermia during resuscitation and surgery; therefore a means of warming the patient should be available.

Warming Devices

Keeping a patient normothermic is very important because hypothermia interferes with normal metabolic functions (leading to problems such as vasodilation, cardiac dysfunction, and interference with coagulation). When the clinician is rewarming a hypothermic patient in hemorrhagic shock, he or she should warm the body core first. Warming the periphery leads to vasodilation and can worsen both core hypothermia and shock. The nonmobile patient should always be monitored closely, because almost any warming device has the potential to cause burns.

Warm-air circulating blankets are an effective means of keeping patients warm. Artificial warming devices and hot-water bottles should not come in direct contact with the patient's skin. Instead, they should be wrapped or covered in a towel before being applied to the patient. A blanket warmer is handy for keeping towels and blankets warm. Warm-water bottles can be kept in an incubator or heated in a microwave. If IV fluid bags are being used as warm-water bottles, then food coloring should be added to the bags so that they can be easily identified for reuse. This also prevents inadvertently using them for parenteral fluids. Homemade warming bags can be made from fabric sacks filled with rolled oats. These can be heated in a microwave and are reusable. Bubble wrap can be warmed in the microwave (in a bowl of water) and wrapped around the patient; the air cells will retain heat well. Bubble wrap or plastic food wrap can be sterilized and used in the operating room to help prevent hypothermia. IV fluids should be kept warm in an incubator or warmed in a microwave. Fluids administered rapidly at room temperature can significantly lower a patient's temperature.

Commercially available infant isolettes and tables can be purchased at reasonable cost through used hospital equipment suppliers. Heat lamps that are either commercially available or even made from an exposed light bulb can provide additional external heat. These always have the potential to overheat the patient, and close monitoring is required. Temperatures should never exceed 106° to 110° F.

Veterinary Team

The veterinary team (i.e., technicians, doctors, receptionists) must be mentally and physically ready to perform the necessary tasks. All team members must be dedicated and trained to do their jobs. Technicians must be familiar with the location and operation of all the equipment needed for diagnostics and treatment. They must be trained to place IV catheters, bandage wounds, and provide anesthesia. Team members must also understand the various procedures involved in preparing instruments and equipment and assist when asked to do so. Familiarity with the techniques, tests, procedures, and treatments means the nurse is able to help monitor for complications and for efficacy.

Drills are the most effective way to prepare the team for emergencies. These drills can be performed on stuffed animals or cadavers. This encourages teamwork and the chance to practice psychomotor skills. It allows each individual to know exactly what his or her responsibility is during an emergency situation. Through practice sessions, recognition, assessment, and treatment become more automatic during a true emergency.

Protocols

It has been shown in human hospitals that the implementation of protocols for treating patients significantly decreases morbidity and mortality. These protocols should be readily available for everyone to use. Charts for drug doses for cardiopulmonary resuscitation should be posted in a visible location. Resuscitation algorithms should be posted so that under the stress of the emergency situation, resuscitation is undertaken in an orderly fashion and important treatments are not overlooked.

First Aid and Safety

Initial treatment often begins at the scene of the accident, and prehospital care may influence outcome significantly. Safety and first aid information can be provided to owners during the initial telephone contact to help both at the scene of the accident and en route to the hospital. Most owners will be stressed and frightened because a pet has just been hurt. Calming the owner is important to gain accurate information so that appropriate first aid instructions can be given. A calm owner also is much more capable of following instructions. The tone of voice that the technician uses may be as important as the information dispensed. If the owner has not had any previous first aid experience, then it may be best to advise him or her to confine the injured pet to a box, strap it to a board, or otherwise limit the animal's movement and transport it to the clinic as rapidly as possible.

All team members should follow several basic rules:

- Ensure that the scene is safe. This means watching for other vehicles, broken glass, spilled chemicals, and other hazards.
- Ensure that the owner and staff are safe while working directly with the animal. Blood on the patient may be human blood. To prevent contact with contagious diseases such as hepatitis and human immunodeficiency virus, direct contact with blood should be prevented until the source of the blood is determined. At the scene, towels or clothing should be used to apply direct pressure on wounds. In the hospital, gloves should always be worn before handling animals with blood on their fur. Injured animals often are frightened and in pain. Appropriate precautions for restraint should be used. Muzzles should be placed when available. Plastic muzzles that cover the entire nose and mouth and contain multiple holes to enable breathing and drainage of oral secretions are often easier to place, less painful, and more comfortable for the trauma patient than the standard muzzles that fit tightly over the bridge of the nose. If a muzzle is not available, a tie or belt can be wrapped around a dog's muzzle. If facial hemorrhage or making a muzzle is not possible, then a blanket or large jacket can be used to cover the patient's head.
- Minimize movement of the patient until the full extent of the injuries is known. The pet should be transported on a board or in a box if it is nonambulatory. If ambulatory, then the animal should not be allowed to jump in and out of the vehicle and walking should be kept to a minimum. This will help to prevent making any potentially minor problem into major problem. For example, a partial body wall hernia may become a complete hernia if the animal jumps.

- Apply direct pressure to wounds with a clean cloth whenever possible. Alternatively, with bleeding from extremities, hands can encircle and squeeze the limb or tail proximal to the wound to help control hemorrhage. Newspaper, large sticks, or pieces of wood can be used as splints for lower limb fractures.

Patient Assessment

Triage

Triage is the sorting of patients according to the severity of injury or illness to ensure that the most critical patients are treated first. The technician, who quickly evaluates each patient on arrival and determines how rapidly each needs to be seen by the doctor, usually does triage. Patients who have been involved in any serious accident should be triaged immediately to the ready area of the hospital for evaluation.

Primary and Secondary Survey

When the patient arrives at the hospital, gloves should be worn, animals should be muzzled, and movement of the patient should be kept to a minimum. The animal should be approached from the rostral direction and quickly surveyed for level of consciousness, breathing and respiratory pattern, abnormal body or limb posture, the presence of blood or other materials in or around the patient, and any other gross abnormalities. The patient should be brought immediately to the ready area for assessment. A primary survey should be completed within 30 to 60 seconds. The primary survey assesses level of consciousness and the *ABCs*. The level of consciousness can be rapidly evaluated using a simple scoring system such as AVPU—alert (A), verbally responsive (V), responsive to painful stimuli (P), or unresponsive (U). If the animal is unconscious, then the head and neck should be extended to help provide a clear airway. The airway is checked for patency. If visual examination of the oral cavity and oropharynx is required, the clinician should make sure appropriate precautions are taken to ensure no one is bitten.

Once the level of consciousness has been evaluated, the clinician assesses the patient's airway by looking, listening, and feeling. If the patient shows signs of an exaggerated inspiratory effort, the airway may not be patent. The presence of increased respiratory effort, paradoxical chest wall movement, abdominal wall movement with respiration, nasal flare, open mouth, extended head and neck, abducted elbows, and cyanosis are all indicators of respiratory distress that require immediate treatment. Airway assessment is followed immediately by breathing assessment done by watching chest wall motion and ausculting the trachea and lung sounds bilaterally. The clinician should auscult lung sounds bilaterally, because the animal may have a significant unilateral injury. He or she should also listen to lung sounds before listening to heart tones, because the ear is much less discerning of softer sounds once it has adjusted to louder sounds. Percussion of the thorax may be indicated to help rule out a pneumothorax or hemothorax. The clinician assesses circulation by checking mucous membrane color and capillary refill time and ausculting for heart tones at the same time as central (femoral) and peripheral (dorsal metatarsal) pulses are palpated. Finally, a very rapid assessment and palpation of the abdomen, flank, pelvis, spine, and limbs is carried out (Technical Tip Box 14-2).

Vital signs are taken *after* the primary survey is completed. Vital signs include heart rate, pulse rate and strength, respiratory rate, mucous membrane color, capillary refill time, and temperature. Temperature should always be checked last for several reasons. Patients with extremely slow heart rates can have a vagally induced arrest with stimulation of the rectum. In these patients an axillary or ear temperature should be taken. In addition, most patients will have an elevation of respiratory and heart rates once a cold thermometer is inserted.

BP measurement is very important and should be considered one of the vital signs that should be monitored in all trauma patients. For example, the combination of a high heart rate and a high BP is consistent with pain. The presence of a high heart rate and low BP indicates hypovolemic shock. Jugular veins should be clipped and assessed for distention, filling time, and relaxation time. A mildly distended jugular vein will be noted when the animal is in lateral recumbency. A highly distended jugular vein or one that is distended with the animal standing or in sternal recumbency indicates a high central venous pressure (CVP) (usually associated with a severe pneumothorax or pericardial effusion in the patient in shock). A flat jugular is consistent

BOX 14-2

Technical Tip: Percussion—Method and Interpretation

Method
1. Lay the hand on the chest wall or body surface being examined.
2. Tap firmly (using the top of the middle finger of the hand) on the patient, with the middle and ring finger of the opposite hand.
3. Strike or tap several times until consistency is reached (interpreting the strength of the tap, the sound, and the vibration generated).

Interpretation
1. A very low-pitched resonant sound (hollow sound) indicates an air-filled structure under the body wall.
2. A moderate-pitched sound with slight resonance (solid sound) indicates fluid- or tissue-filled structure under the body wall.
3. A high-pitched sound with significant resonance indicates solid structure (possibly under pressure) or a fluid-filled structure under pressure under the body wall.

with hypovolemia, as is a jugular vein that takes a long time to fill (i.e., longer than 3 to 4 seconds) when pressure is placed at the thoracic inlet to occlude the vein (as if one was doing a jugular venipuncture). Peripheral vein distention can be assessed in some dogs. When the patient is in lateral recumbency, mild distention of the lateral saphenous vein should occur if the vein is below the level of the right atrium. Raising the limb should cause the vein to flatten. The difference in the height of the leg from when the vein is distended to when it becomes flat can be measured. During resuscitation this can be remeasured as a crude assessment of improving venous volume during resuscitation.

Cyanosis may be difficult to detect in patients with severe hemorrhage because 5 g/dl of hemoglobin (Hb) (equivalent to a hematocrit of 15%) is required for the eye to be able to discern cyanosis. Fluorescent lights also interfere with accurate evaluation of mucous membrane color in the face of pallor; therefore penlights should be used in these patients.

Once vital signs are measured, baseline data can be collected. This includes a lead II ECG and baseline lab work. A minimum laboratory database should include a PCV and total solids (TS), blood urea nitrogen via Azostix, and blood glucose. If point-of-care testing is available, then the blood urea nitrogen and glucose along with electrolytes and a blood gas often can be assessed simultaneously. Although point-of-care testing will provide a hematocrit, assessment of a PCV and TS is recommended always. The technician can collect the blood sample by inserting hematocrit tubes into the hub of the catheter stylet. A more extended database should include electrolytes, serum albumin, activated clotting time (or prothrombin time) and activated partial thromboplastin time, and a platelet estimate. A complete database includes a complete blood count with evaluation of a blood smear for the differential, red cell morphology and platelet estimate, chemistry panel, urinalysis, and arterial blood gas. Usually the minimum or extended database is collected initially, and further tests are considered once the patient has been fully examined and resuscitation has been started. Treatment for arrhythmias or laboratory abnormalities should be instituted as indicated.

Resuscitation is started as the primary survey is being completed. Analgesics should be provided to the patient once airway and circulatory resuscitation has been initiated. If the primary survey indicates severe abnormalities such as an inadequate airway, then the airway is immediately established before the physical examination is completed and diagnostics or other treatments are performed.

Hemorrhage also is controlled at this time. Sterile gauze, sterile laparotomy pads, and sterile towels can all be used as pressure bandages. If strike-through occurs, then the initial dressing should not be removed; a second dressing should be placed over the top of the first one. In some cases applying digital pressure to superficial major arteries supplying the hemorrhaging area can control bleeding. Pressure to the deep area adjacent and ventral to the mandible controls maxillary artery flow and will help control hemorrhage to the head. Pressure to the axillary area will help control brachial artery blood flow, and pressure applied to the inguinal and femoral canal region controls femoral artery blood flow. In smaller animals, pressure can be placed on the caudal abdomen, thus occluding external iliac blood flow. If significant bleeding occurs from a distal extremity, BP cuffs can be placed proximal to the wound and inflated to 20 to 40 mm Hg above systolic pressure. This will effectively control most serious hemorrhage while more definitive treatment is being instituted. Tourniquets should not be used whenever possible, because they can cause permanent neurologic and vascular damage within minutes.

In cases of severe hemorrhagic shock or ongoing significant abdominal or pelvic hemorrhage, limited external counterpressure using a wrap incorporating the pelvic limbs, pelvis, and abdomen will be needed. Pressure is applied indirectly to blood vessels under the bandage. Because flow is proportional to the radius of the vessel to the fourth power, any decrease in the radius of the vessel will significantly decrease flow (and hemorrhage) through that vessel. If the pelvic limbs are not included in the bandage, then blood may pool in the pelvic limbs and a risk exists of occluding the caudal abdominal vena cava. The wrap can be made of towels and duct tape or rolled cotton and a full bandage. A towel is placed in between the pelvic limbs. A second large towel is used to wrap the patient in a spiral fashion, starting at the tip of the toes of the pelvic limbs and extending to the diaphragm. The towels are held in place with duct tape. Respiration must be monitored closely, because incorporation of the cranial abdomen will compromise movement of the diaphragm. If this occurs, then a decision will need to be made to either loosen the bandage, which may lead to further hemorrhage, or to place the patient on a ventilator. Two fingers should be able to be placed easily under the wrap when completed. If desired, then a BP cuff can be partially inflated and incorporated into the bandage. The wrap then is secured placing approximately 30 mm Hg pressure on the abdomen. Higher pressures can lead to serious compromise of the circulation to the gastrointestinal tract and the kidney and can lead to irreversible damage. A urinary catheter should be inserted rapidly in male dogs before placement of the wrap so that urine output can be monitored.

The wrap is left in place until the patient is hemodynamically stable, usually 6 to 24 hours. BP is monitored constantly during removal. The wrap is removed slowly from the cranial extent proceeding caudally. If systolic BP drops by more than 5 mm Hg, then removal is stopped and fluids are infused. If pressure continues to drop, then the wrap is replaced.

Once the primary survey is completed and an initial database has been collected, a secondary survey is usually completed. This entails a complete examination of the patient in a systematic fashion from nose to tail.

History

Once the secondary survey is completed, the history is taken. If the patient is stable, then a capsule history can be taken at the time the patient arrives at the hospital. A useful mnemonic is AMPLE:

A Allergies—Does the animal have any known allergies?
M Medications—Is the animal on any medications? If so, then what drugs and what doses?
P Past history—Has the animal had any past medical problems?
L Lasts—When was the pet's last meal, defecation, urination, medication?
E Events—What is the problem now? Details should be given.

Important historical facts relating to the injury include the time elapsed since the injury, the cause of the injury (e.g., fall, hit by car, gunshot), the speed of the car if the animal was hit, evidence of loss of consciousness at the scene, approximate amount of blood lost at the scene, and deterioration or improvement in the patient since the time of injury. The technician should also find out if the patient has other underlying medical diseases or is currently being treated with any medication. Having the owner fill out a history sheet helps provide complete information on the pet, as well as giving the owner something to do while the preliminary evaluation and resuscitation is being completed.

Additional Diagnostic Tests

Once the patient has been completely examined, a history has been taken, and resuscitation has been initiated, further tests may be instituted as indicated. Trauma radiographs are survey radiographs taken of the entire body. If the patient is on a wooden or Plexiglas board, then radiographs should be taken through the board, and the patient should not be moved into dorsal recumbency until spinal injury has been ruled out. If the patient is stable, then lateral and ventrodorsal views should be taken. Survey

---

BOX 14-3 ⊕

Intensive Care Unit List of Concerns

Airways, lungs, ventilation (work of breathing, dead space, SpO_2, $ETCO_2$, Pco_2)
Cardiac contractility, relaxation and rhythm (ECG, CO)
Vascular volume, flow, pressure (arterial and central venous), and tone
Oxygen (O_2) delivery (including Hb and Pao_2)
Substrate delivery and use (glucose)
Fluid balance (water, albumin, colloid, osmotic pressure)
Electrolyte balance (Na, K, Cl, Ca, Mg, P)
Acid-base balance (pH, HCO_3, BE)
Renal function, urine output, USG, sediment
Energy-protein balance (enteral and parenteral nutrition)
Mentation, LOC, cranial and peripheral nerves
Pain and anxiety control
Gastrointestinal function, motility, and integrity
Skin, muscle, and joint care
Immune function (WBCs)
Coagulation (platelets, BT, ACT, FDPs, coagulation panels)
Drugs (doses, metabolism, compatibility, and route)
Catheter and tube sites
Surgical incisions, bandages, splints
General nursing care (physical therapy, mobility)
Assurance and communication (patient and owner)
Charting complete

SpO_2, Oxygen saturation by pulse oximetry; $ETCO_2$, end-tidal carbon dioxide; Pco_2, partial pressure of carbon dioxide; *ECG*, electrocardiogram; *CO*, cardiac output; *Hb*, hemoglobin; Pao_2, partial pressure of oxygen in arterial blood; *Na*, sodium; *K*, potassium; *Cl*, chloride; *Ca*, calcium; *Mg*, magnesium; *P*, phosphorus; HCO_3, bicarbonate; *BE*, base excess; *USG*, urine specific gravity; *LOC*, level of consciousness; *WBCs*, white blood cells; *BT*, bleeding time; *ACT*, activated clotting time; *FDPs*, fibrin degradation products.

radiographs should be taken and assessed before radiographing extremities or other more localized injury. Once again, treatment should be instituted as abnormalities are detected. Contrast studies may be indicated.

If abdominal hemorrhage or rupture of an abdominal viscus (i.e., ruptured urinary bladder, ruptured bowel) is a possibility, then ultrasound and ultrasound-guided abdominocentesis should be performed. Four-quadrant abdominocentesis can be performed, but a high incidence of false-negative results are possible if only small amounts of abdominal fluid are present. If ultrasound is not available, then diagnostic peritoneal lavage should be performed. Diagnostic peritoneal lavage requires a multiholed catheter, warm 0.9% saline, and a collection bag. The patient is placed in left lateral recumbency, and the ventral midline of the abdomen is surgically prepared. Local anesthetic is infused, and the catheter is inserted approximately 2 cm caudal to the umbilicus on the midline or just lateral to the midline. Fluids are infused into the abdomen (20 ml/kg), the abdomen is gently massaged to mix the fluid, and a sample is collected. If the patient's respiration becomes compromised during infusion of the fluids, then infusion should be discontinued. Fluid is analyzed for PCV, TS, potassium, and creatinine (if the clinician believes the patient has a ruptured urinary bladder), and cytology. The catheter can be left in and the PCV can be reassessed at 5- to 10-minute intervals for signs of ongoing hemorrhage (Box 14-3).

Resuscitation

Goals of Resuscitation

To be able to resuscitate the patient in shock, the signs of shock must be recognized. Signs include increased respiratory rate and effort; tachycardia with weak or bounding pulses; pale or muddy mucous membranes; delayed capillary refill; and low body temperature, cool extremities, or both.

The goal of resuscitation is to reverse the signs of shock and provide effective O_2 delivery to the cells. This means that O_2 must be delivered to the alveoli; once there, the pulmonary circulation must take it up. Adequate Hb to transport the O_2 must be present, because the content of O_2 in the blood (Cao_2) is far more dependent on Hb than the dissolved O_2 ($Cao_2 = 1.34 \times$ Hb $\times$ saturation of Hb in the arterial blood [Sao_2] $+ 0.003 \times$ partial pressure of O_2 in arterial blood [Pao_2]). Once the O_2 is taken into the blood it must be able to be transported to the peripheral tissues. This requires adequate circulating volume and a heart that can pump effectively. Preload, or the amount of venous volume that returns to fill the heart, should be maximized. Treatment is aimed at restoring O_2 levels and blood flow to all tissues.

Oxygen

The clinician should provide O_2 immediately at high flow rates, either by flow-by, mask, baggie, or O_2 collar. An unconscious patient without a good gag reflex should be intubated immediately, and O_2 should be provided via the endotracheal tube. Nasal O_2 provides an inspired fraction of O_2 of 0.4 to 0.6, whereas O_2 collars and baggies provide an inspired fraction of O_2 closer to 0.8 to 0.9. Therefore nasal O_2 may not be the ideal initial means of providing O_2. The clinic should not use O_2 cages, because patients cannot be monitored adequately. Every time the door to the O_2 cage is opened, significant fluctuations occur in inspired O_2 concentration. In addition, most O_2 cages do not allow the inspired fraction of O_2 to exceed 0.4.

If the respiratory rate and effort and mucous membrane color are not improving with O_2 supplementation, then the patient either has an injury that is interfering with ventilation or inadequate pulmonary circulation is the problem. Injuries leading to impaired ventilation include pneumothorax, hemothorax, fractured ribs (causing pain that leads to hypoventilation), diaphragmatic hernia, or severe pulmonary contusions. Thoracentesis is indicated if lung sounds are dull and hemothorax or pneumothorax is a possibility. Thoracentesis always should be performed in the patient with possible pneumothorax before taking radiographs, because the distress caused by positioning for radiographs may cause the patient to arrest. If negative suction is not obtained during thoracentesis, then a chest tube must be placed immediately. If the clinician believes the patient has significant intrapulmonic hemorrhage and the site of the hemorrhage is known, then the patient should be placed in lateral recumbency with the affected side down (to allow for more effective ventilation). If the patient has severe pulmonary contusions and is decompensating despite O_2 supplementation, then the patient may need to be rapidly anesthetized, intubated, and started on positive pressure ventilation. Some of these patients require ventilatory support for up to several days until the contusions resolve.

Patients should be intubated in lateral recumbency. Technicians should be able to intubate patients in both lateral and dorsal recumbency and to use a laryngoscope proficiently. If a patient is significantly hypotensive, then raising the head may cause a sufficient decrease in cerebral blood flow to lead to cardiac arrest. Laryngeal stimulation that can occur with blind intubation can cause a vagal response potentially leading to cardiac arrest in the severely hypotensive or bradycardic patient. Once the patient is intubated, the lungs should be ausculted bilaterally to ensure the trachea has been intubated and that the tube is not in a bronchus. If lung sounds cannot be ausculted, then the esophagus may have been intubated (or the patient may have either an airway obstruction or disruption). If the patient cannot be orotracheally intubated because of oral, pharyngeal, or laryngeal injuries, then a tracheotomy is indicated.

Fluids

IV fluids must be provided to the patient in shock at the same time as O_2 is being supplemented. One or more large-bore IV catheters must be placed (14 to 16 gauge in medium and large dogs; 18 to 20 gauge in small dogs and cats). A vascular cutdown may be required for those patients in severe shock. Because flow is directly proportional to the radius to the fourth power and inversely proportional to the length of the catheter, a short large-bore catheter will be more effective for rapid fluid administration than a long small-bore catheter. Peripheral catheters are suitable in most cases. Ideally, a jugular catheter should be placed if large volumes of fluids are to be administered; this allows for measurement of CVP, which is the only way of measuring preload.

A combination of crystalloids and colloids should be delivered at whatever rate is needed to improve the patient's hemodynamic status. The patient that is dying from hypovolemic shock requires fluids at a much faster rate than the patient showing mild signs of shock. Patients in shock require intravascular volume resuscitation, not interstitial resuscitation; therefore large volumes of crystalloid should be infused with caution. Crystalloids are administered in 20 to 30 ml/kg increments. To maintain adequate intravascular volume, colloids should be infused if response to the initial bolus of crystalloids is limited or not seen. Synthetic colloids such as dextran 70 or hetastarch should be administered in 5 ml/kg increments to a maximum volume of 20 ml/kg. Synthetic colloids can be bolused to dogs but should be infused over 10 to 20 minutes in cats. Because many of these patients are in shock from blood loss, the most effective colloid for resuscitation is whole blood. Blood products should be infused as indicated to maintain a PCV of approximately 30% and an albumin greater than 2.0 g/dl.

Because the goal of IV fluid therapy is to restore an effective circulating volume, fluids should be administered incrementally until hemodynamic parameters have normalized. The clinician can most effectively monitor this by ensuring the heart rate returns to a more normal level (in dogs) and that BP is a minimum of 100 mm Hg systolic.

Patients who are not responding to fluid therapy may have ongoing serious internal abdominal hemorrhage. Serious intraabdominal hemorrhage can come from blunt liver trauma, which leads to liver fractures, splenic lacerations, and renal avulsion. Hypotensive resuscitation, placement of limited external counterpressure, or both may be needed in these patients. Alternatively, surgery may be required as part of the resuscitation.

Resuscitating the Patient with Severe Hemorrhage

Hypotensive resuscitation is reserved for those patients in whom hemorrhage will worsen if the BP is restored to normal. It may be appropriate in these patients to restrict fluid resuscitation until the source of the hemorrhage is controlled. Fluids are infused to reach a systolic BP of 85 to 100 mm Hg. Elevations in BP are controlled in an effort to prevent disrupting soft clots that are starting to form. In addition, decreasing the amount of fluids administered reduces the chance that the patient will develop a dilutional coagulopathy and minimizes the risk of iatrogenic hypothermia. For patients with severe intraabdominal hemorrhage, the use of limited external counterpressure also is needed.

Wounds, Bandages, and Splints

As problems are discovered during the secondary survey, specific treatments may be needed. These treatments include controlling external hemorrhage through the use of direct pressure, placing splints, and keeping the patient warm. Most wound infections in acute trauma patients occur after the patient enters the hospital. Hospital bacteria and bacteria from human hands often are the cause. Whenever possible, sterile dressings (e.g., sterile bandage material, laparotomy pads, towels) should be placed initially to help prevent secondary complications. Ideally, wounds should be clipped and cleaned before dressings are placed. The wound must be kept moist and protected from further injury, contamination, and infection. When time permits, the wounds can be cleaned and treated properly.

All wounds should be clipped and cleaned once resuscitation is complete. Placing sterile water-soluble jelly (i.e., KY jelly) in wounds before clipping helps prevent hair from getting lodged in the wound and prevents wound desiccation. Wounds should be cleaned with a surgical disinfecting solution and should not be irrigated in the awake patient that has not received analgesia (because this is a painful procedure). However, irrigation of the wound using a 35 cc syringe and an 18-gauge needle is a most effective means of cleaning wounds. Puncture-type wounds should not be flushed under pressure, because this may force dirt and debris deeper into the wound.

Once the wound has been cleaned, a sterile dressing is placed. Wet-to-dry dressings are used if residual contamination occurs or necrotic tissue is seen that requires débridement. In some cases sterile water-soluble jelly is placed in the wound, and the wound is covered with a nonadherent dressing such as a Telfa pad. The wound dressing then is covered with a padded layer followed by cling and a water-repellent outer wrap.

Bandages must be kept clean and dry; if they become wet or soiled, then they must be changed immediately. This is especially important if urine gets into the bandage, because urine is very caustic to tissues. Bandages must be changed as soon as strike-through occurs to prevent wicking of external contaminants and bacteria into the wound through the wet bandage. To prevent infection, gloves should be worn whenever dressings on an open wound are changed.

Effective temporary splints can be placed on distal extremity injuries before radiographs are taken. Splinting can prevent a closed fracture from becoming an open fracture; helps stabilize fractures, preventing further injury from bone fragments that may create shearing injury to the soft tissue; and promotes patient comfort by immobilizing the injury. Temporary splints can be placed using newspaper and white porous tape or duct tape. Bubble wrap also makes a very effective lightweight splint.

A properly placed splint stabilizes the joint above and below the fracture. Bandages always should be placed from the digits proximally and should incorporate the lateral two digits. Toes must be monitored to ensure they stay warm and do not start to swell. If either problem is noticed, then circulation to the foot is compromised (the splint or bandage should be removed immediately).

Surgical Resuscitation

Surgery may be required to resuscitate and stabilize some trauma patients. Examples of patients to whom this applies include those with severe external hemorrhage (e.g., lacerated artery), severe ongoing internal hemorrhage, and diaphragmatic hernias. Anesthesia in these patients can be challenging, and a dedicated anesthetist is essential for these patients. The severely hemorrhaging patient will need large volumes of warmed fluids and blood products intraoperatively (Box 14-4).

Basic Monitoring

The trauma patient should be monitored closely during resuscitation, during any intraoperative period, and in the intensive care unit after resuscitation. The frequency of monitoring depends on the severity of the patient's condition and should range from as frequently as every 15 minutes in the more critical animal to as infrequently as every 4 to 8 hours in the more stable one. Trends of change often are more

---

BOX 14-4

Surgical Trauma Pack

Saline bowls (small and large)
Scalpel handle and No. 10 and No. 11 blade
Towel clamps (minimum of eight)
Mayo scissors (curved)
Metzenbaum scissors (curved)
Sharp blunt scissors
Kelly hemostatic forceps (eight curved)
Halsted mosquito forceps (eight curved)
Rochester-Carmalt hemostatic forceps (six curved)
Sponge forceps (curved)
Allis tissue forceps (four)
Right-angle forceps (small and large)
Debakey or Cooley tissue forceps (short and long)
Russian thumb forceps
Brown-Adson tissue forceps
Serrefine forceps (two bulldog clamps)
Balfour retractor (small and large)
Mayo-Hegar needle holders (small and large)
Yankauer, Poole, and Frazier suction tips
Silastic tubing
Bulb syringe
Laparotomy pads (eight)
Rumel tourniquet (umbilical tape, silastic or red rubber tubing)
Cotton towels (four small and four large)

---

important than the exact numbers. Basic monitoring includes measuring level of consciousness, respiratory rate and effort, heart rate, pulse rate and strength, jugular venous distention (as an estimate of CVP), BP, and temperature. Monitoring the difference between rectal and toe web temperature can help assess peripheral perfusion. The temperature difference under normal circumstances should be no more than 7° F. The lungs should be ausculted frequently (every 2 to 4 hours) to check for the presence of pneumothorax, hemothorax, or pulmonary contusions. Variation in pulse quality or detection of pulse deficits is consistent with ventricular premature contractions (VPCs) or rarely pericardial effusion.

BP should remain as close to 120/80 mm Hg as possible, unless the patient's BP is being kept deliberately low (as in hypotensive resuscitation). Three main methods for monitoring BP exist: (1) direct, (2) oscillometric, and (3) Doppler. Direct BP

TABLE 14-1

Goals for Measured Parameters for Trauma Patients

Parameter	Goal
Respiratory rate	>18 and <36/min
Heart rate	>60/min and <130/min
Heart rhythm	Sinus: If ventricular premature contractions (VPCs)—unifocal, no significant pulse deficits, heart rate <160/min, no R on T phenomenon
Temperature	Normal; delta T* < 7° F
Blood pressure (BP)	Systolic >90 and <130 mm Hg Diastolic >60 and <100 mm Hg
Blood flow	Doppler sounds good
Central venous pressure (CVP)	>5 and <10 cm water
Urine output	>0.5 ml/kg/hr
Pulse oximetry	>94%
Packed cell volume (PCV)	>25% and <50%
Total solids (TS)	>4.5 and <7.5 g/dl
Albumin	>2.0 g/dl
Platelet estimate	>5-8/hpf (high powered field)

*Delta T, Difference between rectal and axillary or rectal and toe web temperature.

monitoring is ideal and the most accurate method. However, direct BP is rarely monitored in the emergency situation because of the time needed to place an arterial catheter and the lack of necessary monitoring equipment. A Doppler BP monitor is preferred in most trauma patients, because both BP and flow to distal extremities can be assessed. Arrhythmias such as VPCs can be heard once the operator's ear has been trained to listen for irregularities in the flow signal.

Urine output of 0.5 ml/kg/hr (minimum) helps ensure adequate renal perfusion. Fluid intake and output should be monitored and fluids adjusted every 4 to 6 hours as indicated.

Analgesics should be administered regularly and supplemented based on whether the animal appears to be in pain (rather than based on a set schedule). Pain has detrimental effects both physiologically and psychologically and should be controlled as much as possible.

Basic laboratory monitoring should include measuring the PCV and TS. In cases of possible active hemorrhage, the PCV may need to be monitored every 30 minutes; in the more stable patient the PCV can be checked at 2 hours and then every 4 to 8 hours (Table 14-1).

Advanced Monitoring

More advanced monitoring includes the use of electrocardiography, CVP, and pulse oximetry. VPCs and ventricular tachycardia are the most common arrhythmias seen in trauma patients. The VPCs should be treated if they are multifocal or affecting perfusion (significant pulse deficits), if the heart rate is elevated (usually above 160 beats per minute), or if evidence of R on T phenomenon is seen. Treatment includes the use of supplemental O_2, ensuring tissue perfusion is being maximized, analgesia, and a constant rate infusion of antiarrhythmic drugs (i.e., lidocaine, procainamide).

Pulse oximetry can monitored on the awake patient; however, measurements are subject to technical errors. If perfusion is poor, then the pulse may not be strong enough for the oximeter to provide an accurate measurement. Strong ambient light and motion also can cause artifacts; O_2 saturation normally should read about 97% on room air. If the patient has O_2 saturation readings of 90% to 92% on supplemental O_2, then an arterial blood gas should be checked because the patient may require mechanical ventilation.

CVP monitoring should be performed in all patients in whom fluid overload is a potential complication. Monitoring trends may be more important than exact numbers. Ideally, the CVP should be kept between 5 and 8 cm water. CVP does not reflect circulating venous volume if the patient has a pneumothorax, an abdominal counterpressure wrap, or right ventricular heart failure. If CVP is normal and none of the previously mentioned conditions exists but BP is still low, then cardiac function likely is inadequate and positive inotropic support may be indicated.

Advanced laboratory monitoring includes regular assessment of electrolytes and blood gas parameters. Venous blood gases can be used for accurate assessment of acid-base status and carbon dioxide tension, but arterial blood gases are required to monitor oxygenation. Albumin levels, coagulation parameters, and platelet numbers also should be assessed. If the patient has an indwelling urinary catheter, then daily urine sediments should be evaluated, because urinary tract infections can be a complication of indwelling catheters. The frequency of laboratory monitoring depends on how critical the patient's condition is; typically parameters are assessed every 8 to 24 hours.

Postresuscitation Care: The First 24 Hours

The severely traumatized patient is at risk for developing the systemic inflammatory response syndrome. Respiratory and cardiovascular parameters must be maintained as close to normal as possible. In addition, laboratory parameters should be monitored and values kept as close to normal as possible.

Patients with significant blood loss have lost a significant amount of endogenous clotting factors. In addition, tissue trauma is a trigger for activating the coagulation cascade and, if left uncontrolled, may lead to disseminated intravascular coagulation. Patients in shock frequently are hypothermic and acidotic, which can cause dysfunction of the coagulation system. Infusion of large volumes of crystalloids or synthetic colloids can dilute out the remaining coagulation factors, thus leading to a dilutional coagulopathy.

Many of these patients will have multiple tubes in place. All tubes should be carefully labeled to ensure that O_2 does not get delivered into a nasogastric tube and enteral feedings are not infused intravenously. If nasal tubes are in place, then the patient should be monitored for signs of skin irritation at the suture site (at the naris) and signs of rhinitis. If adhesive tape gets wet, then it can lead to a moist dermatitis. Both complications are usually mild and self-limiting; however, if the patient is experiencing discomfort, then the tube may need to be switched to the other nostril or removed. Feeding tubes such as esophagostomy, gastrostomy, and jejunostomy tubes should have daily to twice-daily bandage changes during the initial healing period (3 to 5 days). Ostomy sites should be examined visually for signs of inflammation or discharge and should be palpated for signs of pain. Any abnormalities should be reported because infection may be present.

Bandages on chest tubes should be changed daily to twice daily, and the ostomy site should be inspected visually and by palpation. The site should be cleaned with an antibacterial solution, and a sterile dressing should be placed. Broad-spectrum antibiotic ointment should be used in generous quantities at the exit site to help form a seal. Patients should wear Elizabethan collars as needed to prevent them from chewing or removing the tubes. Urinary catheter care includes cleaning of the vulva or prepuce with an antibacterial solution and application of a broad-spectrum antibiotic ointment around the tube entry site. Closed collection systems, like IV fluid administration systems, should be replaced every 48 to 72 hours.

Many of these patients will be inactive or have trouble ambulating. Patient comfort is very important; therefore analgesics should be administered as frequently and at as high as dose as necessary to keep the patient comfortable. Uncontrolled pain can cause harmful physiologic effects such as tachycardia, vasoconstriction, and compromised ventilation. Pain should never be used as a means of restricting an animal's movement. For instance, if a patient has a possible soft tissue injury to a limb, then controlling the pain and supporting the limb in a padded bandage or splint is better than keeping the animal immobile through pain. Analgesics ideally should be administered parenterally (locally or regionally). Epidural catheters provide an alterative route that is very effective. Fentanyl patches are effective; however, in some severely injured patients, the sedation and cardiovascular depression caused by the fentanyl can be excessive and the patch may need to be removed.

Patients should be kept on padded bedding and turned every 2 to 4 hours. Larger patients should be monitored closely for the development of decubital ulcers. Gentle physiotherapy should be performed on all possible limbs when the patient is recumbent. This not only will improve patient comfort but also stimulate circulation; once the patient is able to ambulate, it will allow it to do so more rapidly. This becomes especially important in more geriatric animals or animals with arthritis.

Nutrition

Nutritional support is vital to trauma patients because they are in a hypermetabolic state. Patient morbidity can be altered significantly if enteral nutritional support is provided within the first 12 to 24 hours. Enteral nutrition is preferred over parenteral nutrition; enteral nutrition helps preserve the gastrointestinal barrier, thus decreasing bacterial translocation, as well as helping to preserve immune function, and normal intestinal, pancreatic, and biliary secretions.

Enteral nutritional support can be provided most easily by tube feeding if the patient will not eat. Nasoesophageal or nasogastric tubes can be placed. If longer-term nutritional support is anticipated, then an esophagostomy or gastrostomy tube may be indicated. Feedings tubes can be placed easily at the time of any exploratory celiotomy for use postoperatively. Microenteral nutrition (i.e., the provision of small amounts of glucose and a balanced electrolyte solution) may be beneficial. Rates start at 0.1 to 0.5 ml/kg of body weight per hour. If the patient cannot tolerate full enteral nutrition, then this can be slowly increased and liquid enteral diets can be added to the infusion. It can be delivered by a constant rate infusion or as intermittent boluses. Parenteral nutrition should be supplemented if enteral access is not available, and it is anticipated that the patient will not be eating for 2 to 3 days. Caloric intake initially should be estimated based on resting energy requirements. Overfeeding the respiratory patient should be prevented, because excess carbon dioxide will be produced, which requires a compensatory increase in respiratory rate.

Assessment and Management of Specific Injuries

The degree of tissue trauma varies with the type of trauma and the velocity and mass of the impact. Force is equal to the mass multiplied by the velocity squared ($F = MV^2$). The greater the force, the more significant is the tissue trauma. For instance, a dog hit in the head with a baseball bat will suffer a significantly different injury than one shot in the head; a dog hit by a bicycle will suffer much less force of injury than one hit by a car.

Trauma is generally divided into two types: (1) blunt and (2) penetrating. Blunt trauma, which involves crushing forces, usually occurs from collision with an object. This can occur if the animal falls, is stepped on, or is hit by an object such as a car or baseball bat. Penetrating injuries generally are those inflicted by knives, arrows, bullets, and larger objects that cause impalement (e.g., sticks, metal rods). Bite wounds can cause both penetrating and blunt trauma. Significant shearing forces can be applied after penetration, especially with bite wounds. The seriousness of the injury often will depend on what is penetrated. A better understanding of the mechanism of injury allows for greater appreciation of possible internal injuries, which can enable the team to minimize patient morbidity and mortality.

Several types of traumatic injury can lead to death rapidly if the injury is not assessed accurately and treated immediately. These include airway disruptions or obstructions, tension pneumothorax, severe pulmonary contusions, and massive internal thoracic or abdominal hemorrhage. A high index of suspicion should be maintained for these injuries.

In the following sections, injuries are grouped by anatomic location. These injuries can be caused by the animal being hit by a car, colliding with a solid object (e.g., jumping off a balcony), being bitten by another animal, being bitten and shaken, being hit by a penetrating missile (e.g., gunshot, arrow), or being impaled by objects such as sticks, iron rods, and fencing. A description of how to assess, manage, and monitor these patients during the resuscitation period is provided. In all cases it is assumed that O$_2$ will be provided, as well as IV fluid support and analgesics. It is also assumed that basic diagnostics and monitoring as outlined previously are being performed. The list is not all-inclusive, but it is designed to provide an overview of the more common injuries that will arrive at the emergency department. A word of caution: No impaled object should be removed until the wound tract is explored. The object may have passed through or may be lodged in a major vessel such as the heart or the abdominal aorta. Premature removal may lead to rapid exsanguination. The only exception to this rule is any object that is thought to be compromising respiration to the point of impending arrest (generally through obstruction).

Head and Facial Trauma

Assessment. Patients with head trauma have varying levels of consciousness from normal mentation to coma. Head trauma can lead to traumatic brain injury. Trauma to the brainstem is life threatening and can lead to alterations in respiratory pattern and cardiovascular derangement. Facial fractures may lead to intraoral and intranasal hemorrhage and subsequent respiratory difficulty. Blood can pool in the oropharynx, leading to an effective airway obstruction.

Management. A clear airway is the first priority. The airway should be cleared of as much of the blood, vomitus, or other secretions as possible; however, extreme care should be taken to ensure no one is bitten. A gagging response should be avoided in the patient with traumatic brain injury, because this will elevate intracranial pressure and decrease cerebral blood flow. Suction using a Yankauer suction tip may be necessary. If patients are unconscious with no gag reflex, then they must be intubated rapidly without lifting the head (because the decrease in blood flow to the brain caused by this maneuver may lead to a cardiac arrest). A laryngoscope should be used, because excessive manipulation of the larynx may cause a vagally mediated bradycardia with subsequent hypotension and even arrest. Nasal tubes should not be used, because sneezing may elevate intracranial pressure.

The second priority is to ensure adequate cerebral blood flow. The intracranial volume is comprised of the brain tissue, the cerebrospinal fluid, and the blood vessels. Because the skull contains the brain, any change in one of the compartments will affect the other two. Pressure on the jugular veins during venipuncture or placement of catheters should be avoided, because this may raise intracranial pressure and decrease perfusion to the brain. Fluids should be administered to maintain normal BP. These patients must not be volume overloaded or allowed to become hypertensive, because this may exacerbate intracranial hemorrhage; however, hypotension is even more detrimental. Sedatives may be needed if the patient is severely disoriented or hypertensive. Corticosteroids do not improve (and may even worsen) outcome and should not be used. Although mannitol has the potential to worsen active intracranial hemorrhage, its benefits generally outweigh its potential disadvantages. If a compressed skull fracture is seen or the patient's neurologic status is worsening, then intracranial pressure monitoring and emergency surgery for a decompressive craniotomy may be required. Hyperbaric O$_2$ therapy delivered within 2 to 6 hours of the head injury has been shown to be effective in ameliorating ongoing secondary neuronal ischemia caused by edema and swelling, as well as to decrease ongoing hypoxic injury to the brain. Recumbent patients should be kept in a horizontal position (with mild elevation of the head up to 30 degrees) and turned every 2 to 4 hours. When placing the patient in a cage, care must be taken to ensure the neck is not flexed, which may potentially lead to a compromised airway and compromised venous outflow via the jugular veins (leading to increased intracranial pressure). Elevating the head slightly may decrease the risks for silent regurgitation and aspiration.

Severe epistaxis may necessitate the use of intranasal epinephrine or nasal packing. Surgery is rarely required. Sneezing and hypertension will worsen the epistaxis and should be controlled. These animals must be kept very quiet and often require sedation.

Monitoring. Level of consciousness, pupil size and symmetry, respiratory pattern, heart rate, mucous membrane color, BP, CVP, PCV, and TS should be monitored. Blood gases and an ECG should be evaluated as indicated. Platelet numbers, a buccal mucosal bleeding time to check for platelet dysfunction, and a coagulation screen are indicated if epistaxis persists or the clinician is concerned about an underlying coagulopathy.

Cervical Soft Tissue Injury

Assessment. Cervical trauma can lead to airway avulsion or disruption, airway obstruction from hemorrhage or swelling, esophageal laceration, and laceration of major vessels. These animals can experience varying degrees of respiratory distress. Blood loss is highly variable, as is injury to other soft tissues including muscle, subcutaneous tissue, and skin.

Management. The animal's respiratory rate and pattern must be closely observed. Any animal that has noisy breathing has a compromised airway and must be monitored closely, because an obstruction may develop. Exaggerated chest movement without airway sounds is a hallmark for an airway obstruction. The animal that is struggling to breathe and has pronounced respiratory efforts may have an avulsed larynx or trachea. These patients require immediate anesthesia and intubation or an awake tracheostomy; transtracheal or nasotracheal O_2 may help in the interim. The trachea should be ausculted and the entire area carefully palpated and thoroughly clipped of hair to evaluate the wounds, extent of hemorrhage, and swelling. Any wound should be cleaned and a sterile bandage placed unless a tracheal injury is possible. Bandaging a tracheal laceration may cause subcutaneous emphysema and a pneumomediastinum. Extreme care should be taken when placing a cervical bandage, because patient movement often tightens these bandages.

If the clinician is concerned about associated spinal injury, then the patient must not be moved before stabilizing the injury. Cervical spinal injuries at or above the level of C4-C6 can lead to loss of diaphragm function and subsequent respiratory compromise.

Monitoring. Mucous membrane color, respiratory rate and effort, heart rate, BP and pulse oximetry should be monitored. The PCV, TS, blood gases, and ECG should be evaluated as indicated. Neck bandages should be checked every 4 to 6 hours and loosened as needed.

Chest Injury

Assessment. Chest trauma can lead to musculoskeletal injuries such as fractured ribs, lacerated muscles, and bruising. Intrathoracic trauma most commonly leads to pneumothorax, hemothorax, pulmonary contusions, and cardiac contusions. These patients will have varying degrees of respiratory distress. Hypoventilation caused by pain from fractured ribs is a significant concern.

Management. The technician should provide O_2 immediately if he or she believes the animal has a chest injury. Respiratory rate and effort should be assessed rapidly. Rapid shallow ventilation often indicates pain from fractured ribs and pleural space abnormality (pneumothorax or pneumohemothorax). Tension pneumothorax should be considered if the patient has shallow rapid respiration, an expanded thorax, limited movement of the chest wall with ventilation, and distended jugular veins. Deep gasping breaths often indicate severe pulmonary contusions. Auscultation and percussion of the thorax should be performed. Dull lung sounds and dull or hyperresonant areas on percussion are consistent with pleural space abnormalities, and thoracentesis is indicated. Thoracentesis always should be done bilaterally and precede radiographs. A chest tube may be indicated. Analgesia should be provided early with intrapleural analgesia, intercostal nerve blocks, or frequent parenteral injections of opioids. All wounds should be clipped and cleaned, and sterile dressings should be placed. The exception may be a large wound into the pleural space. If this is sealed, then a tension pneumothorax may result. A chest tube may need to be placed through this hole or an occlusive dressing placed that is sealed on three sides only, with the fourth side acting as a pop-off valve. If the patient has a possible flail chest and is in lateral recumbency, then the flail side should be placed down. A flail chest is a segment of chest wall that moves paradoxically with each breath (*in* when the patient inhales and *out* when the patient exhales). The cause of this condition is three or more fractured, adjacent ribs in more than one location, which create a free-floating segment of chest wall. Fluids should be administered to maintain normal BP. In the case of severe intrathoracic hemorrhage, hypotensive resuscitation may be indicated until surgery to definitively control the hemorrhage can be performed.

Monitoring. Patients with chest injuries must be monitored on a continuous basis until they are stable. Vital signs, including respiratory rate and effort, mucous membrane color, heart rate, and BP, should be assessed frequently. In the severely hypoxic patient, rectal temperatures may cause vagally mediated bradycardia and hypotension, and axillary temperatures should be monitored instead. Blood gases are ideal but may stress the patient excessively. In this case, pulse oximetry should be performed on a continuous basis if possible. Patients with chest trauma frequently develop VPCs and ventricular tachycardia secondary to traumatic myocarditis. These patients should have continuous ECG monitoring, and pulses should be palpated routinely for deficits. In most patients who require chest tubes, continuous underwater suction is indicated. If the patient is on continuous underwater suctioning, then the tubing should be stripped every 4 to 6 hours and intermittent hand aspiration should be performed. Connections should be checked frequently for signs of loosening or dislodgment.

Chest dressings must be changed once or twice daily initially (more frequently if strike-through is evident). Bandages that are placed too tightly can lead to compromised ventilation and should be checked every 4 to 8 hours. Two fingers should be able to be slipped beneath the bandage easily. If the bandage is too tight, then it can be cut along the dorsum until the outer layers no longer spread, and then the edges can be taped together using elastic tape. Although opioids can depress ventilation, this is rarely a problem clinically if appropriate doses are administered.

Abdomen

Assessment. Intraabdominal injury can lead to significant hemorrhage from solid visci (e.g., liver, spleen), vascular injury to major vessels, and lacerations to the bowel leading to peritonitis. Persistent vomiting, increasing abdominal pain, and abdominal distention all are indicators of a significant intraabdominal injury. Percussion may indicate areas of dullness, fluid waves, or areas of resonance, suggesting intraabdominal air accumulations. Splenic injuries frequently are associated with VPCs. Retroperitoneal injuries can be more difficult to diagnose. However, if the patient is becoming more anemic and no other known source for the blood loss is found, then the bleeding may be coming from the retroperitoneal space.

Management. Patients with abdominal injuries often have multiple injuries; airway and breathing should always be assessed and managed before dealing with abdominal injuries. Nasogastric decompression is important to decrease vomiting from gastric distention (either from aerophagia or fluid) and to encourage the stomach to return to normal motility. This is especially important if the patient has had surgery for abdominal injuries or has an open abdomen. Pharmacologic control of vomiting may be required. Vomitus should be checked for hemorrhage—either frank blood or digested blood ("coffee grounds")—using an occult blood test if not grossly apparent. Urine should be assessed for the presence of hemorrhage grossly (using a dipstick test) and microscopically. If the patient is not producing urine within the first 4 hours of hospitalization, then the possibility of a ruptured urinary bladder should be considered. The stool should be monitored for signs of hemorrhage and melena. The hair covering the ventral and lateral aspects of the abdomen and caudal rib cage should be clipped and the area examined for the presence of a wound and bruising.

Monitoring. These patients require monitoring of all vital signs including mucous membrane color, respiratory rate and effort, heart rate, and BP. Ongoing hemorrhage always is a concern; therefore serial PCV and TS should be assessed. The abdomen should be monitored closely for signs of distention or excessive bruising. Serial circumferential measurements of the abdomen using a tape measure are more sensitive than direct observation. Urine output should be monitored hourly during initial resuscitation, then every 4 hours.

Musculoskeletal System

Assessment. All areas of possible trauma should ideally be kept as nonweight bearing and as immobilized as possible until the clinician completely evaluates the injury. To accomplish this, the animal should be restricted in lateral recumbency or confined to a small space. Some musculoskeletal injuries are readily apparent because of the soft tissue trauma surrounding the injury. Nonweight-bearing lameness usually indicates luxation, fracture, or severe ligament injury, whereas partial weight bearing usually indicates a less severe injury. Severe hemorrhage into muscle compartments can lead to compartment syndrome. This occurs when the pressure rises within the muscle belly to the point that circulation to the affected area is obstructed. Because compartment syndrome rapidly leads to tissue necrosis, the condition must be recognized early. Clinical signs can include severe swelling, signs that the affected area is becoming more painful than would be expected, decreased temperature of the toes of the affected limb in comparison to a normal limb, and increasing loss of movement or sensation. Fractures can lead to laceration of underlying soft tissue. For instance, rib fractures can be associated with a lacerated lung and pneumothorax, femoral fractures can lead to laceration of major femoral vessels, and pubic fractures can lacerate the urethra. Patients with possible spinal fractures should be immobilized (taped to a board with duct tape or similar material). These patients must be radiographed before they are allowed to move, because movement may cause a significant worsening of the injury.

Management. All distal limb fractures should be splinted before radiographs are taken or the patient is moved, and patients should be kept as immobile as possible until the full extent of the injuries is known. Pain should not be used as a way of immobilizing patients, and analgesics always should be administered. As discussed previously, wounds should be protected with sterile dressings or covered with sterile towels. If it suspected that compartment syndrome is present, then pressure must be released immediately. The clinician does this by performing a fasciotomy in the operating room under aseptic conditions.

Monitoring. The patient should be monitored closely for evidence of soft tissue injury under fracture sites (i.e., monitored for urination with pubic fractures, pneumothorax with rib fractures, and compartment syndrome with long bone fractures).

Communication

Communication with the owner is one of the technician's most important responsibilities. When the critically injured patient arrives and the doctor cannot leave the patient, the technician often can relay basic information on the status of the pet, reassure the owner, and gain permission for procedures or treatment. Because technicians work with patients more closely than doctors do, they are often much more informed about the nuances of the pet's condition and can provide information about the patient's comfort, urination and defecation habits, appetite, and water intake. Owners need to feel that their pets are being well looked after—not only from a medical perspective but also from a psychologic and emotional perspective. The veterinary technician is the patient and owner's advocate. If any part of the patient's care is not being addressed adequately, then the technician's responsibility is to inform the veterinarian and make recommendations to resolve the issues.

Conclusion

The severely injured patient's survival depends on a well-equipped facility and an educated and trained staff. The technician plays a vital role in ensuring the ready area is properly prepared to receive any emergency, in triage (which ensures the seriously injured patient is recognized immediately), and in being able to assist with resuscitation. The technician must be able to use a wide variety of monitors and monitoring techniques. An understanding of the pathology that can occur with different injuries helps ensure the patient is monitored and treated appropriately. Good communication between team members is essential to minimize patient morbidity and mortality.

CHAPTER 15

Hematologic Emergencies

Donna A. Oakley

Hematologic Emergencies

Hemostasis

When a patient has abnormal bleeding, its cause must be determined. Animals may bleed after injury or trauma, but they may also suffer from either an inherited or acquired hemostatic defect. Although the veterinarian is responsible for diagnosing and choosing an appropriate therapy for each patient, the veterinary technician should be knowledgeable and anticipate the needs of the veterinarian and, most importantly, the patient. This requires a basic understanding of the physiology of hemostasis.

Hemostasis is the body's balancing mechanism of arresting hemorrhage while simultaneously maintaining blood flow within the vascular compartment. It occurs through a complex series of events involving the vessels, platelets, plasma coagulation factors, and the fibrinolytic system. The role that each component plays in hemostasis is dependent on the size of the vessel and the amount of damage that has occurred. Bleeding in smaller vessels may be controlled by a simple response involving the vasculature and platelets, known as *primary hemostasis*. With larger vessel injury, plasma coagulation factors are needed to form a stable clot, a process known as *secondary hemostasis*.

The first response to blood vessel injury is vasoconstriction, which allows for diversion of blood flow around the injured area. Once the endothelial lining of the vessel is disrupted, the subendothelial connective tissue (i.e., collagen) is exposed. Circulating platelets pool to the area of injury and adhere to the endothelial lining with the help of adhesive proteins like collagen and von Willebrand's factor (vWF) (i.e., platelet adhesion), acting to arrest the initial episode of bleeding. Once the platelets adhere to the subendothelium, they change shape and secrete certain biochemical substances that enhance platelet layering in the injured area (i.e., platelet aggregation). The platelets form a complete but unstable plug. This portion of the hemostatic process is referred to as *primary hemostasis*.

TABLE 15-1

Coagulation Factors

Coagulation Factor	Name	Vitamin K Dependent
I	Fibrinogen	
II	Prothrombin	X
III	Tissue factor	
IV	Calcium	
V	Proaccelerin	
VI	No factor VI	
VII	Proconvertin	X
VIII	Antihemophilic	
IX	Christmas factor	X
X	Stuart factor	X
XI	Plasma thromboplastin antecedent	
XII	Hageman factor	
XIII	Fibrin-stabilizing factor	

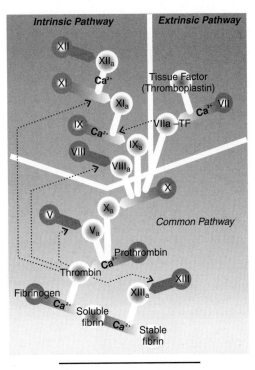

Fig. 15-1 Coagulation cascade.

As previously stated, with greater damage to larger vessels, coagulation factors are needed to form a stable fibrin clot (i.e., *secondary hemostasis*). Plasma coagulation factors (denoted by Roman numerals) are produced in the liver, many with the help of vitamin K. They circulate in the blood in the inactive form and, when exposed to certain substances, become activated (denoted by the letter *a*) in a cascade-like effect (Table 15-1). Blood coagulation involves a complex process by which the multiple coagulation factors contained in blood interact in three major pathways: (1) intrinsic, (2) extrinsic, and (3) common pathways (see Table 15-1).

Tissue factor (thromboplastin) is released from the injured vessel wall and initiates the extrinsic clotting pathway. This is an extravascular process in that tissue thromboplastin is not normally found in blood and must gain entry to the vascular system. Clotting via the intrinsic pathway begins when blood comes into contact with a foreign substance or surface (i.e., damaged endothelium). Activated platelets release a phospholipid, allowing coagulation factors in this pathway to activate one another. In the intrinsic pathway, all factors necessary for clot formation

are within the intravascular compartment. Both the extrinsic and the intrinsic pathways merge into the common pathway, where the end result is the creation of fibrin, a threadlike protein (Fig. 15-1). The fibrin threads form an insoluble meshwork over the site of the platelet plug, consolidating and stabilizing the clot.

For simplicity of presentation, the pathways are reviewed as divided processes. The reader must realize that the classic cascade presentation of fibrin formation has many underlying complexities and interrelationships that go beyond the scope of this chapter (see Fig. 15-1).

The final step in the hemostatic process is fibrinolysis. Once the vessel is healed, fibrinolytic enzymes break down the clot that has been formed. Clot lysis produces small pieces of fibrin, referred to as *fibrin split products (FSP)* or *fibrin degradation products (FDP)*, which are cleared from circulation by the liver. After clot digestion, vessel wall endothelium is reestablished and returned to its original state. Small levels of FSP always appear in the circulation as a result of bleeding and clotting secondary to normal wear-and-tear on vessels. Fibrin split product levels may increase during episodes of excessive bleeding with diffuse coagulation (i.e., DIC) and in patients with compromised liver function.

Disorders of Primary Hemostasis

Platelet Disorders. Patients with a low platelet count, known as *thrombocytopenia*, experience bleeding when inadequate numbers of platelets are available to form a platelet plug. Many things may potentially affect platelet production in both the dog and the cat (e.g., drugs, bone marrow neoplasia, infection). Massive transfusion may also cause thrombocytopenia because of the rapid consumption of platelets for hemostasis and the dilution of the platelets by fluid solutions and blood component replacement. Thrombocytopenia can also result from an increased consumption of platelets due to DIC, infection, neoplasia, inflammation, immune-mediated disorders, and drug interactions.

Immune-mediated thrombocytopenia (IMT) is one of the most common causes of increased platelet sequestration and destruction with subsequent thrombocytopenia. IMT is a disorder in which antibodies are bound to the surface of the platelet, resulting in premature removal by the reticuloendothelial system. IMT can be classified as a *primary disorder*, referred to as *idiopathic thrombocytopenia purpura (ITP)*, in which the production of antiplatelet antibodies has no apparent cause. It can also be classified as a secondary disorder in which antibodies are produced in response to antigenic stimuli (e.g., drugs, vaccines, infections, neoplasia). A complete medical history, including recent vaccinations, medications, and tick exposure, as well as recent or concurrent illness, is important in identifying a potential antigenic stimulus. IMT may be acute, chronic, or recurrent, and can range from mild to severe in presentation.

Thrombopathia. Platelets must have adequate function and number to participate optimally in hemostasis. A platelet function defect, or thrombopathia, is considered in patients with a history of bleeding (especially surface bleeding) and a normal platelet count. When the platelet quality is compromised, platelet adhesion or aggregation (or both) at the site of endothelial damage may be abnormal. Thrombopathias may be classified as *inherited* or *acquired* defects.

Congenital disorders of platelet function have been recognized in small animals but are rare. Some

TABLE 15-2

Common Hereditary Bleeding Disorders

PLATELET DYSFUNCTION	
Disorder	**Breed**
Delta storage pool disease	Cocker spaniel
Glanzmann's thrombasthenia	Otterhound, Great Pyrenees
Chediak-Higashi syndrome	Persian cat
Other thrombopathias	Basset hound, boxer, spitz, domestic shorthair
COAGULOPATHIES	
Disorder	**Breed**
Prothrombin deficiency	Cocker spaniel, boxer
Factor-VII deficiency	Beagle, malamute
Factor-VIII deficiency (hemophilia A)	Many canine breeds, cats
Factor-IX deficiency (hemophilia B)	Many canine breeds, cats
Factor-X deficiency	Cocker spaniels, cats

of the more common inherited thrombopathias are listed in Table 15-2. Certain drugs may have a pronounced adverse effect on platelets. Some drugs may induce thrombocytopenia (e.g., heparin), whereas others inhibit platelet function (e.g., aspirin, nonsteroidal antiinflammatory drugs). Drug-induced hemostatic abnormalities usually resolve when the drug is discontinued. However, after aspirin exposure, platelet inhibition persists throughout the life span of the platelet. Bleeding abnormalities may also be a clinical manifestation of patients with acute or chronic renal failure. Platelet dysfunction secondary to uremia is the primary cause of hemorrhage in these patients.

The major indication for platelet transfusion is to stop bleeding in patients with decreased platelet number, function, or both. Platelet preparation is difficult in regard to the volume needed to measurably increase platelet numbers in larger breed dogs. In some patients, however, cessation of bleeding after platelet transfusion has been achieved without a measurable increase in platelet number. In situations

TABLE 15-3

Canine von Willebrand's Disease

Type	Plasma von Willebrand's factor (vWF)	Examples of Breeds with Known Mutation
1	Variably reduced vWF levels; all multimer sizes proportionately reduced; most common—recognized in >70 breeds; hemorrhage tendency variable, often with surgery or trauma	Doberman pinscher, German shepherd, golden retriever, rottweiler, Manchester terrier, Cairn terrier, Pembroke Welsh corgi, Bernese mountain dog, Kerry blue terrier, poodle, papillon
2	Disproportionately low vWF activity; deficiency of high molecular weight multimers; larger more effective multimers absent; bleeding can be severe	German shorthair pointer, German wirehair pointer
3	Complete vWF deficiency (<1% plasma vWF); most severe in that all multimers absent	Scottish terrier, Shetland sheepdog, Chesapeake Bay retriever, kooiker

Enzyme-linked immunosorbent assay results: normal = >70%, borderline = 50% to 69%, affected = 0% to 49%.

of platelet destruction, such as IMT, the survival of transfused platelets is a matter of minutes rather than days. In patients with IMT, the veterinarian must treat the underlying disease (e.g., ehrlichiosis) or remove the triggering agent (e.g., drugs) immediately.

Platelet transfusion may be warranted if the patient is acutely bleeding into a vital structure (i.e., brain, myocardium, pleural cavity) or in severe, uncontrolled bleeding. In veterinary medicine, treatment of thrombocytopenia and thrombopathia with active bleeding is more practical using fresh whole blood, from which the patient will receive both platelets and oxygen-carrying support. In most instances, however, medical management is the treatment of choice.

von Willebrand's Disease. The most common hereditary bleeding defect in the dog (recognized in more than 60 breeds) is von Willibrand's disease (vWD), a deficiency of vWF (a large plasma protein produced by and stored in endothelial cells). As mentioned previously, vWF facilitates platelet adhesion and aggregation, as well as act as a carrier for factor VIII. The size of vWF multimers varies, with the larger multimers being more hemostatically active. Assays are available to determine the amount of vWF in the circulation; however, they do not determine the multimeric distribution. Multiple measurements of vWF may be necessary because of a daily variation in the concentration of this protein.

The three major types of vWD are differentiated by the amount of vWF and multimer pattern: (1) moderate vWF deficiency (type 1), (2) lack of higher molecular weight multimers (type 2), and (3) complete absence of vWF (type 3).

Mucosal surface bleeding and hemorrhage characterize the bleeding tendency in vWD after surgery or trauma. Severity of bleeding is variable in dogs with type 1 vWD and may not correlate with plasma vWF concentration in each dog. Dogs with type 2 and 3 vWD generally experience the most severe bleeding episodes (Table 15-3).

Blood component therapy is generally indicated preoperatively in dogs with clinically severe forms of vWD and a history of bleeding. Cryoprecipitate, a byproduct of fresh frozen plasma (FFP) that has a high concentration of vWF, factor VIII, fibrinogen, and fibronectin, is the blood component of choice in managing bleeding as a result of vWD. FFP or fresh whole blood may also be used based on product availability.

Desmopressin (DDAVP), a synthetic analog of vasopressin, may be sufficient to control minor bleeding in some (but not all) dogs with type 1 vWD. In humans, DDAVP causes a significant increase in plasma vWF concentration; however, the plasma vWF concentration increases only marginally in dogs, despite improvement in hemostasis. The beneficial hemostatic effects of DDAVP are evident within 30 minutes after administration and may last for up to 4 hours.

Disorders of Secondary Hemostasis

When a deficiency of a coagulation factor or factors is present, fibrin stabilization of the platelet plug cannot occur and hemostasis is impaired. Clotting defects may result from decreased factor synthesis, factor loss or consumption, factor molecular defects interfering with function, and factor inactivation by inhibitors (e.g., warfarin) or antibodies resulting from certain drugs. Coagulation factor deficiencies may be inherited or acquired.

Hereditary Coagulopathies. A hereditary disorder should always be considered when a bleeding patient arrives at the emergency service given a variety of coagulation factor deficiencies have been described in small animals.

Hemophilias are the most common severe hereditary coagulopathies in the dog. Hemophilia A is caused by a factor VIII deficiency, whereas hemophilia B is due to a factor IX deficiency. They are sex-linked autosomal recessive disorders carried on the X chromosome; therefore, both hemophilia A and hemophilia B are expressed only in males (although females may be asymptomatic carriers). Hemophilia A and B have also been identified in cats.

Affected animals usually have cavity type bleeding (e.g., hematoma, hemarthrosis, hemoperitoneum) after trauma or surgery. These animals often experience recurrent bleeding episodes that require transfusion support. Both hemophilia A and hemophilia B can be treated with FFP. Based on component availability, fresh whole blood may be used, especially if the patient is anemic as well. Patients with hemophilia A can also be treated with cryoprecipitate.

Many other hereditary coagulopathies have been identified in the dog and cat but occur less frequently (see Table 15-2).

Acquired Coagulopathies

Vitamin-K malabsorption. Vitamin K is required for the hepatic synthesis of coagulation factors II, VIII, IX, and X. In vitamin K deficiency, the liver produces inactive factors known as *proteins induced by vitamin-K antagonism* (PIVKA). The plasma coagulation factors need to be activated to be functional, but cannot do so in the absence of vitamin K. In small animals, a dietary deficiency of vitamin K is not likely to be encountered, but intestinal malabsorption and biliary obstruction may lead to a deficiency state.

Liver disease. The liver is the site of synthesis of all coagulation factors. In patients with severe liver disease, coagulopathies frequently occur because of impaired coagulation factor synthesis and vitamin K malabsorption. Bleeding tendencies will vary from mild to severe hemorrhage.

Coagulation factor replacement is achieved by administering plasma products. The whole blood-derived components include FFP, frozen plasma, and cryoprecipitate. Before receiving transfusion support, patients must be evaluated to determine whether they need multiple coagulation factor replacement or just an isolated component.

Anticoagulant rodenticide toxicity. Anticoagulant rodenticide poisoning is commonly encountered in the veterinary emergency setting. Anticoagulant rodenticides act as antagonists to vitamin K; therefore, biologically active coagulation factors II, VII, IX, and X cannot be produced. The body does not contain an excessive store of vitamin K, so vitamin K1 must be administered to allow vitamin K-dependent factors to function. First generation rodenticides (e.g., warfarin, indandione) have a relatively low toxicity and generally require repeated ingestion. Second-generation rodenticides (e.g., bromadiolone, brodifacoum) are more potent and have longer half-lives (weeks); therefore, the type of anticoagulant rodenticide ingested determines the duration of vitamin K therapy. Removing the toxic substance and supplementing vitamin K is key, but patients may need coagulation factor support in the form of FFP, frozen plasma, cryopoor plasma, or fresh whole blood transfusion to stop hemorrhage.

Disseminated intravascular coagulation. In certain pathologic situations, the coagulation response may become accelerated and the fibrinolytic system overwhelmed. Clot formation begins to appear not only at the site of endothelial damage but also randomly throughout the circulation. Many stimuli may trigger the coagulation cascade in this way (e.g., sepsis, neoplasia, massive trauma). This imbalance between bleeding, coagulation, and fibrinolysis is called disseminated intravascular coagulation *(DIC)*. Clinical signs are highly variable and depend on the underlying disease. DIC often manifests as diffuse hemorrhage resulting from the ultimate consumption of coagulation factors and platelets.

No single diagnostic test for DIC exists; however, the presence of schistocytes, thrombocytopenia, hypofibrinogenemia, elevated fibrin split products, decreased antithrombin III, and prolonged prothrombin time (PT), partial thromboplastin time (PPT), and activated clotting time (ACT) are evaluated in conjunction with clinical signs.

Therapy for DIC is treatment of the underlying disease process. Administration of fresh whole blood or replacement of specific blood components (e.g., packed RBCs, FFP, platelet-rich plasma, cryoprecipitate) may be necessary to maintain blood volume and to support hemostatic function in patients who are actively bleeding. The administration of heparin is thought to slow or stop the coagulation process by partnering with antithrombin III, thereby inhibiting critical substances of hemostasis. This treatment modality remains controversial, and a wide range of doses has been suggested. Regardless of the dose, patients receiving heparin require careful monitoring for the duration of therapy.

Clinical Assessment

An accurate history, thorough physical examination, and certain laboratory tests must be performed to evaluate a bleeding patient, reach a diagnosis, determine a prognosis, and define an appropriate therapeutic plan.

History

A complete history is critical in beginning a workup for a hemostatic defect. Obtaining and assessing a complete and detailed history will help define the nature, severity, and duration of bleeding and other clinical signs, as well as aid in making a correct diagnosis. Attention to detail will help in establishing probability for each possible differential early in the diagnostic process.

Questions should be clear, nonleading, and thought provoking. Devising a list of questions for owners to review should help to stimulate them to think of some very important (most likely, not obvious) facts. For example, does the animal have any previously diagnosed diseases? Is the animal currently on any medication?

A list of any prescription or over-the-counter medications should be included, because many drugs have potentially harmful or complicating side effects (resulting in a toxic effect on RBCs, WBCs, and platelets, as well as the vasculature and coagulation factors). Complete vaccination history should not be overlooked, since a relationship between recent vaccination and

onset of IMHA has been suggested. The animal's environmental history is important, because it may suggest potential exposure to toxic or organic substances such as anticoagulant rodenticide, poisons, or zinc. Tick exposure should also be investigated.

Evaluation of the current bleeding episode is vital, and the bleed should be characterized as localized or multifocal. Is this the animal's first bleeding episode, or is there a history of bleeding tendency? The answers to these questions may help to differentiate between an acquired and hereditary bleeding disorder. Although hereditary coagulopathies may occur in any breed, each coagulopathy has thus far only been reported in certain breeds. Because specific breeds may suggest a specific coagulopathy, any information the owner may have regarding breed history could provide helpful clues.

Physical Examination

A complete physical examination and multiple monitoring procedures may be required to properly assess the patient in a bleeding crisis. Optimal assessment cannot be based on the result of a single parameter but more so on the results of several physical examination findings and monitored parameters that should always be evaluated in relation to one another.

Certain clinical signs found on physical examination may help determine the origin of the bleeding episode. Small surface bleeds (e.g., petechiation, ecchymosis, epistaxis, hematuria) are usually suggestive of platelet or vascular abnormalities. Larger bleeds or bleeding into body cavities (e.g., hematoma formation, hemarthroses, deep muscle hemorrhage, hemothorax, hemoabdomen) are suggestive of clotting factor deficiencies. A combination of these clinical signs is not uncommon.

Mucous membrane color, capillary refill time, pulse rate and quality, and respiratory rate and effort should also be evaluated to determine bleed severity and the presence of possible life-threatening complications.

Laboratory Tests

Hemostatic tests are indicated whenever an animal is bleeding excessively, before surgery when an increased bleeding tendency is possible, to monitor therapeutic interventions, and for genetic screening in certain breeds with a known bleeding disorder.

To summarize the status of the hemostatic mechanism, the difference between primary and secondary hemostasis must be understood. Information obtained from the history and specific clinical signs may suggest a diagnosis, but certain laboratory tests are necessary for a definitive diagnosis. All laboratory tests should be performed as soon as possible, and therapy should be instituted promptly after test samples are obtained.

Primary Hemostatic Tests

A platelet count should be performed on any patient who arrives at the clinic in a bleeding crisis. A normal platelet count is 150,000 to 400,000/µl. Abnormal bleeding may occur in animals with platelet counts below 40,000/µl; however, each patient varies and some animals may not exhibit clinical signs associated with bleeding with a platelet count of 2000/µl. In an animal exhibiting signs of surface bleeding with a normal platelet count, platelet function should be evaluated.

Because vWD is such a common mild primary hemostatic defect in dogs, plasma vWF measurements (most often by enzyme-linked immunosorbant assay) are indicated. The reference range depends on assay method and laboratory used (see Table 15-3).

The following are simple, in-house tests requiring no specialized equipment. They are quick, inexpensive, practical tests that allow recognition of primary hemostatic defects. These tests are often referred to as *cage-side*, in that they provide results almost immediately.

Platelet Estimation

A quick, reasonably accurate estimation of platelet number can be made from a stained blood smear and is much quicker than an actual platelet count. After routine preparation and staining, the blood smear is scanned to ensure even platelet distribution with no evidence of platelet clumping. The average number of platelets in approximately five to 10 oil immersion fields is counted to estimate platelet numbers. One platelet per oil immersion field represents approximately 20,000 platelets. Approximately eight to 15 platelets per oil immersion field are considered normal.

Although platelet estimation helps determine the presence of thrombocytopenia in an emergency situation, a true platelet count is necessary to classify the severity of depletion. After obtaining baseline values, ongoing platelet quantitation can be helpful in monitoring the course of a disease or the patient's response to certain therapies.

Bleeding Time Test

Bleeding time is the time it takes for bleeding to stop after severing a vessel. The most commonly used bleeding time test in veterinary medicine is the buccal mucosal bleeding time (BMBT). The buccal mucosal bleeding time assesses platelet and vascular contribution to hemostasis, thereby evaluating primary hemostasis. A disposable template with two spring-loaded blades is used to produce standardized incisions in the buccal mucosal surface of the upper lip. The blades create 5 mm long × 1 mm deep incisions. The duration of bleeding from these incisions is monitored.

The materials needed for this test are as follows:

- Bleeding time device
- Gauze strip
- Filter paper or gauze sponges
- Timing device

When performing a buccal mucosal bleeding time test, the veterinary technician should do the following:

1. Place animal in lateral recumbency.
2. Expose the mucosal surface of the upper lip. Position a gauze strip around the maxilla to fold up the upper lip. Tie the strip gently, just tightly enough to partially block venous return.
3. The incision site should be void of surface vessels and slightly inclined so that shed blood from the incision can flow freely toward the mouth. Place the bleeding time device flush against mucosal surface, applying as little pressure as possible; press the tab to release scalpels.
4. Let the stab incisions bleed freely, undisturbed; time the bleeding until it stops. Excessive blood should be blotted as often as necessary to prevent blood flow into the patient's mouth. Place either filter paper or gauze sponge approximately 3 to 4 mm below the incision, taking care not to disturb the incision site and any clot that may be forming.
5. The end point is recorded when the edge of the filter paper or sponge does not soak up free-flowing blood. The bleeding time is the mean bleeding time for the two incisions. Normal bleeding time is less than 4 minutes.

The buccal mucosal bleeding time is a screening test. As with any screening test, sensitivity is not 100%. Therefore not all primary hemostatic defects will be discovered. This test also will not differentiate between vascular defects or platelet function defects. The buccal mucosal bleeding time is prolonged in cases of thrombocytopenia and thrombopathia, vWD, uremia, and aspirin therapy. Obviously, the BMBT should not be performed on any patient known to be thrombocytopenic.

Patients seem to tolerate the procedure well, eliminating the need for chemical restraint. The incisions produced are well above the concentrated pain fibers in the lip. Sometimes the animal will reflex on hearing the noise the scalpels make when released from the device, but the procedure itself is not painful. Although the BMBT does have limitations, several advantages to the test exist:

- Commercial bleeding time devices are readily available
- The templates are standardized and therefore results are reproducible
- The test is simple and quick to perform, and the results are almost immediately available

Secondary Hemostatic Tests

Several standardized coagulation screening tests are useful to define coagulopathies in clinical practice. Blood samples for hematologic testing must be collected using a vacutainer system and processed carefully to prevent potential test errors. Atraumatic venipuncture and smooth blood flow into collection tubes are necessary to prevent extraneous clotting mechanism activation. Samples should be processed immediately after collection and testing performed without delay. If samples are to be sent to an outside laboratory, the plasma should be frozen before shipment. Extra plasma should be saved in case further individual factor analysis becomes necessary.

The clinician assesses the extrinsic and common pathways by either the prothrombin time (PT) or PIVKA test. The PIVKA test detects any coagulation factor deficiency of the extrinsic and common pathways and is not specific for the detection of anticoagulant rodenticide poisoning. The intrinsic and common pathways are assessed by activated partial thromboplastin time (aPTT). Prolongation of PT and aPTT will be seen when clotting factors are depleted below 30% of normal. Each test should be interpreted in terms of what pathway or pathways it specifically evaluates. Although hereditary coagulopathies can be suggested based on the pattern of coagulation test abnormalities, specific factor analyses are needed to confirm a diagnosis.

Activated Clotting Time Test

The activated clotting time (ACT) test is a simple, inexpensive screening test for severe abnormalities in the intrinsic and common pathways of the clotting cascade. It evaluates the same pathways as aPTT, but is less sensitive at detecting factor deficiencies (because factors must be decreased to less than 5% of normal to prolong ACT). The ACT is a useful diagnostic test because results are available within minutes.

The materials needed for this test are as follows:

- Vacutainer sleeve
- Vacutainer single-collection needle
- ACT tube containing diatomaceous earth
- Electric heat block of 37° C (can substitute hot water bath or hold in hand)

When conducting an ACT test, the veterinary technician should do the following:

1. Warm the ACT tube in the heat block to 37° C for approximately 3 minutes.
2. Perform clean venipuncture on an unthrombosed vessel. Discard the first few drops of blood to eliminate tissue thromboplastin, the tissue factor responsible for activation of the extrinsic pathway.
3. Puncture the ACT tube with the distal needle and collect approximately 2 ml of blood. Begin timing as soon as blood enters the tube.
4. After collection, invert the tube several times to mix with diatomaceous earth and place it in the heating block.
5. After 30 seconds from the start of timing, gently tilt the tube and examine the blood for clot formation. Return the tube to heat block and repeat the procedure every 10 seconds.
6. The ACT time is the time from collection of the blood in the tube to initial clot formation. In the dog, the normal ACT time is 60 to 110 seconds. In the cat, the normal ACT time is 50 to 75 seconds.

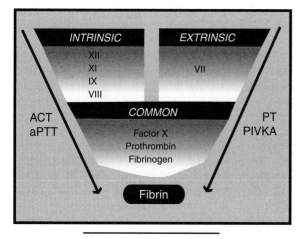

Fig. 15-2 Coagulation testing.

Prolongation of ACT occurs with severe factor deficiency in the intrinsic or common clotting pathway (e.g., hemophilia) in the presence of inhibitors (e.g., heparin, warfarin). Prolongation may also occur in cases of severe thrombocytopenia because of the lack of platelet phospholipid (mild prolongation of 10 to 20 seconds). The ACT is inexpensive, easily learned, quick to perform, reproducible, and provides immediate results. In addition, it provides a useful measurement of coagulation in emergency situations. When compared with the PTT, the role that technical and laboratory error can have on the test results must be taken into consideration. This is not to suggest that one should rely solely on the ACT. In most situations, the ACT should be followed with an aPTT.

Synbiotics Coagulation Analyzer (SCA 2000)

The SCA 2000 is a point-of-care instrument that allows immediate assessment of PT and aPTT. A fresh citrated whole blood sample is recommended; fresh nonanticoagulated blood yields less reliable results (Fig. 15-2).

Anemia

Anemia, a reduction in the number of circulating red blood cells (RBCs), is confirmed by a decrease in red cell count, hemoglobin (Hb), or packed cell volume (PCV). Anemia is a clinical sign or laboratory test abnormality, not a diagnosis for a specific disease.

Clinical signs and a patient's history indicate the possibility of anemia. The severity of signs depends on the rapidity of onset, the degree and cause of the anemia, and the extent of the animal's physical activity. Once anemia is confirmed, its cause should be thoroughly investigated to determine proper therapeutic management of the patient.

Anemia may result from increased loss (acute or chronic) (i.e., hemorrhage), increased destruction (i.e., intravascular or extravascular hemolysis), or decreased production (i.e., hypoplasia or aplasia of the bone marrow) of red blood cells. The red cell life span is usually normal in blood loss anemias and hypoproliferative anemias but is characteristically reduced in hemolytic anemias. Based on the erythropoietic response seen in peripheral blood, anemias may also be classified as *regenerative* or *nonregenerative*. Classification is helpful in differentiating blood-loss and hemolytic anemias (which are generally responsive) from bone marrow depression anemias (which are generally nonresponsive).

Hemorrhage

Normal blood volume is 8% to 9% of body weight in dogs and 6% to 8% in cats. The relative blood volume is determined by the animal's age, splenic reserve, and hydration status.

A significant loss of blood over minutes to hours results in hypovolemia and potential cardiovascular collapse. Healthy animals can tolerate as much as 20% reduction in blood volume, but signs of shock generally develop when blood volume is reduced to 60% to 70% of normal. The therapeutic goal in the treatment of acute hemorrhagic hypovolemia is to stop hemorrhage and support the cardiovascular system. Aggressive, rapid restoration of vascular volume must be instituted while preventing further blood loss if possible. In cases of external hemorrhage, direct pressure can be applied to the bleeding site or sites; however, the veterinary technician should watch for continued blood loss from uncontrolled sites after intravascular volume resuscitation. Although internal hemorrhage may not be evident on presentation, it should be considered if shock occurs after trauma.

When choosing resuscitation fluid for vascular space replacement, volume and composition are critical in determining the effectiveness of volume expansion and duration of its effect. After blood loss, the intravascular space is depleted; only later does interstitial fluid shift from the extravascular into the intravascular space, providing much needed volume. In the early stages of hemorrhage, replenishing intravascular space losses is a priority and can be accomplished easily using crystalloid fluid solutions. Crystalloid solutions also enter the extravascular space; consequently, administering two to three times the amount of crystalloid as volume lost is necessary. Risk of fluid overload is of concern when a large volume of crystalloids are administered, especially in older patients or patients with some degree of cardiovascular compromise. Colloid solutions should be considered when a need exists to maintain intravascular oncotic pressure without administering large volumes of fluid, as well as when blood loss continues and a substantial portion of the blood volume is depleted.

The symptoms that occur immediately after hemorrhage are a result of blood volume depletion, not a decrease in RBC mass. Although fluid administration will improve tissue perfusion, patient assessment is necessary to help determine whether enough Hb is present to provide oxygen to vital organs. The need for transfusion should be based on clinical assessment of the signs of anemia, because no magic laboratory value exists at which a patient must be transfused. Red cell replacement may not be necessary during initial therapy of acute blood loss. The aggressiveness of therapy will depend on the volume of blood lost, the rate at which it was lost, and the patient's condition.

Patients may also present with a chronic blood loss anemia resulting from gastrointestinal bleeding, ectoparasites, endoparasites, neoplasia, and chronic thrombocytopenia. Clinical signs of chronic blood loss anemia may not be obvious because of the body's compensatory mechanisms and ability to adapt to this compromised state.

Hemolysis

Hemolytic anemia is caused by accelerated destruction of RBCs. Whether hemolysis occurs in the intravascular space or, more commonly, in the extravascular space, depends on several factors, including the cause and severity of the disease process. *Extravascular hemolysis* refers to RBC destruction through phagocytosis by macrophages. *Intravascular hemolysis* refers to lysis of RBCs within the circulation. Hemolytic anemias can be classified as *immune-mediated hemolytic anemia (IMHA)*,

inherited RBC defects, hemolysis associated with chemical ingestion, and hemolysis associated with infection.

IMHA may be a primary disease, also known as *idiopathic* or *autoimmune hemolytic anemia*, in which autoantibodies are produced against the unaltered RBC membrane. The specific stimulus provoking an individual to develop antibodies to its own tissue remains unidentified. Researchers hypothesize that a change in antigenicity of the red cells or in an individual's immune status may cause the immune system to recognize and attack its own RBCs. Complement (intravascular hemolysis) or macrophage (extravascular hemolysis) recognition leads to destruction of the RBCs.

IMHA can also be a secondary immune response directed toward a foreign antigen, ultimately leading to inadvertent damage to normal patient cells. Causes of secondary IMHA include neoplasia, infectious disease (i.e., parasitic, viral, bacterial, rickettsial), toxin exposure, and drug therapy. Neoplasia is reported to be the most frequent cause of secondary IMHA.

Although IMHA is the most common cause of hemolytic disease in dogs, other important causes of hemolysis exist. Differentiation of the cause of hemolysis is important given the wide variability between therapy and prognosis. Additionally, immunosuppressive drugs used in the treatment of IMHA may be associated with significant side effects that are far from benign.

Several inherited defects in erythrocyte metabolism that cause hemolysis have been described in a number of canine breeds. The most common are phosphofructokinase deficiency in the English Springer Spaniel and pyruvate kinase deficiency in the Basenji, Beagle, and West Highland White Terrier. Pyruvate kinase deficiency is usually more severe, with myelofibrosis, osteosclerosis, and death occurring before the age of 4. Phosphofructokinase deficiency tends to be associated with mild-to-moderate, intermittent intravascular hemolysis, often exacerbated by exercise. Both disorders exhibit marked reticulocytosis associated with chronic hemolytic disease. Hereditary RBC disorders should be included as a differential for any dog belonging to an affected breed that arrives with regenerative anemia and even mild signs of hemolytic disease. Special laboratory tests are required to definitively diagnose an inherited erythrocyte defect. Additionally, carrier detection can be used in breeding programs to limit the frequency of these genetic disorders in the affected breeds.

Many compounds have been reported to cause damage to the RBC. For example, an oxidizing agent found in onions, n-propyl disulfide, may cause hemolysis. Oxidation results in structural changes to the RBC (i.e., Heinz bodies), leading to hemolysis that may range from subclinical to severe. A single ingestion of large quantities of onion or repeated meals containing small amounts of onion can produce marked hemolysis and anemia in both dogs and cats. Heinz bodies, as well as eccentrocytes (RBC with Hb shifted to one side), appear within 24 hours after onion ingestion. When stained with new methylene blue, Heinz bodies appear as blue to purple refractile bodies on the periphery of the RBC. The key to diagnosing onion-induced hemolytic disease in dogs rests on patient history of onion ingestion and specific laboratory tests.

Zinc toxicosis in dogs is often associated with a hemolytic crisis of rapid onset. Zinc-induced hemolytic disease in dogs occurs most commonly after ingestion of zinc-containing materials (e.g., coins, nuts and bolts, skin ointments). All pennies minted in the United States after 1983 contain 96% zinc and represent the most common source of zinc intoxication in dogs. Signalment and history help establish an index of suspicion of zinc intoxication; many of these dogs are young and may have a history of repeated foreign body ingestion. Although the exact mechanism of zinc-induced hemolysis is unknown, intravascular hemolysis often occurs, thereby causing hemoglobinemia and hemoglobinuria.

Various forms of microangiopathic diseases, including DIC, hemangiosarcoma or metastatic tumors, snake bites, and heartworm infestation, may result in direct red cell damage occurring in the microvasculature, causing clinical signs of hemolysis. In microangiopathic hemolytic anemias, RBCs are mechanically fragmented because of fibrin deposition in small blood vessels.

Reduced or Ineffective Erythropoiesis

All blood cells develop from early stage cells in one of the largest organs in the body, the bone marrow. The bone marrow is stimulated to differentiate cells into RBCs, platelets, and specific types of WBCs according to the requirements of the body. As the cells mature, they proceed through developmental stages before being released from the bone marrow into the circulation where they become fully functional. The development of mature red blood cells is referred to as erythropoiesis.

Anemia caused by reduced or ineffective erythropoiesis may result from nutritional deficiencies (e.g., iron, B$_{12}$, gastrointestinal malabsorption), drugs, infection (e.g., feline leukemia virus, feline immunodeficiency virus), chronic disease, bone marrow infiltration (e.g., leukemia, multiple myeloma), and organ disorders (e.g., renal, liver, and endocrine disease). These anemias are chronic and usually nonregenerative or poorly regenerative.

Anemia of chronic disease is probably the most common form of nonregenerative anemia and is associated with a variety of chronic diseases (e.g., chronic infections, inflammation, neoplasia). The most common example is chronic renal disease of dogs and cats. The degree of anemia is roughly proportional to the degree of uremia and can be more severe in young animals. A variety of conditions (e.g., uremic toxins, blood loss from GI ulcers) can cause anemia; however, decreased erythropoietin production is the main cause. Erythropoietin is a hormone produced by the kidney that stimulates the bone marrow to increase its production of RBCs.

Nonregenerative anemia can be clinically classified according to the number of cell types involved. When only erythrocytes are decreased, this is considered a *refractory anemia*, which may be the result of chronic disease, iron deficiency, or other organ disorders (i.e., external effects that influence bone marrow). When other cell types are involved (pancytopenia), the anemia is called *aplastic anemia*, which can be caused by disease within the marrow, exposure to radiation or chemicals, infection, leukemia, other tumors, or it can be idiopathic. A bone marrow examination is usually necessary to distinguish these two classifications.

Clinical Assessment

An accurate history, thorough physical examination, and appropriate laboratory tests must be performed to properly evaluate an anemic patient, determine a diagnosis, and define a therapeutic plan.

History. All pertinent information regarding patient history must be gathered from the owners. Obtaining and assessing a complete and detailed history will help define the nature, severity, and duration of clinical signs and aid in making a correct diagnosis. Attention to detail allows the clinician to establish probability for each possible differential early in the diagnostic process. For example, an anemic English Springer Spaniel with pigmenturia, especially after physical exertion, should alert the clinician to the possibility of phosphofructokinase deficiency. When a puppy has signs of hemolytic disease, the owner should be questioned about the possibility of foreign body ingestion of certain zinc-containing metallic objects.

Complete vaccination history should not be overlooked, because a relationship between recent vaccination and onset of IMHA has been demonstrated. One study showed that 25% of all IMHA cases were vaccinated within 1 month of presentation and that this complication occurred independent of the type of vaccine used.

The animal's environmental history may suggest possible exposure to toxic and organic substances that will create hemolytic conditions (e.g., onions, zinc). Tick exposure should also be investigated given various infectious agents may cause a hemolytic anemia (e.g., hemobartonellosis, babesiosis, ehrlichiosis, leptospirosis).

Information regarding previously diagnosed diseases and any recently or currently administered medication is very important. Many drugs have potentially harmful or complicating side effects, resulting in a toxic effect (i.e., drug-induced IMHA) on RBCs, WBCs, and platelets.

Physical Examination. A complete physical examination and multiple monitoring procedures may be required to properly assess the patient in an anemic crisis. Optimal assessment cannot be based on the result of a single parameter but on the results of several physical examination findings and monitored parameters that should always be evaluated in relation to one another.

In anemic patients, the development and progression of clinical signs depends on the rapidity of onset of the anemia, the degree and cause of anemia, and the animal's physical activity. Common physical findings are those associated with a decrease in red cell mass: lethargy, weakness, pale mucous membranes, tachycardia, tachypnea, and bounding pulses. Anorexia, exercise intolerance, and collapse may also be seen. The cardiovascular and respiratory system should be carefully evaluated. Assessment of perfusion is based on mucous membrane color, capillary refill time, heart rate, as well as pulse rate, strength, and character. In a severe anemic state, a low-grade systolic flow murmur may occur secondary to decreased blood viscosity. Assessment of respiratory rate and effort, as well as careful auscultation, may help differentiate between decreased oxygen carrying capability and possible pulmonary thromboembolism. Tachypnea and dyspnea may be evident but are not typical signs unless the anemia is severe. Fever is sometimes observed and may be caused by red cell destruction, or secondary or underlying inflammation and infection. Monitoring all parameters in unison with one another will lend information regarding bleed severity and potentially life-threatening complications.

Patients should be evaluated for signs of underlying or concurrent disease. For example, dogs with IMHA should be carefully examined for signs of other immune-mediated disease, such as concurrent IMT (i.e., Evans syndrome). If petechiation is present, then IMT or other coagulopathies, such as liver disease or DIC, should be investigated.

Other common physical findings in dogs with hemolytic disease are those relating to an accumulation of bilirubin or Hb (or both), in blood, urine, and soft tissue. As a result of extravascular RBC destruction, increased quantities of bilirubin are presented to the liver for conjugation and excretion. Bilirubin begins to accumulate in blood, urine, and soft tissue when the quantity of bilirubin present exceeds the liver's capacity to excrete it in the bile. Consequently, dogs with severe extravascular hemolysis have icterus and pigmenturia, caused by the presence of bilirubin or Hb in the urine. Given the low threshold for urinary excretion of conjugated bilirubin, in dogs, bilirubinuria develops early in the disease process and precedes hyperbilirubinemia and icterus. Icterus is easily recognized on all skin surfaces when severe. When more subtle, icterus is best recognized on the gingiva, sclera, conjunctiva, and inner pinnae. If intravascular hemolysis occurs, hemoglobinemia with or without hemoglobinuria may be present.

Splenomegaly, hepatomegaly, or both may be discovered on abdominal palpation. This occurs as a result of increased RBC clearance by the monocyte phagocytic system in these organs, by extramedullary hematopoiesis, and by hemosiderosis (accumulation of iron in the liver). Dogs with IMHA may also develop hepatopathy, particularly after glucocorticosteroid therapy.

Laboratory Tests. Although information obtained from the history and specific clinical signs can suggest a diagnosis, certain laboratory tests are necessary for a definitive diagnosis. Laboratory tests will help define the severity of the anemia, classify the anemia, and identify the underlying disease process.

Anemia is suggested when one or more of the red cell parameters (i.e., RBC count, PCV, hematocrit) are below normal for the age, sex, and breed of the species concerned. Of these three parameters, PCV provides a simple, quick, and accurate means of detecting anemia, and it allows for classification of the anemia as *mild, moderate,* or *severe.* Dehydration and splenic contraction may mask anemia, whereas hemodilution may cause a temporary reduction in red cell parameters; therefore, determination of both PCV and total plasma protein (TP) level may help in differentiating these variables. Dehydration is associated with increases in PCV and TP, but splenic contraction only elevates PCV. Hemodilution after acute blood loss or fluid therapy is associated with decreases in both PCV and TP, whereas hemolytic anemias are usually associated only with a reduction in PCV. TP is usually normal in anemia secondary to decreased production or increased destruction of erythrocytes, compared with blood loss, in which PCV and TP may be decreased because of loss of erythrocytes and plasma proteins and a compensatory shift of fluid from the interstitial space to the intravascular compartment.

Reticulocyte count. The reticulocyte count is the best indicator of the effectiveness of bone marrow activity. The reticulocyte count during regenerative anemia generally varies with the degree of anemia; the greater the stimulation of marrow erythropoiesis, the greater the reticulocytosis. This is not the case with nonregenerative anemias; therefore the degree of reticulocytosis must be viewed in concert with the degree of anemia. The nurse can do this by calculating a corrected reticulocyte count (percent [%]) or an absolute reticulocyte count (numbers/microliters [µl] blood). The absolute reticulocyte count is calculated by multiplying the percentage of reticulocytes by the RBC count. Alternatively, the percentage of reticulocytes can be corrected for the degree of anemia by the following formula:

Corrected reticulocytes %
= (observed reticulocyte count)
× (PCV of patient/mean normal PCV for species)

The mean normal PCV is 45% and 37% for dogs and cats, respectively. A corrected reticulocyte count greater than 1% in the dog and cat indicates a regenerative anemia. An absolute reticulocyte count of greater than 60,000/µl of blood in the dog is evidence of a regenerative response.

The degree of reticulocytosis is generally greater in hemolytic anemia and is evident earlier than in blood loss anemia. Usually it takes about 3 or 4 days for a significant reticulocytosis to be found in blood after an acute hemolytic or hemorrhagic episode, and a maximum response may take 1 to 2 weeks or longer. Thus reticulocytosis in an anemic patient indicates increased red cell destruction or blood loss. Conversely, the absence of reticulocytosis in an anemic patient suggests reduced erythropoietin production, marrow depression or failure, defective iron use, or ineffective erythropoiesis. Bone marrow evaluation is necessary to assess the production of RBCs in these patients.

Blood smear. Much information can be gathered from a complete blood count (e.g., Hb concentration, cell counts, RBC indices). On careful microscopic examination of a stained blood film, RBC indices and morphology can help characterize an anemia. The mean corpuscular volume (MCV), which represents the average size of the RBC, classifies erythrocytes as *normocytic* (normal), *macrocytic* (larger than normal), and *microcytic* (smaller than normal). For example, an increased MCV may result from cells being released from the bone marrow before they reach full maturity. This is called a *macrocytic anemia.* The mean corpuscular Hb concentration (MCHC) is represented by the terms *normochromic* (normal Hb content) and *hypochromic* (less than normal Hb content). For example, a decreased MCHC may result from increased numbers of circulating immature red cells. This is called a *hypochromic anemia.*

The blood smear can also show appropriate morphologic features, such as spherocytosis, polychromasia, and anisocytosis. Marked spherocytosis is indicative of IMHA in dogs. During the IMHA episode, macrophages bind to the RBC membrane and remove a piece. The RBC escapes complete phagocytosis, but its membrane is tightened, creating a small, swollen, densely stained erythrocyte. A small number of spherocytes may also be observed in microangiopathic hemolytic anemia, DIC, zinc intoxication, and heartworm disease.

Platelet count. IMHA and IMT may occur concurrently. If thrombocytopenia is present, then a diagnostic workup for IMT should be performed and appropriate treatment instituted. With any clinical evidence of bleeding, other coagulation studies should be performed to rule out concurrent thrombocytopenia, DIC, or other coagulopathies (see discussion in section on hemostatic testing).

Saline agglutination test. RBC autoagglutination indicates anti-RBC antibodies are present and therefore strongly suggests IMHA. Agglutination appears as grapelike clustering of erythrocytes in the blood smear and can be distinguished from rouleaux formation by examining a wet-mount preparation of a blood sample. The veterinary technician should mix one drop of blood with one drop of isotonic saline on a clean microscope slide, cover it with a coverslip, and examine it under the microscope. Rouleaux, unlike agglutination, should be dispersed by the addition of the saline. This test is not infallible, because weak agglutinins may cause false-negative results. Blood should also be evaluated for macroagglutination (seen grossly on the slide). Persistent agglutination precludes any further blood typing, crossmatching, or Coombs' test.

Coombs' test. Serologic diagnosis of IMHA is based on the demonstration of immune-mediated antibody or complement on the surface of red cells or in the patient's serum via Coombs' antiglobulin tests. The direct Coombs' test demonstrates presence of antierythrocyte antibody or activated complement components on the surface of the patient's red cells. The indirect Coombs' test reveals the presence of antierythrocyte antibody in patient serum. A suspension of washed cells of the patient (direct Coombs' test) or of normal washed red cells exposed to the patient's serum (indirect Coombs' test) is allowed to react with species-specific antiglobulin to induce visible agglutination of red cells. In cases of drug-induced IMHA, the offending drug must be incorporated into the test system, or the test may yield negative results. The diagnosis of IMHA is supported by demonstrating the presence of these antibodies or complement (evidenced by the appearance of agglutination).

Chemistry profile and urinalysis. A serum biochemistry profile and urinalysis is important in detecting and assessing concurrent metabolic disease (e.g., renal, hepatic). Electrolyte disturbances should be monitored closely. Decreased bilirubin and albumin or globulin levels may indicate blood loss. Elevated bilirubin levels suggest hemolysis. Bilirubinuria and bilirubinemia are always observed with active hemolysis, but bilirubinemia may be very modest.

Blood sample collection technique is critical, because hemolysis associated with traumatic venipuncture can cause serum bilirubin to be falsely elevated.

Tick titers. Various infectious agents may cause a hemolytic anemia; therefore serology for tick-borne diseases should be performed if tick exposure is a possibility.

Miscellaneous information. With IMHA, the leukocyte count is often elevated with a slight to marked neutrophilia and left shift as a result of maximal bone marrow stimulation. A patient in hemolytic crisis may exhibit a marked neutrophilia (60,000 to 70,000 with increase in banded neutrophils) in the absence of infection; therefore one must evaluate the clinical presentation of each patient and look for other signs that might support infection along with the WBC count.

IMHA is an important risk factor for pulmonary thromboembolus. Acute onset of dyspnea with little or no radiologic evidence of pulmonary disease strongly suggests pulmonary thromboembolus. Unfortunately, confirming a diagnosis of pulmonary thromboembolus antemortem rarely is possible, and distinguishing pulmonary thromboembolus from pneumonia is difficult.

Treatment and Management. Anemic animals often arrive at the emergency service in advanced stages of disease, on the verge of cardiovascular collapse, and in need of immediate therapeutic intervention. Although a definitive diagnosis is important in the ultimate treatment of these patients, stabilizing the patient's emergent clinical problems is critical. This stabilization may include controlling hemorrhage and replacing lost blood volume with the appropriate intravenous fluid solutions, blood components, or both, as well as improving the oxygen-carrying capacity with oxygen and RBC support and taking all necessary measures to combat shock. Once the patient is stabilized, the clinician should classify the anemia, proceed with diagnostic evaluation, determine the underlying cause, and begin appropriate therapy. Clinical laboratory tests should be performed immediately and therapy instituted promptly after test samples are obtained. The goal is to correct the condition responsible for the blood loss (e.g., provide surgery, withdraw offending drug, administer anthelmintics).

In general, heart disease is more prevalent in males. Important exceptions are patent ductus ateriosus and sick sinus syndrome in miniature schnauzers, which are more common in females. Pericardial disease, aortic stenosis, dilated cardiomyopathy, and endocarditis are more common in large breed dogs. Degenerative valvular disease, patent ductus arteriosus (PDA), and pulmonic stenosis are more common in smaller breeds. Sick sinus syndrome is common in miniature schnauzers, West Highland white terriers, and cocker spaniels. Hypertrophic cardiomyopathy is common in cats and rare in dogs.

History

Clients seek emergency treatment because they have observed something that they perceive to be so serious that it requires immediate attention; this is the chief complaint. The physical examination and diagnostic tests will help the team to understand what is happening now, but only the client or the medical record can describe what occurred before presentation unless the veterinary professionals have personal knowledge of the patient. Those working in emergency care are often frustrated by the inability to obtain the medical record and the need to begin treatment of a life-threatening condition without the benefit a complete history. In a life-threatening emergency, the veterinarian may need to begin treatment immediately and have a technician gather the history while the patient is being treated. The presenting signs may lead the veterinarian to consider the possibility of heart disease, which may influence what sort of information he or she seeks in the history. A veterinarian treating a patient suspected of having heart disease might look to the client or medical record for information related to the chief complaint, the patient's history of heart disease, procedures and medication used to treat preexisting heart disease, previous diagnostic procedures and tests, activity level, exercise capacity, edema, difficulty breathing, cough, syncope, changes in weight, and diet. Box 16-1 lists common signs in cardiac emergencies. Tables 16-1 and 16-2 list various heart diseases and the emergencies associated with them.

Physical Examination

Physical examination is the process of gathering information that can be detected with the senses (sometimes aided with simple equipment like a

BOX 16-1

Common Signs in Cardiac Emergencies

> Sudden death
> Cyanosis
> Dyspnea
> Collapse
> Hind limb paresis
> Syncope
> Tachypnea
> Exercise intolerance
> Cough
> Abdominal distention (ascites)

stethoscope and a thermometer). The veterinarian should be notified if a new sign is observed or if a previously observed sign changes. The following list contains signs that are associated with heart disease and grouped by the sense used to detect them.

Sight:

- Cyanotic or pale mucous membranes
- Cachexia
- Dyspnea
- Tachypnea
- Ascites
- Jugular distention
- Edema
- Hind limb paresis
- Syncope
- Posture
- Response to environment, level of consciousness

Sound:

- Murmurs
- Cough
- Gallop sounds
- Irregular heart rhythm
- Bradycardia or tachycardia
- Crackles or other abnormal lung sounds
- Muffled heart or lung sounds

Touch:

- Body temperature
- Temperature of extremities
- Abnormal pulses, pulse deficits
- Precordial thrills

TABLE 16-1

Emergencies Associated with Various Forms of Canine Heart Disease

Heart Disease	Associated Emergencies
Heartworm disease	Caval syndrome, right heart failure, pulmonary hypertension
Chronic valvular disease	Pulmonary edema, ruptured chordae tendineae, left atrial tear, cardiac arrhythmias, right heart failure
Dilated cardiomyopathy	Pulmonary edema, right heart failure, cardiac arrhythmias, cardiac arrest (sudden death)
Pericardial disease	Right heart failure, cardiac tamponade
Patent ductus arteriosus (PDA)	Pulmonary edema, cardiac arrhythmias, pulmonary hypertension, cyanosis
Subvalvular aortic stenosis	Cardiac arrest (sudden death), cardiac arrhythmias, pulmonary edema (most common with concomitant mitral dysplasia)
Pulmonic stenosis	Right heart failure (most common with concomitant tricuspid dysplasia)
Infective endocarditis	Pulmonary edema, embolism, cardiac arrhythmias
Ventricular septal defect	Left heart failure, pulmonary hypertension, cyanosis, right heart failure
Tetralogy of Fallot	Cyanosis, polycythemia
Tricuspid dysplasia	Right heart failure
Atrial septal defect	Right heart failure, pulmonary hypertension, cyanosis

TABLE 16-2

Emergencies Associated with Various Forms of Feline Heart Disease

Heart Disease	Associated Emergencies
Hypertrophic cardiomyopathy	Thromboembolism, pulmonary edema, pleural effusion, cardiac arrhythmias, sudden death
Restrictive cardiomyopathy	Thromboembolism, pulmonary edema, pleural effusion, cardiac arrhythmias, sudden death
Dilated cardiomyopathy	Thromboembolism, pulmonary edema, pleural effusion, cardiac arrhythmias, sudden death
Cardiomyopathy secondary to hyperthyroidism	Thromboembolism, pulmonary edema, pleural effusion, cardiac arrhythmias, sudden death
Atrioventricular valve dysplasia	Congestive heart failure
Ventricular septal defect	Congestive heart failure, cyanosis
Patent ductus arteriosus (PDA)	Congestive heart failure
Aortic stenosis	Congestive heart failure, sudden death
Tetralogy of Fallot	Cyanosis

- Fluid in abdomen
- Enlarged liver

Auscultation of the heart is one part of the physical examination that deserves particular attention. Heart murmurs and gallops are some of the most important signs of heart disease. The ability to detect and characterize these sounds is a skill that can only be mastered by careful practice. Auscultation skills can be improved by taking the opportunity to examine any animal that is known to have a murmur or gallop sound.

Murmurs and gallops are sometimes missed because they are soft, intermittent, or only audible in a small portion of the chest wall. The person examining the patient should be systematic when listening—murmurs are sometimes missed because the examiner failed to listen to entire chest. Once a murmur is located, its intensity should be noted. Intensity is most often graded on a scale from 1 to 6. A murmur with an intensity of 1 is barely audible in a quiet room, and murmurs with an intensity of 6 are loud enough to be heard without the stethoscope touching the chest wall.

The point of maximum intensity should be noted; it provides a clue as to the source of the murmur. The person examining the patient should describe the location of the point of maximum intensity by describing the side of the thorax, and the intercostal space where the murmur is loudest and determine whether this point is above, below, or at the costochondral junction.

Murmurs are also described by when they occur in the cardiac cycle. Normally only the first and second heart sounds can be heard in dogs and cats. These *lub dup* sounds mark the beginning and end of systole. Murmurs that occur during this time are systolic murmurs; murmurs that follow the *lub dup* are diastolic murmurs. Diastolic murmurs are less common and generally softer than systolic murmurs. Diastolic gallop sounds occur when the normally inaudible third and fourth heart sounds can be heard. The third heart sound occurs just after systole, and the fourth heart sound occurs just before systole.

Electrocardiogram

The ECG is the most accurate technique available for the diagnosis of arrhythmias. The ECG may also aid in the diagnosis of enlargement of the chambers of the heart, electrolyte abnormalities, and pericardial effusion. The presence or absence of conditions other than arrhythmias should be confirmed with other tests. This is particularly true for enlargement of the heart chambers where the ECG will frequently produce false-positive or false-negative results.

Right atrial enlargement—P wave lead II greater than 0.4 mV in dogs, 0.2 mV in cats
Left atrial enlargement—P wave lead II greater than 0.04 seconds in dogs and cats
Right ventricular enlargement—Deep S waves in leads I, II, III, and aVF in dogs and cats
Left ventricular enlargement—QRS duration greater than 0.06 seconds and R wave greater than 3 mV in leads II, aVF and left precordial leads in the dog; QRS duration greater than 0.04 seconds and R wave greater than 1 mV in lead II in the cat.

Thoracic Radiographs

Heart disease usually changes the size and shape of the cardiac silhouette. In many cases the changes are subtle. Relying solely on radiographs to diagnose heart disease will frequently lead to misdiagnosis. One factor that limits the ability of radiographs to detect heart disease is that only the external borders of the heart are visible unless contrast is used. Some forms of heart disease do not significantly increase the size of the cardiac silhouette. Concentric hypertrophy causes the walls of the ventricles to thicken without increasing the external diameter of the heart. Eccentric hypertrophy and dilation are easier to detect using radiographs, because they increase the external diameter of the heart. As the heart fails, increases in the diameter of the pulmonary veins or vena cava become apparent in thoracic radiographs. Increased opacity of the lungs in dogs with heart disease is a sign of pulmonary edema, which indicates left heart failure. Radiographic signs of pleural effusion and enlargement of the vena cava in a patient with heart disease may indicate right or biventricular heart failure. The ability to examine the lungs and pulmonary vessels makes thoracic radiographs one the most sensitive techniques for detecting congestive left heart failure.

Cardiomegaly is a very reliable sign of heart disease when observed, although it will not be seen in every patient with heart disease. Cardiomegaly can be measured objectively by using the length of the thoracic vertebrae as a reference for determining heart size. The technique, known as the *vertebral heart scale* (VHS), was first used in dogs and was published

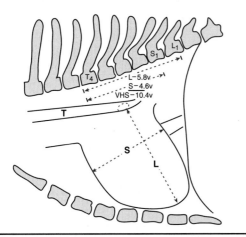

Fig. 16-1 Landmarks for measuring vertebral heart scale (VHS) in dogs. Lateral diagram illustrating the VHS measurement method. The long axis (*L*) and short axis (*S*) heart dimensions are transposed onto the vertebral column and recorded as the number of vertebrae beginning with the cranial edge of the fourth thoracic vertebra. These values are then added to obtain the VHS. *T*, Trachea. (From Buchanan JW, Bücheler J: Vertebral scale system to measure canine heart size in radiographs, *J Am Vet Med Assoc* 206:194-199, 1995).

TABLE 16-3

Normal Range for Vertebral Heart Scale (VHS) in Specific Breeds

Breed	Normal Range
Boxer	10.3-12.6
Cavalier King Charles spaniel	9.9-11.7
Doberman pinscher	9.0-10.8
German shepherd	8.7-11.2
Labrador retriever	9.7-11.7
Whippet (includes dogs trained for racing)	10.3-12.3
Yorkshire terrier	9.0-10.5
Generic (Buchanan)	8.7-10.7

Data from Lamb CR, Boswood A: Role of survey radiography in diagnosing canine cardiac disease, *Compend Contin Educ Pract Vet* 24(4):316-326, 2002; Buchanan JW, Bücheler J: Vertebral scale system to measure canine heart size in radiographs, *J Am Vet Med Assoc* 206(2):194-199, 1995., Bavagems V, Van Caelenberg A, Duchateau L, et al. Vertebral heart size ranges specific for whippets. Vet Radiol Ultrasound 46(5):400-403, 2005.

by Buchanan in 1991. Since then, the VHS has been used in cats and other species, and its use as an aid in the diagnosis of heart disease has been studied extensively. Technicians can assist the veterinarian in diagnosing cardiomegaly by measuring VHS.

To use the VHS technique to measure heart size in dogs, a lateral thoracic radiograph is examined and the distance between the lower margin of the left mainstem bronchus and the cardiac apex is marked on a piece of paper. The paper is then rotated 90 degrees, and the maximal short axis width is also marked on the paper. Then, beginning with the cranial border of the fourth thoracic vertebra (T4), the length and width of the heart is measured in vertebrae (estimating to one tenth of a vertebra). The sum of the length and width is used to determine overall heart size. Buchanan assumed that VHS was relatively unaffected by breed and that VHS values greater than 10.7 were abnormal. Since then, other studies have shown that some normal dogs have higher VHS values than those reported by Buchanan. Dogs with degenerative valvular disease begin to show signs of congestive heart failure when VHS exceeds approximately 12 to 13. Fig. 16-1 shows the landmarks and technique used to measure VHS in dogs. Table 16-3 shows the normal range for VHS in specific breeds.

The technique for measuring VHS in cats is similar to that used in dogs. The vertebrae beginning at the fourth thoracic vertebra in the lateral view are still used as a measuring scale. The anatomic landmarks used to measure the heart are slightly different from those used in dogs. In cats the long axis of the heart is measured in a lateral radiograph, beginning at the point where the most ventral cranial lobar vein meets the trachea and ending at the apex of the heart. The maximal short axis is measured just as it was in the dog. In cats the short axis width of the heart in ventrodorsal or dorsoventral radiographs may be just as useful a diagnostic sign as the sum of the long and short axis measurements in the lateral view. The measurement is made by examining the dorsoventral or ventrodorsal radiograph and drawing a line from the apex to the base of the heart. Next the maximal width of the heart perpendicular to that line is marked on a piece of paper. Then, using the vertebrae starting at fourth thoracic vertebra on the lateral radiograph (not the ventrodorsal or dorsoventral) as a ruler, the distance between the marks on the paper is measured to determine the width of the heart. The combined long and short axis lengths in the lateral view should be less than eight vertebrae, and the short

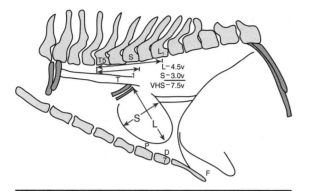

Fig. 16-2 Landmarks for measuring VHS in lateral radiographs in the cat. Diagram of lateral view of the thorax of a cat illustrating the VHS method. The long axis (*L*) and short axis (*S*) dimensions of the heart are transposed onto the vertebral column and recorded as the number of vertebrae beginning with the cranial edge of the fourth thoracic vertebra. These values are then added to obtain the VHS. The depth of the thorax (*D*) is measured from the dorsocaudal border of the seventh sternebra to the closest edge of the vertebral column. Precordial distance (*P*) is the minimum distance from the heart to the sternum. Falciform fat (*F*) is the minimum distance from the dorsocaudal border of the xiphoid cartilage to the liver. *T*, Trachea.

axis width in dorsoventral or ventrodorsal radiographs should be less than four vertebrae in the cat. It may be difficult to measure heart size in obese cats, because fat surrounding the heart may obscure the true cardiac border. Figs. 16-2 and 16-3 show the landmarks and techniques used to measure VHS in cats (Table 16-4).

Echocardiography

Echocardiography allows the beating heart to be examined noninvasively without the need of sedation or anesthesia. With very few exceptions, the technique will provide an accurate diagnosis of heart disease. This is because echocardiography provides information that, in the past, could only be provided by cardiac catheterization or angiography. Patients with heart disease are often referred to veterinary cardiologists or radiologists for an echocardiographic examination. The following discussion is designed to explain how echocardiography is used to diagnose heart disease.

Each echocardiographic mode provides a unique glimpse at the structure and function of the heart. M-mode echocardiography is used primarily to measure the size of structures in the heart. It can also be used to measure certain systolic time intervals. Two-dimensional echocardiography allows the size

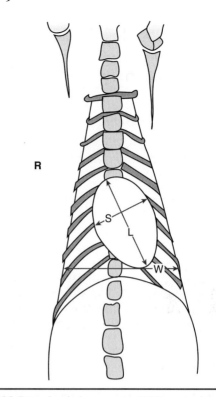

Fig. 16-3 Landmarks for measuring VHS in ventrodorsal or dorsoventral radiographs in the cat.

and relationship of structures that lie in the same plane to be examined; it can also be used to measure the length and area of structures in the heart. Doppler echocardiography is used to detect turbulence and measure the velocity of blood flow. A relationship exists between the increase in velocity and the pressure gradient across an area of stenosis or leaking heart valve. Doppler echocardiography can be used to estimate the pressure in a particular region of the heart by using that relationship. These pressure estimates are useful in determining the severity of pulmonic and aortic stenosis, as well as pulmonary hypertension. The pressure gradient across the stenotic region or a leaking valve can be calculated using the following equation:

$$PG = 4V^2$$

The pressure gradient (PG) in mm Hg is equal to four times the velocity (V) in meters per second squared. The normal velocity across the pulmonic valve is less than about 1.3 m/sec. The normal velocity across the aortic valve is somewhat controversial but should be less than about 1.5 to 2 m/sec. Values greater

TABLE 16-4

Ranges of Severity of Vertebral Heart Scale (VHS) in Dogs and Cats

Severity in Dogs	VHS	Severity in Cats	VHS
Normal	≤11	Normal	6.9 to 8.1
Normal to mild	11 to 12	Mild	8.2 to 8.5
Mild to moderate	12 to 13	Moderate	8.6 to 8.9
Moderate to severe	13 to 14	Severe	9 to 10
Very severe	>14	Very severe	>10

than this indicate stenosis of the valve. If tricuspid or pulmonic insufficiency occurs without stenosis, then the peak velocity can be used to estimate pulmonary artery pressure. A peak velocity equal to or greater than 2.8 m/sec across the tricuspid valve or a peak velocity equal to or greater than 2.2 m/sec across the pulmonic valve is considered abnormal. Tables 16-5 and 16-6 show how the pressure gradient is used to determine the severity of semilunar valve stenosis and pulmonary hypertension.

The diameter of the left ventricular chamber measured during diastole (LVIDd) and systole (LVIDs), the thickness (measured during diastole) of the left ventricular septum and free wall, the diameter of the left atrium and aortic root, and the E point septal separation are some of the most useful measurements that can be made using two-dimensional or M-mode echocardiography. The diameter of the right ventricle measured in diastole also changes in animals with heart disease, but the right ventricle is more difficult to image and measure. Because heart size is related to body size,

these measurements must be compared with values for dogs of the same weight or breed to determine whether or not the measurement is abnormal. Table 16-7 lists normal M-mode values for dogs and cats. Unlike the individual dimensions mentioned previously, the normal ranges of ratios of cardiac dimensions are the same for all dogs regardless of their size. Fractional shortening and the ratio of left atrial diameter to the diameter of the aortic root are particularly useful in diagnosing and determining the severity of heart disease.

Fractional shortening represents the change in diameter that occurs between diastole and systole (LVIDd – LVIDs)/LVIDd. Fractional shortening is decreased in diseases like dilated cardiomyopathy that reduce contractility. The average value for fractional shortening is 33%, and values less than 25% generally indicate myocardial failure, although a few normal dogs may have values this low. Fractional shortening decreases as the severity of the disease increases. Animals with fractional shortening less than 15% have severe heart disease and often show signs of heart failure.

TABLE 16-5

How the Pressure Gradient is Used to Determine the Severity of Semilunar Valve Stenosis

Severity of Stenosis	Pressure Gradient	Velocity
Mild stenosis	20 to 49 mm Hg	2.25-3.5 m/sec
Moderate stenosis	50 to 80 mm Hg	3.5-4.5 m/sec
Severe stenosis	>80 mm Hg	>4.5 m/sec

TABLE 16-6

How the Pressure Gradient is Used to Determine the Severity of Pulmonary Hypertension

Severity of Pulmonary Hypertension	Pressure Gradient (RV to RA)	Velocity (RV to RA)
Mild	30 to 50 mm Hg	2.8 to 3.5 m/sec
Moderate	50 to 74 mm Hg	3.5 to 4.3 m/sec
Severe	≥75 mm Hg	≥4.3 m/sec

RV, Right ventricle; *RA,* right atrium.

TABLE 16-7

Normal M-Mode Measurements

Body Weight (Kg)	LVIDd	LVIDs	LVWd	IVSd	Ao	LA	EPSS
Dogs							
3	2.1	1.3	0.5	0.5	1.1	1.1	0.1
	1.8-2.6	1.0-1.8	0.4-0.8	0.4-0.8	0.9-1.4	0.9-1.4	
4	2.3	1.5	0.6	0.6	1.3	1.2	0.1
	1.9-2.8	1.1-1.9	0.4-0.8	0.4-0.8	1.0-1.5	1.0-1.6	
6	2.6	1.7	0.6	0.6	1.4	1.4	0.1
	3.1-2.2	1.2-2.2	0.4-0.9	0.4-0.9	1.2-1.8	1.1-1.8	
9	2.9	1.9	0.7	0.7	1.7	1.6	0.2
	2.4-3.5	1.4-2.5	0.5-1.0	0.5-1.0	1.3-2.0	1.3-2.1	
11	3.1	2.0	0.7	0.7	1.8	1.7	0.2
	2.6-3.7	1.5-2.7	0.5-1.0	0.5-1.1	1.4-2.2	1.3-2.2	
15	3.4	2.2	0.8	0.8	2	1.9	0.2
	2.8-4.1	1.7-3.0	0.5-1.1	0.6-1.1	1.6-2.4	1.6-2.5	
20	3.7	2.4	0.8	0.8	2.2	2.1	0.3
	3.1-4.5	1.8-3.2	0.6-1.2	0.6-1.2	1.7-2.7	1.7-2.7	
25	3.9	2.6	0.9	0.9	2.3	2.3	0.3
	3.3-4.8	2.0-3.5	0.6-1.3	0.6-1.3	1.9-2.9	1.8-2.9	
30	4.2	2.8	0.9	0.9	2.5	2.5	0.4
	3.5-5.0	2.1-3.7	0.6-1.3	0.7-1.3	2.0-3.1	1.9-3.1	
35	4.4	2.9	1.0	1.0	2.6	2.6	0.4
	3.6-5.3	2.2-3.9	0.7-1.4	0.7-1.4	2.1-3.2	2.0-3.3	
40	4.5	3.0	1.0	1.0	2.7	2.7	0.5
	3.8-5.5	2.3-4.0	0.7-1.4	0.7-1.4	2.2-3.4	2.1-3.5	
50	4.8	3.3	1.0	1.1	3.0	2.9	0.6
	4.0-5.8	2.4-4.8	0.7-1.5	0.7-1.5	2.4-3.6	2.3-3.7	
60	5.1	3.5	1.1	1.1	3.2	3.1	0.7
	4.2-6.2	2.6-4.6	0.7-1.6	0.8-1.6	2.5-3.9	2.4-4.0	
Cats							
	1.5	0.72	0.41	0.42	0.90	1.17	0.06
	1.1-1.9	0.42-1.02	0.27-0.55	0.28-0.56	0.62-1.18	0.83-1.51	

Data from Cornell CC, Kittleson MD, Della Torre P et al: Allometric scaling of M-mode cardiac measurements in normal adult dogs, *J Vet Intern Med* 18(3):311-321, 2004; Kittleson MD, Kienle RD: *Small animal cardiovascular medicine*, St Louis, 1999, Mosby, p 104; Sisson DD et al: Plasma taurine concentrations and M-mode echocardiographic measures in healthy cats and in cats with dilated cardiomyopathy, *J Vet Intern Med* 5(4):232-238, 1991.

LVIDd, Diameter of the left ventricular chamber measured during diastole; *LVIDs,* diameter of the left ventricular chamber measured during diastole and systole; *LVWd,* thickness (measured during diastole) of the left ventricular free wall; *IVSd,* thickness (measured during diastole) of the left ventricular septum; *Ao,* aortic root; *LA,* left atrium; *EPSS,* E point septal separation.

The left atrium/aortic root ratio is useful in determining the likelihood of congestive heart failure. Several echocardiographic techniques are used to measure left atrial size. Each technique has slightly different normal ranges. When the M-mode technique is used, the upper limit of normal in dogs is 1.3 and about 1.6 for cats. Another technique that uses two-dimensional echocardiography to measure the atrium and aorta in dogs has a higher upper limit of 1.57. Animals begin to develop signs of left heart failure when left atrial diameter is about one and a half to two times the size of the aorta.

Despite its usefulness as a diagnostic technique, the results of an echocardiographic examination should be interpreted in conjunction with other diagnostic findings. Just as with most other diagnostic tests, an overlap is often seen between echocardiographic measurements of normal animals and animals with heart disease. The technician should remember that a measurement that falls within the normal range does not always eliminate the diagnosis of heart disease, and a value outside the normal range does not always confirm the diagnosis of heart disease.

The following diseases cause LVIDd to increase:

- PDA
- Mitral regurgitation
- Dilated cardiomyopathy
- Aortic insufficiency

The following diseases cause the diameter of the right ventricle measured in diastole to increase:

- Tricuspid regurgitation
- Heartworm disease

The following diseases cause the left ventricular free wall or left ventricular septum to increase:

- Subaortic stenosis
- Hypertrophic cardiomyopathy
- Hypertension and hyperthyroidism (primarily in cats)
- Hypovolemia (LVIDd should also be decreased)

The following diseases cause LVIDs to increase:

- Dilated cardiomyopathy and other diseases that cause myocardial failure

The following diseases cause E point septal separation to increase:

- Dilated cardiomyopathy and other diseases that cause myocardial failure

Overview of Cardiac Physiology and Pathophysiology

Systolic Function

The heart is a complex organ that contributes in many ways to maintaining homeostasis. Despite this complexity, the heart's main function, pumping blood, can be explained by looking at four determinants of systolic function. Three of the factors—preload, afterload, and contractility—determine how much blood is pumped with each beat of the heart (i.e., stroke volume). Multiplying stroke volume by the heart rate, the fourth factor, determines the volume of blood pumped in 1 minute (i.e., cardiac output).

Preload

Preload is a measure of how much the ventricle is stretched at the end of diastole. Central venous pressure (CVP), pulmonary capillary wedge pressure, or the left ventricular end diastolic diameter is commonly used to evaluate preload. Increasing any of these parameters usually results in increased preload and increased stroke volume. Increasing preload is an important mechanism to compensate for the reduced cardiac output caused by heart disease. Initially small increases in ventricular filling pressure, caused by fluid retention and venoconstriction, can increase preload and return cardiac output to near normal levels. If the heart disease continues to progress, then increasing preload to improve cardiac output causes congestive failure.

Afterload

Afterload is the force that resists the flow of blood from the heart. Increases in afterload make it harder for blood to leave the heart, causing a decrease in stroke volume. Arterial blood pressure (BP) or systemic vascular resistance generally increases along with afterload, and they can be used to evaluate and monitor it. The body is intolerant of hypotension; when BP drops below normal, the body responds by vasoconstricting.

Vasoconstriction improves BP, but it also tends to increase afterload and reduce cardiac output. Animals with poor myocardial function are very sensitive to changes in afterload; a small change in afterload can lead to a much greater change in cardiac output.

Contractility

Contractility is a change in stroke volume that is independent of changes in preload or afterload. Increases in contractility occur when the amount of calcium in the cells of the heart muscle is increased by chemicals produced by the body, such as epinephrine, or by drugs such as digoxin or dobutamine. Contractility is more difficult to evaluate than the other determinants of systolic function; however, if preload and afterload remain constant, then changes in cardiac output and fractional shortening can be used to assess changes in contractility.

Heart Rate and Rhythm

Preload, afterload, and contractility determine stroke volume. The last determinant of systolic function is heart rate. Abnormal heart rhythms can alter the normal sequence and duration of atrial and ventricular contraction (dyssynergy). Changes in heart rate have much more of an effect on the duration of diastole than on the duration of systole. Increases in heart rate usually increase cardiac output. Very fast heart rates can reduce cardiac output by not allowing the ventricle to fill adequately during diastole. Bradycardia also reduces cardiac output. The heart normally maintains adequate cardiac output as the heart rate slows by taking advantage of the increase in preload caused by the extra time spent in diastole. At some point, however, the heart is unable to accept enough blood, and cardiac output decreases.

Diastolic Function

During diastole the ventricle relaxes and fills with blood. Diseases that cause systolic dysfunction often interfere with relaxation and filling, but heart failure caused by diastolic dysfunction can occur even when systolic function is normal. Diastolic dysfunction probably leads to heart failure in many of the cardiac diseases that affect cats, such as hypertrophic cardiomyopathy, hyperthyroidism, and restrictive cardiomyopathy. These diseases can cause the ventricle to become so noncompliant that the filling

---

> **BOX 16-2** ⊕
>
> ### New York Health Association Classification
>
> CLASS I—Signs of heart disease but no signs of failure
> CLASS II—Signs of heart disease and signs of failure with vigorous activity
> CLASS III—Signs of heart disease and signs of failure with minimal activity
> CLASS IV—Signs of heart disease and signs of failure at rest

pressure required to produce a normal end diastolic volume may be high enough to cause signs of congestive failure.

Heart Failure

Most forms of heart disease cause heart failure. Heart failure can be defined as the inability of the heart to supply adequate blood flow to meet the metabolic needs of the body or to provide adequate blood flow only by excessive increases in ventricular filling pressure. This definition allows heart failure to exist in three forms: (1) forward or low-output failure when perfusion is inadequate, (2) congestive failure when filling pressures are excessive, or (3) a combination of forward and congestive failure. Heart failure takes different forms and varies in severity. Commonly used scales for classifying the severity of heart failure, such as the New York Heart Association classification (Box 16-2), are often based on the level of activity that produces signs of failure. Animals with mild failure can tolerate some exercise without showing signs of failure, and severely affected animals show signs of failure while at rest. Because most pets are not required to exercise vigorously, many owners do not recognize heart failure until it affects everyday activities.

Low-Output or Forward Failure

Low-output failure occurs when the heart cannot pump enough oxygenated blood to the tissues. Severe low-output failure, especially when accompanied by hypotension, is called *cardiogenic shock*. A healthy dog that weighs 30 kg has a cardiac output of about 4 L/min at rest, with each liter of blood containing 200 ml of oxygen (O_2). The dog's tissues consume 25% of the O_2 in the blood. If heart disease forces the dog's cardiac output to drop, then the volume of O_2 delivered to the tissues will also drop. Because O_2 consumption has not changed, the body must somehow compensate if normal function is to be maintained. If the change in cardiac output is not too severe, then the body can compensate by extracting more O_2 from the blood. The limit to this form of compensation is usually reached when cardiac output drops to 2 L/min. Delivery of O_2 has now been cut in half, and the tissues consume 50% of the O_2 in the blood. When blood flow drops below this limit, cardiac output may not be adequate to meet the metabolic needs of the body, resulting in inadequate O_2 delivery and low-output failure. Exercise increases the body's demand for O_2. If the heart cannot pump enough blood to supply the increased demand, then the animal's ability to exercise will be reduced.

Congestive or Backward Failure

Congestive heart failure occurs when increased pulmonary or systemic pressure causes fluid to leak from the capillary beds and accumulate in tissue (edema) or in body cavities (effusions). Congestive heart failure is generally categorized as right or left heart failure, according to whether systemic or pulmonary venous pressure is increased. Normally the pressure in the venous system is low, about 0 to 3 mm Hg in the right atrium and 2 to 5 mm Hg in the left atrium. Right heart failure is usually evident when right atrial pressure reaches 10 to 12 mm Hg, and left heart failure generally occurs when left atrial pressure exceeds 20 to 25 mm Hg. When a disease increases venous pressure equally on both sides of the heart, as in pericardial effusion, right heart failure develops first. This is because signs of congestive failure occur at lower pressure on the right side. Left heart failure develops more quickly than right heart failure. This is because the systemic veins have the capacity to hold much more blood than the pulmonary veins.

Relationship Between Hemodynamic Measurements and Clinical Signs of Heart Failure

Cardiac output and right atrial or left atrial pressure indicate whether heart function is adequate or whether heart failure exists. Patients who are not in failure should have a cardiac output that is greater than 2 L/min/m^2 and right and left atrial pressures less than 5 and 12 mm Hg, respectively. Forward

failure occurs if the patient's cardiac output is less than 2 L/min/m^2 at rest. Congestive failure should be present if the right atrial pressure exceeds 10 mm Hg or the left atrial pressures exceeds about 20 mm Hg. A patient suffering from both forward and congestive failure would be expected to have a cardiac output of less than 2 L/min/m^2 at rest and a left or right atrial pressure greater than 10 or 20 mm Hg, respectively. Patients with arteriovenous fistulae or hyperthyroidism may have congestive heart failure and higher than normal cardiac output at rest. This type of heart failure is known as *high-output failure*. Measuring cardiac output or left atrial pressure rarely is necessary (or possible in most practices) to diagnose heart failure. The physical examination, chest radiographs, and echocardiography generally provide enough information to make an accurate diagnosis of the type of heart failure and its cause. Fig. 16-4 shows the relationship between signs of heart failure and hemodynamic measurements.

Identifying Patients Who May Have Heart Failure

Client Complaints

In emergency practice, dyspnea, tachypnea, syncope, weakness, and collapse are the most common client complaints associated with heart failure. Heart failure should be considered when a client seeks help for a pet with a cough (coughing is much more common in dogs with heart disease than in cats), weight loss, exercise intolerance, or abdominal distention.

Physical Findings

Systolic murmurs greater than 3 on a scale of 1 to 6, precordial thrills, diastolic murmurs, and diastolic gallop sounds are generally reliable signs of heart disease. The arterial pulse tends to be weak or normal in most types of heart disease, but animals with patent ductus arteiosus or aortic insufficiency may have a prominent pulse. Irregular pulses, pulse deficits, and changes in the quality of the heart sounds may be present in animals with cardiac arrhythmias. Animals in left heart failure show signs of dyspnea, tachypnea, exercise intolerance, cyanosis, and weakness. Animals with right heart failure show signs of venous distention, hepatomegaly, ascites, weakness, and weight loss. Patients with biventricular failure

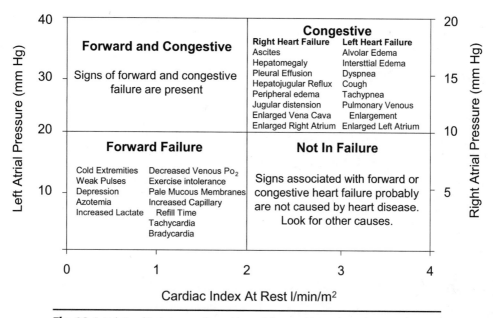

Fig. 16-4 Relationship between signs of heart failure and hemodynamic measurements.

often develop pleural effusion in addition to signs of both right and left ventricular failure. Box 16-3 lists diseases that can cause heart failure. The diseases are listed in decreasing order of prevalence.

Diagnostic Imaging and the Electrocardiogram

Thoracic radiographs will show an increase in the size of the pulmonary veins and increased opacity of the lungs in patients with left heart failure. In most cases, signs of left atrial enlargement are seen. Echocardiography will usually show signs of a disease that is associated with left heart failure. Left atrial enlargement is the most reliable echocardiographic sign of left heart failure. An enlarged vena cava, right heart enlargement, and a globoid heart suggestive of pericardial effusion are radiographic signs associated with right heart failure. The appearance of the pulmonary arteries may suggest heartworm disease in some dogs with right heart failure. Echocardiography usually allows diagnosis of a disease that is associated with right heart failure. The ECG may provide evidence of enlargement of the atria or ventricles. Cardiac arrhythmias are often seen in conjunction with the severe heart diseases that cause heart failure. Electrical alternans and low-amplitude ECG complexes are often seen in patients with pericardial effusions.

Emergency Treatment of Congestive Heart Failure

Pulmonary edema, pleural effusion, and severe ascites are the most common emergencies caused by congestive heart failure. Patients with pleural effusion or ascites can be treated very effectively for the short term by simply removing fluid from the thorax or the abdomen. Care should be taken to prevent stress in patients who are hypoxic or dyspneic because of their effusions. These effusions will return unless proper medical treatment is started to reduce venous pressure.

Pulmonary edema is more difficult to treat. Treatment consists of the use of several different therapies that reduce pulmonary venous pressure while providing adequate O_2 delivery; O_2 therapy maximizes the O_2 content of arterial blood, which provides some increase in O_2 delivery. Avoiding the use of physical restraint, providing a calm quiet environment, and using sedatives minimizes O_2 consumption and reduces the work of the heart. Furosemide and venodilating drugs decrease pulmonary venous pressure by eliminating fluid from the body and by dilating capacitance vessels (large veins). Arterial dilators reduce the regurgitant fraction in patients with

BOX 16-3

Common Causes of Heart Failure

Left Heart Failure in Dogs
Chronic degenerative valvular disease (mitral regurgitation)
Dilated cardiomyopathy
Patent ductus arteriosus (PDA)
Infective endocarditis
Subaortic stenosis (usually with concomitant mitral dysplasia)

Right Heart Failure in Dogs
Pericardial disease
Tricuspid regurgitation
Pulmonic stenosis (usually with concomitant tricuspid dysplasia)
Heartworm disease (may be the most common cause of right heart failure in areas with high infection rates)

Generalized (Biventricular) Heart Failure in Dogs
Dilated cardiomyopathy
Some dogs with severe left heart failure

Heart Failure in Cats
Hypertrophic cardiomyopathy
Restrictive cardiomyopthy
Dilated cardiomyopathy
Cardiomyopathy secondary to hyperthyroidism

TABLE 16-8

Goals in Emergency Heart Failure Treatment

Goal	Solution
Reduce oxygen (O_2) consumption, minimize stress	No physical restraint, calm quiet environment, sedatives
Increase O_2 content of blood	O_2 Therapy
Decrease venous pressure	Lasix, nitroglycerine paste
Decrease regurgitant fraction, decrease afterload	Arterial dilators
Improve contractility and cardiac output	Positive inotropic drugs
Eliminate the work of breathing, improve oxygenation	Positive pressure ventilation
Improve the ability to identify problems and target therapy	Hemodynamic, arterial, and central venous blood gas monitoring

Table 16-8 lists the goals of therapy for pulmonary edema and the therapies used to achieve them.

Diuretic Therapy

Water and salt retention is an important compensatory mechanism in heart failure. Diuretics are drugs that act on the kidneys to promote the elimination of water and salt. Furosemide is a potent diuretic that can be used to eliminate fluid from the body quickly. Furosemide's ability to decrease pulmonary venous pressure rapidly makes it one of the most effective emergency treatments for life-threatening pulmonary edema caused by congestive heart failure. Overzealous administration of furosemide can cause decreased cardiac output and azotemia, as well as electrolyte abnormalities.

Oxygen Therapy

Congestive heart failure often causes hypoxia and hypoventilation because of hydrothorax and pulmonary edema. Therapy using O_2 can improve oxygenation and reduce the work of breathing. However, the

mitral regurgitation and improve cardiac output by decreasing afterload. Positive inotropic drugs improve contractility and cardiac output in patients who have low-output failure in addition to congestive failure.

When the simpler therapies already mentioned have failed, other options are available if clients have the desire and the financial resources and if the necessary facilities exist. Positive pressure ventilation can eliminate the work of breathing and improve oxygenation. Pulmonary artery catheterization can be used to measure cardiac output, pulmonary artery wedge pressure, and central venous blood gases. Arterial catheterization can be used to measure BP and arterial blood gases. This type of intensive monitoring can be used to identify the cause of treatment failure and to allow treatment to be targeted at the problem.

technician should remember that O_2 therapy may only cause a small increase in the O_2 content of the blood; O_2 therapy can lead to death if the method of administering O_2 increases patient stress or causes the patient to struggle. Many methods of O_2 administration are available; if one method does not work, then the technician should try another. The success of therapy is measured by improved patient comfort and oxygenation, not by whether the patient has been forced to breathe increased concentrations of O_2.

Almost every practice has the equipment needed to administer O_2 by facemask. A tight-fitting facemask with adequate O_2 flow can deliver 100% O_2. Unfortunately, facemasks are poorly accepted by most patients and cannot be used for long periods of time.

Nasal insufflation can be used to deliver high concentrations of O_2 for long periods of time. The veterinary professional should use the following three-step technique to insert the catheter:

1. Make a mark on a soft flexible catheter to indicate the distance from the tip of the nose to the medial canthus of the eye.
2. Instill a little lidocaine solution in one nostril, apply some lubricant to the catheter, and insert it into the nostril, stopping when the mark is reached.
3. Suture the catheter to the skin to keep it in place.

The following rule can be used to determine the flow of O_2:

Every 50 ml/kg/min of O_2 flow increases the inspired O_2 concentration by 7%. For example, an O_2 flow of 1.5 L/min administered to a patient breathing room air (20% O_2) should provide an inspired concentration of 41% for a 10 kg dog.

The O_2 should be humidified when using a nasal catheter. The gas in an O_2 cylinder contains virtually no moisture and may cause severe drying of the mucous membranes in the upper respiratory tract.

Most patients tolerate O_2 cages well, but they require high O_2 flows and do not allow hands-on monitoring of the patient. A well designed oxygen cage should remove exhaled carbon dioxide and lower the temperature in the cage when necessary.

Vasodilator Therapy

Vasodilating drugs are effective in treating both congestive and low-output heart failure. Venodilating drugs expand the capacity of the circulatory system by dilating veins, which reduces preload and venous pressure. Venodilation can reduce congestion but will not improve cardiac output. Arterial vasodilators decrease systemic vascular resistance, which reduces afterload, improves cardiac output, reduces the regurgitant fraction in animals with valvular disease, and decreases the work of the heart. The main disadvantage of arterial vasodilators is that they lower BP. Selecting a vasodilator that acts on veins, aterioles, or a combination of the two is possible. Drugs that block the enzyme that converts angiotensin I to angiotensin II (angiotensin-converting enzyme inhibitors) are the most commonly used vasodilators. They also benefit the patient by decreasing the sodium and water rentention seen in heart failure by decreasing the plasma concentration of aldosterone. However, these drugs do not take effect quickly enough to be useful in emergency heart failure treatment.

Positive Inotropic Therapy

Positive inotropic drugs increase stroke volume by increasing contractility. With the exception of drugs like digoxin, positive inotropes are most useful for improving cardiac output or BP for short periods of time. Sympathomimetic drugs such as dopamine and dobutamine lose their effectiveness over time, because their use causes a decrease in the number of receptors. In addition, positive inotropes can cause tachycardia and arrhythmias, increase afterload, and increase the work of the heart.

Sympathomimetic Drugs

Sympathomimetic drugs mimic the effect of stimulating the sympathetic nervous system and work by stimulating adrenergic receptors on the cells of the heart and blood vessels. Dopamine and dobutamine are the sympathomimetic drugs used most often in the treatment of heart failure. Dobutamine increases contractility without causing a significant increase in heart rate or vascular resistance. This combination of properties makes dobutamine a good choice for treating heart failure in patients with myocardial failure or mitral regurgitation. Dopamine is useful in situations in which poor contractility is associated with hypotension.

Bipyridine Derivatives

Amrinone and milronone are positive inotropic drugs that work by inhibiting phosphodiesterase. Both amrinone and milronone cause vasodilation

TABLE 16-9

Drugs Used to Treat Heart Failure

Drugs Used to Minimize Stress	
Morphine	0.5 mg/kg SQ IM in dogs
Oxymorphone	0.05 mg/kg SQ IM dog and cats
Acepromazine	0.03 mg/kg SQ IM dogs or cats
Drugs Used to Decrease Venous Pressure or Preload	
Furosemide	2-8 mg/kg IM, IV, SQ dog 2-4 mg/kg IM, IV, SQ cat
Nitroglycerin	4-15 mg topically dog 3-4 mg topically cat
Drugs Used to Decrease Afterload	
Hydralazine	0.5-3 mg/kg PO dogs
Sodium nitroprusside	0.5-10 µg/kg/min IV
Drugs used to Increase Contractility	
Dobutamine	2-10 µg/kg/min IV
Dopamine	2-10 µg/kg/min IV
Amrinone	1-3 mg/kg IV followed by 10-100 µg/kg/min IV

SQ, Subcutaneously; *IM,* intramuscularly; *PO,* orally.

in addition to increased contractility, and both can be used in situations where sympathomimetic drugs such as dopamine and dobutamine are no longer effective. These drugs are rarely used in veterinary medicine because they are expensive and most of their effects can be achieved with other drugs. Table 16-9 lists drugs used to treat heart failure.

Monitoring Therapy for Heart Failure

Animals suffering from dyspnea caused by heart failure appear anxious and are often unwilling to sit or lay down. Affected animals often assume a characteristic posture, with the feet spread apart, elbows abducted, and the head and neck extended. Tachypnea is usually evident, with respiratory rates greater than 60 breaths per minute. If therapy has been effective in treating pleural effusion or pulmonary edema, then the patient's attitude should improve, the

respiratory rate should decrease, mucous membrane color should improve, and the animal may be able to lie down or sleep. Improvement of pulmonary edema on chest radiographs usually takes longer than improvement of clinical signs.

Monitoring Vasodilator Therapy

Vasodilator therapy should improve cardiac output or improve pulmonary edema. Improved cardiac output may be monitored by looking for signs of increased perfusion such as warming of the extremities, increased venous O_2 tension, and a decreased blood lactate. Whenever arteriolar vasodilating drugs are used, BP should be monitored to maintain mean BP around 70 mm Hg. Venodilating drugs reduce venous pressure and should therefore decrease central venous and pulmonary capillary wedge pressure.

Monitoring Positive Inotropic Therapy

Positive inotropic therapy should improve cardiac output. Most commonly this is monitored by looking for the signs of improved cardiac output. Decreases in blood lactate, increased venous O_2 tension, or measured cardiac output provide a more objective assessment of therapy. In addition to increasing contractility, positive inotropic agents can cause vasoconstriction, vasodilation, increased heart rate, or cardiac arrhythmias. Vasoconstriction generally causes an increase in CVP, pulmonary capillary wedge pressure, and arterial blood pressure. Vasodilation may cause a decrease in CVP, pulmonary capillary wedge pressure, or arterial blood pressure depending on the increase in cardiac output. The ECG is helpful in detecting cardiac arrhythmias or sinus tachycardia. Safe, effective use of sympathomimetic drugs requires monitoring of at least the ECG and BP and assessment of perfusion.

Monitoring Diuretic Therapy

Diuretic therapy should quickly produce an increase in urine production when furosemide is used. This elimination of fluid should result in a decreased respiratory rate and improved oxygenation and ventilation. Weighing the patient and palpating the urinary bladder to determine its size may be useful for establishing a baseline before diuretic therapy is started. The loss of volume can be estimated by measuring the volume of urine, by measuring the increase in weight caused by urine soaked up in a disposable diaper, or by noting the patient's weight loss during treatment. Electrolyte and acid-base disturbances can be caused by diuretic therapy, so these values should be monitored. The loss of pre-load may cause a decrease in cardiac output. This can result in prerenal azotemia or signs of low-output failure.

Cardiac Arrhythmias

Client Complaints

Cardiac arrhythmias should be considered when-ever an animal experiences syncope, weakness, or collapse. Some clients may detect tachycardia, bra-dycardia, or an irregular heart rhythm. Cardiac ar-rhythmias should not be considered a primary disease. Instead cardiac arrhythmias occur as a result of some other disease that affects the heart. Box 16-4 lists several diseases that are common in emergency medicine and have a high incidence of cardiac ar-rhythmias.

Physical Findings

An ECG should be recorded to determine if a car-diac arrhythmia is present whenever changes in the character of heart sounds, tachycardia, bradycardia, irregular heart rhythm, pulse deficits, or changes in arterial or jugular pulses are present.

Diagnostic Imaging and the Electrocardiogram

The ECG is the gold standard for the diagnosis of cardiac arrhythmias. Many cardiac arrhythmias can be diagnosed using echocardiography, but this is rarely useful. The main use of radiographs and echocardiography is to provide evidence of a disease that may be the underlying cause of the arrhythmia.

Medical Treatment of Cardiac Arrhythmias

The efficacy of antiarrhythmic therapy has not been determined in most forms of heart disease found in dogs and cats. In humans the use of certain

---

BOX 16-4

Emergencies in which Cardiac Arrhythmias are Common

Trauma
Splenic tumors
Gastric dilatation volvulus
Canine dilated cardiomyopathy
Urethral obstruction in cats
Heat-induced illness
Feline cardiomyopathies

---

antiarrythmic drugs was found to decrease survival in patients with certain forms of heart disease. The following five principles should be considered be-fore deciding whether to use antiarrhythmic drugs to treat an arrhythmia:

1. Treating the primary disease may eliminate the arrhythmia.
2. Generally arrhythmias that cause hypotension or perfusion should be treated.
3. Prolonged tachycardia can damage the heart, even when BP and cardiac output are adequate.
4. The arrhythmia should be treated if it has the risk of progressing to a more severe arrhythmia or cardiac arrest. Multiform ventricular premature contractions, R on T phenomenon, more than 20 to 30 ventricular premature contractions per minute, ventricular flutter, and ventricular tachy-cardia greater than 130 per minute are generally considered to be rhythms that have the potential to become more dangerous.
5. When the decision is made to treat an arrhythmia, the technician should select an antiarrhythmic drug based on its ability to eliminate the arrhyth-mia balanced against the risk of proarrhythmic effects, hypotension, decreased contractility, al-tered atrioventricular conduction, and interac-tions with other drugs.

Role of Electrolytes and Drug Interactions in Antiarrhythmic Therapy

Electrolyte and acid-base abnormalities can cause arrhythmias, increase their severity, and influence the effect of antiarrhythmic drugs. Hyperkalemia is one of the more common and easily recognized electrolyte abnormalities that cause arrhythmias. Hyperkalemia causes characteristic changes on the ECG: low amplitude or absent P wave, prolongation of the QRS complexes, and increased amplitude of the T wave.

Hypomagnesemia has been associated with ventricular arrhythmias, and magnesium administration may be useful as a treatment for some forms of ventricular tachycardia. Hypokalemia, hypomagnesemia, and hypercalcemia can increase the risk of toxicity in patients on digoxin therapy. Restoration of these electrolytes to appropriate levels plays an important role in treating digoxin toxicity. Lidocaine is most effective in regions of the heart in which pH is decreased and potassium levels are increased. A lack of efficacy in lidocaine therapy of arrhythmias may be a result of hypokalemia. Quinidine is highly bound to protein. Changes in blood pH can change the amount of active drug. Alkalosis decreases the concentration of active drug, whereas acidosis can increase it. Some of the toxic effect of the accidental ingestion or overdose of calcium-blocking drugs (e.g., diltiazem) can be treated by administration of calcium chloride or calcium gluconate.

Interaction between antiarrhythmic drugs is common. In some cases the interaction is additive or synergistic; in others it may be antagonistic. Synergistic or additive interaction is usually beneficial when it applies to antiarrhythmic effects, but adverse effects may also be synergistic. Both calcium-blocking drugs and beta-blocking drugs are effective in the treatment of supraventricular arrhythmias; however, when they are combined the risk of adverse effects such as hypotension, worsening congestive heart failure, and bradycardia is increased.

Treatment of Ventricular Fibrillation

The use of a defibrillator is the only effective method of treating ventricular fibrillation. Successful treatment of ventricular fibrillation depends on diagnosing and treating the patient as soon as possible after ventricular fibrillation occurs. Current recommendations for treating ventricular fibrillation in adult humans are to attempt to defibrillate as soon as possible for a witnessed arrest. In the case of an unwitnessed arrest, cardiopulmonary resuscitation should be performed for 2 minutes before the initial shock. Cardiopulmonary resuscitation should be continued while the defibrillator

charges if a second and third shock are required. If the first three attempts are unsuccessful, then three more attempts should be made after 2 minutes of cardiopulmonary resuscitation. This pattern is continued until the patient is no longer in ventricular fibrillation. If a monophasic waveform defibrillator is used, then a dose of 360 J is recommended for each shock. Manual biphasic defibrillator doses are device specific; however, if the specific dose for a device is unknown, then a dose of 200 J is recommended. This method of treating ventricular fibrillation can be used in dogs or cats if the electrical dose is modified to account for the smaller body size. The initial dose, for the electrodes placed externally on the body wall, should be 5 J/kg, with subsequent attempts made at 5 J/kg. For electrodes placed directly on the heart, the initial dose should be 0.2 J/kg, with subsequent attempts made at 0.2 to 0.5 J/kg. The use of excessive electrical doses for defibrillation can result in death or damage to the heart. The preceding recommendations are for a monophasic defibrillators. Biphasic defibrillators are beginning to be used in some veterinary practices, and this will require an adjustment in the energy used. In humans, defibrillators using biphasic waveforms are as effective using 150 to 200 J as monophasic defibrillators using up to 360 J. This fact implies that energies of 2 to 3 J/kg for defibrillation using a biphasic waveform will be effective in veterinary patients.

Treatment of Ventricular Tachycardia

Lidocaine, procainamide, and quinidine are the drugs used most often in the emergency treatment of ventricular arrhythmias in the dog. Lidocaine and beta-blockers such as propranolol or esmolol are the drugs used most often in treating cats. Lidocaine is considered the drug of choice for treating ventricular tachycardia in the dog. Lidocaine has very little effect on myocardial function. BP and cardiac output usually are unaffected when lidocaine is used. Discontinuing the drug treats adverse reactions such as depression or twitching, and seizures are treated by discontinuing the drug and giving diazepam. Rapid IV administration of quinidine (and to a lesser extent procainamide) can cause dangerous hypotension and decreased cardiac output. Beta-blocking drugs can exacerbate heart failure and cause bradycardia and bronchospasm. Esmolol has an extremely short duration of action, and any adverse reaction

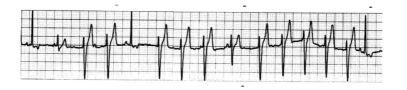

Fig. 16-5 Accelerated idioventricular rhythm.

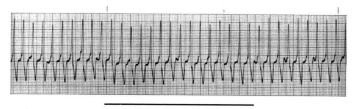

Fig. 16-6 Ventricular tachycardia.

caused by the drug should stop soon after the drug is discontinued. Ventricular tachycardia that causes cardiac arrest should be treated like ventricular fibrillation.

Accelerated idioventricular rhythm is a unifocal ventricular rhythm with a rate that falls within the range of normal sinus rhythm and is sometimes mistaken for ventricular tachycardia. Accelerated idioventricular rhythm rarely causes any hemodynamic dysfunction, is usually benign, and is commonly associated with many diseases. This rhythm probably has a different cause than ventricular tachycardia and usually does not respond to lidocaine treatment. Usually the rhythm disappears when the underlying disease is controlled (Figs. 16-5 and 16-6) (Table 16-10).

Treatment of Atrial Fibrillation

Reestablishing normal sinus rhythm in patients with long-standing atrial fibrillation, particularly atrial fibrillation coexisting with other forms of heart disease, usually is impossible. Most often, therapy consists of using digoxin and a beta-blocker to slow the ventricular rate and improve cardiac function. Animals who have recently developed atrial fibrillation and do not have significant heart disease are the best candidates for conversion to normal sinus rhythm. Quinidine is the most common drug used for cardioversion. Electrical cardioversion has also been used successfully to convert atrial fibrillation

into sinus rhythm. Defibrillators using monophasic waveforms may achieve cardioversion using shocks in the 1 to 5 J/kg range (Fig. 16-7). Biphasic defibrillators would be expected to achieve the same results using less energy.

Treatment of Supraventricular Tachycardia

Beta-blocking drugs, such as esmolol, or propranolol, or calcium channel–blocking drugs such as diltiazem are the most frequently used therapies for supraventricular tachyarrhythmias (Fig. 16-8). If drug therapy

TABLE 16-10	
Drugs Used to Treat Ventricular Arrhythmias	
Lidocaine	2-4 mg/kg IV over 1 to 3 min followed by 40-100 µg/kg/min IV for dogs 0.5 mg/kg IV slowly for cats
Procainamide	5-15 mg/kg IV, IM q6h for dogs
Esmolol	0.05-0.5 mg/kg IV, 50-200 µg/kg/min IV for dogs and cats
Quinidine	5-15 mg/kg IM q6-8h for dogs
Propranolol	0.01-0.1 mg/kg IV slowly titrated to effect for dogs and cats

IM, intramuscularly.

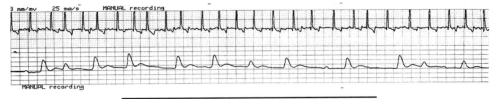

Fig. 16-7 Atrial fibrillation and arterial pressure waveform.

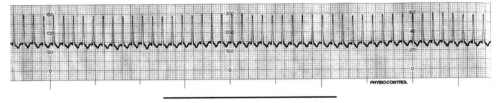

Fig. 16-8 Supraventricular tachycardia.

is not effective, then nonpharmacologic therapies can be tried. Electrical cardioversion and mechanical methods (e.g., precordial thump) are often effective, and vagal maneuvers (e.g., ocular pressure, carotid sinus massage) sometimes are effective (Table 16-11).

Treatment of Bradyarrhythmias

Sinus bradycardia, sinus arrest, and second-degree atrioventricular block often respond to treatment with anticholinergic drugs like atropine or glycopyrrolate. Anticholinergic drugs are not usually effective in treating third-degree atrioventricular block, but sympathomimetic drugs like epinephrine or dopamine can often be used to increase the ventricular rate to an acceptable level. Drug therapy is ineffective in treating the bradycardia associated with sick sinus syndrome (Fig. 16-9). Anticholinergic and sympathomimetic drugs can worsen the tachyarrhythmias in patients with bradycardia-tachycardia syndrome. Pacemaker implantation is the best long-term therapy for most patients with bradyarrhythmias (Table16-12).

Treatment of Hyperkalemia

Hyperkalemia can be treated by giving drugs that cause potassium to move from the vascular space to the intracellular space, such as bicarbonate or insulin, or by giving calcium, which antagonizes the effect

of potassium on the heart. Definitive treatment for hyperkalemia should be started as soon as possible, because the effect of calcium, bicarbonate, or insulin therapy is short lived. To prevent hypoglycemia, glucose must always be given when insulin is used to treat hyperkalemia (Fig. 16-10) (Table 16-13).

Monitoring Treatment of Cardiac Arrhythmias

Continuous ECG monitoring increases the safety and effectiveness of antiarrhythmic therapy. Arterial BP and clinical signs of perfusion should be monitored to determine whether antiarrhythmic therapy has improved cardiac function. Changes in the P-R interval, QRS duration, and Q-T interval on the ECG may be important signs of toxicity for some

TABLE 16-11

Drugs Used to Treat Supraventricular Arrhythmias

Propranolol	0.01-0.1 mg/kg IV slowly titrated to effect for dogs and cats
Esmolol	0.05-0.5 mg/kg IV 50 to 200 µg/kg/min IV for dogs
Diltiazem	0.05-0.2 mg/kg IV titrated to effect for dogs and cats

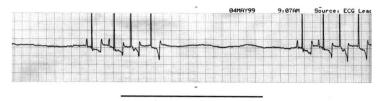

Fig. 16-9 Sick sinus syndrome.

antiarrhythmic drugs. Vomiting, twitching, seizures, and syncope are a few of the physical signs that can be associated with toxicity from antiarrhythmic drugs. Electrolytes and glucose should be monitored in patients being treated for hyperkalemia.

Pacemaker Therapy

A permanent implantable pacemaker can be used to treat a variety of bradyarrhythmias and restore near-normal quality of life to patients. Temporary pacing is used to treat cardiac arrest caused by asystole or other bradyarrhythmias and improve cardiac function in patients before or during permanent pacemaker implantation. Several modes of temporary pacing are available. Specific types of equipment are required for each mode of pacing, and each technique has advantages and disadvantages. Transvenous and transcutaneous techniques are the safest, most commonly used, and most reliable methods (although transesophageal and transmyocardial techniques are possible). One advantage of transvenous pacing is the ability to insert the lead and use the pacemaker in a conscious animal. A 3.5-French transvenous pacing lead (Fig. 16-11)

can be inserted into the right ventricle via a percutaneous introducer placed in the jugular vein or the lateral saphenous vein. Transcutaneous pacing has advantages when a patient requires immediate treatment for a life-threatening bradyarrhythmia, because pacing can be started quickly, without the need for vascular access. Adhesive pacing electrodes are attached to the left and right sides of the chest over the heart (Fig. 16-12). A disadvantage of transcutaneous pacing is the need to use more energy, which increases discomfort and muscle stimulation. The discomfort caused by transcutaneous pacing makes it difficult or impossible to use in a conscious animal. The electrical stimulus applied to the muscles of the chest causes movement, which can interfere with surgery. Esophageal pacing is not commonly used in dogs or cats, but it has potential advantages that could be useful in certain situations. Inserting a transesophageal pacing electrode in the esophagus is simple. Because the electrode is close to the heart, pacing can be achieved with less energy than a transcutaneous electrode. In the author's one experience with transesophageal pacing, it was possible to capture the atrium but not the ventricles in a dog with third-degree atrioventricular block. The clinician performs transmyocardial pacing by inserting a special pacing lead through the thoracic wall, and then the ventricular wall using an introducing needle. Although the technique is reliable and can be performed quickly, the risk of injury to the heart makes its use rare.

Precordial Thumps in the Treatment of Arrhythmias

The precordial thump is a controversial technique. Some studies have shown that the precordial thump can produce a perfusing rhythm in some patients, whereas other studies show deterioration in the rhythm. The 2005 *American Heart Association Guidelines* discuss the technique but make no recommendation for or against its use for ventricular

TABLE 16-12	
Drugs Used to Treat Bradyarrhythmias	
Atropine	0.01-0.04 mg/kg IV, IM, SQ for dogs and cats
Glycopyrrolate	0.005-0.01 mg/kg IV, IM, SQ for dogs and cats
Dopamine	2-10 µg/kg/min IV for dogs and cats
Epinephrine	0.03-0.15 µg/kg/min IV for dogs and cats

IM, intramuscularly; *SQ,* subcutaneously.

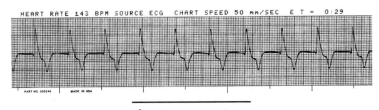

HEART RATE 143 BPM SOURCE ECG CHART SPEED 50 mm/SEC E T = 0:29

Fig. 16-10 Hyperkalemia.

tachycardia or ventricular fibrillation. When synchronized electrical cardioversion, defibrillation, and temporary pacing are available, they should be used; they are consistent, reliable and controllable. Situations occur in which drugs are not effective, electrical pacing or a defibrillator are not available, and a precordial thump may be life saving. A precordial thump is administered by striking the chest wall over the heart with the side of the fist. Precordial thumps can injure a patient from the force of the blow or cause ventricular fibrillation if the thump occurs during the vulnerable period on the ECG (i.e., R on T phenomenon). Precordial thumps are often effective in converting supraventricular tachycardia into sinus rhythm and are also effective in treating certain bradyarrhythmias. In these cases a thump on the intact chest wall or the flick of the surgeon's finger against the ventricle during a thoracotomy will not convert the patient to a normal rhythm, but each thump can effectively stimulate one or more heart beats. When a thump is able to stimulate a heart beat in a bradycardiac patient, much less force is usually required to stimulate a heart beat with a thump than is required

to generate an effective pulse using the chest compression techniques normally used for cardiopulmonary resuscitation. Thumps may be effective in keeping bradycardic patients alive while waiting for temporary pacing to be started. A human patient was kept alive for 1 hour using only this technique (Box 16-5).

Heartworm Disease

Caval Syndrome

Caval syndrome is complication of heartworm disease that can occur in both dogs and cats. Caval syndrome occurs when large numbers of heartworms enter the right atrium and entwine themselves in the tricuspid valve apparatus, causing acute and severe tricuspid regurgitation. The heart is not the only organ to be affected. Hemolysis occurs when red blood cells shear as they are forced through the entangled worms. This also causes hemoglobinuria.

Analysis of the complete blood count and serum chemistry in dogs with caval syndrome may indicate

TABLE 16-13

Drugs Used to Treat Hyperkalemia

Calcium gluconate 10%	0.5-1 ml/kg given over 15 min for dogs and cats
Sodium bicarbonate	0.5-2 mEq/kg IV given over 20 min for dogs and cats
Regular insulin	0.1-0.25 U/kg IV followed by 1-2 g/U glucose to prevent hypoglycemia for dogs and cats

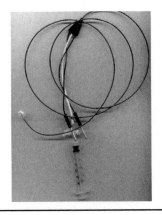

Fig. 16-11 Transvenous pacing lead.

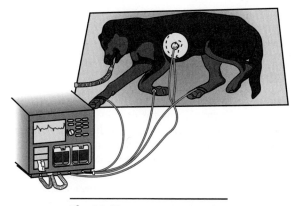

Fig. 16-12 Transcutaneous pacing.

BOX 16-5

Bradyarrhythmias that Often Require Permanent Pacing

Second- or third-degree atrioventricular block
Sick sinus syndrome
Persistent atrial standstill

liver and renal dysfunction and signs of disseminated intravascular coagulation.

Client Complaints

Owners of dogs with caval syndrome typically notice anorexia, weakness, and depression. Some owners may complain that the animal has hemoglobinuria (dark brown urine), dyspnea, or cough. Many animals with caval syndrome will arrive at the clinic in a state of shock.

Physical Findings

Pale mucous membranes, prolonged capillary refill time, weak pulses, distended jugular veins, ascites, icterus, and dyspnea may be identified on a physical examination. Auscultation of the chest may reveal a systolic murmur split second heart sound or a gallop sound.

Diagnostic Imaging and the Electrocardiogram

Thoracic radiographs will often show right heart enlargement and enlargement of the main pulmonary artery. Peripheral pulmonary arteries are often enlarged relative to the corresponding pulmonary veins. The pulmonary arteries may show other changes characteristic of heartworm disease, such as tortuousity, blunting, or uneven diameter. These radiographic signs are seen in both dogs and cats with heartworm disease, but they tend to be more subtle and difficult to interpret in cats. Using echocardiography, heartworms can be seen as parallel lines about 2 mm apart that look like "equal signs" or "railroad tracks" if heartworms are present in the right heart or main pulmonary artery. Doppler echocardiography may show evidence of pulmonary hypertension. The ECG may show cardiac arrhythmias or signs of right heart enlargement.

Surgical Treatment of Caval Syndrome

The presence of heartworms in the right atrium and vena cava is associated with high mortality. Patients with caval syndrome often arrive at the clinic in shock and must be stabilized before heartworm removal is attempted. Fluid therapy is usually needed to improve poor perfusion, but care must be taken to avoid exacerbating preexisting right heart failure. The anesthetic protocol selected should minimize further depression of the cardiovascular system. In severely affected patients the procedure can be performed with local anesthesia. For general anesthesia, the lowest possible concentration of inhalational anesthetic and 100% O_2 should be used, and positive pressure ventilation can be used to improve oxygenation and eliminate hypercapnia. The procedure is usually performed with the patient in lateral or dorsal recumbency. After the surgical site is prepared, an incision is made over the jugular vein. The jugular vein is then dissected free from the surrounding tissue. An incision is made in the jugular vein and alligator forceps are inserted. This technique allows one or more worms to be removed from the right atrium and vena cava (Fig. 16-13). Two-dimensional echocardiography can be used to visualize the heartworms and direct the forceps.

Monitoring

Even with treatment, mortality is high in caval syndrome. CVP monitoring is useful for managing fluid therapy and as a prognostic sign. CVP of 20 cm of water or greater is associated with a poor prognosis. Arterial BP, mucous membrane color, capillary refill

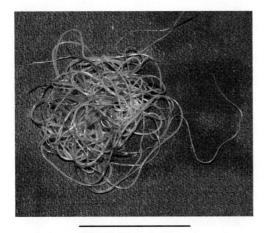

Fig. 16-13 Heartworms.

time, extremity temperature, and urine production should be monitored to evaluate perfusion. Doppler echocardiography or a catheter can be used to determine pulmonary arterial pressure.

Complications of Adulticide Therapy

Embolization of dead or dying worms after adulticidal therapy is another emergency that can occur as a consequence of heartworm disease. Lethargy, cough, right heart failure, dyspnea, shock, and sudden death may occur 7 to 10 days after treatment to kill adult heartworms. Therapy with O_2 and prednisone (as well as cage rest and careful fluid therapy) is generally considered to be effective. The use of heparin, aspirin, and vasodilators is more controversial.

Cardiac Tamponade and Pericardial Effusion

Fluid can accumulate in the pericardial sac for many reasons. Neoplasia and percarditis are the most common causes of pericardial effusion and generally produce signs of right heart failure as a result of chronic pericardial effusion that accumulates slowly. Trauma, atrial tears, and some cases of right atrial hemangiosarcoma are the most common causes of acute cardiac tamponade. When fluid accumulates slowly in the heart, the pericardium stretches and the heart has time to compensate for the increased pressure on the heart. Effusions that develop slowly tend to produce large volumes of pericardial fluid and cause signs of right heart failure. When fluid accumulates quickly, no time exists for compensation (even a small volume of fluid in the pericardial sac can cause signs of shock).

Client Complaints

Lethargy, dyspnea, anorexia, and collapse are the most common reasons for owners to seek help for dogs with acute signs of pericardial effusion. Abdominal distension, lethargy, anorexia, and cough are common client complaints for dogs with chronic signs of pericardial effusion. Sudden death, collapse, or a history of trauma may be the presenting complaint for animals with cardiac tamponade.

Clinical Signs

Ascites, jugular venous distention, cachexia, tachycardia, and weak pulses are common findings. An exaggerated weakening of the arterial pulse during inspiration is often associated with pericardial effusion. Auscultation may reveal muffled heart sounds, murmurs, or friction rubs. Signs of shock accompanied by signs of increased systemic venous pressure should raise the possibility of cardiac tamponade.

Diagnostic Imaging and the Electrocardiogram

When fluid accumulates slowly, thoracic radiographs will usually show a large globoid heart. Acute traumatic cardiac tamponade is unlikely to be detected with radiographs because of the small amount of fluid in the pericardium. Echocardiographic examination of the heart is very sensitive in detecting even small amounts of pericardial fluid. Diastolic collapse of the right atrium is a characteristic sign of tamponade. Echocardiography may also detect a mass, which is frequently the cause of the effusion. Tachycardia, low amplitude ECG complexes, and electrical alternans are almost pathognomonic signs of pericardial effusion.

Treatment of Cardiac Tamponade and Pericardial Effusion

Pericardiocentesis will rapidly relieve the signs caused by increased pressure in the pericardium. The patient should be prepared by shaving the hair on the right side of the chest over the region of the heart. After scrubbing the shaved area, local anesthetic is infiltrated into the tissues between the fourth and fifth intercostal spaces at the level of the costrochondral junction. Ultrasound imaging can be used to determine the best location. A 16-gauge over-the-needle catheter is recommended for the typical patient, which is usually a large breed dog. Many clinicians will cut several side holes near the end of the catheter before insertion. If this is done, then the technician must be sure that the holes do not weaken the catheter so much that the tip can tear off in the pericardium. The catheter is inserted through the chest wall and into the thoracic cavity. The catheter may be felt to contact the pericardium as it is advanced. Once the catheter has entered the pericardium, fluid flashes into the stylet and the catheter can be advanced over the needle. The ECG should be monitored during the procedure to help determine if the needle has contacted the myocardium. Contact with the myocardium is indicated by ventricular premature beats. A small sample of the fluid can be taken to see if it will clot and to check the hematocrit. Clotting of the fluid sample after collection indicates active bleeding. As the pericardial fluid is removed, the heart rate may decrease and the ECG may show increased amplitude.

Monitoring

Most animals improve rapidly after the fluid is removed from the pericardium. If the patient does not improve or worsens, then it may be because of active bleeding (in the case of cardiac tamponade) or because of a complication of pericardiocentesis (e.g., laceration of a coronary artery). Monitoring the CVP may help with the initial diagnosis of cardiac tamponade or pericardial effusion. BP should be monitored if cardiac tamponade is a possibility.

Feline Aortic Thromboembolism

Feline aortic thromboembolism (FATE) is a devastating complication of myocardial disease. Thrombi develop in the heart and then break free and travel into the systemic arteries. These thromboemboli most frequently lodge in the distal aorta where they often cause posterior paresis, paralysis, and pain. Mortality is very high in aortic thromboembolism, with about two thirds of the patients being euthanized or dying during the initial episode. Animals that survive sometimes lose skin, toes, or even a leg

to ischemic necrosis. Survivors of the initial episode will require treatment of their underlying heart disease, which is often severe. Survivors are also at increased risk for recurrence.

Client Complaints

Clients are motivated to seek help quickly because many of the signs seen in patients with FATE (e.g., vocalizing, apparent pain, inability to walk, dyspnea, urinary and fecal incontinence) are very distressing. The majority of clients will be unaware of any problem with the patient's health before embolism occurs.

Diagnostic Imaging and the Electrocardiogram

Thoracic radiographs often show signs of heart enlargement pleural effusion or pulmonary edema. Although angiography is usually not needed to make the diagnosis, it can be used to show the location of the thrombus. Echocardiography usually shows signs of heart disease. Left atrial enlargement and spontaneous contrast (smoke) are frequently seen in cats with FATE. In some cases a thrombus may be seen in the left atrium. The majority of cats with FATE will have some abnormality in the ECG.

Clinical Signs

In about 70% of patients the embolus will affect blood flow to both hind limbs. In 15% a single front limb will be affected, and in 15% a single hind limb is affected. In addition to paralysis and pain, the affected limbs will be cold and pale or cyanotic. Pulses in the affected area will be nonexistent or very weak. A heart murmur, gallop sound, or irregular heart rhythm may be heard. Some cats may show signs of dyspnea or tachypnea. It is very important to measure the patient's rectal temperature (an important prognostic sign). The odds favor survival when the temperature is greater than 98.9° F.

Treatment

The prognosis for patients with aortic thromboembolism is poor, but many animals can regain an acceptable quality of life after treatment. To make an informed decision regarding treatment, clients should be educated about what to expect and the

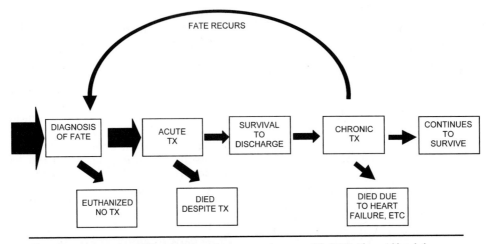

Fig. 16-14 Survival at different points of treatment for cats with FATE. The width of the arrow correlates with the number of cats surviving.

role they must play in the patient's care should they decide proceed. About one third of clients decide to euthanize the patient after the diagnosis is made. Although many of the patients who are euthanized are moribund, some of those euthanized would probably have survived, at least for the short term. Clients should be advised that about one half of the patients who receive treatment survive. Patients with higher rectal temperatures and only one affected limb appear to have the best chance of survival. Patients with taurine deficiency or hyperthyroidism may show significant improvement in their heart disease when these conditions are treated. Clients that elect to treat their cat should be aware that the patient may need some level of nursing care for weeks or months while it recovers from nerve damage or ischemic necrosis. Survivors usually need to receive medication for the rest of their lives to treat their heart disease and prevent another episode of thromboembolism. The client must be prepared to give injections if low molecular weight heparin is prescribed to prevent formation of another clot. Fig. 16-14 illustrates possible outcomes for a patient with FATE. The width of the arrows correlates with the number of patients.

Patients should be handled carefully, because many have severe underlying heart disease. In one study, 66% of the animals had radiographic signs of congestive heart failure. The treatment of pleural effusion and pulmonary edema may be as urgent as the treatment of the aortic embolus. Three forms of treatment are available: (1) supportive, (2) extraction of

the clot using catheter techniques or surgery, and (3) elimination of the clot with thrombolytic agents.

In supportive treatment the patient is treated for its heart disease and pain. Drugs such as heparin are used to prevent the growth of the clot. Some clinicians also advocate the use of vasodilating drugs to improve circulation, although the benefit of this therapy is unproven. Some clients may be interested in having the embolus removed. This usually requires referral to an institution capable of providing this type of care.

Clots have been successfully removed by using one of several different catheter techniques, as well as surgery. Anesthesia for aortic embolectomy in a cat with severe heart disease is particularly challenging and should be performed in an environment in which the patient can be intensively monitored and supported during the procedure. Thrombolytic therapy is expensive, requires careful patient monitoring, and may be contraindicated in patients known to have thrombi in the heart; however, it does not require anesthesia.

In theory, surgical, catheter, and thrombolytic therapies are most likely to be effective when they are started as early as possible in the course of the disease. Although new methods of removing clots and preventing recurrence have been developed during the last few years, the evidence does not show that therapies that eliminate the clot are better at reducing mortality than supportive therapy or that recurrence can be substantially reduced. Therapy to

BOX 16-6 ⓣ

Goals of Therapy in Feline Aortic Thromboembolism (FATE)

Stabilize preexisting heart disease.
Administer analgesics for pain.
Consider the use of vasodilators to improve collateral circulation (the effectiveness of this therapy is unproven).
Administer heparin to prevent the growth of the clot.
Consider using tissue plasminogen activator, streptokinase, surgery, or catheter techniques to remove the clot.
Treat the injuries caused by ischemic necrosis.
Use warfarin, aspirin, or low molecular weight heparin to prevent the formation of clots in the future.

remove the clot appears to improve circulation in the majority of patients, but complications resulting from the use of this type of therapy also appear to have contributed to the deaths of some patients. The therapies used to prevent recurrence also appear to be relatively ineffective or risky. Box 16-6 lists the goals of therapy for FATE.

Suggested Readings

Abbott JA: Traumatic myocarditis. In Bonagura JD, editor: *Kirk's current veterinary therapy XII small animal practice*, Philadelphia, 1995, WB Saunders Co, 846-850.

American Heart Association: 2005 American Heart Association guidelines for cardiopulmonary resuscitation and emergency cardiovascular care, *Circulation* 112(24)(suppl):IV-1-IV-211, 2005.

Atkins CE: Caval syndrome in the dog, *Semin Vet Med Surg (Small Anim)* 2(1):64-71, 1987.

Boon JA: *Manual of veterinary echocardiography*, Baltimore, 1998, Williams & Wilkins.

Bright JM, Martin JM, Mama K: A retrospective evaluation of transthoracic biphasic electrical cardioversion for atrial fibrillation in dogs, *J Vet Cardiol* 7(2):85-96, 2005.

Buchanan JW, Bücheler J: Vertebral scale system to measure canine heart size in radiographs, *J Am Vet Med Assoc* 206(2):194-199, 1995.

Cole SG, Otto CM, Hughes D: Cardiopulmonary cerebral resuscitation in small animals—a clinical practice review, II, *J Vet Emerg Crit Care* 13(1):13-23, 2003.

Cornell CC et al: Allometric scaling of M-mode cardiac measurements in normal adult dogs, *J Vet Intern Med* 18(3):311-321, 2004.

DeFrancesco TC, Hansen BD, Atkins CE: Noninvasive transthoracic temporary cardiac pacing in dogs, *J Vet Intern Med* 17(5):663-667, 2003.

Fox PR, Sisson D, Moïse NS: *Textbook of canine and feline cardiology: principles and clinical practice*, ed 2, St Louis, 1999, WB Saunders Co.

Gelzer ARM, Kraus MS: Management of atrial fibrillation, *Vet Clin North Am Small Anim Pract* 34(5):1127-1144, 2004.

Gidlewski J, Petrie JP: Therapeutic pericardiocentesis in the dog and cat, *Clin Tech Small Anim Pract* 20:151-155, 2005.

Johnson L, Boon J, Orton EC: Clinical characteristics of 53 dogs with Doppler-derived evidence of pulmonary hypertension: 1992-1996, *J Vet Intern Med* 13(5):440-447, 1999.

Kienle RD, Thomas WP: Echocardiography. In Nyland TG, Mattoon JS: *Small animal diagnostic ultrasound*, ed 2, Philadelphia, 2002, WB Saunders Co, 354-423.

Kittleson MD, Kienle RD: *Small animal cardiovascular medicine*, St Louis, 1999, Mosby.

Knight DH: Reason must supersede dogma in the management of ventricular arrhythmias. In Bonagura JD, editor: *Kirk's current veterinary therapy XIII small animal practice*, Philadelphia, 2000, WB Saunders Co, 730-733.

Lamb CR, Boswood A: Role of survey radiography in diagnosing canine cardiac disease, *Compend Contin Educ Pract Vet* 24(4):316-326, 2002.

Litster AL, Buchanan JW: Vertebral scale system to measure heart size in radiographs of cats, *J Am Vet Med Assoc* 216(2):210-214, 2000.

Reimer SB, Kittleson MD, Kyles AE: Use of rheolytic thrombectomy for the treatment of feline distal aortic thromboembolism, *J Vet Intern Med* 19(3):424, 2005 (abstract).

Rishniw M, Thomas WP: Bradyarrhythmias. In Bonagura JD, editor: *Kirk's current veterinary therapy XIII small animal practice*, Philadelphia, 2000, WB Saunders Co, 719-725.

Scherf D, Bornemann C: Thumping of the precordium in ventricular standstill, *Am J Cardiol* 5:30-40, 1960.

Sisson DD et al: Plasma taurine concentrations and M-mode echocardiographic measures in healthy cats and in cats with dilated cardiomyopathy, *J Vet Intern Med* 5(4):232-238, 1991.

Smith SA, Tobias AH: Feline arterial thromboembolism: an update, *Vet Clin North Am Small Anim Pract* 34(5):1245-1271, 2004.

Wright KN: Assessment and treatment of supraventricular arrhythmias. In Bonagura JD, editor: *Kirk's current veterinary therapy XIII small animal practice*, Philadelphia, 2000, WB Saunders Co, 726-733.

Zoll PM et al: External mechanical cardiac stimulation, *N Engl J Med* 294(23):1274-1275, 1976.

17

Respiratory Emergencies

ANDREA M. BATTAGLIA, DON SHAWVER

The animal that has difficulty breathing could have a problem in any area of the respiratory system. Observing the animal's stance, auscultating lung sounds, and observing the respiratory pattern can help the veterinary team localize the affected area (Fig. 17-1).

The affected area almost always can be localized through physical examination and observation. Once it has been determined what the primary problem is, life-saving procedures can be performed.

Equipment list:

- Devices for oxygen (O_2) administration
- Endotracheal tubes (multiple sizes)
- Tracheostomy tubes (multiple sizes)
- Thoracic drainage tubes (multiple sizes)
- Grasping forceps for foreign body retrieval
- Laryngeal scopes
- Thoracic drainage pumps
- Three-way stopcocks
- Butterfly catheters
- Bronchoscopes

Upper Airway Disease

Larynx

Obstruction can be caused by edema from trauma, tumors, and foreign bodies, as well as by structural deformities of the airway. Laryngeal paralysis can result from interrupted innervation to the intrinsic muscles of the larynx. The arytenoid cartilages and vocal folds fail to abduct, thus creating an airway obstruction. The cause can be congenital or acquired. The congenital form has been noted in the Bouviers des Flandres, dalmatians, Siberian huskies, and rottweilers. The acquired form can be idiopathic, traumatic, polyneuropathic, or iatrogenic. The most common form of laryngeal paralysis is idiopathic and is usually seen in large, older dogs.

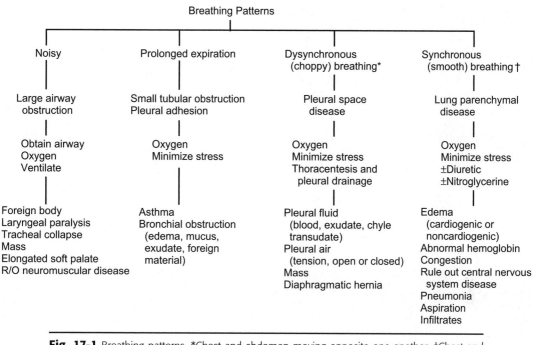

Breathing Patterns

Noisy	Prolonged expiration	Dysynchronous (choppy) breathing*	Synchronous (smooth) breathing†
Large airway obstruction	Small tubular obstruction Pleural adhesion	Pleural space disease	Lung parenchymal disease
Obtain airway Oxygen Ventilate	Oxygen Minimize stress	Oxygen Minimize stress Thoracentesis and pleural drainage	Oxygen Minimize stress ±Diuretic ±Nitroglycerine
Foreign body Laryngeal paralysis Tracheal collapse Mass Elongated soft palate R/O neuromuscular disease	Asthma Bronchial obstruction (edema, mucus, exudate, foreign material)	Pleural fluid (blood, exudate, chyle transudate) Pleural air (tension, open or closed) Mass Diaphragmatic hernia	Edema (cardiogenic or noncardiogenic) Abnormal hemoglobin Congestion Rule out central nervous system disease Pneumonia Aspiration Infiltrates

Fig. 17-1 Breathing patterns. *Chest and abdomen moving opposite one another. †Chest and abdomen moving together in same direction. (Courtesy Rebecca Kirby. From Murtaugh RJ: Acute respiratory distress, *Vet Clin North Am Small Anim Pract* 24(6):1043, 1994.)

Presentation. A history of exercise intolerance, gagging while eating or drinking, and laryngeal stridor may be seen. The condition usually worsens and can include episodes of severe dyspnea, including cyanosis.

The animal with laryngeal paralysis may have dyspnea, respiratory stridor, and hyperthermia. Many animals collapse with severe respiratory distress. The first priority is to establish an airway. Sedation may be necessary before intubation; O2 and fluid therapy are necessary to stabilize the animal before further tests can be performed.

Diagnosis. Once the animal is stabilized, the team should confirm the cause of the problem. Laryngeal paralysis is diagnosed through laryngoscopic examination on a lightly anesthetized patient. The vocal folds should abduct on inspiration in the normal animal. The affected animal shows little or no movement of one or both of the folds. The team can then determine whether the condition is congenital or acquired. If the animal is less than 1 year old, then the condition probably is congenital.

Treatment. Treatment initially is accomplished through medical therapy and O2 administration. Corticosteroids are administered intravenously (dexamethasone 0.2 to 1.0 mg/kg twice daily) to reduce the inflammation and edema. Fluid therapy is used with caution. Some animals with upper airway obstruction can develop pulmonary edema.

Surgical treatment is recommended once the animal has been stabilized and involves removing or repositioning the laryngeal cartilages. Intensive postoperative care is necessary because of the possible complications, and animals should be placed under 24-hour observation for 1 to 3 days. Antibiotics should be continued; corticosteroids may be necessary if inflammation occurs, obstructing the airway postoperatively. The dogs should be offered a small amount of water 12 to 24 hours postoperatively; careful observation will help determine if it is able to swallow normally. Owners must be instructed to keep the animal quiet and avoid excessive exercise for 6 to 8 weeks. Tranquilizers are recommended for the very active animal.

BOX 17-1

Establishing an Airway

The following procedures are performed when an endotracheal tube cannot be placed. These situations include head or facial trauma, spinal injuries, and upper airway obstructions.

Transtracheal Catheterization

A 14- or 16-gauge over-the-needle catheter or commercially available transtracheal catheter is placed through the tracheal rings. Commercially available transtracheal catheters are made with guarded tubing to prevent kinking once they are advanced into the trachea. This is a temporary solution until a more permanent airway can be established (see Box 1, Fig. 1).

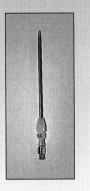

Procedure

Note: When possible and appropriate, the anterior neck of the animal should be surgically prepared.

- Identify the cricothyroid membrane between the cricoid and thyroid cartilages.

- Stabilize the trachea with the thumb and index finger.
- Insert the catheter between the rings in the midcervical region, directing it caudally. A loss of resistance is felt once the trachea is punctured.
- Aspirate air to ensure proper position.
- Administer O_2 at 50 ml/kg/min.
- Administer O_2 at 100 ml/kg/min if airway obstruction is present. Watch for chest expansion, then press on the chest and abdomen in an attempt to dislodge the foreign body.

Note: Tracheotomy is necessary if cyanosis does not resolve. Maintain control of the catheter position at all times. High O_2 pressures can dislodge the catheter from the airway.

Possible Complications

- Barotrauma
- Pneumomediastinum
- Bleeding
- Catheter dislodgement
- Subcutaneous emphysema
- Hematoma
- Tracheoesophageal fistula

To perform a tracheotomy, an incision is made through the skin and muscles of the neck overlying the trachea. A tube 1- to 1.5-sizes smaller than what would be used for orotracheal intubation is placed through the incision. Although commercially made tubes are available, tracheostomy tubes can be made out of endotracheal tubes by using the following method:

Foreign bodies partially blocking the upper airway in the form of sticks, balls, or other objects can be removed manually using forceps after sedation. The animal should be placed in a quiet environment and given flow-by O_2. Trying to restrain the animal can cause additional stress and possibly dislodge the foreign body, allowing it to move further down into the airway. Once the foreign body is removed, the airway must be examined for possible trauma to any of the structures. The animal must be monitored for any other complications, which can include swelling or pulmonary edema.

Trachea

Tumors, tracheal stenosis and collapse, and intraluminal occlusion can cause tracheal obstructions. An acute onset of coughing and dyspnea is observed, and high-frequency rales can be heard where the foreign body is lodged (if only a partial obstruction). Collapse and respiratory arrest occur in animals with complete obstructions. These animals need a tracheostomy (Box 17-1).

The ideal presentation allows the time to preoxygenate the animal, sedate it, and then perform

BOX 17-1

Establishing an Airway—cont'd

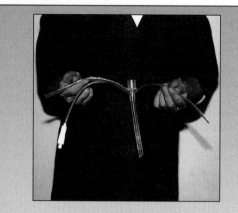

- Remove 15-mm adapter from the endotracheal tube.
- Estimate how long the tube should be, and mark the length on the tube.
- Cut the tube in two places, starting proximally, down to the center of the tube. Do not cut the airline and stop at the mark.
- Replace the 15-mm adapter at the junction of the cut.
- Shorten the split ends and place two holes at either end to be used for stabilizing.

Procedure

- Administer general anesthesia or sedation with a local block around the site of the incision.
- Surgically prepare the area.

- Position the animal in dorsal recumbency with the neck extended backward. Place a rolled towel under the neck to cause dorsal flexion of the cervical region. (Placing tape over the jaw can stabilize the animal's head.)
- Make a ventral midline incision from approximately the first to the eighth tracheal ring.
- Part the two sternohyoid muscles on the midline. Continue blunt dissection down to the tracheal rings.
- Elevate the trachea using hemostats or fingers.
- Make a transverse incision between the fourth and fifth ring.
- Place stay sutures through the skin and tracheal cartilage adjacent to the transverse incision on either side of the opening.
- Insert the tube into opening and tie it into place.

Note: Slash tracheostomy is necessary for animals in respiratory arrest because of a complete upper airway obstruction or severe head trauma. This procedure is performed without surgical preparation. Scissors or a blade rather than blunt dissection is used to expose the trachea.

Complications

- Obstruction from excessive secretions
- Nosocomial pneumonia
- Laryngeal stenosis
- Tube dislodgement
- Subcutaneous emphysema

---

the technique. However, many times an emergency tracheostomy (i.e., slash tracheostomy) is needed to save the animal's life. Once the airway has been established and the animal has been stabilized, further diagnostic procedures can be performed.

Tracheal collapse is a common condition that often affects toy breeds and middle-aged to older dogs. It occurs when the tracheal ring does not maintain its rigidity. The trachea collapses dorsoventrally to form a flattened oval or slitlike lumen.

Presentation. Animals with a collapsed trachea usually have a history of coughing and signs of respiratory distress. Exercise intolerance is noted. Radiographs and bronchoscopy can confirm the condition.

Treatment. Medical therapy (including bronchodilators, cough suppressants, and antiinflammatory drugs) often is successful. Some animals with severe collapse need surgical intervention. Ring prosthetics made out of syringe cases, surgical stents, or a tracheal ring resection and anastomosis are a few of the techniques used to repair a collapsed trachea.

Postoperative care includes 24-hour observation and antibiotics. Cage rest with only light exercise is recommended.

Trauma to the trachea can result from dogfights, poor intubation or extubation techniques, and cords or chains placed around the animal's neck. Establishing a functional airway is the primary goal in all these situations. Once this has been accomplished, further stabilization techniques can be performed.

Lower Airway Disease

Feline Bronchial Disease

Bronchitis is a common cause of respiratory distress in cats. It has also been called *feline asthma*, which can be misleading. Many forms of bronchial disease exist, and feline asthma is one of those forms. It most often affects young to middle-aged cats of any breed. Allergens, irritants, and infectious agents can cause the bronchitis, but often the cause cannot be determined.

Presentation. Common clinical signs include respiratory distress characterized by prolonged expiration, coughing episodes, and wheezing. Vomiting and retching can occur after a severe coughing episode. Expiratory wheeze may be noted on auscultation. No breath sounds may be noted in the more severe cases because of airway obstruction.

Diagnosis. Cardiac disease can cause very similar clinical signs and must be ruled out before treatment is administered. Bronchial disease is confirmed by evaluating a complete blood count, thoracic radiographs, and a tracheal or bronchoalveolar lavage. A fecal float should be evaluated to rule out a lungworm infestation.

Treatment. The cat in respiratory distress must be stabilized before any procedures can be performed. Therapy with O_2 can begin immediately, using a stress-free technique. Short-acting glucocorticoids (prednisolone sodium succinate 10 to 20 mg/kg intravenously) is highly recommended. This can be given intramuscularly if the intravenous injection is too stressful. Bronchodilators are used in conjunction with the steroids and antibiotics if indicated.

Parenchymal or Gas Exchange Disease

Pneumonia

Pneumonia is an inflammation of the lungs with accompanying consolidation. More than one agent can cause pneumonia. Viral, bacterial, aspiration, fungal, and chemical causes are possible. Pneumonia can be self-limiting, but some forms can be life threatening. Isolation may be necessary to prevent infecting other patients (depends on the type of pneumonia present).

Presentation. An animal with pneumonia has a fever, severe cough, rapid respiration, and possibly bloody mucus. Chest sounds consist of rhonchi, rales, and diminished breath sounds. Vomiting and lethargy also can be present.

Pneumonias cause inflammation of the parenchyma of the lung, primarily the bronchi. Exudate forms and flows into the alveoli, plugging the alveoli and small airways. Chemical pneumonias can be caused by exposure to inhalants containing substances such as ammonia, nitrogen dioxide, cadmium, and fat or oil aerosol. Aspiration pneumonia is the aspiration of stomach content.

Diagnostic Testing. Microbiologic testing is used to determine the particular type of pneumonia that is present. A tracheal wash can be performed to collect the necessary specimen. Radiographic examination also is a valuable tool for evaluating the effects of specific types of pneumonia. Radiographs will reveal collapsed lobes or atelectasis, pleural effusion, and other effects of various pneumonias. Blood work and electrocardiography are helpful in determining the physiologic effects, and blood gas analysis is also performed to determine treatment protocols.

Treatment. Specific treatment depends on laboratory and radiographic diagnostic tests and physical assessment, because so many types of pneumonia exist. The primary treatment for early-onset pneumonia is antibiotic therapy. Which antibiotic is appropriate depends on the type of pneumonia. In more advanced stages of pneumonia, standard treatment for respiratory emergencies is needed. This could consist of basic O_2 support or ventilation support and control. For minor respiratory distress such as tachypnea, flow-by O_2 is started with 100% O_2. The results of arterial blood gas analysis indicate the severity of the respiratory distress and will also assist in determining if ventilatory support is needed.

Fluid administration is important in these animals. Septic shock can occur in more advanced cases of pneumonia. The patient should be monitored for fluid input and output, blood pressure, cardiac function, and acid-base status. Nebulization and coupaging also is performed. Specific antibiotics can be selected based on laboratory cultures and titers.

Pulmonary Contusion

One of the most common types of pulmonary parenchymal injury in household pets is pulmonary contusion caused by chest trauma. The problem results from blood inside the alveolar and interstitial space. This blood interferes with the adequate exchange of O_2 and carbon dioxide at the alveolar capillary membrane.

Presentation. Depending on the degree of contusion, symptoms can vary from mild pain and dyspnea to total inability to move air in and out of the lung. Other complications of pulmonary contusion could be laceration, broken ribs, pneumothorax, hemothorax, pneumomediastinum, diaphragmatic hernia, and shock caused by fluid loss.

Treatment. Because so many conditions include pulmonary contusions, each condition must be evaluated individually, with emphasis on respiration, circulation, and fluid volume. As with all trauma conditions, careful examination is imperative.

The patient is monitored on a 24-hour basis. Blood pressure, electrocardiogram, pain management, and arterial blood gas are critical aspects of adequate patient care. Wounds must be dressed and evaluated regularly, and splints and supports must be checked at regular intervals.

Pulmonary Edema

Pulmonary edema is defined as an abnormal accumulation of fluid in the extravascular tissues and lungs. This problem can be caused by increased pulmonary capillary pressure, leaking of the alveolar capillary membrane caused by trauma, or low plasma protein levels. Increased capillary permeability is the cause of edema. The most common cause of pulmonary edema is left heart failure. Trauma, sepsis, O_2 toxicity, hypoalbuminemia, airway obstruction, chemical inhalation, and pancreatitis are only a few of the conditions that can lead to pulmonary edema.

Presentation. The patient may have blood tinged frothy mucus (may not be observed in the earlier stages). Restlessness, labored respiration, crackling breath sounds on auscultation, and rapid, irregular heart rate also can be noted. Radiography shows pulmonary venous congestion and airspace edema. Vascular markings are very clear in upper lung fields, and pleural effusion can be present. The heart shadow usually indicates an enlarged heart, particularly the left ventricle. A mixed acidosis might also be seen (respiratory and metabolic). One of the classic symptoms of pulmonary edema is engorgement of the neck veins.

The cause of the edema must be determined before proper treatment can begin. Fluid overload, hyperalbuminemia, upper airway obstructions, and increased membrane permeability as the result of shock are possible causes of pulmonary edema.

Treatment. The patient with pulmonary edema needs oxygenation to help alleviate the dyspnea. Assisted ventilation with positive end-expiratory pressure may be necessary for severe cases.

Airway care is especially challenging. Frequent airway suctioning may be needed to remove the fluid that usually accumulates with this disease. Suctioning must be performed carefully and for short duration. Suctioning for long periods further reduces interalveolar pressure, increasing the permeability of the alveolar capillary membrane.

Two physiologic forces work to maintain positive pressures in the alveolar capillary network: (1) plasma oncotic pressure and (2) transcapillary pressure. Plasma oncotic pressure usually is higher than transcapillary pressure; this higher pressure is what keeps fluid from entering the airspace of the alveoli through leakage from the capillaries. Fluid regulation usually can be managed with diuretics. Furosemide (Lasix) is a common diuretic recommended at 2 to 4 mg/kg intravenously. When using diuretics, one must be careful to avoid hypovolemia. Bronchodilators may also be helpful for reducing the work of breathing.

Airway care and monitoring physiologic parameters for O_2 saturation, blood pressure, and cardiac status with electrocardiogram are necessary. Ventilator use also may be indicated. Specific anesthesia and sedation monitoring is of particular importance, because many anesthetics and sedatives can increase the potential for edema, hypoxia, and complete respiratory failure.

Pleural Cavity Diseases

Pneumothorax

Pneumothorax is the presence of air in the pleural space. The condition is divided into two categories: (1) spontaneous and (2) traumatic pneumothorax. Spontaneous pneumothorax usually occurs in the absence of known pulmonary disease. This condition could be a congenital lesion, lung abscess, or any other condition affecting the lung parenchyma. Traumatic pneumothorax is caused by some injury to the chest (e.g., a broken rib) that punctures the thoracic wall or a piercing wound made by a sharp object (e.g., an arrow or a piece of glass or metal) that penetrates the thoracic wall. Traumatic pneumothorax also may result from an iatrogenic source (e.g., a subclavian catheter or esophagostomy feeding tube placed too low in the neck).

A pneumothorax occurs when air from the surrounding environment is sucked into the thoracic cavity by the negative pressure within the cavity (when the integrity of the thoracic wall or pleural cavity is breached). Sometimes this air moves in and out with the expansion and contraction of the lung. When air enters the pleural cavity and the wound acts as a one-way valve, not allowing the air to escape back to atmosphere, the pressure in the thoracic cavity continues to rise, exerting increasing force on the lungs, heart, and great vessels. This pressure can become higher than atmospheric pressure. This condition, called *tension pneumothorax*, is life threatening. Any wound to the chest or neck should be considered a sucking chest wound until proven otherwise.

Presentation. The onset in most cases of traumatic pneumothorax is abrupt. The respiratory symptoms can emerge gradually, particularly in spontaneous pneumothorax. The degree to which air enters the pleural space determines the degree of symptoms. If the pneumothorax is very small, then symptoms may not be present at all.

The patient may be restless and wincing from pain. During breathing, less chest movement may occur on one side than on the other. Chest auscultation reveals hyperresonance or diminished breath sounds. On chest percussion, hyperresonance also is noted. The patient may be cyanotic and show signs of increased dyspnea. Cough and hemoptysis often are not present. Subcutaneous emphysema may be present over the neck and chest. The quickest way to diagnose pneumothorax is through examination and thoracentesis. Radiographic studies also can be used to confirm the pneumothorax. Radiographs would indicate collapsed lung or lungs and possible mediastinal shift opposite the pneumothorax. Free air between the parietal and visceral pleura and, in more severe cases, deviation of the heart opposite the point of pneumothorax can be seen.

Treatment. Thoracentesis should be performed immediately in all animals suspected of having a pneumothorax (Box 17-2). A chest tube is necessary for animals with tension pneumothorax or a pneumothorax that will not resolve. The general rule is to use the largest chest tube that will fit between the ribs. A chest tube with larger fenestrations can be used when exudate and air are being removed from the thoracic cavity, as in pyothorax and hemothorax. The length of the chest tube should be measured from the point of insertion just to the thoracic inlet. The chest tube should be equipped with a three-way stopcock and additional connecting tubing and clamps so that it can be attached to a Heimlich valve or active sealed drain of some sort (e.g., a water seal drain). A Heimlich valve used for humans should not be used in small animals (< 40 lb). If the duckbill flaps inside the Heimlich valve become wet, then they may stick together, preventing air from escaping the thoracic cavity and exacerbating the condition. This malfunction could result in respiratory arrest.

General monitoring of the patient's ventilatory pattern is necessary. Heart rate, respiratory rate, blood pressure, and blood gas should be monitored. If a chest tube is in place, then it should be checked frequently to ensure that the tube is not dislodged or obstructed. Lidocaine 1.5 mg/kg and bupivacaine 1.5 mg/kg can be used as a block to alleviate the discomfort. Air is removed periodically by a syringe or removed continually by a thoracic drainage system or pump. Active airflow is determined by observing the bubbles in the water seal drainage system. As the pneumothorax begins to heal, the bubbles become less frequent.

A light chest wrap is used for additional support. An Elizabethan collar is used to prevent the animal from pulling the tube out.

Supplemental O_2 can be given via face tent or in an O_2 cage if hypoxia is present. Pulse oximetry can be used to determine O_2 saturation.

BOX 17-2

Thoracentesis

Placing a needle or catheter into the thoracic cavity is necessary for removing air or fluid from the chest cavity for diagnostic or therapeutic reasons.

Procedure

- The area over the seventh to ninth intercostal space in the midsection of the chest should be surgically prepared.
- The area to tap if fluid is present is the ventral third of the fourth to seventh intercostal space in an animal that is standing or in sternal recumbency.
- The area to tap if air is present is the midthorax in an animal in lateral recumbency or the dorsal third of the chest in an animal that is standing or in sternal recumbency.
- A 18- or 20-gauge butterfly catheter can be used. A drop of saline is placed in the hub of the catheter or needle.
- The needle is advanced slowly into the pleural space, in front of the rib and at a 45-degree angle. The saline will be sucked inward once the pleural space is entered.
- At this point, advancement of the needle should stop and the angle of the needle made level with the chest wall.
- A three-way stopcock is attached and aspiration is started.

Complications

- Lung laceration

Thoracostomy Tube Placement

Placing a tube in the thoracic cavity is necessary if large amounts of air or fluid are present. A chest tube should be placed if more than two thoracenteses are needed in the first few hours of presentation. Chest tubes are commercially available. Red rubber feeding tubes can be used as an alternative. Three or four holes must be made large enough for fluid to flow through easily.

Procedure

- Sedation and local intercostal nerve blocks are used for the critically ill animal.
- A large section of the lateral thorax is surgically prepared.
- The tube chosen should be approximately the same size as the mainstem bronchus (as estimated from a thoracic radiograph).

- The skin is grabbed at the level of shoulder blade and pulled cranially.
- A stab incision is made (slightly larger than tube) into the seventh or eighth intercostal space.
- The clinician bluntly dissects through the incision into the thorax with hemostats. The hemostats are held so that the dominant hand is grasping near the tip of the hemostats to prevent overpenetration.
- Air is allowed to enter the thoracic cavity (to allow some lung deflation).
- The chest tube is placed in a cranioventral direction for fluid and craniodorsally for air (a stylet will help guide the tube).
- The skin is released to create a subcutaneous tunnel.
- The tube is twisted 180 degrees in each direction to confirm that it is not kinked. Radiographs can be used to confirm proper placement.
- The tube is secured to the periosteum of ribs (using additional local anesthetic).
- A purse-string suture is tied around the tube as it exits the skin to seal the chest.
- The tube is anchored by placing a suture through the skin and around the tube at about the level of the eighth or ninth rib. A Chinese fingertip is placed around the tube to prevent it from slipping out of the chest.
- Triple-antibiotic ointment is placed at the insertion site to create a better seal.
- A wrap is placed around the chest to provide better stability.
- The tube can be connected to a thoracic drain pump for continual suction, or a three-way stopcock can be stabilized to the tube for intermittent suction.
- Lidocaine is infused into the chest tube (1.5 mg/kg). The chest tube is then flushed with saline (1-3 mls depending on the size of the chest tube). The patient is gently rocked and rolled for a complete coating of the area. Bupivicaine is then infused into the chest tube (1.5 mg/kg) and the chest tube is again flushed with saline. The patient is once more gently rocked and rolled for a complete coating of the area. This treatment can be repeated every 6 hours for pain management. The dose may need to be adjusted in cats if the animal becomes too sedate.
- Heimlich valves can be used for animals with pneumothorax who weigh more than 15 kg.

Pleural Effusion

The lining of the thoracic cavity and the outer surface of the lung are called the *pleural lining*. The lining covering the outer portion of the lung is called the *visceral pleura*, and the lining covering the diaphragm and the mediastinum is called the *parietal lining*. A thin layer of fluid usually separates these two linings and eliminates friction between the two surfaces. A collection of excess fluid between the visceral and parietal pleura is known as *pleural effusion*. Normally the fluid in the pleural space flows from the interstitial tissue on the parietal side to the interstitial tissue of the lung by an absorptive force. An imbalance in this force impedes the flow of water, electrolyte, and protein. Some causes of pleural effusion are cancer, heartworm, congestive heart failure, chylothorax, hemothorax, hypoalbuminemia, infections, trauma, and idiopathic conditions.

Presentation. Clinical signs can include dyspnea, restlessness, cough, and lethargy. Respiration is labored with abdominal contraction. Lung auscultation indicates increased bronchial sounds. Cardiac sounds may be decreased. The degree of symptoms depends solely on the amount of fluid present and the rate of fluid formation.

Radiographic examination is the best way to diagnose pleural effusion. Determining whether the effusion is unilateral or bilateral (and the extent of the effusion) is possible. The type of fluid can be determined by obtaining a sample. This is accomplished by performing a pleural tap. The tap also can be performed to relieve the pressure caused by the fluid accumulation. A chest tube may be necessary, with a continual closed-suction system attached.

Treatment is based on what is found in the fluid analysis. Blood, chyle (milky-looking aspirate), and protein can indicate conditions such as pyothorax, hemothorax, or chylothorax. The cause should be determined so that appropriate treatment can be administered. Pleural biopsy may be necessary if cancer is suspected.

Continual monitoring and assessment of the animal's status is essential during stabilization and treatment. Pulse oximetry is monitored to determine O_2 saturation; O_2 therapy and maintenance of a thoracic drainage tube also may be necessary.

Diaphragmatic Hernia

Diaphragmatic hernia occurs when the contents of the abdomen herniate into the thoracic cavity. Blunt trauma to the chest or abdomen is the usual cause. A congenital form has been noted but rarely is seen in emergency cases.

Animals with a diaphragmatic hernia have varying degrees of dyspnea, abdominal breathing, cyanosis, and shock. (The degree of respiratory distress depends on the degree of trauma and displacement of the organs.) Many other forms of trauma to the chest and abdominal wall also can be noted.

Radiographs and ultrasound can be used to diagnose the diaphragmatic hernia. Radiographic diagnosis can be challenging if pleural effusion or pulmonary contusions are present. The abdomen may feel empty on physical examination. Heart and lung sounds may be diminished on auscultation.

Treatment. Diaphragmatic hernia usually is secondary to trauma. The ideal would be to stabilize the animal before the hernia repair is done, but many times the surgery is necessary as part of the stabilization. Assisted ventilation is required during the entire procedure, and the animal should be surgically prepared as much as possible before anesthetics are administered.

The animal must be monitored closely for signs of deterioration and respiratory distress before the corrective surgery. Elevating the animal's front end may move the abdominal contents out of the thoracic cavity toward the abdominal cavity. This alleviates some of the pressure in the thoracic cavity.

Flail Chest

Flail chest occurs after severe trauma to the thoracic wall. A rib segment is broken off and becomes a free-floating segment. Pain and dyspnea are observed.

The animal must be maintained on O_2 and analgesics. Cage rest is necessary. Surgical intervention may be necessary to stabilize the flail segment.

Smoke Inhalation

Handling the animal that has survived a fire involves many factors. The owner can be experiencing a severe level of stress (having lost everything but the beloved pet). Often organizations are available to assist people in financial distress after such a catastrophe.

Some veterinary facilities have established funds and specific protocols for this type of situation.

The type of injury is dependant on many factors (e.g., how long the exposure, what was burning, heat and the intensity of the exposure). Hypoxemia, pulmonary damage, and thermal injury are the three major concerns. The upper airway most commonly is affected by the thermal injury. Swelling and irritation to the mucosa can be severe. Lower airway complications are also common. A full physical is performed, including examination of the skin for burns or irritation, the eyes for corneal ulcers, and the nervous system for signs of abnormalities.

Once the animal arrives, immediate O_2 therapy is necessary. Usually a high flow of flow-by O_2 can be administered while the necessary stabilization procedures and tests are performed. The animal may also have burn injuries that need to be addressed and ash that needs to be removed from its coat to prevent further inhalation injury. Radiographs are taken initially so that damage to the lungs can be reassessed during the days after the initial injury.

Continued therapy includes fluid therapy, O_2 support, pain management, and care of abrasions and burn injury. Antibiotics are not recommended unless an infection develops. Nebulizing and coupaging may be indicated. Hyperbaric O_2 therapy has also been used to treat this injury.

The animal suffering with smoke inhalation can recover well with rapid and appropriate supportive care.

Conclusion

Respiratory emergencies require a skilled team of veterinary technicians who can quickly assess breathing patterns, interpret their findings, and provide appropriate stabilization. Gentle handling techniques and creating a stress-free environment is also crucial for a positive outcome. Hospitals need to be equipped with the tools necessary to assist the small animal patient with respiratory compromise. When one cannot breathe, nothing else matters.

Suggested Readings

Braund KG et al: Laryngeal paralysis polyneuropathy complex in young dalmatians, *Am J Vet Res* 55:534, 1994.

Buback JL, Booth HW, Hobson HP: Surgical treatment of trachea collapse in dogs: 90 cases (1983-1993), *J Am Vet Med Assoc* 208:308, 1996.

Burbridge HM: A review of laryngeal paralysis in dogs, *Br Vet J* 151:71-82, 1995.

Cole RB: *Essentials of respiratory disease*, ed 2, Philadelphia, 1975, JB Lippincott.

Farzan S: *A concise handbook of respiratory disease*, Reston, VA, 1978, Reston Publishing Co.

Fingland RB: Treatment of tracheal collapse. In Bojrab JM, Ellison GW, Slocum B, editors: *Current techniques in small animal surgery*, Baltimore, 1998, Williams & Wilkins.

Ford RB, Mazzaferro EM: *Kirk and Bistner's handbook of veterinary procedures and emergency treatment*, ed 8, St Louis, 2006, WB Saunders.

Hedlund CS: Tracheostomies in the management of canine and feline upper respiratory disease, *Vet Clin North Am Small Anim Pract* 24:873, 1994.

Moise NS et al: Clinical, radiographic and bronchial cytologic features of cats with bronchial disease: 65 cases (1980-1986), *J Am Vet Med Assoc* 194:1467, 1989.

Murtaugh RJ: Acute respiratory distress, *Vet Clin North Am Small Anim Pract* 24(6):1041, 1994.

Wilkins RL, Stoller JK, editors: *Egan's fundamentals of respiratory therapy*, ed 8, St Louis, 2003, Mosby.

CHAPTER 18

Gastrointestinal Emergencies

JENNIFER J. DEVEY, DENNIS T. CROWE, JR.

Gastrointestinal (GI) emergencies are a common problem in veterinary medicine. Because nausea (in the form of drooling or retching), vomiting, and diarrhea are very apparent, GI emergencies are easy to diagnose. Some of the signs, such as restlessness, shivering, abnormal posture, and crying, are subtler. Anorexia may be the only sign some animals, especially cats, show to indicate a GI problem. Pain on abdominal palpation, which may or may not be present, typically indicates a more serious problem.

This chapter addresses the common emergency conditions affecting the GI system, including problems affecting the esophagus, stomach, small intestine, large intestine, and pancreas. Close attention to history (including accurate questioning of the owner) and physical examination are vital to early diagnosis, as well as to choice of appropriate diagnostic tests and treatment and prevention of unnecessary expenses.

The technician's responsibilities for the patient with GI emergencies may include taking the history, performing physical examination and laboratory analyses, taking radiographs, assisting with ultrasound examination, setting up endoscopy equipment, readying the operating room, monitoring anesthesia, assisting in the operating room, and providing postoperative care.

Vomiting

Vomiting (the active expulsion of GI contents) is preceded by signs of nausea (e.g., restlessness, salivation, repeated swallowing attempts), followed by forceful contractions of the abdomen and diaphragm and expulsion of food or fluid. The act of vomiting ultimately is initiated in the medullary vomiting center, which receives input from the chemoreceptor trigger zone, higher central nervous system centers, vestibular system, and peripheral sensory receptors. Knowing which of these mechanisms is responsible enables practitioners to treat the vomiting patient appropriately. For instance, if a dog were vomiting because persistent gastric distention was stimulating the peripheral sensory receptors, then it would be far better to place a nasogastric (NG) tube for

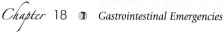

BOX 18-1

Assessment of Vomiting

- Is it regurgitation (no nausea or active expulsion of GI contents)?
- Is it vomiting (nausea and abdominal contractions/ active expulsion of GI contents)?
- Is it projectile vomiting?
- Is it nonproductive?
- What color is it (white, yellow, green, brown, red)?
- Is there blood present (red, black, or chemistry strip evidence)?
- How frequently is it occurring?
- How much volume is being vomited?
- What is the consistency (fluid, foam, fluid)?
- When does it occur (after drinking, after eating, after medication)?

BOX 18-2

Assessment of Diarrhea

- How frequently does the diarrhea occur?
- How much volume is being produced?
- What is the consistency (watery, soft, undigested food, foreign material)?
- Is there blood present (red, black)?
- Does the animal have tenesmus?
- Is there an odor?

stomach decompression than to treat the patient with a phenothiazine derivative.

Vomiting must be differentiated from regurgitation. Regurgitation indicates an esophageal disorder, and close attention must be paid to the possibility of underlying aspiration pneumonia. Signs of nausea do not precede regurgitation, and no active expulsion of food or fluid occurs. It often occurs very soon after drinking or eating (food present in the vomitus is undigested).

Projectile vomiting is associated most commonly with a pyloric outflow obstruction or a complete proximal intestinal obstruction. This can be either mechanical, as in the case of a foreign body, or functional, as in the case of pyloric thickening or a mass (benign or malignant) compressing the pylorus. Vomiting of white fluid suggests a disorder of gastric or esophageal origin, and yellow fluid suggests gastric vomiting mixed with bile from the duodenum. Green fluid indicates bile and duodenal vomiting or evidence of a significant amount of bile that has been refluxed into the stomach and immediately vomited. Both yellow and green fluid can be associated with pancreatitis. Brown fluid suggests reflux of fecal-like material from further down the small intestine. It usually has a fecal odor as well. Frank blood in the vomitus (hematemesis) typically indicates esophageal, gastric, or duodenal bleeding from erosions or ulceration, whereas "coffee grounds" or black flecks indicate gastric or duodenal vomitus with the presence of digested blood (where hydrochloric acid has denatured the hemoglobin). Frank blood can be seen on occasion with jejunal lesions.

Vomiting should be characterized as precisely as possible in all patients (Box 18-1). The frequency and amount of vomitus being produced is important to note, because fluid therapy is dictated largely by ongoing losses. In addition, the timing of the episodes (as related to food or water ingestion or administration of medications) is important to note. The presence of blood or foreign material also should be noted, because this may determine the need for specific therapy.

Diarrhea

As with vomiting, characterizing diarrhea is important in determining the underlying cause (Box 18-2). The team should note whether the diarrhea is frequent, whether straining accompanies the passage of feces, and whether frank blood (hematochezia) or black digested blood (melena) is present. High-frequency diarrhea usually is associated with the large intestine, as is straining. The presence of frank blood usually indicates colitis; however, patients with hypermotility disorders may have blood in the stool that is coming from the distal jejunum or ileum. The color of the stool, the presence of odor, and the presence of undigested food or foreign material should be noted, because these provide important clues about the health of the GI tract.

First Aid Measures

Owners often call veterinary hospitals indicating that their pet has evidence of a GI disorder. They may report vomiting or retching, diarrhea, or ingestion of foreign material. Some descriptions are very obvious emergencies, such as nonproductive retching and abdominal distention in a 2-year-old dog, indicating a high likelihood of gastric dilation and volvulus; however, some problems are not so easy to diagnose. In almost all situations the patient should be seen (because many patients who seem to have a minor problem based on the owner's description may actually have a serious or even life-threatening problem).

If the owner declines to bring in the pet on an emergency basis, he or she should remove food for at least 12 to 24 hours and water for at least 4 hours. When water is reintroduced, ice cubes or several teaspoons to tablespoons of water (depending on the size of the patient) or electrolyte solution should be offered every 1 to 2 hours. The owner should be advised to have the pet reexamined immediately if vomiting recurs. If the pet does well with water for 12 hours, then several teaspoons to tablespoons of a bland diet can be offered every 3 to 4 hours. If the pet vomits again, then examination is highly recommended. If the emergency call comes in at night and the owner refuses to have the pet examined, then it may be appropriate to have the owner withhold all water and food and have the pet examined first thing in the morning.

If the pet has ingested foreign material or a potential toxin, it may be appropriate to have the owner induce vomiting at home and then either bring in the pet for examination and treatment or monitor the pet at home. Vomiting should never be induced if the pet has an altered level of consciousness or is having breathing difficulties. Inducing vomiting is also contraindicated with the ingestion of a caustic toxin, a petroleum-based product, or a foreign body that may get stuck or cause trauma to the stomach, esophagus, or oral cavity as it is expelled.

Physical Examination

Patients with GI emergencies may be stable, critical, or any grade in between. A complete history and physical examination including a complete set of vital signs is performed in stable patients before initiating a diagnostic and therapeutic plan. In critically ill patients, rapid assessment is followed by immediate resuscitative measures, and no time may be available initially to take a full history or to perform a complete physical examination.

Patients with GI diseases may have a concurrent pneumothorax, secondary aspiration pneumonia, or metastatic disease, and close attention should be paid to the ventilatory pattern, the presence of cough, and bilateral auscultation of the thorax. The jugular vein should be clipped and evaluated for distention and filling time (less than 2 to 3 seconds), because this will provide a crude estimate of central venous pressure (CVP).

Blood pressure (BP) should be considered the fourth vital sign. Pulse palpation may provide a very inaccurate assessment of pressure, although monitoring the strength of metatarsal pulses can be used as a crude estimate of BP if indirect or direct BP monitoring is not available. Normal pressure in stable patients provides a baseline to use if the patient's condition deteriorates; if hypotension is present, then it helps identify a more unstable condition that otherwise would have been missed. In critical patients, and in stable patients with hypotension, it helps guide fluid resuscitation. A Doppler ultrasonic blood flow detector or an oscillometric device can be used; the Doppler is preferred, because it allows the clinician to evaluate perfusion or flow and BP. In addition, many arrhythmias can be detected with a Doppler. If the patient has any auscultable evidence of an arrhythmia or is unstable from a cardiovascular standpoint, then a lead II ECG should be assessed. Patients with myocardial hypoxia or ischemia secondary to circulatory shock often have ventricular premature contractions or ventricular tachycardia. These arrhythmias also are common in patients with splenic disease (i.e., gastric dilation and volvulus with concurrent splenic torsion).

Rectal thermometers may induce a vagally mediated arrest in the severely bradycardic or hypotensive patients and should not be used in these patients. Rectal temperatures also should not be used in patients with rectal trauma or bleeding. Instead, axillary or auricular temperatures should be taken. Rectal temperatures in patients with a dilated rectum may be very inaccurate because of the presence of air; the tip of the thermometer must be in contact with rectal mucosa. If concerned about the accuracy of the rectal temperature, then axillary, auricular, or colon temperatures (using a long thermometer probe) can be taken. If significant hypoperfusion is a concern, then toe web temperatures can be taken and compared with rectal temperatures. If the patient is perfusing normally, then the delta temperature (ΔT) should be less than $7°$ F.

The abdomen should be palpated, auscultated, and percussed with the goal of localizing pain and detecting fluid waves, gas-filled organs, or solid masses. A rectal examination should be performed and the presence of blood noted. The ventral abdomen should be clipped, because petechiation or ecchymoses may indicate thrombocytopenia or a coagulopathy. Distended superficial abdominal veins are consistent with increased intraabdominal pressure, which can be associated with decreased preload and decreased cardiac output.

Resuscitation of the Critical Patient

Patients with acute abdomen secondary to GI emergencies may be unstable from a respiratory and cardiovascular standpoint; therefore on presentation a primary survey examination (evaluation of level of consciousness, airway, breathing, and circulation) should be completed within 30 to 60 seconds, and abnormalities should be treated as indicated. For instance, a patient who arrives at the clinic obtunded with shallow respiration should be intubated, and positive pressure ventilation should be instituted. (This will help respiration and protect the airway against aspiration.) Depending on the severity of the patient's condition, fluid resuscitation may be initiated before a complete physical examination is performed. A very brief history is obtained at this time, if possible; however, resuscitation should not be delayed in the critically ill patient while a complete history is obtained. Instead, permission to start treatment should be obtained from the owner immediately (frequently done by the technician). Resuscitation of the critically ill patient also should not be delayed while diagnostic tests are being performed unless those tests are needed to guide resuscitation.

Oxygen (O_2) should be provided (by flow-by) to any patient showing signs of shock (using high flow rates [i.e., 3 to 15 L/min]). One or two large-bore peripheral catheters (14 to 16 gauge in medium and large dogs, 18 to 20 gauge in small dogs and cats) should be placed. A central line should be placed if CVP monitoring is indicated; however, this frequently is not performed until the patient is more stable. In dogs, perfusion abnormalities should be corrected as quickly as possible, with fluids given until BP is greater than 100 mm Hg systolic, heart rate approaches normal for the breed, digital pulses are palpable, and the patient's mentation has improved.

Usually 30 to 90 ml/kg of a balanced electrolyte solution (e.g., lactated Ringer's solution, Normosol-R, Plasmalyte-A) and 10 to 20 ml/kg of synthetic colloid (e.g., dextran 70, hetastarch, pentastarch) are needed. Alternatively, if pressures are almost nonexistent, then 7.5% hypertonic saline (1 ml/kg) with dextran 70 or hetastarch (3 ml/kg) can be given to effect. Because approximately 70% to 80% of crystalloids have left the intravascular space within 1 hour, in most cases IV colloids are needed because the volumes needed to resuscitate these animals with crystalloids alone may lead to tissue edema (peripheral, gut, and pulmonary). Fluid volumes should be reduced by about 30% in cats, and colloids should be given over 10 to 20 minutes. Many patients with sepsis are hypoglycemic and need an IV bolus of 25% dextrose (1 to 2 ml/kg or body weight), followed by dextrose supplementation in the fluids.

Diagnosis

Diagnostic tests are needed to determine the extent of the disease and confirm the diagnosis. The choice of tests may vary, based on the presenting complaint. Laboratory work, including packed cell volume (PCV), total solids (TS), blood urea nitrogen, and glucose should be part of an immediate database. Ideally, electrolytes and a venous blood gas analysis should be included in this initial database, because this information often will confirm the presence or absence of gastric or proximal duodenal obstructions and the degree of fluid loss into the GI tract. A complete blood cell count with microscopic evaluation of a blood smear for the differential, red cell morphology, and platelets provides important information. A more complete workup would include serum chemistries and a urinalysis. A prothrombin time and activated partial thromboplastin time (or activated clotting time) should be assessed in all critical patients and all those requiring surgery. A fecal screen, including a direct smear (to rule out parasites, clostridial spores, and certain pathogenic bacteria) and fecal flotation (as well as evaluation for *Giardia*) should be performed on all patients with diarrhea. A parvovirus test is indicated in all young dogs with hemorrhagic diarrhea, especially if the vaccination status is uncertain.

Survey abdominal radiographs usually are indicated. Chest radiographs ideally should be evaluated preoperatively in every injured patient and in any patient in whom aspiration pneumonia or metastases are a potential concern. Contrast studies including a barium series may be needed. Barium should not be used if the clinician is concerned about GI perforation or aspiration; water-soluble contrast material should be used instead. Abdominal ultrasound can be useful for diagnosis of some GI emergencies, but because ultrasound waves do not pass through air, the usefulness of ultrasound in patients with significant amounts of air in the GI tract can be limited.

Abdominocentesis (four quadrant or ultrasound guided) or diagnostic peritoneal lavage is indicated if peritonitis is a concern. Fluid should be evaluated for PCV, TS, white blood cell count, and chemistries (as indicated) and evaluated microscopically. Elevations in amylase or lipase will help to determine if the animal has a pancreatic or small bowel injury or inflammation. Vegetable fibers, degenerative white blood cells, and those with intracellular bacteria indicate GI content, contamination, and septic peritonitis.

Medical Treatment

Some GI emergencies can be managed medically, and some warrant emergency surgery (within minutes to hours of presentation); therefore the clinician should determine rapidly whether surgery is indicated. Acute abdominal conditions that warrant emergency surgery include a penetrating wound to the GI tract, a GI obstruction (e.g., foreign body, neoplasia), a GI tract accident (e.g., gastric or intestinal torsion or volvulus, intussusception), peritonitis, and vascular accidents (Box 18-3).

Fluids of the appropriate type are the most important therapy for patients with GI emergencies. IV fluids should be continued until the patient is drinking normally. The type of crystalloid to be administered, the use of colloids, and the rate of administration vary depending on the patient's status and underlying disease process. Generally replacement balanced electrolyte solutions (e.g., lactated Ringer's solution, Normosol-R, Plasmalyte-A) are infused; however, normal saline should be infused in patients with gastric obstructions. Fluid deficits should be calculated based on estimated dehydration (percent of dehydration times body weight in kilograms equals the number of liters of fluid deficit). This deficit should be replaced over the first 8 to 12 hours in the stable patient; however, in the unstable patient

---

BOX 18-3

Management of the Patient with Vomiting and Diarrhea

- Monitor vital signs every 4-8 hours (T, RR [and effort], HR, PR, BP, ECG, CVP, MM, CRT).
- Give nothing by mouth until the patient's vomiting is under control.
- Provide crystalloid fluid support:
  Correct dehydration over 2-6 hours if the patient is critical and over 8 to 12 hours if the patient is stable.
  Replace ongoing losses.
  Help to restore euvolemia (CVP between 5-8 cm of water, urine production 1-2 ml/kg/hr).
  Correct electrolyte and acid-base imbalances.
- Provide colloid fluid support:
  Normalize intravascular volume and organ perfusion (BP >110 mm Hg, CVP 5-8 cm of water, urine output 1-2 ml/kg/hr).
  Give fresh frozen plasma if albumin is <2.0 g/dl.
  Give red cells or hemoglobin if PCV <20%-25%.
- Ensure that NG tube is decompressed.
- Increase or decrease antiemetics.
- Increase or decrease antiulcer medications (H_2 blockers, ulcer-coating agents).
- Increase or decrease antibiotics.
- Provide nutritional support.
- Monitor PCV/TS, glucose, BUN, electrolytes, and venous/arterial blood gas every 8-24 hours.
- In critical patients, monitor coagulation parameters and albumin every 12-24 hours.

T, Temperature; *RR,* respiratory rate; *HR,* heart rate; *PR,* pulse rate; *BP,* blood pressure; *ECG,* electrocardiogram; *CVP,* central venous pressure; *MM,* mucous membranes; *CRT,* capillary refill time; *NG,* Nasogastric; *PCV,* packed cell volume; *TS,* total solids; *BUN,* blood urea nitrogen.

---

it may be necessary to replace this deficit in 2 to 6 hours. Ongoing losses are estimated, and both the fluid deficit and the ongoing loss volume are added to the calculated maintenance rate. Glucose and potassium should be supplemented based on laboratory results.

Synthetic colloids or human albumin are indicated if the albumin is less than 2.0 g/dl, if the colloid osmotic pressure is low, or if ongoing protein loss into the intestinal tract is possible. Constant rate infusions (CRIs) of synthetic colloids of up to 20 ml/kg/day may be needed. If the albumin is less than 2.0 g/dl, then human albumin or frozen plasma also is indicated. Fresh frozen plasma should be provided to correct any coagulopathy. Packed red blood cells or whole blood should be administered to keep the PCV at approximately 30%.

Broad-spectrum antibiotics covering aerobic and anaerobic bacteria are indicated if infection is a concern or if patients have hemorrhagic diarrhea. Inappropriate antibiotics use should be avoided, because it can lead to bacterial overgrowth and severe diarrhea, as well as potentially creating bacterial resistance and nosocomial infection problems. Like all medications, they should be given via IV in the vomiting patient.

Antiemetics are indicated if intractable vomiting occurs. Antiemetics are classified based on the mechanism of action; therefore knowing the cause (or possible cause) of the vomiting is important. Several classes of antiemetic medications exist. Phenothiazines (e.g., acepromazine, chlorpromazine, prochlorperazine) act at higher central nervous system centers and at the chemoreceptor trigger zone. They can cause significant hypotension, and BP should be monitored if any of this class of drug is being administered. Metoclopramide acts by enhancing gastric emptying, increasing lower esophageal sphincter tone, and acting centrally at the chemoreceptor trigger zone; clinically, metoclopramide is most effective when given via CRI. Anticholinergics act by decreasing GI secretions and motility; however, these agents are almost never used because even a single dose can lead to prolonged ileus. Serotonin antagonists such as ondansetron hydrochloride or dolasetron are some of the most effective antiemetics; however, they are expensive. Serotonin receptors are present in the chemoreceptor trigger zone, peripherally on vagal nerves, and in the GI tract; however, how the drug controls vomiting is unknown. Butorphanol is a fairly effective antiemetic that counteracts the nausea caused by certain medications (especially chemotherapeutic agents) and may help decrease vomiting caused by pain. Parenteral antiemetics should be used in most vomiting patients, because oral medications can cause vomiting and GI absorption is unreliable.

Ulcer prophylaxis is used in patients with evidence of hematemesis and those considered to be at risk for ulceration. This typically includes the use of an H_2-receptor antagonist (e.g., famotidine, ranitidine) or a proton pump inhibitor (e.g., omeprazole) and sucralfate.

Many patients with GI emergencies will exhibit some degree of pain on abdominal palpation (from very mild to severe). The degree of pain exhibited will vary with the underlying disease or injury and the nature of the animal. Patients who are depressed may not exhibit signs of pain initially; however, once resuscitation has been instituted, the pain will become evident. Typically the more severe the pain is, the more serious the problem. Pain always should be treated. Opioids such as butorphanol, oxymorphone, hydromorphone, morphine, and fentanyl are recommended. Buprenorphine is useful in cats with mild pain. Drugs should be given via IV, because absorption from subcutaneous or intramuscular sites may be unpredictable. In cases of severe pain, CRIs may be required. Alternatively, epidural analgesia using morphine, oxymorphone, or hydromorphone can be administered. This is a very effective means of controlling pain; if an epidural catheter is placed, then repeat doses can be given. In the critical patients, doses of opioids may need to be reduced to 25% to 50% of normal because patients often cannot tolerate normal doses. For those patients who are not responding as desired to systemic analgesics, a peritoneal lavage may provide significant pain relief, especially in patients with pancreatitis or serositis. Nonsteroidal antiinflammatory drugs should not be used because of their negative effects on splanchnic organs (and, in some cases, coagulation). Very small doses of an anxiolytic such as midazolam or acepromazine may be useful if the patient is very anxious. Acepromazine should be used with extreme caution in hypotensive patients because of its α-adrenergic blocking effects.

Patients with an acute abdomen may have hypothermia, or they may become hypothermic during resuscitation secondary to intravascular infusion of large volumes of room temperature fluids. Hypothermia interferes with normal metabolic functions leading to vasodilation, cardiac dysfunction, and interference with the coagulation cascade. Core rewarming should be instituted, because peripheral rewarming may lead to worsening of the vasodilation and subsequent worsening of the hypothermia. Artificial-warming devices should be insulated from the patient because they can cause burns. Means of rewarming patients include the use of warm-water bottles, warm-water circulating blankets, oat bags, warm blankets, and hot-air circulating devices. Fluids should be infused at normal body temperature in the hypothermic patient.

Appropriate catheter care is important in these patients. Peripheral venous catheters should be checked hourly to ensure they are still patent, and veins should be checked several times daily for phlebitis. Central catheter sites should have external bandages changed daily to every 3 days; care should be taken not to manipulate the catheter. If patients have indwelling urinary catheters, then the vulva or prepuce should be disinfected three times daily and antibiotic ointment should be applied around the catheter entry site.

If silent regurgitation and aspiration are concerns, the head and neck should be kept slightly elevated (30 degrees). Patients with limited mobility may require passive range of motion exercises and sling walking. Larger patients who are recumbent should be provided with padded bedding, and all recumbent patients should be turned every 2 to 4 hours.

Nasogastric Tubes. NG tubes are used for both decompression of the stomach and for delivery of enteral nutrition. Decompression is indicated in all patients in whom significant volumes of air or fluid are accumulating. Gastric distention is one of the major triggers for vomiting; if gastric distention can be prevented, then the frequency of vomiting can be reduced. NG tubes should be placed in all patients who are aerophagic, have a tendency to bloat, are vomiting frequently, have gastric motility disorders or megaesophagus, or are at risk for silent regurgitation and aspiration. Suctioning is indicated every hour initially until large volumes of air and fluid are not accumulating. (Fluid volumes of up to 1 ml/kg/hr may be normal.) Continuous suction devices are available if prolonged frequent suctioning is indicated. Once air is no longer being suctioned and volume of fluid being suctioned decreases to less than 1 ml/kg/hr, the frequency of suctioning should be reduced to every 4 to 6 hours. If large volumes of fluid are being aspirated, then electrolytes must be closely monitored.

Nutritional Support. Enteral nutrition should be started as soon as possible based on the patient's underlying condition and clinical status. Initially, microenteral nutrition is recommended. Microenteral nutrition is composed of electrolytes and dextrose (2.5% to 5%) given in small volumes. The fluid is infused via the NG tube starting at rates of 0.1 to 0.25 ml/kg/hr, either as a bolus or CRI. This rate is slowly increased up to 1 ml/kg/hr over 24 to 48 hours

depending on the patient. Once this is tolerated a liquid diet can be provided via the NG tube, or gruel of canned food (small amounts) is offered orally. Microenteral nutrition usually can be started within the first 12 to 24 hours after admission. Glucose solutions delivered to the gastric mucosa have been shown to help prevent gastric ulceration and may help improve splanchnic blood flow, thereby decreasing the chance for bacterial translocation. Clinically the use of microenteral feeding appears to be associated with a quicker return to normal enteral nutrition. This may be because of the microenteral nutrition helping to preserve GI function.

When patients will not tolerate enteral nutrition, parenteral nutrition is indicated. Partial parenteral nutrition (comprised of 3% amino acids and glycerol or dextrose) can be easily and inexpensively administered. These solutions are hyperosmolar and are ideally administered via central venous catheters; however, they can be provided via peripheral IV catheters. These solutions act primarily as protein-sparing solutions and do not provide total nutritional support. As such they should only be used for short-term nutritional support. Total parenteral nutrition is indicated in any patient who is not expected to be able to tolerate enteral nutrition for at least 5 to 7 days. Parenteral solutions should be used with caution in patients who are not completely fluid resuscitated or those not well hydrated.

Monitoring. The number of parameters being monitored and the frequency of monitoring will depend on the patient's underlying condition and status. If the patient's condition is critical, then parameters should be monitored every 30 to 60 minutes; in extremely critical patients, parameters may need to be monitored every 5 minutes or even continuously. In more stable patients, monitoring may be indicated every 4 to 8 hours. The technician often is the person spending the most time with the patient; observations on patient discomfort and how the patient is progressing are vital. As with all hospitalized patients, good communication between the technician and doctor helps ensure patient morbidity is minimized.

All vital signs should be monitored closely, including level of consciousness, respiratory rate and effort, heart rate, pulse rate, pulse strength, BP, temperature, mucous membrane color, and capillary refill time. CVP monitoring is indicated in any patient who has signs of moderate to severe shock, any patient in whom large volumes of fluids are being used for resuscitation, and in any patient in whom fluid overload is a concern. ECG monitoring should be performed in all patients with arrhythmias or those at risk for arrhythmias. Urine output should be quantitated if renal function is a concern, otherwise it should be estimated.

Laboratory work should consist of a minimum of a PCV, TS, glucose, blood urea nitrogen, and electrolytes. Ideally venous blood gas should be assessed at the same time, along with serum albumin. IV fluids (type, rate, and supplements) should be adjusted based on these results. Potassium frequently requires supplementation unless the patient is receiving parenteral nutrition. These tests should be repeated every 12 to 24 hours, more frequently if the patient is extremely critical or if the clinician is concerned about certain parameters such as hypoglycemia. Complete blood cell counts and coagulation parameters should be monitored every 24 to 48 hours depending on the patient's status.

Fluid rates will need to be adjusted based on output, including ongoing losses, NG suctioning, and urine output. Patients receiving IV fluid therapy rarely urinate less frequently than every 6 to 8 hours; if this occurs, then fluid therapy may not be adequate.

Importance of Record Keeping. Continued 24-hour care is ideal and should be strived for in all GI emergency patients. The watchword is *diligent care*, from the time of arrival, through the course of hospitalization. All monitoring and treatments must be recorded. A flowchart should be used to record this information in chronologic order, because remembering what happened hours after the event is difficult. To decrease morbidity from things such as inadequate fluid support, inadequate use of antiemetics, and insufficient nutritional support, accurate and thorough record keeping is essential.

Anesthesia and Surgery

Surgical treatment is indicated in many GI emergencies. The sun should never rise or set on an esophageal or GI obstruction. Valuable time can be saved if the technician has the operating room ready so that an emergency surgery can be done within minutes. Ideally, at least three people—a surgeon, assistant surgeon, and anesthetist—are available to treat these patients. Balanced anesthesia with intensive BP

monitoring (if possible with a Doppler ultrasonic flow detector) and assisted ventilation is essential. In the unstable patient, efforts should be made to use anesthetic agents that have the least effect on the cardiovascular system, and the anesthetist should try to keep the animal at the lightest possible level of anesthesia to minimize cardiovascular depression. Effective use of analgesia with IV or intrathecal opioids minimizes the general anesthetic needed, makes the patient more comfortable, and reduces patient morbidity both preoperatively and postoperatively. Most of these patients do not ventilate well under anesthesia and may need hand ventilation or mechanical ventilation. Positive pressure ventilation will help prevent respiratory acidosis (which can contribute significantly to hypotension), prevent atelectasis, minimize the amount of inhalant that is required, and promote a less complicated recovery. Many currently available anesthetic ventilators are very easy to operate and allow the technician to attend to other important anesthetic tasks. Broad-spectrum antibiotics should be given before the lumen of the bowel is incised.

The entire abdomen, including the inguinal regions and flanks, should be clipped and surgically prepared. The caudal third of the thorax also should be clipped and surgically prepared to provide adequate exposure in anticipation of a full exploratory celiotomy, including the exposure of the inguinal canals for additional venous access and extension into the chest via a parasternal approach if needed. A full exploratory celiotomy consists of a ventral midline incision from the xiphoid to near the pubis; this should be anticipated in every patient with a GI surgical emergency.

Every effort should be made to prevent hypothermia because it promotes vasoconstriction and poor tissue perfusion, decreases immune function, and prolongs coagulation time. Preventing hypothermia is especially important in intestinal surgery, in which the intestine often must be placed outside the abdomen where it cools down to room temperature rapidly. Supplemental heat can be provided by various means; the patient always should be protected to ensure that burns do not occur. Patients should be placed on warmed surgical tables or on warm-water circulating blankets. Warm-air circulating blankets are the most effective at preventing heat loss and actively warming patients. IV fluids should be warmed before administration and kept warm during administration (by keeping them in a commercial warming unit or running the administration tubing through a warm-water circuit or warm-water bath). When the abdomen is open, the exposed contents should be covered with laparotomy pads or towels as much as possible to prevent evaporative heat and water loss.

Occasionally the technician may be assisting with surgery. An attempt should be made to set aside a set of instruments for closing (or a separate pack should be made available), because once the instruments have penetrated the GI tract, they are contaminated. Ideally, radiopaque gauze sponges and laparotomy pads should be used. Sponges and laparotomy pads should be counted at the beginning of the surgery and then immediately before closure. Moistened sponges or laparotomy pads will be needed to isolate the affected area of the GI tract. The assistant inserting a Poole suction tip into the stomach or intestine as soon as the incision has been made will help to minimize spillage of GI contents.

The abdomen should be lavaged adequately with warm sterile saline before closures. Usually 1 to 3 L is needed unless the patient has peritonitis, in which case up to 10 L may be indicated. Lavage helps flush out any contamination, reduce adhesions, and rewarm the patient. The temperature of the irrigation fluid should be 100° F to 105° F.

Ideally an NG tube is placed at the time of surgery, before the abdomen is closed, so that the surgeon can verify its placement. Otherwise a radiograph may need to be taken to confirm placement in the appropriate location. The NG tube allows postoperative decompression and early enteral nutritional support. Animals undergoing an exploratory celiotomy will not have normal gastric motility for at least 24 hours. Suctioning air and excess fluid, not only prevents vomiting but also ensures that gastric motility will return to normal more rapidly. An esophagostomy, gastrostomy, duodenostomy, or jejunostomy tube may be needed for postoperative nutritional support. If it is anticipated that the patient will not be eating normally for at least 3 days postoperatively, then a feeding tube should be placed.

Before extubation the oropharynx should be evaluated for signs of regurgitation. If vomitus is noted, then the oropharynx should be suctioned and strong consideration should be given to lavage and suction of the esophagus. This often is indicated in patients with gastric dilation and volvulus, in whom passive regurgitation is common. Lavage and suction of the esophagus helps prevent silent aspiration and pneumonia. Failure to remove gastric contents from the esophagus and pharynx can lead to inflammation, erosion, and possibly ulceration of these areas.

Postoperative Care

Postoperative monitoring should be performed as described previously except that parameters may need to be monitored more closely until the patient is normothermic and sternal. Patients ideally should not be disconnected from a ventilator until it is confirmed that the patient is able to maintain a normal end-tidal carbon dioxide concentration while spontaneously breathing. High levels of supplemental O_2 should be provided in the immediate postoperative period to all patients (recent research has shown that doing this improves healing in patients who have undergone intestinal surgery). Providing high levels of supplemental O_2 may not be feasible in most veterinary patients; however, supplemental O_2 is definitely recommended in critically ill or injured patients after surgery.

Postoperative laboratory work in the critically ill or injured patient should consist of a minimum of a PCV, TS, and glucose. Electrolytes, blood urea nitrogen, and albumin also should be checked.

Microenteral nutrition is started within 6 hours in the postoperative patient or as soon as the patient is sternal, normothermic, and normotensive.

Jejunostomy Feeding Tubes. Placement of jejunostomy tubes is done in anticipation that the upper GI tract, including the stomach and pancreas, is going to require a rest, with no food being presented to the stomach for at least several days. Liquid diets that are either polymeric (which will require digestion) or monomeric (which will not require digestion) are used as a CRI through these tubes. They allow early and progressive feeding in such conditions as pancreatitis and complicated gastric surgery. Generally 1 to 2 ml/kg/hr is administered throughout the course of the day and tapered off at night. The exit site of these tubes is inspected and cleaned every day, and antibiotic ointment is placed around the tube exit site to help prevent infection.

Specific Gastrointestinal Emergencies

Foreign Bodies

Foreign bodies are some of the most common causes of vomiting in the young dog or cat; however, animals of any age can ingest foreign material. Fortunately many foreign bodies pass or are vomited without serious consequence; however, frequently these materials will cause a partial or complete obstruction of the GI tract, and endoscopic or surgical intervention is required to remove the material.

Esophageal Foreign Bodies. Esophageal foreign bodies are sometimes dealt with in a different manner from GI foreign bodies. Therefore esophageal foreign bodies are discussed first (and the discussion of GI foreign bodies follows).

History and Clinical Signs. History is very important in the diagnosis of an esophageal foreign body. The animal may have signs of salivation, excessive swallowing, dysphagia, and apparent vomiting (which on closer questioning will be determined to be regurgitation). Animals with an upper or midesophageal foreign body may have signs of respiratory distress, because the foreign material may be compressing the trachea. Harsh lung sounds may indicate aspiration pneumonia.

Diagnosis. Some foreign bodies may be palpable. Radiographs and esophagoscopy can be used to locate the material if not readily visible. Barium should not be used if a perforation is possible; instead a low osmolarity nonionic contrast material should be used.

Treatment. Perfusion deficits should be corrected before anesthesia and antibiotics are started. General anesthesia should be used, and a cuffed endotracheal tube must be in place. The degree of hypoperfusion and dehydration present is easy to underestimate, and fluid requirements to maintain normal BP under anesthesia may be higher than expected. Suctioning any esophageal fluid or contrast material will aid in observation and removal of the material, as well as in the prevention of aspiration pneumonia. Frequently the foreign material lodges at the base of the heart, and significant bradycardia may be present. Anticholinergics often are used, both to help decrease salivation and to help prevent severe bradycardia.

Often the clinician can remove the foreign body by the oral route using a rigid or flexible endoscope. A rigid endoscope and a "mechanic's helper" (or mare uterine biopsy forceps) are most useful. Generous amounts of lubrication (water-soluble jelly and water) should be used. The lubrication can be placed at the location of the foreign body using a stiff polyethylene catheter with its tip placed at the junction of the foreign body and the esophageal mucosa. By gentle manipulation after lubrication, the foreign body is bought close to the end of the rigid endoscope, and all three objects (foreign body, grasper, and endoscope) are pulled out together.

If the foreign body cannot be removed orally, then it may be possible to manipulate it into the stomach (where the foreign body is removed via a gastrotomy). If it cannot be manipulated into the stomach, then the foreign material will need to be removed via an esophagotomy. After removal, a gastrostomy feeding tube may be placed to bypass the esophagus (allowing it to heal while providing enteral nutritional support). Some clinicians may prefer to use a small flexible esophagostomy tube (with its tip distal to the site of injury or surgical incision). The authors are not aware of any contraindications for the use of esophagostomy feeding after esophageal surgery.

Gastrointestinal Foreign Bodies

History and Clinical Signs. History gathered from an owner is the most useful factor in early diagnosis of a foreign body. Early signs of a GI foreign body include nausea, vomiting, and inappetance. Vomiting usually persists until the material has passed, been vomited, or is removed. The character of the vomiting may indicate the location of the problem and the degree of obstruction. Abdominal pain may or may not be present, depending on the duration of the problem and the degree of obstruction.

Diagnosis. The GI foreign body may be directly palpable on physical examination. Abdominal pain is a warning sign, and splinting may indicate the presence of a surgical disorder. Vomiting at the time of or at the conclusion of palpation of the abdomen is a significant indicator that the animal has a surgical abdomen. Survey radiographs may reveal radiopaque foreign bodies, and an abnormally gas-distended loop of bowel may indicate an obstruction. Contrast radiographs may be needed to locate the material. Loss of detail on radiographs suggests the possibility of peritonitis, and a sample of fluid should be procured immediately for analysis.

Treatment. The patient with a foreign body may arrive at the clinic in stable condition, in hyperdynamic shock, or in decompensatory (hypodynamic) shock. Fluid therapy should be guided by the patient's status. Many patients with intestinal foreign bodies cannot be stabilized completely until surgery is performed.

Surgery is indicated in the vast majority of these patients and in all patients with significant clinical signs or a radiographic pattern of distended bowel loops. In some patients, rehydration "lubricates" the bowel and allows the lodged material to pass, but this is uncommon. In the critically ill or unstable patient, prompt surgery may be needed, because pressure necrosis can lead to bowel perforation. Operating early is best, even if a foreign body is only a slight possibility. Safety pins, straight pins, and other identifiable gastric or intestinal foreign bodies should be removed if clinical signs are present. The only time a watch-and-wait attitude is taken is if no clinical signs are seen. In these cases, serial radiographs should be taken to monitor the progress of the object. These objects generally pass through the GI tract without any difficulty; however, if the object has a string attached to it, then exploratory surgery should be performed. If any doubt exists regarding the nature of the foreign body or whether it will pass, then surgery should be performed. Significantly radiopaque foreign bodies should be removed immediately, because they may contain zinc, which can cause a hemolytic anemia.

Gastric Dilation and Volvulus

Cause and Pathophysiology. The cause of gastric dilation and volvulus is not yet clearly understood. Gastric dilation and volvulus has been associated with many clinical entities and typically is seen in large deep-chested dogs. However, it can occur in any size of dog, and typically an underlying cause is never discovered. Gastric dilation and volvulus has been observed in patients who ingest foreign material, in patients with chronic debilitating diseases, in patients with altered gastric emptying, in patients with neuromuscular diseases or respiratory difficulty, as well as in animals requiring hospitalization that are very nervous.

Twisting causes a one-way valve effect at the gastroesophageal junction, allowing swallowed air to enter the stomach but not leave. Carbon dioxide also may accumulate secondary to bacterial fermentation, diffusion from trapped blood, and metabolism of gastric acid and bicarbonate from the pancreas and saliva. Normal fluid secretion into

the stomach (as well as transudation from venous congestion) contributes to gastric distention. Subsequent pressure on the diaphragm from the distended stomach can lead to respiratory distress, which also may worsen the aerophagia. The gastric distention causes compression of the vena cava, resulting in a decrease in venous return that negatively affects cardiac output. Gastric distension also compromises gastric circulation, causing ischemia of the stomach. Rotation of the stomach can cause tearing of the short gastric vessels, which can lead to significant blood loss.

The distension and rotation of the stomach, which can also occur to some extent with distension alone, causes partial to complete blockage of the portal vein. The degree of venous obstruction of the portal vein is variable, and the liver, pancreas, small intestine, and stomach all become ischemic to some degree. Portal vein obstruction also contributes to decreased preload.

Toxic and vasoactive substances accumulate secondary to the ischemia. Ultimately hemorrhagic, distributive, and cardiogenic forms of shock can develop. Reperfusion injury during treatment contributes significantly to the tissue damage.

History and Clinical Signs. Patients commonly have a history of attempting to vomit or nonproductive retching. Abdominal distention may or may not be noted by the owner. The onset is usually acute. It also may be associated with dietary indiscretion, such as ingestion of unleavened bread, garbage, or poorly digestible dog treats. A history of GI disease or previous episodes of "bloating" may also exist.

On presentation, dogs are usually showing some degree of circulatory shock. Pressure on the diaphragm caused by a progressively dilating stomach may compromise lung expansion and lead to ventilatory compromise. Salivation, nausea, and nonproductive retching may or may not be present.

Diagnosis. The clinician commonly makes his or her diagnosis using the patient's history, clinical signs, and physical examination. Abdominal distention may or may not be present, based on the degree of gastric distention and the conformation of the breed. The gas-distended stomach will be detectable on percussion of the cranial abdomen. Because the dog may be in hyperdynamic shock or in a stage of decompensatory shock, findings vary from tachycardia, tachypnea, bounding pulses, and injected mucous membranes to collapse, respiratory distress, and weak thready pulses.

A right lateral abdominal radiograph should be taken. On occasion, the volvulus will not be evident on the right lateral view; however, if the clinician believes that the volvulus is still possible, then a left lateral radiograph should taken. A characteristic shelf sign with compartmentalization supports a diagnosis of a gastric volvulus. Chest radiographs should be taken to rule out aspiration pneumonia and metastases.

Treatment. Treatment should be instituted before taking radiographs, unless the presence of a volvulus will lead the owner to make a decision to have the dog euthanized. Immediate treatment should consist of O_2 if the dog is showing any signs of shock, as well as volume replacement with crystalloids and synthetic colloids. BP should be monitored closely. An ECG should be monitored, because these dogs are prone to ventricular arrhythmias. The stomach should be decompressed only after volume replacement has been started because of the potential for worsening the hypovolemic shock. Rapid-onset corticosteroids can be given (dexamethasone sodium phosphate at 4 to 8 mg/kg IV or methylprednisolone sodium succinate at 15 to 30 mg/kg IV), and broad-spectrum antibiotics should be started. Coagulation parameters should be monitored closely, because these patients are at risk for disseminated intravascular coagulation.

Gastrocentesis to decompress the stomach is performed using a 12- to 16-gauge needle or catheter after percussion to identify the best insertion location. This procedure is usually followed by immediate surgery; if the owner declines surgery, then lavage may be indicated. Effluent that is bloody or very dark indicates the possibility of gastric necrosis. Until the clinician confirms that the stomach is back into normal anatomic position, the patient continues to be at high risk.

Immediate surgery for gastric dilation and volvulus is indicated for several reasons. It can be difficult to confirm that the stomach is in its correct anatomic position without surgery. In addition, determining if gastric necrosis or active hemorrhage is present (usually from tearing of the short gastric vessels) or if the spleen is thombosed (secondary to partial or complete torsion) is almost impossible without performing surgery. Gastric lavage can be performed before or during surgery; however, it should

be remembered that passing a stomach tube on a twisted stomach is possible. Passing a stomach tube through the wall of an ischemic stomach is also possible; therefore excessive force should not be used.

Intestinal "Accidents"

Other intestinal disorders requiring rapid surgical intervention include intestinal intussusception and mesenteric volvulus.

History and Clinical Signs. If seen early in the disease process, then these patients may show only signs of possible restlessness and nausea. Late in the disease they may have a history of vomiting, diarrhea (which may or may not be hemorrhagic), abdominal distension, and possible abdominal pain.

Diagnosis. Palpation may reveal an intussusception; however, in the case of a sliding intussusception that may reduce itself intermittently, diagnosis can be challenging. These animals generally are painful on abdominal palpation and significant splinting may be present. Gut sounds may or may not be present. Survey radiographs may reveal gas-distended loops of bowel; however, in some cases a contrast series may be required. Ultrasound is very useful for diagnosing an intussusception. Surgical exploration must be done as soon as possible. In the case of a mesenteric volvulus, endotoxic shock commonly leads to death; therefore surgery is indicated immediately on presentation if the animal is to have any hope of survival. Prognosis with mesenteric volvulus is grave.

Treatment. As with all patients in shock, resuscitation should be initiated immediately. Close monitoring is required, because these patients may have a complicated preoperative, operative, and postoperative course. Surgery is needed as soon as possible. Enteroplication (a procedure in which the small intestine is folded back and forth and sutured together from the duodenum to the colon) may be performed on patients with an intussusception to help prevent recurrence.

Hemorrhagic Gastroenteritis

History and Clinical Signs. The patient with hemorrhagic gastroenteritis usually is unmistakable because of the presence of blood (frank or digested) in the vomitus or diarrhea. Occasionally, especially with cats, no history of vomiting or diarrhea exists. A characteristic foul odor to the stool is identified, most often with rectal examination. Onset may be peracute or may be more chronic. In the peracute cases, profound septic shock may be present. A bleeding ulcer (with or without perforation) may be present if the patient has a history of nonsteroidal antiinflammatory drug use. These patients may arrive at the clinic in severe hemorrhagic shock.

Diagnosis. Because of the multiple causes of blood in the vomitus or stool, many tests may be required to get a diagnosis. A much-dilated rectum is present on rectal examination in almost all parvovirus patients (almost never present in other causes of hemorrhagic diarrhea in puppies). In the emergency patient the most important lab tests include those that assess the degree of anemia or hemoconcentration, a complete blood cell count, fecal parvovirus test, coagulation parameters and radiographs to rule out the presence of a foreign body. Abdominal radiographs usually reveal a small to moderate amount of gas throughout the small and large intestine, but a characteristic obstructive pattern is not observed. Free air indicates a perforation of the GI tract. A contrast series, endoscopy, and possibly exploratory surgery may be required to diagnose and treat the patient. Parvovirus enteritis may appear as a surgical abdomen; fortunately the antigen test is usually positive, negating the need for surgery.

Treatment. IV fluids should be given according to the parameters noted on presentation, the degree of perfusion abnormality, and the underlying disease. In the patient with idiopathic hemorrhagic gastroenteritis, rapid boluses of crystalloids to restore a normal hematocrit and normal rheology may be required. Synthetic colloids frequently are needed because of the low colloid osmotic pressure often associated with this disease. In the poorly perfused parvovirus patient, colloids may be required as part of the initial resuscitation for the same reason. Because of *third spacing* of fluids into the gut in the hemorrhagic gastroenteritis patient, severely underestimating the volume of fluids required is easy to do. Close attention must be paid to maintaining normal heart rate, normal BP, and normal CVP. IV broad-spectrum antibiotics should be used to cover the range of pathogens that could be contributing to endotoxin and exotoxin effects in the seriously ill patient. Ulcer

prophylaxis is indicated frequently. Plasma may be required early on in the disease to replace albumin and clotting factors. Red blood cell transfusions may be required if blood loss is significant.

In the case of severe gastric ulceration and bleeding, lavage of the stomach with ice water may be required. Some cases of GI ulceration may require surgical intervention, especially if perforation is a possibility.

Pancreatitis

Cause and Pathophysiology. Pancreatitis ultimately is a result of activation of the pancreatic enzymes (proteases) within the pancreas, which lead to autodigestion, as well as digestion of the peripancreatic tissues, with subsequent activation of the inflammatory process through neutrophil activation and production of cytokines and free radicals. If the inflammatory cascades persist unabated, then the systemic inflammatory response syndrome can result. Plasma protease inhibitors such as the α-macroglobulins are consumed as the process continues.

Grossly, pancreatitis progresses from that of edema and saponification to abscess formation, followed by hemorrhagic pancreatitis and localized peritonitis. Secondary biliary blockage and necrosis of the ventral aspect of the duodenum can occur.

Multiple causes of pancreatitis have been identified; however, the underlying cause is rarely known, and most cases are diagnosed as idiopathic. Dietary indiscretion appears to be a common predisposing factor in dogs, and cholangiohepatitis and inflammatory bowel disease appear to be involved in many cats.

History and Clinical Signs. These patients may have signs similar to those of other GI emergencies. Anorexia and intermittent vomiting may be the only signs in cats. Dogs typically have a history of dietary indiscretion followed by nausea, vomiting, and anorexia. Diarrhea may be present late in the disease. Abdominal pain is present; in mild cases it can be localized to the upper-right quadrant of the abdomen. If seen early in the disease process, then these patients may only appear to act abnormally, with possible restlessness and nausea. Late in the disease they may have a history of vomiting, diarrhea (which may or may not be hemorrhagic), abdominal distention, and abdominal pain.

Diagnosis. The diagnosis of pancreatitis often is difficult and may be a presumptive diagnosis based on history, clinical signs, and physical examination findings of upper-right quadrant abdominal pain. Pancreatic enzyme elevation is an inconsistent finding. Abdominal radiographs often reveal loss of detail in the right cranial quadrant and displacement of the descending duodenum to the right with gas in the duodenum. Ultrasound can be very useful in diagnosing pancreatitis in dogs, but false negatives are common in cats. Evaluation of abdominal fluid, obtained via abdominocentesis or diagnostic peritoneal lavage, for pancreatic enzyme concentrations and cytology can help confirm the diagnosis and rule out peritonitis.

Treatment. Fluid therapy is the cornerstone of treatment for pancreatitis. Crystalloids, synthetic colloids, and plasma often are indicated. Patients with pancreatitis often are in pain, and opioids should be used as frequently as needed to control the pain. Abdominal lavage clinically appears to help alleviate the pain, probably by diluting enzymes and other factors from the inflamed pancreas. The surgical management of pancreatitis is controversial. If the patient has signs of peritonitis, then a pancreatic abscess (or phlegmon) is not clinically improving after several days of medical management or is deteriorating, and surgery is indicated. Ideally an intestinal feeding tube is placed for nutritional support in all patients who undergo surgery for pancreatitis. Nutritional management of pancreatitis is controversial. In the past it was recommended not to feed patients with pancreatitis for 5 to 7 days. Studies over the past decade in humans have shown that oral feeding can be provided as long as no clinical exacerbation of the pancreatitis is seen. The authors recommend trickle feeding with small amounts of a liquid low-fat diet.

Peritonitis

History and Clinical Signs. Patients who have an acute rupture or perforation of a hollow viscus (usually secondary to trauma) may appear to act abnormally, with possible restlessness and nausea. Late in the disease they may have a history of vomiting, diarrhea (which may or may not be hemorrhagic), abdominal pain, and possibly abdominal distention. These patients arrive at the clinic in varying degrees of shock, depending on the length of time they have been sick and the cause of the peritonitis.

Diagnosis. Peritonitis may be diagnosed definitively by microscopic evaluation of fluid obtained via abdominocentesis (or diagnostic peritoneal lavage). A fluid blood glucose less than 50 mg/dl or a blood to fluid difference of greater than 20 mg/dl is consistent with septic peritonitis. Abdominal ultrasound can be useful in helping to determine the underlying cause. Because patients with peritonitis may have many systemic abnormalities, complete laboratory work is recommended. Chest radiographs may be indicated to rule out concurrent injuries, aspiration pneumonia, or metastases.

Treatment. These patients require fluid resuscitation, antibiotics, and analgesics as with other serious intraabdominal conditions. A complete exploratory surgery is indicated as soon as possible after diagnosis and initial resuscitation. Surgically placed feeding tubes frequently are indicated. Antibiotic therapy is best guided by culture and sensitivity results. Before receiving the results, it should be assumed that a mixed infection is present.

The abdominal cavity is either left open or closed, and closed-suction drains are placed. Open abdominal drainage allows for septic material to drain externally, allows for repeat evaluations of the intraabdominal process to be done easily, and (by permitting air to enter) decreases the survival of anaerobic bacteria. The linea alba is sutured in a continuous pattern; however, the suture is left loose, allowing a gap of approximately 2 to 3 cm. The incision is covered with sterile highly absorbent towels or laparotomy pads followed by an abdominal bandage. To facilitate changing the abdominal dressing, it can be held in place by umbilical tape that has been laced from one end of the incision to the other. Suture loops can be tied on either side of the abdominal incision (approximately 4 to 5 cm from the edges of the incision). The sterile towels or laparotomy pads are placed, and umbilical tape is laced in between the suture loops to hold the dressing in place. When it comes time to change the dressing, the umbilical tape is untied, the dressing is easily removed, and then a new dressing is placed. A urinary catheter and closed collection system definitely is indicated in the male dog and highly recommended in the female dog. Open abdominal drainage typically is required for 3 to 5 days.

The abdominal dressing is evaluated every 6 to 8 hours and changed between one and three times per day or when strike-through is evident. The dressing change is done aseptically and may require light sedation. General anesthesia is provided if the veterinarian intends to perform a second-look laparotomy. A second-look laparotomy typically is performed if the drainage from the abdomen does not begin to decrease in volume, becomes worse in character, when the initial repair performed or tissue viability was believed tenuous, or in cases in which deep intraabdominal abscesses, septic disease processes, or both are present.

The amount of fluid lost through the drainage can be estimated by weighing the dressings removed and comparing this weight to that of a similar amount of dry dressings. The difference in weight of the dressings represents the amount of fluid drained with 1 gram equaling 1 ml of fluid. The amount of protein lost can be estimated by measuring the concentration of total protein in the fluid and multiplying this number by the estimated amount of fluid drained. Fluid can be examined microscopically to trace the cellular changes within the abdominal cavity.

Open abdominal drainage is associated with a number of complications, including significant hypoproteinemia necessitating plasma transfusions, electrolyte abnormalities, hypothermia, ascending infection, evisceration, and additional costs associated with bandage changes and a second surgery.

Closed-suction drainage may provide an alternative to open abdominal drainage. After irrigation, closed-suction drains are placed in the cranial abdomen and the abdomen is closed. The drains are left in place until the amount of fluid being produced is within physiologic limits and the fluid cytology shows no signs of active inflammation or infection. Recent reports, as well as personal experience, suggest this method of drainage is effective and minimizes patient morbidity.

Conclusion

Animals with GI disease can deteriorate very quickly, especially when vomiting, diarrhea, or both are present. Almost all calls from owners involving an animal with some form of GI distress should be considered emergencies. Evaluating this kind of problem over the phone is difficult, and what may be described by the owner as mild discomfort may be life threatening.

Surgery for GI emergencies can be very challenging. Therefore the facility must be equipped with a highly skilled team to stabilize and monitor these patients throughout treatment.

19

Metabolic and Endocrine Emergencies

RICHARD W. REID

Patients with metabolic and endocrine emergencies are some of the most demanding and critical cases who arrive at the intensive care unit. With careful attention to details and patient monitoring, these animals can be some of the most rewarding patients to be treated. This chapter discusses diabetic ketoacidosis (DKA), hypoadrenocorticism, hypercalcemia, hypocalcemia, and hypoglycemia.

Diabetic Ketoacidosis

Definition

DKA (or ketoacidotic diabetes mellitus) is a complicated form of diabetes mellitus that can have fatal consequences in dogs and cats. Patients with insulin-dependent diabetes mellitus have an absolute or relative insulin deficiency. As a result, the body's cells (except the brain and heart) are unable to take up glucose via insulin-dependent insulin receptors located in the cell membrane. Insulin deficiency initiates lipolysis (the breakdown of stored body fat into fatty acids) and promotes the conversion of the released fatty acids into glucose precursors in the liver via a process called *beta oxidation*. Additionally, the body experiences increased secretion of the stress hormones, glucagons, cortisol, catecholamines, and growth hormone. These hormones are gluconeogenic and promote beta oxidation. The by-products of beta oxidation are ketoacids (i.e., acetoacetate, β-hydroxybutyrate, acetone), which cause acidosis.

Presentation

Diabetes mellitus in dogs can occur from 4 to 14 years of age, with most patients 7 to 9 years of age. Females are affected nearly twice as frequently as males. Diabetes seems to be common in poodles, miniature schnauzers, beagles, and dachshunds, and has a genetic basis in keeshonds and golden retrievers. A genetic basis for diabetes mellitus may exist in cairn terriers and miniature pinschers. Diabetes mellitus can be diagnosed at any age in the cat; however, most are 6 years of age or older. No breed predisposition has been identified, but neutered males are predominantly affected.

BOX 19-1

Most Common Clinical Signs Associated with Diabetes and Ketoacidosis

Anorexia
Dehydration
Dry flaky skin
Ketotic breath
Lethargy/depression
Muscle wasting
Panting or Kussmaul's type of breathing
Plantigrade stance (cats, usually)
Polydipsia
Polyphagia (nonketotic)
Polyuria
Vomiting
Weakness
Weight loss

Most cases show typical signs of diabetes mellitus (Box 19-1). Polyuria, polydipsia, weight loss, and muscle wasting are most common. Dermatologic signs include unkempt haircoat and flaky dry skin. Some patients, usually cats, will develop a diabetic neuropathy typically in the form of a plantigrade stance in the pelvic limbs. Careful evaluation for concurrent illness is essential, especially for pancreatitis (in which patients may have a painful cranial or right cranial abdomen). As the acidosis worsens, patients may experience anorexia, vomiting, dehydration, weakness, lethargy or depression, hypotension, coma, panting, and Kussmaul's respiration. The breath will have a distinctive acetone odor. Table 19-1 provides a list of common clinicopathologic abnormalities.

Treatment

The major focus of the treatment of DKA is to replace sufficient amounts of insulin to stabilize the patient's metabolic condition. Electrolyte, mineral, and acid-base status must be corrected concurrently. If an underlying cause of the diabetes is identified or concomitant infection (e.g., urogenital, skin, respiratory, abscess) is found, then it must also be treated.

TABLE 19-1

Common Initial Clinicopathologic Values Associated with Diabetic Ketoacidosis

Complete Blood Count	Serum Chemistry Profile	Urinalysis	Blood Gases
Anemia of chronic disease	Azotemia	Bacteriuria	Acidemia
Leukocytosis (if infection present)	Decreased total carbon dioxide (CO_2)	Glucosuria	Decreased base excess
Polycythemia (if dehydrated)	Hyperamylasemia (if pancreatitis present)	Hematuria	Decreased partial pressure of CO_2
Usually normal	Hypercholesterolemia	Ketonuria	Decreased total bicarbonate (HCO_3)
	Hyperglycemia	Proteinuria	
	Hyperlipasemia (if pancreatitis present)	Pyuria	
	Hyperlipidemia	Submaximal urine concentration	
	Hypertriglyceridemia		
	Hypochloremia		
	Hypokalemia		
	Hyponatremia		
	Increased liver enzyme activities		
	Increased serum osmolality		

The initial insulin therapy of choice is regular IV or intramuscular (IM) insulin. The greatest control can be achieved with a constant rate infusion (CRI) of IV regular insulin at a rate of 0.05 to 0.5 U/kg/hr for dogs and 0.05 to 0.2 U/kg/hr for cats. A CRI pump is required for this technique. Changing the rate of the infusion will change the speed at which the blood glucose deceases in the patient. Regular insulin can be placed in lactated Ringer's solution or 0.9% sodium chloride solution. Insulin adheres to plastic, and 30 to 50 ml of the insulin solution should be allowed to flow through the line to saturate the tubing before starting the infusion to the patient. Insulin is damaged by ultraviolet light, and fresh infusions should be made every 24 hours. Insulin infusions are administered at slower rates than noninsulin-containing solutions used for rehydration. A double-lumen central line or a second IV catheter in another vein is required for this procedure (Box 19-2).

Another method to administer regular insulin is the IM route. The initial dose of 0.2 U/kg is followed by subsequent doses of 0.1 U/kg. The half-life of regular insulin is approximately 2 hours, and redosing will be needed every 3 to 6 hours. However, the clinician must consider the response to the previous insulin dose before determining when the next dose is given (i.e., if the serum glucose concentration is decreasing at an appropriate rate, then it would be inadvisable to redose the insulin, even if the patient is still hyperglycemic).

With both IV and IM dosing, the goal is to have the serum glucose concentration decline 50 to 100 mg/dl/hr. If the glucose declines more rapidly, then significant complications may occur. The brain produces neurogenic osmoles (i.e., small molecules that attract water) in an effort to maintain adequate hydration in a hyperosmolar environment. It takes time for these neurogenic osmoles to be depleted in the brain. Rapid changes in serum glucose concentrations cause marked reductions in the osmolality of the blood. The brain then becomes hyperosmolar and attracts water. This can cause cerebral edema, seizures, coma, and death. If signs coincide with a rapid drop in the blood glucose concentration, then the clinician should add dextrose to the fluids to produce a 5% to 10% solution to maintain the blood glucose in the range of 250 to 300 mg/dl. The cerebral edema should be treated with mannitol.

Once the patient has been stabilized, longer-acting insulin can be used. In dogs the initial dose is

---

BOX 19-2

Basic Supplies Needed for Stabilization

Selection of catheters suitable for long line or jugular vessels
Multilumen catheters
Regular insulin
50% Dextrose
Potassium phosphate
Sodium bicarbonate (NaHCO₃)
Dexamethasone sodium phosphate
Desoxycorticosterone pivalate (DOCP)
Prednisone and prednisolone
Fluidrocortisone acetate
Calcium gluconate 10% solution
Calcium chloride 10% solution
Furosemide
Calcitonin
Electrocardiogram (ECG; HP Pagewriter)
Infusion pumps
Syringe pumps
Blood chemistry analyzers
Blood glucose monitor

0.5 U/kg once or twice daily, based on the glucose curve. An initial dose of 1 to 3 U/kg once or twice daily (depending on the glucose curve) is recommended. Most dogs and cats will ultimately require lifelong, twice-daily insulin injections. Insulin glargine, a new synthetic human insulin analogue, can be used once daily; along with proper nutritional management, it may induce remission of diabetes mellitus in cats.

Table 19-2 provides a comparison of insulin types and administrations. All insulin types (including regular insulin) should be refrigerated to maintain a constant temperature. Regular insulin does not settle, so it does not need to be resuspended. All the other types of insulin will settle out and require gentle resuspension. All insulin should be protected from sunlight and ultraviolet light to prevent degradation. Bottles of insulin should be discarded after 3 months of initiation of use, regardless of the amount left in the bottle. Most insulin comes in the concentration of 100 U/ml (U-100). Insulin syringes designed for U-100 insulin should be used, because they measure 1 U/0.01 ml more accurately than a 1 cc (tuberculin) syringe. Also available are U-40 (40 U/ml) syringes for U-40 insulin.

TABLE 19-2

Insulin Types, Time to Maximal Effect, and Duration of Action for Cats and Dogs

Type	Route of Administration	Time Until Onset of Action	TIME UNTIL MAXIMAL EFFECT		DURATION OF ACTION	
			Cats	Dogs	Cats	Dogs
Regular	IV	Immediate	30 min-2 hr	30 min-2 hr	1-4 hr	1-4 hr
Lente	Intramuscular (IM)	10-30 min	1-4 hr	1-4 hr	3-8 hr	3-8 hr
NPH	Subcutaneous (SQ)	10-30 min	1-5 hr	1-5 hr	4-10 hr	4-10 hr
Ultralente	SQ	15-60 min	2-8 hr	2-10 hr	6-14 hr	8-24 hr
PZI	SQ	30 min-3 hr	2-8 hr	2-10 hr	4-12 hr	6-12 hr
Glargine	SQ	2-8 hr	4-16 hr	4-16 hr	8-24 hr	8-28 hr
	SQ	1-4 hr	3-12 hr	4-14 hr	6-24 hr	6-28 hr
	SQ	1-4 hr	14-18 hr	Not available (n/a)	n/a	n/a

IV fluid therapy is required in all patients for rehydration purposes. Rehydration helps to improve cardiac output and tissue perfusion, provides fluid diuresis to remove ketoacids and other retained organic acids, and helps to correct acid-base and electrolyte imbalances. The use of isotonic crystalloid fluids (e.g., lactated Ringer's solution, 0.9% sodium chloride) is preferred. The fluid rate should be calculated to provide maintenance fluid volume plus dehydration deficit volume (percent of dehydration multiplied by the body weight in kilograms) delivered over a 24- to 48-hour period. In some severely dehydrated and critical patients, the dehydration deficit may need to be delivered more rapidly, over a 6- to 12-hour period. The clinician should monitor lung sounds, respiration rate, and respiratory effort closely to ensure that the patient does not become overhydrated.

Potassium supplementation is required in most DKA patients. Diabetes mellitus and especially ketoacidosis cause total potassium depletion because of a shift of potassium out of the cells into the serum to replenish renal losses and to help offset acid-base imbalances. Treatment of DKA will further decrease potassium concentrations because of the dilution from the fluid therapy, insulin-mediated uptake of potassium by the cells, correction of acidemia, and continued renal losses. The technician should measure serum concentrations of potassium before treatment and follow the recommendations in Table 19-3.

TABLE 19-3

Potassium Supplementation Recommendations for Diabetic Patients

Serum Potassium (mEq/L)	Amount to Supplement	
	mEq Potassium/L* *or* mEq Potassium/kg/hr	
>3.5	20	0.055
3.0-3.5	30	0.083
2.5-3.0	40	0.110
2.0-2.5	60	0.165
<2.0	80	0.220

*Amount supplemented to 1 L of fluids if delivered at a maintenance rate of 30 ml/lb/day.

If in-house serum chemistries are not available, then potassium should be supplemented at a rate of 0.055 to 0.11 mEq of potassium chloride/kg/hr while waiting for pretreatment serum biochemical analysis. Potassium supplementation should be avoided in patients with oliguria or anuria, hyperkalemia, hypocalcemia, or hyperphosphatemia.

Shifts in body phosphorus occur in a similar fashion as potassium. Treatment of DKA also decreases phosphorus via similar mechanisms as it does for potassium. Phosphate bonds are the main energy storage vehicles for the cells (especially red blood cells [RBCs], skeletal muscle, and brain), and phosphorus is important for 2,3-diphosphoglycerol's role in oxygen dissociation in the RBC. Most canine and feline patients have normal serum phosphorus and phosphate concentrations and should be supplemented with 0.01 to 0.03 mmole phosphate/kg/hr (potassium phosphate has 3.3 mmoles phosphate/ml) for 6 to 24 hours in the IV fluids. The calcium in lactated Ringer's will precipitate out some the phosphate, so 0.9% sodium chloride is a better choice in patients who are severely hypophosphatemic. Dogs and cats with a phosphorus concentration of 1.5 mg/dl or less will require 0.03 to 0.12 mmole phosphate/kg/hr. Close monitoring is required for these patients (see following). Phosphate supplementation should be avoided in patients with oliguria or anuria, hyperphosphatemia, hypocalcemia, or hyperkalemia.

IV bicarbonate (HCO_3) therapy is controversial. Most DKA patients will improve with insulin and fluid therapy alone. If the plasma HCO_3 concentration is 11 mEq/L or less, or total venous carbon dioxide (CO_2) is 12 mEq/L or less (total CO_2 − 1 = plasma HCO_3 concentration), HCO_3 therapy can be considered, especially if the venous blood pH is 7.0 or less. The clinician should only use HCO_3 if venous blood gases can be monitored. The amount of HCO_3 (in milliequivalents) needed to correct the acidosis to a plasma HCO_3 of 12 mEq/L over a 6-hour period is as follows:

mEq HCO_3 =
$BW_{kg} \times 0.4 \times (12 - \text{patient's } HCO_3 \text{ [mEq/L]}) \times 0.5,$

where BW_{kg} is the body weight in kilograms. Bolusing HCO_3 is not advised. The acid-base status needs to be rechecked 6 hours after starting the HCO_3 infusion. Additional HCO_3 therapy can be used until the HCO_3 concentration is 12 mEq/L or greater.

Patients who are not eating and have hypoglycemia (<70 mg/dl) from their insulin therapy may require dextrose supplementation to their IV fluid therapy. If a CRI of regular insulin is being used, stop the fluids and recheck the blood glucose in 30 to 60 minutes. If the blood glucose continues to decline or the concentration is below 60 mg/dl, dextrose therapy should be initiated. It should be remembered that dextrose gets converted into glucose, which enters the cells with potassium and phosphorus via insulin-mediated glucose receptors. Dextrose therapy is not required unless hypoglycemia exists or the blood glucose concentration drops too rapidly. If the patient is experiencing signs of insulin shock and has neurologic signs of hypoglycemia, the clinician should bolus 50% dextrose at a dose of 1 ml/kg IV. Next he or she should add enough dextrose to the patient's IV infusion to create a 5% to 10% dextrose IV drip, which can be maintained as needed.

Antibiotics should be used as needed based on signs of infection. Urogenital tract infections are most common; sampling the urine for culture before antibiotic therapy is advised.

Nursing Care and Monitoring

Most of the monitoring involves evaluating the patient's response to treatment and identifying common complications early in the treatment process. These patients should be weighed twice daily to monitor rehydration and to make sure they do not gain too much weight (more than the estimated dehydration, 1 L = 1 kg = 2.2 lb). Monitoring of the respiration rate and effort and of the lung sounds will also assist in preventing volume overload. The urine output should be carefully evaluated. Initially, urine output will be lower than volume input because of dehydration, but once rehydrated, the patient's urine output should closely match intake and input.

Electrolytes should be measured every 4 to 8 hours. If phosphorus cannot be measured as frequently as potassium, changes in the potassium concentration can be correlated with the phosphorus concentration (because they change for similar reasons). Decreases in the potassium or phosphorus concentrations should be addressed promptly to prevent a crisis from occurring. The acid-base status also needs to be closely monitored. In patients with severe disturbances, venous blood gases should be monitored every 6 hours until stable, then evaluated once daily.

Urine color should be monitored continuously, and a packed cell volume (PCV) should be measured once or twice daily. The clinician should take note of the serum color. Severe hypophosphatemia causes the RBC membranes to destabilize and results in acute hemolysis, which will manifest as hemoglobinuria, hemolysed serum, and a rapidly decreasing PCV. The urine should also be checked daily for ketones. The separated serum can be used with a urine dipstick in a similar fashion to check for ketonemia.

Ketones may persist in the urine for 1 to 5 days after resolution of the ketotic state. Because urinary tract infections are very common in patients with diabetes mellitus, sign of bacterial infection should be carefully noted (e.g., foul odor, cloudiness, hematuria, strangury) on a daily basis.

Blood glucose should be monitored every 2 hours. Initially in some severely affected patients, taking measurements every hour will be required to ensure that the blood glucose is not decreasing too rapidly. The ideal rate of decline in the blood glucose is 50 to 100 mg/dl/hr. If blood glucose drops below 50 to 60 mg/dl, then neuroglycopenic signs may occur such as weakness, depression, lethargy, coma, bradycardia, or seizures. If the patient is eating, then it should be fed. If not eating, then IV dextrose therapy can be used (see previous discussion). As previously mentioned, if the blood glucose drops too quickly, then cerebral edema may occur; therefore careful attention must be paid to the animal's mental status.

With careful monitoring and anticipation of complications, these patients can do quite well. No two DKA patients are the same, and nothing is routine about this disease.

Hypoadrenocorticism (Acute Addisonian Crisis)

Definition

Hypoadrenocorticism (Addison's disease) is a deficiency in the production of mineralocorticoids (aldosterone), glucocorticoids (cortisol), or both in the adrenal glands. Destruction of the adrenal gland by immune-mediated causes is the likely cause of most cases of primary hypoadrenocorticism. Iatrogenic primary hypoadrenocorticism occurs if the adrenal cortex is destroyed by mitotane (Lysodren). Secondary hypoadrenocorticism, which is decreased production of adrenocorticotropic hormone (ACTH) by the pituitary gland, causes glucocorticoid deficiency only. Iatrogenic secondary hypoadrenocorticism occurs when a sudden withdrawal of exogenous high-dose or long-term glucocorticoid therapy occurs.

Mineralocorticoids (aldosterone) are important in regulating body electrolyte status. Aldosterone promotes sodium and chloride reabsorption in exchange for potassium and hydrogen ions in the connecting segment and the collecting tubules of the renal nephron. Free water travels with the sodium. A lack of aldosterone results in sodium, chloride, and free water loss in the urine with retention of potassium, hydrogen ions, and calcium. The resultant severe electrolyte imbalances and dehydration cause the shock and cardiotoxic events in an addisonian crisis.

Glucocorticoids (cortisol) are important for many body systems. Gastrointestinal (GI) integrity is the major consequence of cortisol deficiency. Poor vascular perfusion of the intestinal mucosa, decreased mucus production, and GI ulceration has clinical manifestations. Glucocorticoids are also important gluconeogenic hormones and are one of the four primary stress hormones.

Presentation

Hypoadrenocorticism is an uncommon disease of dogs and an extremely rare disease in the cat. Both species are treated similarly. The disease is generally seen in young dogs (mean, 4 to 4.5 years; range, 2 months to 12 years) and middle-aged cats. In dogs, 70% to 85% of those affected are female. There appear to be no breed predilections in the cat; however, with dogs, Great Danes, Portuguese water dogs, rottweilers, West Highland white terriers, and Wheaton terriers are at increased risk. The disease is inherited in standard poodles and Leonbergers.

Clinical signs and symptoms are variable (Table 19-4). They range from mild signs to severe or fatal signs with acute crisis. The history may reveal a waxing and waning course. The most common signs in the dog are anorexia, vomiting, lethargy or depression, and weakness. Some patients also have weight loss, diarrhea, melena, shaking and shivering, polyuria, and polydipsia. In cats, lethargy, anorexia, vomiting, weight loss, polyuria, and polydipsia are the most common clinical signs.

Dogs often arrive at the clinic depressed and dehydrated. Pale, tacky oral mucous membranes with slow capillary refill time are common. In severely affected patients, shock, collapse, coma, and seizures can occur. Weak pulses and bradycardia because of hyperkalemia can be appreciated. An ECG in patients with hyperkalemia may reveal tall and spiked T waves with a narrow base (Fig. 19-1). The QRS complexes become widened and the P-R interval increases. The P waves become smaller and wider and, in severe hyperkalemia, will disappear altogether (i.e., atrial standstill). Severely hyperkalemic patients may have QRS-T fusion resulting in a wide complex idioventricular arrhythmia followed by

TABLE 19-4

Clinical Signs Associated with Hypoadrenocorticism and Addisonian Crisis

Most Common (50% to 100% of Patients)	Frequent (25% to 50% of Patients)	Infrequent (<25% of Patients)
Anorexia	Collapse	Bradycardia
Lethargy/	Dehydration	(<60 beats
depression	Diarrhea	per minute)
Vomiting	Hypothermia	Hair loss
Weakness	Polydipsia	Melena
Weight loss	Polyuria	Painful
	Previous	abdomen
	response	Weak pulses
	to therapy	
	Shaking	
	Slow capillary	
	refill time	
	Waxing/waning	
	course	

ventricular fibrillation and asystole. A similar clinical presentation has been reported in the cat. Because many of these are nonspecific signs, the clinician must rule out severe GI disease, renal disease, and whipworm infestation. Table 19-5 provides a review of common clinicopathologic abnormalities.

Treatment

Patients with acute crisis or a significant number of clinical signs require hospitalization and treatment. Those with subtle or mild signs can be treated at home. The primary goals are to rapidly replace depleted volume, correct electrolyte status, and provide hormone replacement therapy. (See Box 19-2 for a list of supplies required for managing a patient with hypoadrenocorticism in a well-equipped emergency facility.)

Correction of hypovolemia and addressing electrolyte imbalances are the most important primary goals. The fluid of choice is 0.9% sodium chloride administered at a maintenance volume plus dehydration deficit volume (percent of dehydration multiplied by body weight in kilograms) over a 24-hour period. Rapid rehydration of the dehydration deficit over 4 to 12 hours may be required in some severely affected patients.

Initially, parenteral administration of glucocorticoids is advised. Once the patient is stable, mineralocorticoid support can be used. Because dexamethasone sodium phosphate is inexpensive and readily available, most clinicians consider it the glucocorticoid of choice. Dexamethasone sodium phosphate is a water-soluble, rapid-onset steroid, and it does not crossreact with the cortisol assay required for the ACTH stimulation test. Table 19-6 provides glucocorticoid dose recommendations.

Once the patient is more stable, those with primary hypoadrenocorticism can have mineralocorticoids added to their treatment. Desoxycorticosterone pivalate (DOCP) is the most economical way to replace mineralocorticoids. DOCP (Percorten-V, Novartis) is dosed at 1.1 to 2.2 mg/kg IM every 21 to 30 days. It has no glucocorticoid activity, so supplementation with prednisone or prednisolone at a dose of 0.1 to 0.2 mg/kg/day will likely be required. Alternatively, fludrocortisone acetate (Florinef) is dosed at 0.01 to 0.02 mg/kg/day orally (PO) divided twice a day (bid). Because fludrocortisone has some glucocorticoid activity, only about 50% of canine patients will need oral prednisone or prednisolone supplementation. The dose of the mineralocorticoids should be based on clinical signs and electrolyte concentrations. The glucocorticoids should be dosed primarily on the presence of GI signs.

The hyperkalemia in some patients may warrant more than just fluid therapy. Patients with severe bradycardia or serious ECG abnormalities will need to have their serum potassium lowered more rapidly. IV dextrose (1000 mg/kg diluted 1:1 with sterile-water slow IV infusion) with regular insulin (0.5 U/kg IV) will promote cellular uptake of potassium (and phosphorus). Supplementing the fluids with 0.01 to 0.03 mmole phosphate/kg/hr (potassium phosphate = 3.3 mmole phosphate/ml) will help prevent hypophosphatemia. In life-threatening cases of hyperkalemia, the clinician should administer 10% calcium gluconate at a dose of 0.5 to 1.0 ml/kg slow IV over 15 to 30 minutes. Calcium provides important cardioprotective effects. The ECG should be monitored closely while the calcium is administered. Bradycardia and Q-T interval shortening are indications to stop.

Nursing Care and Monitoring

Careful monitoring of the heart rate and ECG is very important because fatal arrhythmias can occur. During initial therapy, the heart rate and rhythm needs

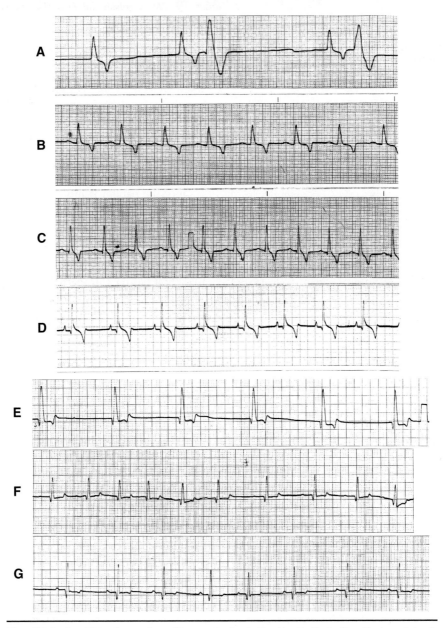

Fig. 19-1 The ECG of two dogs (dog 1: *A, B, C, D*; dog 2: *E, F, G*) with hyperkalemia caused by Addison's disease. In tracings **A** and **E,** the effects of severe hyperkalemia (8.6 mEq/L and 9.4 mEq/L) exhibit a lack of visible P waves, short and wide QRS complexes, and slow heart rate. The reader should note that the T waves are not of excessive amplitude. Tracing **A** also demonstrates ventricular escape beats, which are the wide and bizarre-looking QRS complexes after the more normal-appearing QRS complexes. Hyperkalemia, hypoxia, or both may cause this. Tracings **B** and **F** were obtained after treating each dog for 1 hour with IV 0.9% saline solution as the only treatment, which lowered the serum potassium concentration to 7.6 and 7.9 mEq/L, respectively. The reader should note that the P waves have begun to return, the heart rate has increased, and the ventricular escape beats have disappeared. In addition, the prolonged P-R interval (first-degree heart block) improved, but QRS complexes still widened and Q-T segment shortened. Tracings **C** and **G** were collected when the serum potassium concentrations were 6.2 and 5.9 mEq/L, respectively. The P-R interval and P, QRS, and T waves are of a shorter duration, and the R waves are taller. Tracing **D** demonstrates a more spiked T wave. This serum potassium concentration was 5.6 mEq/L.

TABLE 19-5

Clinicopathologic Findings in Patients with Hypoadrenocorticism

Most Common (50% to 100% of Patients)	Frequent (25% to 50% of Patients)	Infrequent (<25% of Patients)
Azotemia	Anemia	Eosinophilia
Hyperkalemia	Decreased total carbon dioxide (CO_2)	Hyperbilirubinemia
Hyponatremia	Hypercalcemia	Hypoglycemia
Sodium/potassium ratio <27	Hypochloremia	Lymphocytosis
Submaximal urine concentration	Increased liver enzyme activities (alanine amino aminotransferase and aspartate aminotransferase)	

TABLE 19-6

Commonly Used Steroid Replacement Medications and Doses

Drug	Dose, Route, and Frequency
Glucocorticoids	
Prednisolone sodium succinate	11-25 mg/kg IV q2-6h
Dexamethasone sodium phosphate	1-3 mg/kg IV q12h
Hydrocortisone sodium hemisuccinate	1-2 mg/kg IV q8h
Hydrocortisone phosphate	1-2 mg/kg IV q8h
Dexamethasone (Azium)	2-4 mg/kg IV q12-24h
Mineralocorticoids	
Desoxycorticosterone pivalate (DOCP)	1.1-2.2 mg/kg IM or SQ q21-30 days
Fludrocortisone acetate	Dogs: 0.02 mg/kg PO q24h (or divided q12h) Cats: 0.1-0.2 mg/kg PO q24h
Hydrocortisone acetate	1-2 mg/kg PO q12h

to be recorded every 1 to 2 hours while a continuous ECG is monitored. Electrolytes should be measured every 4 to 6 hours, initially. Once stable, the patient can be checked every 12 to 24 hours. Blood work to reevaluate for azotemia, hypercalcemia, and to see if hypophosphatemia is present should be performed daily or every other day.

As with any patient that is dehydrated, weighing the patient twice daily and monitoring skin turgor are important. Measuring urine output is a good way to determine when patients are rehydrated or if renal insufficiency exists.

Fludrocortisone therapy monitoring requires measurement of the serum electrolyte, calcium, blood urea nitrogen (BUN), and creatinine concentrations on a 2- to 4-week basis, until the patient becomes stable. Once the patient is stable, monitoring every 3- to 6-months is sufficient. After the first DOCP injection, the serum electrolyte, calcium, BUN, and creatinine concentrations should be measured 3 weeks and 4 weeks after the injection to establish the duration of action of the DOCP. Most patients require injections every 21 to 30 days. Changes in the dose are based on abnormalities with the blood work. If signs of GI upset (e.g., nausea, anorexia, vomiting) occur, the clinician should supplement with prednisone or prednisolone as previously discussed.

A 3-year-old, 30 kg, spayed female standard poodle was referred for evaluation and treatment of azotemia, polyuria, and polydipsia. The owner had noted vomiting and decreased appetite for 4 days before seeing the referring veterinarian. The referring veterinarian's initial physical examination revealed mild dehydration, and blood was drawn for serum biochemical analysis. The dog was discharged after receiving 500 ml of 0.9% sodium chloride subcutaneously (SQ).

Present on the serum biochemistry analysis was blood urea nitrogen (BUN) concentration of 42 mg/dl (reference range 8 to 33 mg/dl) and a creatinine concentration of 2.1 mg/dl (reference range 0.5 to 1.7 mg/dl). A total serum calcium concentration of 12.1 mg/dl (reference range 8.7 to 11.0 mg/dl) was also seen. The sodium concentration was 148.2 mEq/L (reference range 140 to 161 mEq/L), the potassium concentration was 5.7 mEq/L (reference range 3.8 to 5.4 mEq/L), and the chloride concentration was 112 mEq/L (reference range 105 to121 mEq/L). The referring veterinarian prescribed a low-protein diet for renal impairment. Initially the dog improved within the first 24 hours after the visit, but over the next 2 days it continued to vomit and remained polyuric and polydipsic at home. The dog was then referred for additional diagnostic and therapeutic options.

Physical examination on presentation revealed a very weak, 7% dehydrated patient, with mild bradycardia (heart rate 60 beats per minute). A rectal examination produced dark soft stool. During the examination the dog vomited. The vomitus contained small flecks of blood. Blood and urine samples were submitted for a complete blood count, serum biochemical analysis, and urinalysis. Rapid-analysis biochemical testing providing venous blood gas analysis, electrolytes, and BUN and creatinine concentrations was performed at the time of admission. An ECG was also performed.

The rapid chemistry analysis revealed a worsening azotemia (BUN 69 mg/dl [reference range 7 to 34 mg/dl]; creatinine 4.2 mg/dl [reference range 0.4 to 1.5 mg/dl]), a moderate to marked hyperkalemia (7.1 mEq/L [reference range 3.9 to 5.6 mEq/L]), a mild hyponatremia (136 mEq/L [reference range 142 to 161 mEq/L]), and a mild hypochloremia (99 mEq/L [reference range 104 to 120 mEq/L]). The calculated sodium/potassium ratio was 19.2. Venous blood gas analysis showed a mild acidemia (pH 7.247 [reference range 7.398 to 7.416]) with a reduced bicarbonate (HCO_3) concentration (15.5 mEq/L [reference range 20.5 to 23.9 mEq/L]). The complete blood count produced a mild normocytic, normochromic anemia (hematocrit 35% [reference range 37% to 55%]). Additional biochemical abnormalities besides those identified with the rapid-analysis testing were a total serum calcium concentration of 12.9 mg/dl (reference range 8.6 to 10.8 mg/dl) and a mild increase

in alanine amino aminotransferase activity (121 U/L [reference range 10 to 95 U/L]). The urine concentration was suboptimal at 1.017 (reference range 1.015 to 1.036). The ECG was unremarkable.

A tentative diagnosis of hypoadrenocorticism was proposed, based on the signalment, history, hyperkalemia, hyponatremia, reduced sodium/potassium ratio, hypercalcemia, mild azotemia with suboptimal urine concentration, and mildly increased alanine amino aminotransferase activity. An IV central catheter was placed in the left jugular vein, and a rapid-rehydration protocol was initiated with 0.9% sodium chloride at a rate of 416 ml/hr (7% dehydration deficit plus 6 hours of maintenance fluid requirements) for the first 6 hours of fluid therapy. Dexamethasone sodium phosphate (0.25 mg/kg q12h) was given via IV. Famotidine (1.0 mg/kg slow IV q12h) was administered to treat gastrointestinal (GI) bleeding. After the initial 6 hours, the fluid rate was reduced to 100 ml/hr (approximately 1.5 times maintenance).

An adrenocorticotropic hormone (ACTH) stimulation test was performed and submitted to the laboratory. The electrolytes and venous blood gases were rechecked after 6 hours of fluid therapy. The blood gases were within reference ranges, so HCO_3 therapy was not required. A mild hyperkalemia persisted. The packed cell volume (PCV) was 31%, and a reticulocyte count was submitted.

On day 2 the dog was markedly improved, was no longer weak, and was very vocal. The dog's appetite was improved but still somewhat decreased. Dark formed stools were noted, and no vomiting had occurred in the past 12 hours. The electrolytes were again rechecked. The sodium and chloride were in the upper limits of the reference range (sodium 159 mEq/L; chloride 121 mEq/L), and the potassium was well within the reference range (4.1 mEq/L). A total of 13 mEq of potassium chloride was added to the 0.9% sodium chloride to provide maintenance potassium needs. The reticulocyte count was 158,000/μl (reference range <50,000/μl), indicating a regenerative response. Later in the day the patient was eating and drinking normally, and the fluid rate was reduced to 50 ml/hr.

On day 3 the results of the ACTH stimulation test confirmed hypoadrenocorticism. The dog was discharged after being given desoxycorticosterone pivalate (DOCP, 1.1 mg/kg IM q28 days) for long-term management of the hypoadrenocorticism. Because it can take up to 48 hours for the DOCP to start working, fludrocortisone acetate (0.011 mg/kg PO q12h) was prescribed in addition to the DOCP for the first 2 days. Additionally, prednisone (0.23 mg/kg) was ordered to be given if the dog's appetite waned, vomiting returned, or the owner anticipated a stressful event would upset the dog. Oral famotidine (1 mg/kg PO q12h) was given for 7 days, and an oral hematinic was given for 7 days or until the PCV returned to normal.

Hypercalcemia

Definition and Causes

Hypercalcemia is the state of increased serum total calcium concentrations. If hypoalbuminemia exists, then the calcium concentrations should be corrected in dogs using the following formulas:

Corrected calcium =
    calcium (mg/dl) − albumin (g/dl) + 3.5

or

Corrected calcium =
calcium (mg/dl) − (0.4 × total protein [g/dl]) + 3.3

These formulas do not apply to cats, although hypoalbuminemia also affects their serum calcium. Lipemia and hemolysis will cause artifactual hypercalcemia. In addition, young animals with physiologic bone growth will have benign hypercalcemia.

The most common cause of persistent hypercalcemia is hypercalcemia of malignancy. Lymphoma is by far the most common malignancy causing hypercalcemia. Other neoplasms, such as anal sac adenocarcinoma, multiple myeloma, myeloproliferative disease, and solid tissue tumors have also been reported to cause hypercalcemia. Potentially any neoplastic disorder could cause hypercalcemia. Other important "rule outs" include renal insufficiency (most patients have normal serum calcium concentrations), primary hyperparathyroidism, and hypoadrenocorticism. Less common causes are granulomatous diseases (e.g., blastomycosis, nocardiosis), osteolytic bone lesions (e.g., primary or metastatic neoplasia, septic osteomyelitis), calciferol-containing rodenticide intoxication (e.g., hypervitaminosis D), oral calcium supplements, oral phosphate binders, thiazide diuretics, and plant intoxications (e.g., *Cestrum diurnum, Solanum malacoxylon, Trisetum flavescens*). An ill-defined syndrome of idiopathic hypercalcemia also occurs in the cat that requires further in-depth evaluation. Box 19-3 provides a list of the most frequently reported causes of hypercalcemia.

Presentation

Because hypercalcemia has many causes, no specific signalment is seen at the time of presentation. The reader should refer to the texts and literature to

---

BOX 19-3

Causes of Hypercalcemia in Dogs and Cats

- Calciferol-containing rodenticides
- Chronic granulomatous diseases
  Fungal disease (blastomycosis)
  Nocardiosis
- Hypercalcemia of malignancy
  Lymphoma (most common)
  Anal sac adenocarcinoma
  Multiple myeloma
  Myeloproliferative disease
  Solid tissue tumors
- Hyperalbuminemia
- Hypervitaminosis D
- Hypoadrenocorticism
- Idiopathic
- Laboratory error
- Osteolytic bone lesions
- Plant intoxications
  Cestrum diurnum
  Solanum malacoxylon
  Trisetum flavescens
- Oral calcium supplements
- Oral phosphate binders
- Primary hyperparathyroidism
- Primary renal insufficiency
- Thiazide diuretics

---

review the signalments for the most common causes of hypercalcemia. In addition, Table 19-7 lists the clinical signs associated with hypercalcemia.

Hypercalcemia affects primarily four body systems: (1) renal, (2) GI, (3) neuromuscular, and (4) cardiovascular. Renal signs most commonly seen are polyuria and polydipsia, as well as signs of renal failure. Calcium inhibits vasopressin receptors in the kidney and prevents free water reabsorption, creating nephrogenic diabetes insipidus. Very severe hypercalcemia (>15 mg/dl) can lead to tubular necrosis, renal failure, and mineralization. Vomiting, anorexia, lethargy, and depression are common signs of renal failure. On physical examination, small kidneys would suggest the kidney disease has been chronic and may be the cause of the hypercalcemia. In some patients, signs of urolithiasis are present, and uroliths can be palpated in the urinary bladder or urethra.

Hypercalcemia reduces excitability of smooth, skeletal, and cardiac muscle and causes GI dysfunction.

TABLE 19-7

Clinical Signs Associated with Hypercalcemia

Common	Uncommon
Anorexia	Coma
Dehydration	Constipation
Depression/lethargy	Death
Polydipsia	ECG abnormalities
Polyuria	Prolonged P-R
Vomiting	interval
Weakness	Shortened Q-T
	segment
	Ventricular fibrillation
	Seizures
	Stupor

Anorexia, vomiting, and constipation are most commonly reported. Firm stool may be felt in the colon when examined. Alterations in skeletal muscle function cause generalized weakness (common) and muscle twitching (uncommon). Cardiac conduction abnormalities that can be identified with an ECG are prolonged P-R interval, shortened Q-T segment, and ventricular fibrillation may, but they tend to be uncommon.

The most common direct effect of hypercalcemia on the central nervous system is lethargy. Rarely will this progress to seizures, stupor, or coma.

Careful palpation of the lymph nodes and abdomen is important. Lymphadenomegaly or organomegaly may support lymphoma or other neoplasia. A complete rectal examination to palpate for lymph nodes or pelvic canal tumors is essential. A waxing and waning history may suggest hypoadrenocorticism. Palpation of the neck may reveal a parathyroid tumor.

Because hypercalcemia has many causes, additional laboratory values may help define the cause. Hyperphosphatemia without azotemia suggests a nonparathyroid cause. Hypophosphatemia or low-normal phosphorus is most commonly seen with primary hyperparathyroidism or malignancy. Combinations of hyperphosphatemia with azotemia are difficult to assess, because renal failure is both a cause and a result of hypercalcemia. Renal failure rarely causes calcium concentration to go above 15 mg/dl, in general. Serum ionized calcium is high with primary hyperparathyroidism or hypercalcemia of malignancy. Low or low-normal ionized calcium is seen in patients with renal failure. Intact parathormone concentrations are increased with primary hyperparathyroidism and renal failure, whereas low-normal or low concentrations are seen in hypercalcemia of malignancy. Other electrolyte abnormalities (e.g., hyponatremia with hyperkalemia) are associated with hypoadrenocorticism.

Ancillary diagnostic testing such as radiography and ultrasonography can be used to evaluate for kidney size and architecture, bone lesions, urolithiasis, hepatic and splenic architecture, and lymphadenopathy. Fine-needle aspirates, biopsies, and bone marrow analysis may be required. An ACTH stimulation test can be used to rule out hypoadrenocorticism.

Treatment

Treatment focuses primarily on removing the underlying cause and on volume expansion. The clinician should not allow treatment to inhibit his or her ability to identify the underlying cause. In many cases the cause may be readily identified but not immediately treatable. Therefore supportive care is required. (See Box 19-2 for a list of supplies required to manage a patient with hypercalcemia.)

Volume expansion with IV 0.9% sodium chloride at a rate of 100 to 180 ml/kg/day is recommended. Fluids containing calcium-like lactated Ringer's solution should not be used. Any dehydration deficit should be added into the fluid rate. In conditions of dehydration, the kidneys reabsorb sodium and calcium more effectively. By rehydrating and volume expanding, naturesis and calciuresis can occur. To prevent iatrogenic hypokalemia, potassium supplementation is necessary. Volume expansion is sufficient in most patients to resolve the hypercalcemia; however, some patients require additional supportive care.

Calciuretic diuretics can be used after rehydration and volume expansion have been completed. Furosemide, a loop diuretic, is the diuretic of choice. Thiazide diuretics should not be used. In the acute management of severe hypercalcemia, furosemide can be dosed at 5 mg/kg IV once, followed by a CRI of 5 mg/kg/hr. Alternatively, a dose of 2 to 4 mg/kg IV, IM, or PO given bid to tid (three times a day) can be used. Maintaining adequate hydration while using diuretic therapy is important.

Glucocorticoids increase renal calcium excretion, decrease gut calcium absorption, and decrease bone resorption; they are also cytotoxic to hematopoietic neoplasms like lymphoma. Collecting all diagnostic samples before glucocorticoid administration is important if lymphoid neoplasia is a possibility. If hypoadrenocorticism is possible, then dexamethasone is the preferred glucocorticoid because it will not interfere with the cortisol assay. Glucocorticoids will also help to antagonize the effects of vitamin-D intoxication. In the short term, steroids may reduce inflammation and hypercalcemia associated with granulomatous disease, but high-dose or intermediate- or long-term use may cause a progression of disease, especially fungal disease. Prednisone or prednisolone can be used at a dose of 1 to 2 mg/kg PO, SQ, or IM bid. Dexamethasone can be used at a dose of 0.1 to 0.2 mg/kg IV, IM, SQ, or PO bid.

Bisphosphonates are metal-complexing compounds that also inhibit the production of calcitriol (i.e., active vitamin D) by inhibiting 1α-hydroxylase. Pamidronate is a relatively new bisphosphonate that has been described in veterinary medicine. Recent work with the medication has shown rapid reductions in serum and ionized calcium concentrations with minimal adverse reactions or signs of toxicity. Dosing in dogs is 1.0 to 2.0 mg/kg IV; dosing in cats is 1.5 to 2.0 mg/kg IV. Pamidronate is given as a single-dose, slow IV (in 0.9% sodium chloride, over 4 hours) infusion. The onset of action ranges from 24 to 48 hours, and the duration of action is days to weeks (median, 8.5 weeks). Pamidronate can be given before a definitive diagnosis, because it will not interfere with the results of additional diagnostic testing. Etidronate, another bisphosphonate, has limited use in veterinary medicine; however, oral doses of 2.5 mg/kg PO bid for the dog and 5 mg/kg PO bid for the cat have been reported. Etidronate also is available as an IV solution. No IV dose has been reported, but most believe it to be lower than the oral dose.

Sodium bicarbonate ($NaHCO_3$) therapy is rather controversial. Most clinicians reserve this modality for management of acute crisis in the presence of metabolic acidosis. Ionized calcium concentrations decrease as serum pH rises (because the calcium binds to serum proteins and HCO_3 ions). A dose of 1 to 4 mEq/kg as a slow IV bolus has been recommended. It may take up to 24 hours to see results. Multiple dosing may be required, but generally CRIs are not required. The clinician should refrain from using HCO_3 if calcium and acid-base status cannot be measured. HCO_3 seems to work best in combination with other treatments.

Bone resorption inhibitors such as calcitonin and mithramycin are much less commonly used.

Calcitonin (5 U/kg IV initially, then 4 to 8 U/kg SQ every 6 to 24 hours) is a hormone that antagonizes parathormone and is used as an antidote for calciferol-containing rodenticides. It can also be used as a temporary treatment for primary hyperparathyroidism. Calcitonin is expensive, has a short duration of action, and can cause anorexia and vomiting. Mithramycin is an antineoplastic agent that is also a potent inhibitor of bone resorption. This medication has been used infrequently in veterinary medicine for treating hypercalcemia. A single dose of 25 µg/kg has been recommended, but once- or twice-weekly dosing may be required to effectively treat hypercalcemia. Significant nephrotoxicity, hepatotoxicity, and myelosuppression can occur.

Nursing Care and Monitoring

Weighing the patient twice daily, evaluating skin turgor, and observing urine output should be used to monitor hydration status. Ionized or serum calcium should be measured every 12 to 24 hours during initial therapy. Urinalysis (looking for renal casts) and reevaluation of BUN and creatinine need to be performed to monitor kidney function. Electrolytes should be monitored to identify imbalances caused by fluid therapy. If ECG abnormalities are present, then an ECG must be reevaluated every 12 to 24 hours. Phosphorus concentrations also should be monitored, because persistent hyperphosphatemia with hypercalcemia can result in tissue mineralization, (especially if the product of the calcium multiplied by the phosphorus concentration is greater than 60).

Hypocalcemia

Definition and Possible Causes

Hypocalcemia is the state of decreased serum total calcium concentration. If hypoalbuminemia exists, then the calcium concentrations should be corrected in dogs using the following formulas:

Corrected calcium =
    calcium (mg/dl) − albumin (g/dl) + 3.5

or

Corrected calcium =
calcium (mg/dl) − (0.4 × total protein [g/dl]) + 3.3

These formulas do not apply to cats, although hypoalbuminemia also affects their serum calcium. Hypoalbuminemia is the most common cause of hypocalcemia in dogs and cats. It does not cause clinical signs, because ionized calcium (i.e., physiologically active calcium) concentrations remain normal, in general. Box 19-4 provides a list of causes of hypocalcemia in dogs and cats.

Other common causes of hypocalcemia include chronic and acute renal failure, puerperal tetany (eclampsia), and acute pancreatitis. In renal failure, mass law interactions of calcium with hyperphosphatemia result in hypocalcemia. Additionally, decreased 1-α-hydroxylase activity and subsequent calcitriol (i.e., active vitamin D) production in the kidney significantly contribute to hypocalcemia. Puerperal tetany usually occurs within the first 21 days of lactation, generally in small breed females. Eclampsia causes large amounts of calcium to be diverted into milk production. Acute pancreatitis causes hypocalcemia by mineralization of traumatized tissues and precipitation of calcium salts in saponified fat.

Hypoparathyroidism is an uncommon to rare disease of dogs and cats. It can be a spontaneous primary disease or an iatrogenic result of thyroid surgery (especially in cats). It can also be a result of rapid reversal of chronic hypercalcemia or after removing a functional parathyroid tumor. In all cases the lack of parathormone results in reduced gut absorption of calcium, decreased renal reabsorption of calcium, and unopposed osteoblastic activity (bone production).

Other causes include intestinal malabsorption, which is seen in patients with severe, diffuse GI diseases like lymphangiectasia, inflammatory bowel disease, and infiltrative neoplasia (e.g., lymphoma, mast cell tumor). Ethylene glycol intoxication causes precipitation of calcium salts, usually in the urinary tract and soft tissues. Severely traumatized or necrotic tissue can take up calcium and cause mild hypocalcemia. Phosphate enemas (Fleet enemas) cause severe hyperphosphatemia and subsequent mass law effects with serum calcium. Phosphate enemas affect small dogs and cats more severely. Oversupplementation with $NaHCO_3$ or phosphate IV infusions can cause iatrogenic hypocalcemia. Dietary deficiencies in vitamin D are uncommon, as are chronic consumption of low-calcium, high-phosphorus diets (all meat). Any condition that creates alkalosis will cause a shift from protein-bound (measured total serum calcium) to ionized calcium.

BOX 19-4

Most Common Clinical Signs Associated with Hypocalcemia

- Anorexia (especially in cats)
- Disorientation
- ECG changes
  Bradycardia or tachycardia
  Prolonged S-T segment
  Prolonged Q-T segment
  Wide T waves
- T-wave alternans
- Excitation
- Facial rubbing
- Fever
- Hypersensitivity to stimuli
- Muscle tremor or fasciculation
- Panting
- Polyuria and polydipsia
- Posterior lenticular cataracts (hypoparathyroidism)
- Prolapsed nictitans gland (cats)
- Respiratory arrest
- Restlessness
- Seizures
- Stiff gait/ataxia
- Vomiting (especially in cats)
- Weakness

Laboratory error should be ruled out if the patient's signs do not correlate with the laboratory data. Sampling technique should be reviewed. Citrate, oxalate, and ethylenediaminetetraacetic acid all chelate calcium and will spuriously reduce serum calcium concentrations.

Presentation

Because hypocalcemia has many causes, no specific signalment is seen at the time of presentation. The reader should refer to the texts and literature to review the signalments for the most common causes. A careful history is extremely important in evaluating these patients (e.g., recent parturition, enemas given, toxin exposure, trauma, recent thyroid or parathyroid surgery, historical cues of renal failure).

Hypocalcemia primarily affects the neuromuscular, cardiovascular, GI, and respiratory systems (Box 19-5). Neuromuscular excitability is increased by hypocalcemia. Clinical signs generally do not

BOX 19-5

Causes of Hypocalcemia in Dogs and Cats

- Alkalemia
- Dietary imbalance
- Hypoalbuminemia
- Iatrogenic
- IV phosphate oversupplementation
- Laboratory error
- Pancreatitis
- Phosphate enema administration
- Postoperative thyroid/parathyroid surgery
- Primary hypoparathyroidism
- Primary renal insufficiency (including ethylene glycol intoxication)
- Puerperal tetany (eclampsia)
- Sample handling (collected in calcium-chelating anticoagulant)
- Secondary renal hyperparathyroidism
- Severe intestinal malabsorptive disease
- Sodium bicarbonate (NaHCO₃) oversupplementation

occur unless the calcium concentration is below 6.5 mg/dl in dogs. Acute development of hypocalcemia is associated with more severe clinical signs, whereas chronic hypocalcemia results in adaptation by the body, and patients may show few signs even with calcium concentrations less than 5.0 mg/dl. The most common neuromuscular signs are weakness, facial rubbing, muscle fasciculations or twitching, tetany, ataxia, and seizures. A fever may be recorded in patients who have excessive muscle activity. Common cardiovascular changes are bradycardia and ECG changes (Fig. 19-2). These changes include prolongation of the S-T segment and Q-T segment, as well as wide T waves or T-wave alternans. Anorexia and vomiting are common GI signs (and are the most common clinical signs seen in cats). Panting or respiratory arrest can also be seen. Other signs less commonly seen are polyuria and polydipsia, perhaps because of nephrocalcinosis secondary to conditions that cause hypercalciuria (hypoparathyroidism). A painful abdomen may be a sign of pancreatitis.

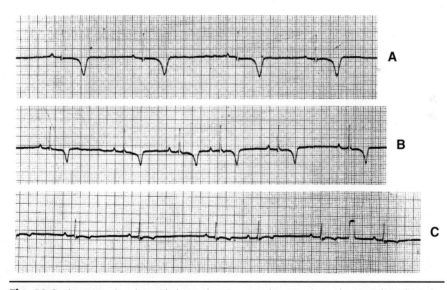

Fig. 19-2 The ECG of a dog with hypocalcemia secondary to primary hypoparathyroidism during various stages of treatment. Tracing **A** demonstrates prolonged S-T and Q-T segments, as well as prolonged (wide) and deep T waves. The serum calcium concentration was 4.0 mg/dl, and the electrolyte concentrations were within reference ranges. Tracing **B** shows improvements in S-T, Q-T, and T-wave duration and amplitude as the serum calcium concentration has been increased to 6.2 mg/dl. Tracing **C** is was taken when the calcium concentration was returned to the reference range (9.7 mg/dl). The S-T, Q-T, and T waves are normal. The three tracings also suggest diminishing R-wave amplitude and increased heart rate as the serum calcium concentration rises to normal.

Treatment

Patients with clinical signs of hypocalcemia should be hospitalized and treated. (See Box 19-2 for a list of supplies required to manage a patient with hypocalcemia.) Hypocalcemia solely caused by hypoalbuminemia does not require treatment; instead the cause of the albumin deficit needs to be identified and treated. Treatment focuses on parenteral calcium salt therapy. Emergency cases with severe hypocalcemia usually have primary or iatrogenic hypoparathyroidism, puerperal tetany (eclampsia), or have been given phosphate-containing enemas. However, any cause could create signs severe enough to require treatment.

The two most commonly used parenteral calcium products are calcium gluconate 10% solution and calcium chloride 10% solution. Calcium chloride is three times more potent than calcium gluconate; however, calcium gluconate is preferred because it causes much less vessel irritation and is not caustic if it extravasates. Table 19-8 contains dosing information that the reader will find helpful.

The clinician should monitor the ECG while the calcium is being administered. Bradycardia and Q-T segment shortening are indications to temporarily stop the infusion. Acute treatment is by slow IV bolus infusion. After stabilizing serious neurologic signs, tetani, and excessive muscle activity, a CRI of calcium can be given to prevent relapse from occurring (relapse can occur from 1 to 24 hours after a bolus infusion). Patients with puerperal tetany should have the puppies removed from the dam. Long-term therapy may include oral calcium and vitamin-D supplements (see Table 19-8).

Laboratory testing (i.e., complete blood count, serum biochemistry profile, urinalysis) is required to fully evaluate these patients. Azotemia and submaximal urine concentration are hallmarks of renal failure and ethylene glycol intoxication. Although both have increased anion gaps, ethylene glycol intoxication usually produces an anion gap of 40 or greater. Increased amylase and lipase activities and an inflammatory leukogram are seen in patients with pancreatitis. These patients may also have a secondary hepatitis as evidenced by increased liver enzyme activities and total bilirubin concentration. Hyperphosphatemia can be seen in patients with renal failure, ethylene glycol intoxication, primary hypoparathyroidism, and those who have

TABLE 19-8

Commonly Used Calcium and Vitamin-D Supplements and Doses

Drug	Dose, Route, and Frequency
Parenteral Calcium	
Calcium gluconate 10% solution (9.3 mg calcium/ml)	Initial: 0.5-1.5 ml/kg slow IV Maintenance: 5-15 mg/kg/hr IV infusion *or* 1-2 ml/kg diluted 1:1 with saline SQ tid
Calcium chloride 10% solution (27.2 mg calcium/ml)	5-15 mg/kg/hr IV infusion
Oral Calcium Supplements	
Calcium carbonate	25-50 mg/kg/day
Calcium gluconate	25-50 mg/kg/day
Calcium lactate	25-50 mg/kg/day
Calcium chloride	25-50 mg/kg/day
Vitamin-D Supplements	
Dihydrotachysterol	Initial: 0.02-0.03 mg/kg/day PO Maintenance: 0.01-0.02 mg/kg PO q24-48h
Calcitriol	2.5-10 mg/kg/day PO
Ergocalciferol	Initial: 4000-6000 U/kg/day PO Maintenance: 1000-2000 U/kg PO q1-7 days

been given a phosphate-containing enema. The presence of increased total CO_2 concentrations supports alkalosis. Blood gases should be evaluated in these patients (the ECG has been previously discussed). Ancillary testing including ethylene glycol testing of the serum, radiography to help evaluate bone density and renal size and shape, ultrasonography of the abdomen to evaluate the kidneys, and intact parathormone concentrations can be additionally helpful.

Nursing Care and Monitoring

During initial management in severely affected patients, calcium concentrations should be measured every 4 to 6 hours, if possible. The ECG should be monitored continuously. Bradycardia, Q-T interval shortening, vomiting, and cardiac arrest are signs to stop calcium administration. Neuromuscular signs may persist for 30 to 60 minutes after adequate correction of serum calcium concentrations. Repeat seizures and excessive muscle activity may cause hyperthermia severe enough to warrant tepid baths. If the patient has kidney disease or ethylene glycol intoxication, then urine production and hydration status (i.e., body weight, skin turgor, PCV) need to be monitored closely. Monitoring the amount of intravenous fluids being administered (the "ins") and changing rates based on what the urine production and insensible losses are (the "outs") may be necessary in patients with acute renal failure or ethylene glycol intoxication. Venous blood gases need to be initially monitored every 12 to 24 hours in patients with alkalosis. Long-term monitoring of the stable patient requires monthly calcium concentration evaluation for the first 6 months, then every 3 to 4 months until the clinician determines the underlying cause has been treated successfully. If the underlying cause does not respond to treatment, life long monitoring may be required.

Hypoglycemia

Definition and Possible Causes

Hypoglycemia is the state of decreased serum glucose concentration. Causes are usually divided into those that accelerate glucose removal and those that cause a failure of glucose production or secretion. The clinician must rule out proper sample handling and processing before pursuing a diagnostic evaluation

---

BOX 19-6

Causes of Hypoglycemia in Dogs and Cats

- Delayed separation of serum from the red cells
- End-stage hepatic disease
- Extrapancreatic neoplasia
- Glycogen storage disease
- Hunting dog hypoglycemia
- Hypoadrenocorticism
- Insulinoma
- Intoxication
  Ethanol
  Salicylates
  Propranolol
  Ethylene glycol
  Oral hypoglycemic agents
- Iatrogenic insulin overdose
- Late-term gestation
- Neonatal hypoglycemia
- Prolonged seizure activity
- Sepsis/endotoxemia
- Severe polycythemia
- Severe primary glucosuria or Fanconi's syndrome
- Starvation/malabsorptive disease
- Toy breed dog hypoglycemia

---

of these patients. Red cells that are allowed to sit in the tube for longer than 1 hour before separation will have artifactual hypoglycemia. Box 19-6 lists the causes of hypoglycemia in dogs and cats.

Many disorders promote more rapid removal of glucose from the plasma. Insulinomas are rare tumors of the pancreatic B cells that have uncontrolled insulin secretion. This is the most common tumor associated with hypoglycemia in the dog. Other tumors (e.g., hepatoma, hepatocellular carcinoma, lymphoma, leiomyosarcoma, plasmacytoid tumors, oral melanoma, hemangiosarcoma, salivary gland adenocarcinoma) produce insulin-like proteins that are biologically active; however, other factors are probably involved with paraneoplastic hypoglycemia. Some patients have such a large tumor burden that it consumes a disproportionately large amount of glucose to sustain the aberrant metabolic needs. Accidental iatrogenic overdose of exogenous insulin is an important consideration in all diabetic patients. Increased RBC mass (i.e., polycythemia) causes hypoglycemia by overuse of glucose to support the metabolic needs of the RBCs. Patients with

Fanconi's syndrome or primary renal glucosuria will lose excess amounts of glucose in their urine. Rarely, females in late term gestation will also experience hypoglycemia because of the demands placed on them by the fetuses. Severe prolonged seizures will cause increased consumption of glucose by the overactive skeletal muscle (Seizures usually cause serum glucose to increase, because they increase cortisol and epinephrine secretion). Intoxications with ethanol, salicylates, propranolol, and oral hypoglycemic agents are also reported causes.

The most common diseases associated with a failure to produce or secrete glucose are neonatal hypoglycemia and toy breed hypoglycemia. With neonatal hypoglycemia, young puppies and kittens have low hepatic glycogen stores and a reduced ability to perform gluconeogenesis. Therefore short periods of fasting can cause hypoglycemia. Starvation or malabsorptive GI diseases are associated with preexisting systemic illness that can deplete the liver of glycogen stores. After prolonged periods of physical exertion and little to no food consumption, hypoglycemia may occur as in hunting dog hypoglycemia. An uncommon cause is end-stage hepatic insufficiency. Glucose homeostasis is one of the last functions to be lost with advanced liver disease.

Some diseases have a combination of causes. Sepsis, endotoxemic shock, and virulent babesiosis promote increased use of glucose by the body by altering metabolism and by increasing insulin release. These problems also deplete hepatic glycogen stores, making less glucose available for release. Patients with hypoadrenocorticism (i.e., Addison's disease) have an absence of counterregulatory cortisol, which facilitates increased insulin action (increased consumption) and decreased gluconeogenesis (decreased glucose secretion). This results in mild to moderate hypoglycemia.

Presentation

No specific signalment is seen in patients with hypoglycemia; however, age, breed, and breeding status (i.e., young puppies and kittens, toy breed dogs, hunting breed dogs, pregnant females) are important in evaluating these cases. Hypoglycemia primarily affects the nervous and musculoskeletal systems (Box 19-7).

Nervous tissue relies on glucose as its primary energy source, and hypoglycemia causes central nervous system depression. Typical signs include lethargy, depression, ataxia, paraparesis and, in some cases, seizures.

BOX 19-7   ⓣ

Most Common Clinical Signs Associated with Hypoglycemia

- Abnormal behavior
  Fly biting
  Stargazing
  Staring at walls
- Ataxia
- Collapse
- Depression/lethargy
- Exercise intolerance
- Muscle fasciculation
- Muscle weakness
- Paraparesis
- Polyphagia
- Seizures

Abnormal behaviors like fly biting, stargazing, and staring at walls also can be seen. Hypoglycemia also stimulates appetite, and polyphagia may be a presenting sign. The skeletal muscle also requires large amounts of energy to maintain normal function. Patients with hypoglycemia will display muscle weakness, collapse, muscle fasciculations, and exercise intolerance.

Many patients will have minimal to no clinical signs. Some animals will adapt to their persistent hypoglycemia and may have few clinical signs, even with blood glucose concentrations as low as 50 mg/dl. Those with paraneoplastic or a large neoplastic burden usually have obvious physical examination abnormalities. Additional laboratory evaluation may show a leukocytosis and abnormalities associated with specific organs that may be affected (e.g., liver, kidneys). Animals with plasmacytoid tumors can have hyperglobulinemia and proteinuria. Additional testing such as urine Bence-Jones protein, bone marrow analysis, and radiographs of the skeleton will be needed to verify the diagnosis. Animals with an insulinoma will have an inappropriately high plasma insulin concentration in the face of hypoglycemia in two thirds to three quarters of patients. A fasted (8 to 12 hours) glucose/insulin ratio should be evaluated. An amended insulin/glucose ratio can be determined using the following formula:

Amended insulin/glucose ratio =
  (plasma insulin [mcU/ml] × 100)/
    (plasma glucose [mg/dl] − 30)

If the plasma glucose is less than or equal to 30, then the denominator for the equation should be 1. Amended ratios above 30 are indicative of insulin-secreting tumors. Ratios between 19 and 30 are difficult to interpret and need to be repeated. If the ratio is below 19, then an insulinoma is unlikely. False-positive results can occur if the patient's blood glucose is below 40 mg/dl.

Patients with end-stage liver disease or portovascular anomaly often have other clinical signs. Dogs and cats with portovascular anomaly frequently have stunted growth, are thin, and have polyuria and polydipsia. Usually they are juvenile to middle-aged. GI signs, icterus, and ascites are signs more commonly seen with end-stage liver disease or severe hepatic dysfunction. Laboratory findings that may be observed include anemia, microcytosis (especially portovascular anomaly), decreased BUN, hypoalbuminemia, and increased serum liver enzyme activities. The fasted and 2-hour postprandial bile acid concentrations will be increased. Urinalysis may reveal urate crystals (especially portovascular anomaly), bilirubinuria, and low urine concentrations.

Septic animals are very ill when they arrive at the clinic. These cats and dogs are shocky, febrile, and have injected mucous membranes when they are in the hyperdynamic phases of septic shock. If presented in the later hypodynamic phase, then hypothermia, pale mucous membranes, and signs of circulatory collapse are seen. The leukogram can be variable from leukopenic to leukocytosis. Evidence of organ failure may be evident (liver, kidneys), and a coagulation profile may reveal disseminated intravascular coagulopathy. Blood cultures should be performed.

Dogs and cats with hypoadrenocorticism (see previous section, *Hypoadrenocorticism [Acute Addisonian Crisis]*) often have a waxing and waning history. In addition to hypoglycemia, biochemical analysis may reveal azotemia, hypercalcemia, hyponatremia, and hyperkalemia. The animal also may develop a *reverse stress leukogram* (lymphocytosis, eosinophilia).

Rarely a dog or cat will develop hypoglycemia from an uncommon cause. Glycogen storage is a rare disease and is most commonly seen in animals less than 1 year of age. Polycythemic patients have dark mucous membranes and are weak, polyuric, and polydipsic, with seizures and a PCV above 65%.

Treatment

The goal of therapy is to increase serum glucose concentrations by administering dextrose via IV. All patients with clinical signs should be treated (see Box 19-2 for a list of supplies required to manage a patient with hypoglycemia). Patients who are able to eat (i.e., alert, not vomiting) should be fed as a part of their therapy. Some causes of hypoglycemia will require treatment of an underlying cause, whereas others will require long-term therapy. The clinician must be sure to perform diagnostic testing required to identify the underlying cause of the hypoglycemia.

IV 50% dextrose at 1 to 4 ml/kg diluted 1:1 with sterile water delivered over a 15-minute period is typically given as an initial treatment for severe hypoglycemia. Patients with an insulinoma may have an increase in insulin secretion in response to the dextrose infusion (thus driving the blood glucose lower). Feeding them frequently using a diet high in complex carbohydrates may better treat these patients. If this is unsuccessful, then a dextrose infusion may prove better than an IV bolus of dextrose. Infusions of 2.5% or 5% dextrose solutions can be delivered at a rate that maintains blood glucose high enough to eliminate clinical signs of hypoglycemia. Some patients may require dextrose concentrations of 10% or higher. Potassium supplementation should be used as needed, based on maintenance requirements or laboratory values.

Insulinomas can be treated with surgery (e.g., partial pancreatectomy) or medically. No location predilection exists for the tumor in the pancreas. Medical management includes frequent feedings, prednisone and prednisolone (0.25 mg/kg PO bid), diazoxide (5 to 30 mg/kg PO bid, starting at the low end of dose, initially), and octreotide (10 to 40 μg SQ bid to tid). Toy breed dogs and young puppies and kittens should be fed frequent meals high in complex carbohydrates. A bottle of corn syrup should be available in case a hypoglycemic event occurs. Hunting dogs should be fed a meal before hunting and offered snacks every 2 to 4 hours while hunting. If these dogs still have hypoglycemic events, then they should not be allowed to hunt again. If the patient is in a late term of pregnancy, then caesarian section and removal of the puppies will be required. Polycythemia requires therapeutic phlebotomy, and chemotherapy (hydroxyurea) may be required for long-term control.

Nursing Care and Monitoring

Monitor the glycemic status of these patients can be difficult because of the production of counterregulatory hormones. Single or intermittent measurement of blood glucose is not recommended. Monitoring the blood glucose every 2 hours will give a better indication of the trends in glucose control. The target blood glucose is 60 to 150 mg/dl. Mental and neuromuscular status should be monitored frequently throughout the day, because they provide early clues to an oncoming hypoglycemic event. Septic patients need to be monitored very closely for signs multiple organ failure syndrome, acute respiratory distress syndrome, and disseminated intravascular coagulopathy. Patients with hypoadrenocorticism should be monitored as previously described (see *Hypoadrenocorticism [Acute Addisonian Crisis]*). PCVs should be monitored on a daily basis in polycythemic patients. Other monitoring should be based on the patient's underlying disease.

Suggested Readings

Chew DJ et al. In Bonagura JD: *Current veterinary therapy XII*, Philadelphia, 1995, Saunders, pp 378-383.

Chew DJ et al. In DiBartola SP: *Fluid therapy in small animal practice*, Philadelphia, 1992, Saunders, pp 116-176.

Crenshaw KL. In Bonagura JD: *Current veterinary therapy XIII*, Philadelphia, 2000, Saunders, pp 348-349.

Feldman EC. In Ettinger SJ, Feldman EC: *Textbook of veterinary internal medicine*, Philadelphia, 1995, Saunders, pp 1437-1465.

Feldman EC, Nelson RW. In Bonagura JD: *Current veterinary therapy XIII*, Philadelphia, 2000, Saunders, pp 345-347.

Feldman EC, Nelson RW. In Bonagura JD: *Current veterinary therapy XIII*, Philadelphia, 2000, Saunders, pp 354-356.

Feldman EC, Nelson RW. In Feldman EC, Nelson RW: *Canine and feline endocrinology and reproduction*, Philadelphia, 1996, Saunders, pp 274-303.

Feldman EC, Nelson RW. In Feldman EC, Nelson RW: *Canine and feline endocrinology and reproduction*, Philadelphia, 1996, Saunders, pp 357-374.

Fox LE. In Bonagura JD: *Current veterinary therapy XII*, Philadelphia, 1995, Saunders, pp 530-541.

Greco DS, Peterson ME. In Kirk RW: *Current veterinary therapy X*, Philadelphia, 1989, Saunders, pp 1042-1045.

Hardy RH. In Ettinger SJ, Feldman EC: *Textbook of veterinary internal medicine*, Philadelphia, 1995, Saunders, pp 1579-1592.

Kintzer PP, Peterson ME. In Bonagura JD: *Current veterinary therapy XII*, Philadelphia, 1995, Saunders, pp 416-420.

Leifer CE. In Kirk RW: *Current veterinary therapy X*, Philadelphia, 1989, Saunders, pp 982-987.

MacIntire DK: Emergency treatment of diabetic crisis: insulin overdose, diabetic ketoacidosis and hyperosmolar coma, *Vet Clin North Am Small Anim Pract* 25:639, 1995.

Meleo KA, Caplan ER. In Bonagura JD: *Current veterinary therapy XIII*, Philadelphia, 2000, Saunders, pp 357-361.

Nelson RW. In Ettinger SJ, Feldman EC: *Textbook of veterinary internal medicine*, Philadelphia, 1995, Saunders, pp 1501-1537.

Nichols R, Crenshaw KL. In Bonagura JD: *Current veterinary therapy XIII*, Philadelphia, 2000, Saunders, pp 384-386.

Peterson ME et al: Pretreatment clinical and laboratory findings in 225 dogs with hypoadrenocorticism, *J Am Vet Med Assoc* 208:85-91, 1996.

Peterson ME. In Kirk RW, Bonagura JD: *Current veterinary therapy XI*, Philadelphia, 1992, Saunders, pp 376-379.

Schulman R: Insulin and other therapies for diabetes mellitus, *Vet Med* 98:334-347, 2003.

Waters CB, Scott-Moncrieff JCR: Hypocalcemia in cats, *Compend Contin Educ Pract Vet* 14:497-507, 1992.

CHAPTER 20

Urologic Emergencies

Andrea M. Battaglia

The editor and pusblisher acknowledge and appreciate the original contribution of Jona Spano, whose work has been incorporated into this chapter.

Urologic emergencies can result from trauma or disease. Animals with abdominal trauma from automobile collisions, fights, or physical abuse should be examined for kidney or bladder damage. Trauma also can occur during treatment for urologic emergencies. Overly aggressive palpation of the bladder or cystocentesis can cause the bladder to rupture. Improper catheterization techniques can cause urethral tears. The veterinary technician must understand the proper techniques for placing urinary catheters and the problems that can occur.

Urinary obstruction is common in small animals and most common in male cats and specific breeds of dogs. Immediate treatment is necessary to prevent further complications, which can lead to renal failure and possibly death.

Renal failure can be acute or chronic. Ischemic or physiologic events, nephrotoxins, or diseases may cause acute renal failure (ARF). Chronic renal failure (CRF) is caused by progressive congenital disease or by renal disease acquired during life. Appropriate treatment depends on the cause and stage of the renal failure.

Stabilization and maintenance of the patient with a urologic emergency are based on an understanding of the signs associated with the various problems that can occur and the types of treatment that can be successful. These animals may need surgical intervention and medical management (Box 20-1).

Urinary Obstruction

Urinary obstruction is the inability of urine to flow normally from the body. An obstruction can either be partial or complete, resulting from a physical or functional condition of urinary outflow.

A space-occupying object in the urethra, urinary bladder, ureters, or renal pelvis can cause a physical obstruction (Fig. 20-1). Examples of these include urethral plugs, uroliths, tumors, and blood clots.

Uroliths are composed of very organized crystals of phosphate, urate, cystine, and oxalate and often are caused by a congenital abnormality in the metabolism or excretion of these minerals. Functional obstructions usually are abnormalities such as congenital strictures or damage to the nerves that control micturition; such nerve damage can result from a traumatic event.

Urinary obstructions can be found in dogs or cats, both male and female. Urinary calculi are the more common causes of outflow obstruction in male dogs and male cats. Although obstruction in dogs is caused by organized uroliths, in cats the debris is much less organized and usually forms a urethral plug at the tip of the penis. The blockage in the male dog usually is found in the bladder neck or the urethra. Whether physical or functional in nature, urinary obstructions must be treated immediately because they can lead to renal failure and possibly death.

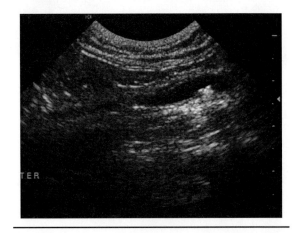

Fig. 20-1 Ultrasound depicting a urinary obstruction caused by a stone in the urethra of a cat.

Blocked Cat

A urethral plug composed of mucus and crystalline material can cause physical obstructions in cats. This condition is most common in male cats, because the lumen of the urethra is small throughout its length and even smaller at the tip of the penis. The urethral plug generally is found at the tip of the penis, where the debris becomes trapped. Female cats rarely have urethral obstructions because of their shorter urethra and wider urethral lumen. Small clumps of crystals, tiny calculi, blood clots, and mucus can pass more easily during urination. Untreated urinary obstructions in the cat can lead to severe metabolic changes and death.

Clinical Presentation. Cats with urethral obstruction may be alert or depressed, depending on the duration and degree of obstruction. Owners may notice episodes of stranguria (straining to urinate) or pollakiuria (passing small amounts of urine frequently) and longer periods in the litter box. They may also find the cat urinating in unusual places outside the litter box. Hematuria (blood in the urine) also may be present in varying amounts, depending on the amount of inflammation and irritation. Cats may appear restless and uncomfortable and lick continuously at the tip of the penis. Owners may perceive these signs as indications of constipation.

Cats with complete obstruction have a distended, painful bladder on palpation. Palpating the bladder may cause the cat to cry out and may induce straining to urinate and the passing of a few drops of blood-tinged urine.

Prolonged obstruction leads to depression, dehydration, vomiting, a low body temperature, and fluid volume and serum electrolyte imbalances caused by an acute onset of uremia.

Diagnosis. A series of diagnostic tests can be performed to determine the severity of an obstruction. If the cat is stable, then the bladder can be compressed carefully to check for resistance in urine outflow. Excessive or localized pressure should not be put on the bladder because it can rupture. Compressing the bladder can dislodge a urethral plug if located at the tip of the penis, and normal outflow can be obtained.

If resistance is excessive and urine outflow is not adequate, a urinary catheter and irrigation of the urethra may be necessary to dislodge the plug back into the bladder. Before placing the urinary catheter, the clinician may find it necessary to sedate the cat with ketamine and Valium or propofol (especially true if the cat is very active). The treatment orders include placement of an IV catheter and a check for azotemia and serum electrolyte imbalances. An ECG should be obtained to identify cardiac arrhythmias caused by hyperkalemia (Fig. 20-2). If a urinary catheter cannot pass easily into the bladder because of a urolith, plug, swelling, or stricture in the proximal urethra, then further diagnostic tests including ultrasound or radiographic imaging, including contrast, may be indicated to define the lesion.

Cystocentesis can be performed on a palpable bladder to collect urine for urinalysis and culture or to provide decompression if the bladder cannot be catheterized. This specimen allows a more accurate assessment of bacteria, cells, crystals, the presence of blood or protein, specific gravity, and pH in the bladder. A cystocentesis should be performed with the cat in a ventral-dorsal position. The cat should be well restrained to prevent movement and possible trauma.

The collection site should be free of hair and prepared aseptically with soap and water and alcohol or a dilute solution of a tincture of benzalkonium chloride. A sterile 23- to 22-gauge needle 1- to 1½-inches long (depending on the size of the animal) is attached to a 5-ml or 10-ml sterile syringe. A larger needle should not be used because it can cause leakage from the bladder wall. The bladder is then palpated and immobilized to direct needle insertion and to ensure an adequate volume for collection. The needle is inserted into the ventral midline about midway between the pelvis and dome of the bladder, with the tip of the needle pointing caudally at a 45-degree angle. If urine collection is unsuccessful because of misinsertion of the needle, then the needle should be removed and both the needle and the syringe should be replaced before the procedure is repeated.

On presentation, if the cat appears very depressed or dehydrated and has a low body temperature, then blood work should be performed immediately. These results determine the rest of the diagnostic workup and in what order treatment should be initiated, because the cat has begun to show signs of uremia.

Treatment. Treatment begins almost in conjunction with the diagnostic procedures and the efforts to relieve the obstruction. If the cat is showing signs of depression or dehydration and has a low body

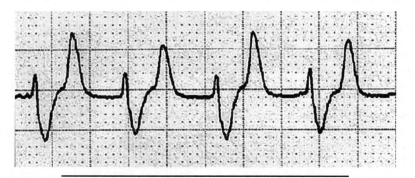

Fig. 20-2 ECG showing hyperkalemia in a severely uremic animal.

temperature, then the animal is probably uremic; if so, an IV catheter should be placed and therapy started to correct fluid volume deficits, metabolic acidosis, and identified electrolyte disturbances. An ECG should be evaluated for evidence of arrhythmias and hyperkalemia. Hyperkalemia can cause bradycardia, diminished P waves, widened QRS complexes, and increased T waves. If abnormalities are recognized, then sodium bicarbonate ($NaHCO_3$) or dextrose with or without regular insulin can be administered to drive potassium into the cells and transiently correct the hyperkalemia and cardiac disturbances. Metabolic acidosis also should be treated with IV $NaHCO_3$ if serum pH is less than 7.2 or the base deficit is greater than 10. IV fluids should be given at a rate of 40 to 60 ml/kg/hr to correct existing fluid deficits. Using 0.9% sodium chloride to minimize potassium administration is best.

Catheterization. The decision to use an indwelling urinary catheter should be made with an understanding of the rationale and therapeutic goals in mind. Catheters should not be placed haphazardly because they can cause injury, induce urinary tract infections, cause urethral strictures, and potentially rupture the bladder. The therapeutic goals of urinary catheterization are to document the rate of urine formation in critically ill patients, prevent reobstruction during the first 24 hours after the initial obstruction has been relieved, and keep the bladder decompressed to facilitate reestablishment of normal bladder wall contractility. A cystocentesis can be performed with a 22-gauge or smaller needle to relieve excessive pressure while attempts of urinary catheterization are implemented (Technical Tip Boxes 20-2 and 20-3).

Managing Indwelling Urinary Catheters. Once an indwelling catheter has been placed, the cat must be monitored and the urinary catheter must be maintained properly. Elizabethan collars are often necessary to prevent the cat from pulling the catheter out.

After the catheter is placed, the cat may undergo a postobstructive diuresis in which fluid administration must match the rate of urine production. The amount of a 0.9% sodium chloride solution to administer can be estimated from the urine produced during the previous 2 hours; fluid input must equal urine output. While the diuresis is occurring, serum electrolytes should be measured every 2 to 4 hours in a severely ill animal and every 6 to 8 hours in a stable patient. Cats should be weighed

accurately every 12 hours to document net fluid balance. Serum potassium may drop quickly during the postobstructive diuresis, and potassium supplementation may be needed to prevent hypokalemia. Guidelines for parenteral potassium supplementation used at the Veterinary Medical Teaching Hospital intensive care unit at the University of California at Davis are listed in Table 20-1.

Cats with cardiac problems may not tolerate fluid administration and may be predisposed to fluid overload (uscultate the chest for heart murmurs or gallop rhythms, listen for lung sounds and possible crackles, and monitor changes in central venous pressure when fluid is given). Continuous ECG recording is useful to monitor heart rate and rhythm and to detect potassium oversupplementation.

Urine output should be measured and recorded every 2 hours, and hematuria or excessive sediment should be noted.

For cats with prolonged obstruction, serum electrolytes and venous blood gases should be measured every 1 to 12 hours to detect ongoing electrolyte and acid-base abnormalities. Blood glucose concentrations should be measured every 1 to 4 hours if the cat is being treated with dextrose and insulin, and the packed cell volume and total protein concentration should be measured in animals receiving fluid therapy every 6 hours. Azotemia (blood urea nitrogen, serum creatinine) should be documented every 6 hours. Obtunded cats must be turned every 4 hours.

Other medications that may be indicated are antibiotics to prevent urinary tract infections from the indwelling catheter, phenoxybenzamine to decrease urethral resistance, and bethanechol to manage atonic bladder by increasing detrusor muscle contractility. Corticosteroids should not be used in these patients because they can impair the immune system and make the patient susceptible to bladder infections.

The patient's bladder should be palpated every 2 to 4 hours to assess its volume. If the bladder is not emptying, then the catheter and urinary collection system should be checked for kinks or plugs. If none are noted, then the bladder may be compressed carefully to dispel urine. If the bladder remains distended, then the catheter may be obstructed and should be flushed retrograde with sterile saline. Hydrogen peroxide, antiseptic soap and water, a 1:60 dilution of Betadine solution, and Betadine ointment are used to maintain urinary catheters (Box 20-4).

BOX 20-2

Technical Tip: Placing the Male Cat Urinary Catheter

Items needed:

- A sterile, soft, flexible catheter (For maximum benefit, the catheter should be the largest diameter and most flexible that will pass readily through the urethra. This prevents urine leaking around the catheter insertion site. If urine is leaking from the site, then the rate of urine production and the amount of urine collection cannot be calculated accurately. The preferred catheters are a 5-French feeding tube and urethral catheter (Sovereign) or a 3.5-French infant feeding catheter (Mallinckrodt Medical, St. Louis, MO.)
- Betadine ointment
- Cotton-tipped swabs
- Suture: 3-0 Ethilon (Ethicon, Inc)
- 1-inch tape
- Antiseptic soap or Betadine surgical scrub (The Purdue Fredrick Company, Norwalk, CT)
- Small sterile urinary collection bag (Sherwood Medical, St. Louis, MO)
- Sterile connecting adapters (Sherwood)
- Sterile KY jelly (Carter Products, NY) or 2% lidocaine jelly (Abbott Laboratories, North Chicago, IL)
- Sterile gloves
- 12 cc syringe with a solution consisting of 4 ml Betadine and 250 ml sterile water
- Sterile needle holder and soft tissue thumb forceps
- Sterile drapes
- Cable ties and cable tie gun (Cole-Parmer, Vernon Hills, IL)

An indwelling urinary catheter should be placed aseptically to prevent a urinary tract infection as follows:

1. With the cat in a ventral-dorsal position, clip the hair from the prepuce and from a small area on the perineum around the preputial orifice.
2. Clean the preputial orifice with antiseptic soap and water or flush the orifice with Betadine solution.
3. Retract the prepuce to extrude the penis. Gently prepare the tip of the penis with antiseptic soap and water using soft cotton balls.
4. Place a sterile barrier drape under the penis to prevent contamination of the catheter with hair.
5. Put on sterile gloves.
6. Lubricate the sterile urinary catheter with sterile KY jelly or lidocaine jelly.
7. Retract the penis caudally to straighten the urethra, insert the catheter into the tip of the penis, and advance the catheter gently and carefully into the bladder using an aseptic technique.
8. Once the catheter is in the bladder, urine should flow into the catheter. Cap the catheter opening and allow the prepuce to return to a normal position.
9. Apply 1-inch tape to the catheter (making a butterfly around the catheter with the tape). Place two stay sutures on opposite sides of the prepuce, and suture each flap of the butterfly to its corresponding stay suture.
10. Apply Betadine ointment with cotton-tipped swabs to the urethral orifice.
11. Using a sterile adapter, connect the catheter to a urinary drainage bag.
12. Make sure all joints are tight and secured with cable ties to prevent them from disconnecting or leaking.
13. Tape the extension tubing to the tail to prevent traction on the prepuce.
14. Place the collection bag lower than the patient so that urine will flow only into the bag. If urine does not flow properly, then it will increase the risk of urinary tract infection.

Response to Treatment. The indwelling urinary catheter should be removed after the first 24 hours of treatment if no complications occur (e.g., hematuria, atonic bladder). The next 24 hours are devoted to careful monitoring of the cat for urine production and ability to void urine. If production is normal, all other clinical signs are stable, and the cat is eating and drinking normally, then it can be sent home. The owner is instructed to watch the cat for straining to urinate and for frequent trips to the litter box. He or she should observe the amount of urine produced and note whether blood is present.

BOX 20-3

Technical Tip: Placing the Female Cat Urinary Catheter

The list of preparatory supplies is the same as needed for male cats (see Box 20-2), with the exception of a 3.5-French infant feeding tube, a nasal speculum or otoscope, and a light source.

The sedated cat is placed in sternal recumbency with the hind legs hanging over the edge of the table, and the tail is retracted back toward the head. Once the patient is positioned, the following procedure is recommended:

1. Clip hair from the vulvar area.
2. Gently clean the vulvar area with antiseptic soap.
3. Using a sterile syringe, gently flush the vestibule with a 1:60 dilution of Betadine solution.
4. Place a barrier drape around the perivulvar area.
5. Put on sterile gloves.
6. Lubricate the urinary catheter with sterile KY jelly or lidocaine jelly.
7. Gently insert a nasal speculum or otoscope in the vagina and locate the papilla and urethral orifice. Insert the catheter into the urethra, and gently pass it into the bladder. (Note: A blind technique includes gently inserting a finger 2 cm into the rectum. Apply gentle pressure to the floor of the rectum. This will reposition the urethral opening and allow passage of the urinary catheter.)
8. Once the catheter is in the bladder, it should fill with urine. Cap the catheter closed.
9. Attach 1-inch tape to the catheter, making a butterfly. Place two stay sutures on opposite sides of the vulva, and suture each flap of the butterfly to its corresponding stay suture.
10. Attach a sterile urinary collection system.
11. Attach the extension tubing to the tail to prevent tension on the catheter while allowing enough slack for a full range of tail movement.
12. Make sure all connections are secure and tight.

TABLE 20-1

Guidelines for Parenteral Potassium Supplementation

Plasma Protein K	Potassium Chloride (Added to Sufficient Quantity of Fluids)
≥3.5	Should not add potassium chloride
3.0-3.5	20 mEq/L
2.5-3.0	30 mEq/L
2.0-2.5	40 mEq/L
<2.0	50 mEq/L

The cat's diet must be monitored. Dietary recommendations include feeding canned food to increase water intake and feeding acidifying diets (e.g., Hill's Prescription Diet C/D, Waltham pH Control, Iams, Low pH/S, and CNM UR), which are low in phosphate and magnesium, to decrease the production of struvite crystals.

The cat may also be continued on antimicrobials to reduce the incidence of urinary tract infections secondary to catheterization, phenoxybenzamine to reduce internal urethral sphincter tone, propantheline to decrease spasm of the urethra, and bethanechol to increase detrusor muscle tone.

If the patient does not void urine for 24 hours after catheter removal, a new indwelling catheter is placed and indwelling catheter procedures are started again. Recatheterization usually is attempted three times. If normal urine voiding is not achieved after the third catheterization, then the urethra may be damaged and the prognosis is guarded.

Because urinary obstructions are most common in male cats, a urethrostomy, in which the penile urethra is amputated, may be performed as a salvage procedure to provide urethral patency. The urethrostomy removes the narrowest, scarred portion of the urethra to expose a larger urethral lumen, which usually prevents future obstruction.

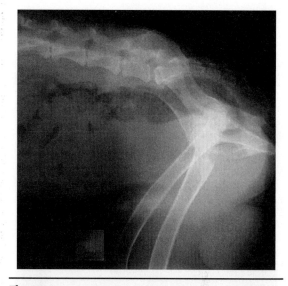

Fig. 20-3 Urinary obstruction in the penile urethra of a male dog.

Blocked Dog

Urinary obstruction in the male dog usually results from a physical blockage of urinary outflow by a urolith; in the female dog the causes usually are associated with bladder tumors.

Functional outflow obstruction occurs secondary to a traumatic event affecting the nerves that control the detrusor muscles of the bladder for micturition.

Urinary calculi are the most common causes of male dog outflow obstruction, followed by scarring in the urethra and bladder neck tumors. Usual sites of obstruction are in the middle to distal end of the penile urethra (Fig. 20-3).

Uroliths form in urine supersaturated with minerals, which precipitate to form microaggregates. These aggregates can fuse together, forming stones of a variety of shapes, sizes, and composition that can build in the kidney or bladder and move down the urinary tract. Some examples of these mineral aggregates are magnesium ammonium phosphate (struvite), calcium oxalate, silica, and purines. Many different minerals can form uroliths, so when a urolith is removed from a site of obstruction, it should be analyzed to determine its composition. The exact composition of the stone dictates the course of medical or surgical treatment.

Clinical Presentation. Signs of urinary obstruction vary greatly and depend on the degree and location of the obstruction. Urethral obstruction can be associated with dysuria or anuria. If obstruction has been complete for a long time, then signs of uremia can occur, including depression, dehydration, and vomiting. The dog also may have a distended or turgid bladder. When an obstruction is located in the bladder, the dog may have signs similar to those of cystitis. Hematuria can be present, and micturition can be characterized by the frequent passage of small amounts of urine. Ureteral obstruction can lead to hydronephrosis and cause cranial abdominal pain.

Diagnosis. The diagnosis of urinary obstruction is established on the basis of a complete history and physical examination, as well as a series of diagnostic tests to determine the location and severity of the obstruction. If the dog has signs of uremia, then a complete blood cell count and serum chemistry profile should be performed to identify fluid, acid-base,

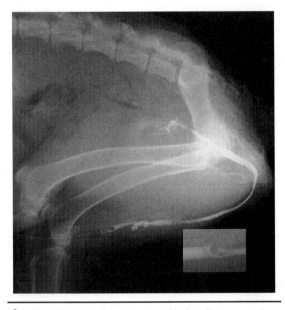

Fig. 20-4 The use of a contrast medium to diagnose a urinary obstruction in the penile urethra of a male dog.

and electrolyte imbalances. A cystocentesis can be performed to collect a sterile sample for urinalysis and culture and to alleviate bladder distention. The technique is similar to that described for the cat. In large breed dogs, cystocentesis can be performed more easily in a standing position or in lateral recumbency as long as the bladder is palpable and the procedure is performed aseptically. Once the urine is obtained, a careful analysis of the crystals can aid in determining urolith composition.

Urethral obstruction should be considered if a urinary catheter of appropriate size cannot be passed up the urethra into the bladder.

Radiographic evaluation and ultrasound can be useful in diagnosing obstructions of the kidney ureters, bladder, or urethra. The use of contrast medium may help determine whether the obstruction is intralumenal or extralumenal (Fig. 20-4).

Treatment. If the dog is weak, hypotensive, dehydrated, and uremic, treatment should be initiated to correct these conditions before the obstruction is corrected. An IV catheter should be placed and therapy should be started to correct fluid volume deficits, metabolic acidosis, and electrolyte disturbances. An ECG should be used to monitor cardiac arrhythmias and evidence of hyperkalemia.

Catheterization. Once the patient is stabilized, passage of an indwelling urinary catheter should be attempted to relieve the obstruction. If a catheter cannot be passed into the bladder because the urolith is blocking the urethra, then urohydropropulsion can be used in an attempt to push the stone or stones back into the bladder.

When urine outflow has been established, an indwelling urinary catheter may be placed to keep the urethra from reobstructing (Technical Tip Boxes 20-5 and 20-6).

Urohydropropulsion. The disposition of the animal may necessitate sedation or general anesthesia for this procedure. If the animal is an anesthetic risk because of a uremic crisis, then a topical application of lidocaine and a small dose of analgesia may be adequate to keep the animal comfortable.

With the animal in lateral recumbency, inject a liberal quantity of a 1:1 mixture of sterile saline solution and aqueous lubricant through a flexible catheter into the urethral lumen to facilitate movement. An assistant should be asked to insert an index finger into the patient's rectum and firmly occlude the lumen of the pelvic urethra by applying digital pressure. Sterile saline is then injected into the urethra through the catheter; the pressure builds rapidly and the assistant releases the digital pressure placed on the pelvic urethra. Pressure should be maintained in the urethral lumen by forcing more saline forward after the assistant has released digital pressure. This technique should force the fluid and usually the uroliths into the urinary bladder. Sometimes the urolith returns quickly to the bladder; it may be necessary to repeat the procedure a couple of times to get the urolith to reach the bladder.

Response to Treatment. Once urine outflow has been established, management is directed at surgical or medical removal of the uroliths and medical therapy to prevent reoccurrence.

Struvite is the most common mineral detected in canine uroliths. The urine must be supersaturated with magnesium, ammonium, and phosphate for struvite uroliths to form. In contrast to cats, struvite urolith formation in dogs generally is associated with urinary tract infections with urease-producing microbes, which cause alkalization of the urine. Resolution of the urinary tract infection with antibiotics is the foundation of therapy. Dietary modifications that reduce phosphorus and magnesium excretion

BOX 20-5

Technical Tip: Male Dog Urinary Catheter Insertion

Equipment:
- Sterile soft flexible catheter such as a male infant feeding catheter sizes 5, 8, or 10 French (Mallinckrodt Medical, St. Louis, MO).
- Betadine ointment
- Cotton-tipped swabs
- Suture: 3-0 Ethilon (Ethicon, Inc)
- 1-inch tape
- Antiseptic soap or Betadine scrub (The Purdue Fredrick Company, Norwalk, CT)
- Sterile urinary collection bag (Sherwood)
- Sterile connecting adapters (for the male urinary collection system) (Sherwood)
- Sterile KY jelly (Carter Products, NY) or lidocaine jelly 2% (Abbott Laboratories, North Chicago, IL)
- Sterile gloves
- 12 cc syringe with a solution of 4 ml Betadine and 250 ml sterile water
- Sterile needle holder and soft tissue thumb forceps
- Sterile barrier drape
- Cable ties and cable tie gun (Cole-Parmer, Vernon Hills, IL)

Procedure:
1. Place the dog in lateral recumbency.
2. Clip hair from the prepuce and around the preputial orifice.
3. Clean the preputial orifice with antiseptic soap and water.
4. Retract the sheath to expose the entire shaft of the penis. Disinfect the tip of the penis with tincture of zephirine or chlorhexidine solution.
5. Put on sterile gloves.
6. Lubricate the sterile urinary catheter with sterile KY jelly or lidocaine jelly.
7. Insert the lubricated catheter into the urethra using an aseptic technique and gently pass retrograde along the urethra into the bladder.
8. Once the catheter is in the bladder, urine should fill the catheter. Cap the catheter opening and allow the prepuce to return to a normal position.
9. Apply tape to catheter using 1-inch tape to make a butterfly. Place two stay sutures on opposite sides of the prepuce, and suture both flaps of the butterfly to the stay sutures.
10. Using a sterile adapter, connect the catheter to a urinary drainage bag.
11. Make sure all joints are cable-tied together to prevent them from disconnecting or leaking.
12. Tape the tubing to the hind leg or tail to prevent traction on the prepuce.

and urinary acidification are recommended. Hill's Prescription Diet S/D is one such diet that is low in protein, phosphorus, and magnesium. Surgical removal of existing uroliths is the preferred method of treatment, but medical dissolution with antibiotics and dietary modification has been advocated and may be indicated in animals with recurrent disease or those who are poor surgical risks.

Ammonium urate uroliths are most common in dalmatians and are managed medically. The manage these uroliths with dietary modifications that reduce urine concentrations of uric acid and ammonium and hydrogen ions. The diet should be a purine-restricted, nonacidifying diet that does not contain supplemental sodium (Hill's Prescription Diet U/D or Hill's Prescription Diet K/D). Besides diet changes, xanthine oxidase inhibitors (Allopurinol) are given to block uric acid formation in the serum and urine. The urine should be alkalinized by the administration of $NaHCO_3$ or potassium citrate orally to achieve a urine pH of 7.0. Documented urinary tract infections are treated with appropriate antibiotics.

BOX 20-6

Technical Tip: Female Urinary Catheter Insertion

Equipment:
The list of preparatory supplies is the same as needed for male dogs (see Box 20-5), with the addition of Foley catheters sizes 5, 8, and 10 French (Sherwood, St. Louis, MO) and a vaginal speculum.

Procedure:
1. Clip hair from vulvar area.
2. Gently clean the vulvar area with antiseptic soap or Betadine solution.
3. Using a sterile syringe, gently flush the vestibule with a 1:60 dilution of Betadine solution.
4. Put on sterile gloves.
5. Lubricate a sterile Foley catheter with sterile KY jelly or lidocaine jelly.
6. Gently insert a gloved finger, sterile speculum, sterile laryngoscope blade, or sterile otoscope into the vagina. Locate the papilla and urethral opening and insert the catheter.
7. Once the catheter is inserted, fill the balloon of the Foley catheter with the indicated amount of sterile water.
8. Gently retract the catheter to ensure that the balloon is within the bladder.
9. Attach a sterile urinary collection system.
10. Apply a piece of 1-inch tape around the hind legs. Tape the catheter or tubing to the tape on the leg or tail, allowing enough slack for the animal to stand and walk without tension on the catheter.
11. Make sure all connections are cable-tied together to prevent leaking.

Calcium oxalate uroliths are managed very differently. Surgery appears to be the most effective treatment because they are very difficult to dissolve. Some dietary modifications can be effective. A diet moderately restricted in protein, calcium, oxalate, and sodium such as Hill's Prescription Diet U/D may be considered to help prevent recurrences. Ideally the diet should not be restricted or supplemented with phosphorus or magnesium. Attempts should be made to alkalinize the urine.

Some dog breeds are more susceptible to urolith production than others, and some breeds are predisposed to particular urolith types. According to the Minnesota Urolith Center, where extensive studies of canine uroliths were performed, the following uroliths were matched to a particular breed of dog. Calcium oxalate uroliths were prominent in male dogs, especially miniature schnauzers, Lhasa apsos, Yorkshire terriers, miniature poodles, and Shih Tzus. Struvite uroliths were more common in female dogs, possibly because of the higher prevalence of urinary tract infections. Common breeds associated with these uroliths are the miniature schnauzer, bichon frise, Shih tzus, Yorkshire terriers, Lhasa apsos, cocker spaniels, and miniature poodles. Uroliths composed of purines were found mostly in male dogs, dalmatians, Yorkshire terriers, and English bulldogs. These breeds have normal serum uric acid concentrations but high urine uric acid concentrations.

Renal Disease

Renal failure is the inability of the kidneys to perform their numerous functions of excretion, metabolic regulation, and hormone production. As the disease progresses, the animal begins to show signs of multiple-organ dysfunction, a syndrome called *uremia*. Conventional and specialized treatments are available. If the disease is treated early and aggressively, then the kidney can regenerate and recover. If left untreated, then the patient will deteriorate and eventually die.

Kidney

The kidneys are located in the lumbar region of the abdomen, enveloped in peritoneum and loosely attached to the body wall.

Each kidney is made up of a variety of structures that are responsible for several functions, such as fluid regulation, electrolyte balance, excretion of metabolic waste products, and hormone production.

The functional unit of the kidney is the nephron, made up of a glomerulus, proximal tubule, loop of Henle, distal tubule, and collecting duct. As blood passes through the kidney, an ultrafiltrate is formed containing water and very small molecules. This filtrate is later modified by the nephron to form final urine. Water balance and electrolyte balance is maintained in these tubules, and nitrogenous waste is excreted.

The kidneys also produce the hormones erythropoietin, renin, and calcitriol. Erythropoietin is

Causes of Acute Renal Failure

- Ischemia
- Shock
- Hypovolemia
- Hemorrhage
- Decreased cardiac output
- Heart failure
- Renal thrombosis
- Nephrotoxins
- Organic compounds such as ethylene glycol (antifreeze) and pesticides
- Antimicrobials such as cephalosporins, aminoglycosides, and tetracyclines
- Anesthetics
- Heavy metals such as lead
- Analgesics or nonsteroidal antiinflammatory drugs, including aspirin and phenylbutazone
- Snake venom
- Infectious diseases
  Leptospirosis
  Bacterial infections, including pyelonephritis
  Immune-mediated diseases (e.g., glomerulonephritis, systemic conditions, hypercalcemia)

responsible for producing red blood cells, renin is involved in controlling blood pressure (BP), and calcitriol stimulates calcium absorption from the small intestine.

Renal Failure

When the kidneys are injured, resulting in their inability to maintain excretory function, they are considered to be in failure. Renal failure can be an acute or chronic condition.

ARF is a sudden decrease in renal function, usually less than a week. ARF is classified as either prerenal, intrinsic renal parenchymal (functional element), or postrenal. Prerenal ARF is a functional consequence of reduced blood flow to the kidneys and is completely reversible with restoration of adequate renal perfusion. Hemorrhage, vomiting, diarrhea, dehydration, poor fluid intake, and systemic diseases such as heart failure can cause it. Intrinsic ARF results from damage to the cellular structure of the kidney by ischemic or toxic events. Postrenal

ARF results from an obstruction or diversion of the outflow of urine from the animal. Obstructions can be located in the urethra, bladder, ureter, or renal pelvis, and urine can be diverted into the abdominal cavity or soft tissue with rupture of the ureters, bladder, or urethra. All of these conditions are potentially reversible if diagnosed early and treated aggressively, and they constitute a urologic emergency.

CRF develops over an extended period of time, usually several months to years. The renal injury is not reversible; however, in its early stages the animal can be supported with proper diet and medication; CRF rarely is considered an emergency condition.

Causes of Intrinsic Acute Renal Failure. ARF most commonly results from ischemic or physiologic (prerenal) events, nephrotoxins, or other diseases. Ischemic injury occurs with profound or prolonged decreases in renal blood flow. Prolonged ischemia causes the epithelial cells of the kidney to be deprived of oxygen, lose cellular function, and die (Box 20-7).

Clinical Presentation of Acute Renal Failure in Animals. The presenting complaints typically are vague and nonspecific for renal disease and may include the following:

- Anorexia
- Vomiting
- Listlessness
- Diarrhea
- Halitosis
- Ataxia
- Seizures
- Known toxin exposure
- Oliguria
- Anuria
- Polyuria

The physical examination may demonstrate the following:

- Normal body condition and hair coat, which helps differentiate ARF from CRF.
- Dehydration or overhydration. Dehydration is most commonly from a decrease in fluid intake, vomiting, or diarrhea; overhydration may be seen if the animal has been given parenteral fluids.
- Oral ulceration or necrosis of the tongue, halitosis, hypothermia or fever. Most uremic animals

have low body temperature proportional to their azotemia; however, if the condition is caused by infection, then the temperature may be elevated. A normal temperature in a uremic animal may suggest the presence of fever and infection.

- Scleral infection; nonpalpable urinary bladder; tachypnea; bradycardia; large, painful, firm kidneys.

Causes of Chronic Renal Failure. Because this injury to the kidney is long standing, little or no potential for repair exists. Surviving nephrons compensate maximally for those that have been lost. As the CRF progresses and renal function deteriorates, the animal becomes polyuric and progressively azotemic and eventually develops uremia. CRF results from congenital diseases that progress or from renal diseases acquired through life. The animal may be able to compensate for the loss of renal function initially, but over time, as more renal function is lost, the signs of renal failure materialize.

Clinical Presentation of Patients with Chronic Renal Failure. Some telltale signs of CRF include weight loss, prior episodes of illness, polyuria, polydipsia, pale mucous membranes, small irregular kidneys, low body temperature, and poor hair coat and body condition.

Diagnosis of Acute and Chronic Renal Failure. The diagnosis of renal failure is confirmed with laboratory tests that document the extent of renal impairment and distinguish between ARF and CRF. These tests may include the following:

A complete blood cell count may reveal changes in hematocrit depending on hydration levels. If the renal failure is caused by an infectious state, then an increase in the white blood cell count will be seen. A complete blood cell count can distinguish regenerative from nonregenerative anemia. Anemia usually is not present in ARF but is present in CRF.

A chemistry panel demonstrates progressive increases in serum urea nitrogen, creatinine, phosphate, and potassium. Serum bicarbonate usually is decreased, and serum calcium may vary. The chemistry panel also helps determine whether other organ systems are involved.

Urine specimens should be obtained by cystocentesis to prevent contamination by the lower urogenital tract and to provide a clearer interpretation. In ARF, urine specific gravity ranges from 1.007 to 1.017, representing an inability to concentrate urine.

A more concentrated urine predicts a prerenal component. Mild proteinuria usually is present. Casts, white blood cells, red blood cells, bacteria, and crystals usually are present. The presence of calcium oxalate crystals suggests ethylene glycol toxicity.

Radiographs typically reveal normal to large kidneys with smooth contours or may show small, irregular kidneys in animals with decompensated CRF. Ultrasound may confirm ethylene glycol toxicity, which appears as brightness of the cortex secondary to calcium oxalate crystal deposition. Ultrasound can further define the shape and size of the kidneys and alterations in intrarenal architecture.

Renal biopsy confirms the diagnosis of ARF and may establish its cause. Renal histopathology can define the severity of the disease and its potential reversibility and is an excellent indicator to distinguish between ARF and CRF. The procedure is invasive, with inherent risks such as hemorrhage and further renal damage.

Ethylene glycol levels should be assessed in cases of known antifreeze exposure or when calcium oxalate crystals are present in the urine of an animal with ARF.

Leptospirosis titers must be evaluated in animals with ARF. Leptospirosis is highly suspected in young dogs with ARF of unknown origin. Animals with signs of systemic infection including fever and an increase in white blood cells also must be evaluated for this disease. Leptospires are spirochetes that infect humans and animals; urine from the infected host is the common source of contamination. The staff working with these animals should wear gloves and use other measures to prevent contamination.

Treatment of Acute Renal Failure

Once the diagnosis of ARF or CRF has been established, the goals of treatment are to minimize further injury to the kidney, quickly correct renal hemodynamics, and reestablish water and solute balances. The sooner treatment is implemented, the greater the chances for renal regeneration and recovery.

If a patient arrives to the clinic after a nephrotoxin has been ingested, gastric lavage should be instituted or vomiting induced, and activated charcoal should be administered within 30 to 60 minutes to absorb any residual toxin. When the toxin has been identified, specific treatments or antidotes can be given to reverse the effects. For example, ethanol or methylpyrazole is given to treat ethylene glycol toxicity.

ARF treatment can be divided into three areas: (1) fluid therapy, (2) drug therapy, and (3) nutritional support.

Fluid Therapy

Animals with ARF can be dehydrated because of vomiting, diarrhea, and anorexia or overhydrated if they are anuric and have no way to excrete excessive fluid loads. If a fluid deficit is present, then fluid volume to be replaced is calculated by multiplying the estimated percentage of dehydration by the body weight in kilograms. Fluids should be given via IV catheter (peripheral or central venous catheter). Using a jugular catheter is preferable, because other diagnostic sampling or testing can be performed easily through this site. During the period of rehydration, the animal should be monitored to determine urine output and detect signs of overhydration (i.e., changes in body weight, arterial pressure, and central venous pressure, packed cell volume, and total solids). If blood losses also are detected, then transfusion should be given to restore packed cell volume and BP.

Animals who are oliguric or anuric must be monitored closely because they have a greater potential of becoming fluid overloaded, hypertensive, and edematous.

Drug Therapy

If oliguria or anuria persists, additional treatment is needed to induce diuresis. Some agents used to induce diuresis are furosemide (Lasix, Hoechst) and mannitol (Osmitrol). These drugs often are used in combination to enhance diuresis. Urine output should improve within 1 to 2 hours if treatment is likely to be effective.

BP should be monitored with changes in fluid balance. Oscillometric techniques or ultrasonic Doppler can measure BP indirectly. Normal BP of the dog should be 148 mm Hg systolic, 87 mm Hg diastolic, and 102 mm Hg mean. Normal BP of the cat should be 125 mm Hg systolic, 75 mm Hg diastolic, and 100 mm Hg mean. Systemic hypertension develops from either fluid overload or uremia and may warrant antihypertensive therapy to prevent retinal detachment and cerebral hemorrhage.

Animals with ARF also have severe hyperkalemia and acidosis. Hyperkalemia is the most life-threatening electrolyte abnormality associated with ARF.

Acidosis may resolve with fluid therapy, but if serum bicarbonate is less than 15 mEq/L, then treatment with $NaHCO_3$ should be initiated. Blood gases and total carbon dioxide should be reevaluated to determine whether additional therapy is needed.

Hyperkalemia can cause cardiac disturbances such as bradycardia, ventricular tachycardia, and fibrillation. ECG changes include peaked T waves, loss of P waves, and wider QRS complexes. If the ECG changes are severe, then immediate therapy is needed to decrease serum potassium. $NaHCO_3$ helps correct serum potassium concentrations by exchanging intracellular hydrogen for extracellular potassium. The effects on the heart can be counteracted with calcium gluconate, which antagonizes the cardiotoxicity of high serum potassium concentrations. Glucose and insulin can be given in an emergency to promote the shift of potassium into the cells, where it is safe. If this therapy is used, then monitor the animal for hypoglycemia.

Gastrointestinal complications such as vomiting, diarrhea, anorexia, and severe ulceration of the gastrointestinal tract and mouth are some of the most common signs of ARF. Histamine blockers such as cimetidine, ranitidine, or famotidine can control vomiting. Gastrointestinal protectives such as sucralfate can be given to promote gastric ulcer healing. Oral ulcerations are managed effectively by rinsing the mouth frequently with a 0.1% chlorhexidine solution.

Nutritional Support

Many animals with ARF cannot tolerate oral food intake because of vomiting, nausea, or ulcerations. Their diet should be low in protein, phosphorus, and sodium while providing adequate amounts of calories, vitamins, and minerals. The basal energy expenditure in kilocalories per day can be determined by the following formula: 70 × body weight in kilograms to the 75th power. If an animal is critically ill, the basal energy expenditure should be multiplied by 1.5. If the animal is under minimal stress and has a low activity level, the basal energy expenditure is multiplied by 1.25. When the patient is catabolic or has a very severe disease, the basal energy expenditure should be multiplied by 1.75 to 2.0.

Animals that will not eat enough can be fed by a nasogastric tube or through a percutaneous endoscopically placed gastric tube. Feeding can be achieved by blending therapeutic diets (Hill's

Prescription Diet K/D, Waltham Low Protein Diet) or by using formulated liquid diets (Renal Care). Percutaneous endoscopically placed gastric tube feeding should be provided three or four times daily. Each meal should not exceed one half the animal's stomach volume (60 ml/kg in cats, 90 ml/kg in dogs).

Response to Treatment

Appropriate therapy should improve renal hemodynamics and water and solute imbalances as predicted by a decrease in azotemia, normalization of serum potassium and serum bicarbonate, control of vomiting, resolution of oral and gastric ulceration, and a stabilization of body weight.

If medical management fails to increase urine production and the clinical complications associated with ARF cannot be controlled, alternative approaches must be initiated to stabilize the animal.

Treatment of Chronic Renal Failure

CRF is irreversible and progressive. No cure exists, but medical and dietary management can minimize the progression of CRF.

Fluid Therapy

In CRF, urine production is increased. Therefore to maintain fluid balance and prevent dehydration, water consumption must be increased orally, subcutaneously, or intravenously. Some owners are able to give their pets fluids subcutaneously at home.

Drug Therapy

Animals with prolonged CRF become progressively azotemic and eventually develop uremia. Laboratory tests reveal changes in the serum blood chemistry, complete blood cell count, and fluid and electrolyte balances. These can include increases in serum bicarbonate, increases in serum phosphorus concentrations, and a nonregenerative anemia caused by the failure of the kidney to synthesize erythropoietin. BP monitoring can reveal systemic hypertension.

Metabolic acidosis can be treated with oral $NaHCO_3$. Hyperphosphatemia can be controlled with a dietary phosphate restriction and oral phosphate binders (aluminum hydroxide). Nonregenerative anemia can be supported with blood transfusions of compatible packed red blood cells or recombinant human erythropoietin (Epogen, Amgen). Epogen stimulates red blood cell production.

Systemic hypertension can be treated with a combination of sodium-restricted diets (e.g., Hill's Prescription Diet K/D) and antihypertensive drugs such as enalapril, hydralazine, or diltiazem. Treatment depends on the severity and causes of the systemic hypertension.

Nutritional Support

Dietary therapy plays an important role in managing CRF. Some of the benefits of appropriate diet for animals with CRF include preventing clinical signs of uremia, minimizing the excess or loss of electrolytes and minerals, slowing the progression of CRF, and maintaining adequate nutrition.

Diets should be low in protein, phosphorus, and sodium. Examples of renal diets are Hill's Prescription Diet K/D, Waltham Low and Medium Protein Diets, and Purina CNM NF. The diets should be fed according to the animal's caloric needs. Appropriate measures should be taken if the animal is showing signs of an acute onset of uremia such as vomiting and anorexia.

Response to Treatment

The animal with CRF should be reevaluated at regular intervals to check for therapeutic response. Monitoring these animals regularly allows treatment of the changing needs that develop over time. If conservative medical management cannot support the patient with CRF, then alternative treatments are available.

Alternative Treatments

When conventional therapy fails to restore renal function or the clinical consequences of uremia, hemodialysis or renal transplantation must be considered.

Hemodialysis

Hemodialysis is a sophisticated renal replacement therapy instituted on a temporary or permanent basis when conventional therapies fail. In ARF, dialysis is initiated at an early stage to stabilize the animal and provide excretory supplementation until

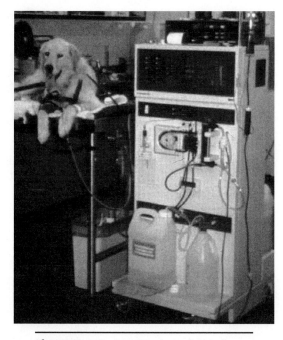

Fig. 20-5 Animal receiving hemodialysis therapy.

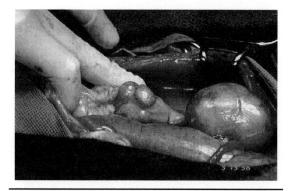

Fig. 20-6 Kidney transplant. The left organ is a diseased kidney; on the right is the newly transplanted kidney. (Photograph courtesy of Dr. Lili Aronson, University of California–Davis, Veterinary Medical Teaching Hospital, 1997.)

renal injury is repaired and adequate renal function returns. Hemodialysis also can be used in combination with conventional medical therapy in animals with severe CRF that cannot be managed with medications and diet alone (Fig. 20-5).

Hemodialysis incorporates an artificial kidney or dialyzer to reduce the azotemia and correct life-threatening fluid, electrolyte, and acid-base imbalances. The artificial kidney uses a biocompatible membrane that removes nitrogenous waste products, excess water, and other solutes from the animal's blood down gradients from high to lower concentrations without permitting diffusion and ultrafiltration of larger constituents such as blood cells and proteins.

To perform hemodialysis, a special double-lumen catheter is surgically placed into the external jugular vein for access to the animal's blood for delivery to the dialysis machine. Blood is carried to and from the dialysis delivery system and dialyzer by extracorporeal tubing. Liters of blood, many times the total blood volume of the animal, are processed to normalize the serum creatinine and the blood urea nitrogen, concentrations of electrolytes, and water balances.

Many therapeutic options are available for animals with ARF. If treatments are initiated early enough, then the chances of kidney regeneration and recovery increase. The animal may go on to lead a normal life with or without supportive care and nutritional management for many months to years.

Renal Transplantation

Renal transplantation can be used to treat cats with ARF or CRF if regeneration and recovery of the existing kidneys is unlikely (Fig. 20-6).

The owners of the transplanted animal must be dedicated to treating their pet for life with medications to prevent donor kidney rejection. These medications are immunosuppressive drugs that are combined for optimum effect, such as cyclosporine and prednisone. Transplant recipients must be examined periodically to assess their renal function and cyclosporine levels. Transplanted patients can lead a normal life, and the new kidney can function for many years.

Conclusion

Treatment of the urologic emergency depends on the stage of disease or degree of trauma that has occurred. Monitoring equipment and blood analyzers must be available.

The veterinary technician plays a very important role in treating these patients by recognizing the progression of symptoms in the declining patient and understanding the tools used to evaluate the patient's condition.

Suggested Readings

Cowgill LD: Renal failure, acute. in Tilley LP, Francis WK, Smithe JP, editors: *The five minute veterinary consult, canine and feline*, Baltimore, 1997, Williams & Wilkins.

Cowgill LD, Langston CE: Role of hemodialysis in the management of dogs and cats with renal failure, *Vet Clin North Am Small Anim Pract* 26(6):1347, 1996.

Finco DR: Obstructive uropathy and hydronephrosis. In Osborne CA, Finco DR, editors: *Canine and feline nephrology and urology*, Baltimore, 1995, Williams & Wilkins.

Lees GE: Management of voiding disability following relief of obstruction. In August JR, editor: *Feline internal medicine*, ed 2, Philadelphia, 1994, WB Saunders.

Ling GV: *Lower urinary tract diseases of dogs and cats. Diagnosis, medical management and prevention*, St Louis, 1995, Mosby.

Osborne CA et al: Feline lower urinary tract disease: relationships between crystalluria, urinary tract infections and host factors. In August JR, editor: *Feline internal medicine*, ed 2, Philadelphia, 1994, WB Saunders.

Osborne CA et al: Canine and feline urolithiasis: relationships of etiopathogenesis to treatment and prevention. In Osborne CA, Finco DR, editors: *Canine and feline nephrology and urology*, Baltimore, 1995, Williams & Wilkins.

Polzin D, Osborne C, Adams L: Nutritional management of chronic renal failure, *Semin Vet Med Surg (Small Anim)* 5(3):187, 1990.

21

Reproductive Emergencies

ANDREA M. BATTAGLIA, HAROLD DAVIS

Emergencies of the reproductive tract occur most often in the female animal during pregnancy or estrus. The pregnant patient creates a unique challenge, because many lives can be threatened at one time.

The male animal also is susceptible to diseases or trauma of the reproductive tract. In both male and female patients, stabilization and treatment depend on disease severity, age, and breeding potential.

Equipment list:

- Oxytocin
- Calcium gluconate
- Antimicrobials
- Dextrose (50%)
- Antibiotics
- Lubricant
- Doxapram
- Naloxone
- Ear syringe for suction
- Small endotracheal tubes
- Feeding tubes (3.5, 5 French)
- Towels
- Hemostats
- Tincture of iodine
- Incubator
- Small bottles and different sizes and shapes of nipples

Reproductive Emergencies in the Female

Dystocia is defined as abnormal labor or birth. Normal parturition is the delivery by the bitch or queen of full-term, healthy puppies or kittens, respectively, without outside assistance of any sort. Dystocia occurs in almost all breeds of dogs and is not uncommon. Dystocia is not common in most cats; however, it does occur in purebred cats such as Persians and breeds with large heads and wide shoulders (Fig. 21-1).

321

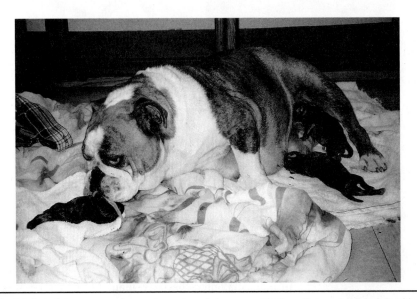

Fig. 21-1 Bull dogs commonly experience dystocia because of the breed's large head and shoulders.

Stages of Parturition

The demarcation between the three stages of labor is not always obvious. The onset of stage 1 is heralded by increased maternal behavior. The bitch displays nesting behavior, restlessness, panting, and shivering, and she may seek seclusion. Vomiting may be observed. Lactation and a transient temperature drop of approximately 2° F, in conjunction with luteolysis, occurs 24 to 36 hours before stage 1. Toward the end of stage 1 the cervix is dilated. The duration of the first stage is approximately 12 to 24 hours.

Increased strength and frequency of uterine contractions, visible abdominal contractions, and movement of the fetus through the cervix into the vagina are indicative of stage-2 parturition. The time between the onset of straining and the delivery of the first fetus varies (should be less than 1 hour). Both resting and straining phases occur between individual deliveries. The resting phase may last up to 3 hours. It may take up to 30 minutes of maximum straining before subsequent fetuses are delivered. The size of the litter and the quality of the labor are factors in the length of time between delivery of the first and last fetus. The time from the first to the last birth is variable and can be as long as 24 hours, but this is undesirable. Stage 3 is the delivery of the allantochorion (placenta). This stage actually is interspersed with stage 2. Passage of the allantochorion

may occur after each fetus or after two or three fetuses. The bitch should be monitored for delivery of an allantochorion for each fetus. Retained allantochorion can lead to endometritis. Stages 2 and 3 alternate until all fetuses have been delivered. A green to reddish-brown vaginal discharge can occur for up to 2 weeks after whelping, and light spotting can occur for 8 weeks.

Dystocia

Dystocia should be considered when the bitch experiences prolonged gestation and can be characterized as active straining for more than 60 minutes without delivery of a fetus, resting without straining for more than 4 hours between deliveries with known retained fetuses, intermittent weak contractions for more than 2 hours, or maternal or fetal stress.

Although definitive diagnosis of dystocia requires a complete physical examination, thorough history, and positive or negative diagnostic tests as indicated, identifying potential dystocias (usually by telephone) is the first step. Immediate examination is recommended if dystocia is considered a possibility.

Experienced, reputable breeders generally know when a problem exists; often they telephone to alert the hospital to the nature of the problem and explain when the animal is arriving. Unfortunately, these are not the typical dystocia cases. Typically the owner is an inexperienced breeder or an owner with a pet with an unplanned pregnancy. These owners usually have no experience with the delivery of a litter and no reference point for what is normal. Many, if not most, callers will not have educated themselves regarding the care of the female or the newborns. Often the hospital personnel attempt to not only identify potential dystocias and encourage immediate examinations but also to counsel callers on what to expect during a normal delivery. Deciding when intervention is necessary or what warrants another call for additional advice is difficult to do over the phone. The following section provides questions that can be asked to help determine if the bitch is experiencing dystocia; however, the owner should be encouraged to bring the pet to the clinic if he or she remains concerned or confused at the end of the call.

Screening for Potential Dystocias. Questions to ask the owner (in order of importance) are as follows:

- What is the bitch doing now, and what concerns prompted the owner to call?
- What is the age and breed of pet?
- What is the breed of father?
- Is the due date known? If not, then when was the dog bred, and when was the last time the dog was in season?
- Does the owner know how many puppies exist (by radiograph or ultrasound)?
- Does the bitch have any foul discharge? If so, what is the color of the discharge? Is there a foul odor?
- Have any fetuses been delivered? How many were born alive? How many were stillborn?
- Is the bitch actively pushing now? If so, for how long?
- If the bitch is not pushing, how long has it been since the last fetus was born?

Causes. The causes of dystocia can be maternal or fetal. Maternal causes include uterine inertia or anatomic abnormalities. Uterine inertia is poor strength or frequency of myometrial contraction efforts. An inherited predisposition, overstretching (large litters), insufficient stimulation (small litters), systemic disease (e.g., obesity, hypocalcemia, hypoglycemia, septicemia), age-related changes, exhaustion, stress, and anxiety cause uterine inertia. Anatomic abnormalities

---

BOX 21-1 ⓜ

Questions to Ask as Part of an Obstetric History

- Is this the first litter? If not, then have there been problems with previous litters?
- How long has it been since the last mating? Was any ovulation timing done?
- Did stage 1 of labor occur? How long did it last?
- Has an amnion or fetus been seen at the vulva? How long ago was this observed?
- How long has the straining lasted? Did it produce a neonate? What was the length of time between neonates?
- What was the condition of the neonates at birth?
- Was there any vaginal discharge? If so, then what was the color and consistency?
- Have all the placentas been accounted for?

---

include narrowing of the pelvic canal (congenital, neoplasia, or trauma related), uterine malposition, and developmental abnormalities of the genital canal. Fetal causes of dystocia include abnormally large, malpositioned, or dead fetuses.

Diagnosis. The normal variations of parturition make recognizing dystocia difficult. Diagnosis and therapy are based on thorough history and physical examination. In addition to the normal patient history, an obstetric history (Box 21-1) must be obtained.

As part of the physical examination, a digital examination (using aseptic technique) should be performed to ascertain the presence and position of a fetus in the birth canal. Bone or soft tissue abnormalities of the pelvis or vaginal vault (e.g., strictures, masses) also should be noted during the digital examination.

Diagnostic aids such as radiography, ultrasonography, and Doppler examination of the fetal heart may help in decision making. Radiographs can reveal the presence, number, size, location, and possible viability of fetuses. Spinal collapse and malposition, intrafetal gas patterns, and overlapping cranial bones are suggestive of past fetal death (Fig. 21-2). Assessment of the abdomen and pelvis also is aided by radiography. Ultrasonography can detect fetal movement, heartbeats, and heart rate, which are useful in assessing fetal stress.

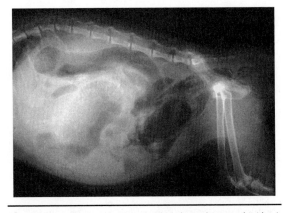

Fig. 21-2 Evidence of a fetus within the pelvic canal with air surrounding the fetus. Three additional fetuses were found, with evidence of abnormal position, suggesting fetal death.

Treatment. Management options depend on several factors, including the value of the offspring and bitch, the owner's wishes, and the availability of personnel and equipment. Three treatment options are available: (1) medical intervention, (2) manual manipulation, and (3) surgical management.

Medical intervention may be as simple as administering a tranquilizer to calm a stressed bitch. After obstruction has been ruled out and the quality of uterine contractions assessed, ecbolic agents may be given to stimulate uterine contractions. Oxytocin is the most common ecbolic agent used. The emergence of fetal monitoring in the veterinary patient is beginning to be seen. Fetal monitors help to guide medical therapy by revealing the frequency and strength of contractions. One of the benefits of fetal monitoring is a reduction in the amount of oxytocin given. Lower doses (0.25 to 0.5 U/dog intramuscularly) have been used in the female with success. Previously, recommended doses for oxytocin ranged from 1.1 to 2.2 U/kg intramuscularly. Oxytocin overdose can lead to tetanic uterine contractions, which can result in impaired placental blood flow. Calcium gluconate or dextrose can be administered when hypocalcemia or hypoglycemia has been confirmed and uterine inertia is a problem. If the initial dose of oxytocin is ineffective, then calcium gluconate can be administered (even if serum calcium is normal) subcutaneously 15 to 20 minutes before subsequent oxytocin doses. Intravenous calcium should be given with caution, and heart rate and rhythm should be monitored. Intravenous calcium

administration should be slowed or discontinued if bradycardia and arrhythmias develop. Veterinarians experienced in this area have suggested that calcium gluconate be given subcutaneously 15 minutes before oxytocin administration and that intravenous calcium be reserved for cases of eclampsia; they believe that the oxytocin will stimulate contractions and the subsequent dose of calcium will strengthen them.*

In the case of obstructive dystocia caused by fetal malposition or slightly oversized or dead fetuses, manual manipulation may be of benefit. Vaginal manipulation may be attempted digitally or by careful use of instruments. Obstetric instrumentation is difficult to use except in very large dogs. Lubrication may help, but the veterinarian must proceed cautiously to avoid injuring the fetus or bitch.

Surgical intervention is needed in the case of uterine inertia that is unresponsive to medical therapy or obstructive dystocia that cannot be corrected by manipulation. If a cesarean section is to be performed, then an anesthetic protocol should be selected that provides adequate analgesia, muscle relaxation, and sedation or narcosis to the bitch with minimal depression or compromise to the fetuses. Steps should be taken to minimize anesthesia time, such as clipping and preparing the patient and surgeon before anesthetic induction. Fluid support should be provided to the patient to prevent hypovolemia.

Hypotension may be a problem when the patient is placed in dorsal recumbency (and may be caused by compression of the caudal vena cava by the gravid uterus). If hypotension is a problem, then the patient can be repositioned (tilted slightly toward the surgeon). Hypoxia is a potential problem because the diaphragm is impinged by the abdominal contents.

Once the neonates are delivered, the technician may be responsible for resuscitation. Resuscitation includes removing fetal membranes, clearing the airway with gentle suction, administering oxygen by a small face mask, or stimulating breathing with intramuscular doxapram or naloxone (if opioids are used). The umbilical stumps are tied off and swabbed with a tincture of iodine solution. The neonates should be placed in a prewarmed environment

---

*Personal communication with Autumn P. Davidson, DVM, Dip ACVIM.

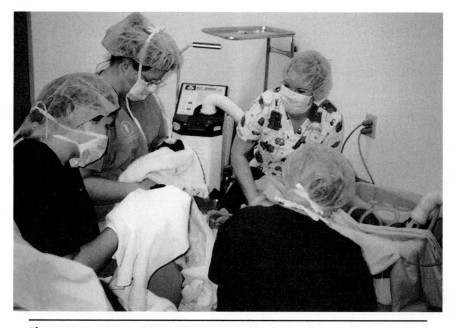

Fig. 21-3 Often a team is required to resuscitate large litters delivered by cesarean section.

(i.e., incubator) until they can be placed with the bitch. Routine postoperative care is provided to the patient (Fig. 21-3).

Care of the neonates. Puppies that remain in the hospital to be with the bitch are considered separate patients. Color-coded neck bands or ribbon can be used to differentiate between multiple puppies and will eliminate confusion when attempting to maintain records of assessments on individual puppies.

Owners are encouraged to take the bitch home soon after recovery (owners sometimes choose to take puppies home while the bitch recovers). Instructing owners on how and when to feed their animals, as well as how and when to stimulate them to urinate and defecate is important. Puppies are not to be fed unless the temperature is 96° F or higher.

Puppies that remain in the hospital are not to be left in the cage with the bitch unsupervised (having one of the puppies fall through the bars of the cage or become trapped in a blanket is too great to risk). The bitch must be introduced to the puppies slowly and cautiously. She is a postoperative patient and uncomfortable; therefore the technician should assume that she is unpredictable. To ensure their safety, puppies should be placed in an incubator between feedings.

The clinician should do the following when filling out the patient's treatment sheet:

- Document behavior, strength, nursing ability, and increase or decrease of urine and/or defecation when stimulated.
- Assess ventilatory nature, respiration rate, heart rate, and environmental temperature every 30 minutes for the first 90 minutes postoperatively, then every 2 hours afterward. (The doctor will order rectal temperatures if necessary.)
- Encourage puppies to latch on every 1 to 2 hours; stimulate the animals to urinate and defecate.
- Check the umbilical cord site for excessive bleeding.
- Record examination on the puppy's individual form when the doctor examines for cleft palate and heart murmurs (Fig. 21-4).

Pyometra

Pyometra is an infection in the uterus that is most common in middle-aged to older female dogs and cats during diestrus, 45 days after estrus. It can also be seen up to 10 weeks after estrogen therapy for mismating in female dogs and in cats or dogs receiving

Neonate Record

Neonate Evaluation Form

Date: _____   Name/ ID Number: _____
                                      Weight: _____

Time:	RR	Vent. Pattern	HR	E Temp	Latching on	Eating	U/D	Activity Level

Date: _____   Name/ ID Number: _____
                                      Weight: _____

Time:	RR	Vent. Pattern	HR	E Temp	Latching on	Eating	U/D	Activity Level

Date: _____   Name/ ID Number: _____
                                      Weight: _____

Time:	RR	Vent. Pattern	HR	E Temp	Latching on	Eating	U/D	Activity Level

Fig. 21-4 Neonate record. Neonate evaluation form.

progestins. Hormonally induced changes (progesterone or exogenous estrogens) cause pyometra.

Clinical Presentation. Patients may be depressed and septic or clinically normal. Clinical signs include lethargy, anorexia, dehydration, vomiting, diarrhea, polyuria, polydipsia, and vaginal discharge (with open pyometra). Clinical signs may be subtle in cats. Because of their grooming habits, vaginal discharge may not be seen.

Diagnosis. Diagnostic workup may include complete blood cell count, chemistry, urinalysis (clinician should not attempt cystocentesis if pyometra possible), cytology of discharge and culture, blood gases, and electrolytes. Additional diagnostic techniques include radiography and ultrasonography. Leukogram may show a leukocytosis with or without a left shift, or it may be normal. Nonregenerative anemia and hyperglobulinemia are common. Prerenal azotemia may be attributed to endotoxins elaborated by coliforms. Vaginal cytology and culture may be helpful in diagnosing pyometra and selecting antibiotics. Blood gases and electrolytes will help in developing a fluid therapy plan.

Radiography is used to confirm the presence of an enlarged uterus. Loss of abdominal detail may suggest peritonitis secondary to uterus rupture. Ultrasonography is used to differentiate pyometra from pregnancy or hydrometra.

Treatment. Treatment options are based on the condition, age, and breeding value of the animal. Pyometras can be surgically (treatment of choice) or medically managed. Medical management in the case of open pyometras involves prostaglandin administration. Patients receiving prostaglandin therapy should be observed in the hospital. Transient side effects such as anxiety, vomiting, diarrhea, tachypnea, and tachycardia may be seen shortly after prostaglandin administration. The therapeutic index of prostaglandins is narrow. All patients should be treated with intensive fluid therapy, antibiotics, and supportive care.

Uterine Torsions

Uterine torsions are very uncommon in the dog and in the cat. A partial or complete torsion can occur during pregnancy. Possible causes include jumping or running late in the pregnancy, active fetal movement, premature contractions, partial abortions, or abnormalities of the uterus.

Clinical signs may include pain, collapse, and abdominal distention. Severe hemorrhage can occur if the uterine artery is damaged.

Differentiating between uterine torsion and dystocia is difficult. Radiographs may indicate a large fluid- or air-filled tubular structure in the abdominal cavity; however, often the problem is not diagnosed until surgery. Ovariohysterectomy is recommended.

Reproductive Emergencies in the Male

Acute Bacterial Prostatitis

Acute bacterial prostatitis is acute inflammation of the prostate gland with gram-positive or gram-negative bacteria. The infection commonly results from bacteria ascending through the urethra. The bacteria also can be introduced through the bloodstream or reproductive tract. Older, intact male dogs are most commonly affected.

Clinical signs include lethargy, fever, dehydration, purulent or bloody discharge from the urethra, and caudal abdominal pain. The dog may walk with a stiff gait and arched back because of the pain. A diagnosis usually is made based on the examination, routine laboratory evaluation, and response to treatment. Caudal abdominal radiographs may show an enlarged prostate. Evaluation of the prostatic fluid including culture and cytology would be another tool for diagnosing bacterial prostatitis. Obtaining prostatic fluid from a dog experiencing prostatitis is painful and difficult, because ejaculation is necessary. Prostatic washes are an option but must be performed very carefully because of the risk of sepsis.

An antimicrobial is chosen based on the urine culture and administered for 4 to 6 weeks. Stabilization and fluid therapy may be necessary for more severe cases. Castration is recommended once the animal is stabilized.

Prostatic Abscess

Prostatic abscess occurs in dogs with an acute or chronic form of prostatitis. Clinical signs include lethargy, fever, vomiting, dysuria, abdominal pain, and urethral discharge. The animal may also experience signs of shock if the abscess has ruptured. A prostatic abscess can be confirmed by the use of radiography, ultrasonography, and prostate fluid analysis.

Surgical drainage of the prostatic abscesses or prostatectomy is performed once the dog has been stabilized. Castration also is recommended. Antimicrobials are continued postoperatively.

Paraphimosis

Paraphimosis, the inability to retract the penis within the prepuce, most commonly occurs after copulation. Treatment includes cleaning and lubricating the penis before attempting to replace it manually into the prepuce. Hyperosmotic agents (50% dextrose) applied on the penis may help decrease swelling. Sedation may be needed. Surgical intervention may be necessary if the penis cannot be returned to the normal position or if the penile vessels have been thrombosed.

Testicular Torsion

Testicular torsion is most common in dogs with retained testicles. Clinical signs include acute abdominal pain, anorexia, vomiting, and occasionally collapse. A dog with scrotal testes will have a stiff gait and testicular swelling if a testicular torsion is present. Treatment involves excision of the testicle.

Conclusion

Understanding the breeding potential of the animal with a reproductive emergency is important. Owners must understand the treatment options and relative risks. The veterinary technician can provide information to help the owner make the best decision for the patient.

Suggested Readings

Grotter AM: Diseases of the ovaries and uterus. In Birchard SJ, Sherding RG, editors: *Saunders manual of small animal practice*, Philadelphia, 1994, WB Saunders.

Macintire DK: Emergencies of the female reproductive tract. In Kirby R, Crow DT, editors: *Veterinary Clin North Am*, Philadelphia, 1994, WB Saunders.

Ocular Emergencies

PAM DICKENS

The eye is a sensitive organ that, when irritated, can cause the animal much discomfort. This discomfort may cause the animal to rub and scratch at the area. A mild inflammation or infection may change to a serious condition in a short period of time. When an owner calls with a concern involving a pet's eye, the animal should be seen to rule out a serious condition and provide pain relief as soon as possible. All brachycephalic breeds should be seen as soon as possible when any signs of blepharospasm are present.

Problems can occur in various parts of the eye. The globe, eyelids, cornea, anterior chamber, and lens are the areas covered in this chapter (Fig. 22-1).

Equipment list:

- OptiVISOR for magnification
- Tono-Pen for glaucoma
- Mannitol
- Topical ointments
- Ophthaine
- Nonsteroidal antiinflammatory drugs (Voltaren)
- Steroid (prednisolone acetate)
- Combination steroid and antibiotic (Maxitrol)
- General antibiotic
- Atropine 1%
- Phenylephrine 2.5%
- Suture materials
- 4-0 or 5-0 Silk with P-3 or G-3 needle
- 8-0 Vicryl
- Surgical pack with the following instruments:
  - Nasolacrimal cannula (23 gauge)
  - Bishop-Harmon dressing forceps
  - Barraquer cilia forceps
  - Troutman-Barraquer cornea utility forceps
  - Hartman curved hemostatic mosquito forceps
  - Barraquer eye speculum (pediatric and adult sizes)
  - Catalano needle holder, curved with or without lock (8-0 Vicryl)

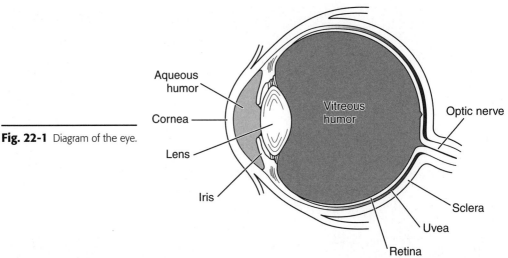

Fig. 22-1 Diagram of the eye.

Labels: Aqueous humor, Cornea, Lens, Iris, Vitreous humor, Optic nerve, Sclera, Uvea, Retina

- Westcott curved or straight tenotomy scissors
- Stevens straight tenotomy scissors
- Derf needle holder

Globe

Exophthalmos (i.e., the protrusion of a normal-sized globe from its usual position) may be seen with retrobulbar abscesses, tumors, as well as trauma from proptosis and some immune-related diseases. Exophthalmos should not be confused with buphthalmos, which is actual globe enlargement.

Patients with glaucoma can have dilated pupils, corneal edema, and conjunctival congestion, and the pupillary light reflex may or may not be present. Glaucoma can be caused by inherited predisposition, trauma, anterior luxating lens, or infection (Fig. 22-2, Color plate 4).

Treatment begins by determining whether vision is present and whether the glaucoma is a chronic or acute condition. If the condition is chronic and vision is not apparent, then pain relief is the goal. Pain relief is accomplished medically or surgically. Medical therapy can include topical drugs such as Xalatan (increases the uveoscleral outflow of the aqueous humor) and Alphagan (increases uveoscleral outflow and decreases production of aqueous humor). Other topical drugs (Timoptic, Trusopt) and oral medications (methazolamide) are used to decrease fluid production. Surgical procedures used to relieve the pain

in the blind eye include enucleation, ciliary body ablation, and intrascleral prosthesis (Table 22-1).

If the glaucoma is acute, the vision may be saved with immediate treatment. IV mannitol is administered (1 g/lb) to shrink the vitreous humor. Topical drugs are used concurrently. Laser or surgical treatment may be necessary.

- Cyclophotoablation (laser therapy) and gonio implants are used to decrease intraocular pressure.
- Surgical removal of the lens is an option to relieve the pressure and preserve vision if a luxated lens is the cause of the glaucoma.

Intraocular tumors may present as an acute onset of pain. Hyphema, melanosis (a change in the iris, most common in cats), buphthalmia, inability to retropulse the eye, and medial or lateral strabismus are other signs associated with tumors. Pupillary light response may or may not be present. Cats may have a history of a previous trauma to the affected eye (sometimes years earlier) and have a sudden onset of these signs. Treatment usually involves orbital enucleation or exenteration to relieve pain.

Panophthalmitis is inflammation of all structures or tissues of the eye. It presents as an acute onset of pain, conjunctival congestion, or hypopyon (i.e., pus in the chamber). Panophthalmitis can be a secondary sign of a systemic illness, especially if hypopyon is present. Aggressive oral and topical antibiotic therapy is necessary. Antiinflammatory

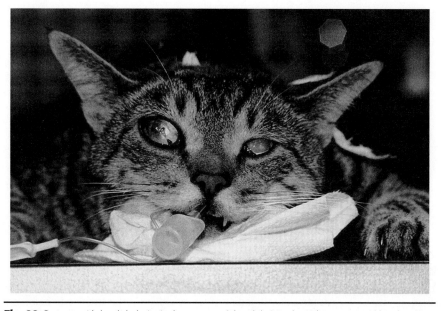

Fig. 22-2 A cat with buphthalmia (enlargement of the globe) in the right eye caused by glaucoma.

medications also are used. Enucleation often is necessary to relieve the pain.

Retrobulbar mass can be caused by trauma, tumors, or abscess. Skull radiographs, chemistry profiles, and a complete blood cell count are performed to determine the underlying cause. The protrusion of the globe, inability to blink, and inability to retract the eye are common presenting signs. Once the underlying cause is determined, treatment can begin. The cornea must be protected from drying with a lubricating ointment.

Animals with proptosis, the forward displacement of the globe, may have conjunctival hemorrhage, hyphema, or both. The common causes include trauma or tumors. IV dexamethasone is used to decrease inflammation in the optic nerve. The eye can be replaced with or without a lateral canthotomy; then a temporary tarsorrhapy is performed to protect the cornea. Topical antibiotic is used to protect the cornea. Oral antibiotics and cortisone are continued after surgical intervention. Lids are closed for 2 weeks minimally, and an Elizabethan collar is used to prevent rubbing. Lateral strabismus may be observed after proptosis.

Animals with enophthalmos, the backward displacement of the globe into the orbit, have a retracted eye, prolapse of the third eyelid, blepharospasm, miotic pupil, or epiphoria. Corneal ulcers, a foreign body, Horner's syndrome, acute glaucoma, trauma, and entropion are possible causes of this condition.

Determining the underlying cause is important (if possible). Topical anesthetic (Ophthaine) is used to relieve the blepharospasm. Horner's syndrome should be considered a possibility if the topical anesthetic provides no relief.

Horner's syndrome involves the sympathetic nervous system. The sympathetic nerves are located close to the surface of the skin, and consistent pressure applied to this area (e.g., by a choke collar) can damage these nerves. Drops of 2.5% to 10% phenylephrine are used to test for this disorder. If a positive response occurs, then the pupil dilates, the third eyelid goes down, and the eyeball comes forward. If the underlying disorder is not determined, then this treatment can be used as needed. Some animals recover without treatment; however, when the underlying disorder is determined, it must be treated appropriately.

Eyelid

The animal with entropion (i.e., inward displacement of the lid) experiences squinting, third-eyelid protrusion, epiphoria, and blepharospasm. An inherited form and a spastic form of entropion exist. The spastic form usually is caused by trauma or corneal ulceration. If a corneal ulcer is present, then enophthalmia can result from pain, relaxing

TABLE 22-1

Common Medications Used for Ocular Emergencies

Drug	Effect	Treatment Protocol
Acetylcysteine 10% (topical)	Assists in stopping collagenic activity	1 drop every hour on melting ulcers, usually mixed with equal amount of an antibiotic
Alphagan	Increases uveoscleral outflow and reduces production of aqueous humor	3 times a day
Atropine 1% (topical)	Dilates pupils, relieves pain, prevents synechia	1 drop as needed to dilate; effect is long lasting
Cosopt	Combination of timolol and Trusopt (less expensive than both drugs alone)	3 times a day
Dexamethasone (IV)	Decreases inflammation of optic nerves, uvea, anterior chamber	0.25 mg/lb
Gentocin (topical)	Antibacterial medication	1 drop three to four times a day (up to every hour for severe ulcer)
Mannitol (IV)	Decreases pressure by shrinking vitreous humor	1 g/lb IV given slowly over 20-30 min (if solution is crystallized, dissolve crystals by immersing bottle in hot water)
Maxitrol (topical)	Controls inflammatory response; steroid/antibiotic combination	1 drop every 2-8 hr depending on severity of infection
Methazolamide (oral)	Decreases fluid production	0.25-0.5 mg/lb twice a day
Muro 128 ointment 5%	Assists in attachment of new epithelial cells	Applied every 8 hr for ulcers; always applied 30-60 min after any other medication
Mydriacyl 1% (topical)	Dilates pupils; short acting (4-6 hr)	Can be toxic to the epithelium; should use 1-3 drops only as needed to relieve pain to perform necessary tests

the eyelids to cause entropion. Treatment for spastic entropion includes temporary tacking of the eyelids and applying lubricating ointment. Antibiotic ointment may be necessary if an infection is present.

Age is an important factor in the inherited form of entropion. Many dogs grow out of the defect, and surgical intervention in young dogs is to be avoided if possible. Temporary eyelid tacking may be necessary until the animal is fully grown (Table 22-2).

Ectropion, the outward displacement of the lids, can cause epiphora and mucopurulent discharge.

Horner's syndrome, enophthalmia caused by trauma, and lagophthalmos can cause this condition. Ectropion is an inherited disorder. Lubricating ointment is used to protect the corneal surface, and an Elizabethan collar is placed to prevent further trauma.

Meibomian gland abscess or adenoma (chalazion) is the chronic or acute swelling of one or more meibomian glands along the upper and lower eyelids. Crusting or bleeding along the eyelids may be observed. Inflammation caused by an abscess or benign growth of the glands is a common cause of this

TABLE 22-1

Common Medications Used for Ocular Emergencies—cont'd

Drug	Effect	Treatment Protocol
Ophthaine (topical)	Anesthetic; relieves blepharospasm	Can be toxic to the epithelium; should use 1-3 drops only as needed to relieve pain to perform necessary tests
Optimmune ointment	Tear stimulant	¼ inch three times a day
Tacrolimus 0.02%	Tear stimulant	1 drop twice a day
2.5% Phenylephrine (topical)	Dilates pupils; usually for Horner's syndrome as needed to bring third eyelid down	1 drop once or twice a day
Pred Forte 1% (topical)	Controls inflammatory response	1 drop every 2-8 hr depending on severity of inflammation
Propine 0.1%	Decreases aqueous production and enhances outflow	3 times a day
Timolol/Timoptic (topical)	Decreases fluid production	1 drop every 8 hr
Trusopt (topical)	Decreases fluid production; topical does the same as the oral methazolamide	1 drop every 8 hr
VIRA-A ointment	Antiviral medication	¼ inch every 6 hr; decreases weekly
VIROPTIC (topical)	Antiviral medication	1 drop every 6 hr initially; usually decreases weekly
Diclofenac (Voltaren) (topical)	Nonsteroidal antiinflammatory drug	1 drop twice a day
Xalatan (topical)	Increases uveoscleral outflow of the aqueous humor; human drug used only at bedtime, when pressure usually rises; may cause severe miosis and have to be discontinued	Can be used once or twice a day

condition. Treatment includes lancing the swelling if an abscess is present and surgical excision of the growth if a tumor is present. Topical antibiotic ointment is applied after the surgical intervention, and an Elizabethan collar is placed on the animal to prevent rubbing.

Symblepharon is the adhesion of the conjunctiva to the lid and the eyeball. This condition occurs in utero and is caused by a virus (i.e., herpes, calici, chlamydia). Treatment includes surgical correction by removing the conjunctiva from the corneal surface and treating the underlying virus with an ophthalmic ointment (VIRA-A Ophthalmic Ointment, VIROPTIC Ophthalmic Solution).

Cherry eye, or prolapsed gland of the third eyelids, can appear very red and irritated. Trauma and breed predisposition are the common causes of this condition. The gland can be replaced manually after the use of a topical anesthetic. Cortisone ointment (Maxitrol) controls the inflammatory response. Surgical intervention may be necessary if the gland continues to prolapse. Removing the gland is not recommended because of the risk of keratoconjunctivitis sicca (KCS). Suturing it in place is preferred.

TABLE 22-2

Breed Predisposition for Ocular Disease

Breed	Condition
Dogs	
Akita	Entropion
Alaskan malamute	Glaucoma
American Staffordshire terrier	Entropion
Australian cattle dog	Anterior luxating lens
Basset hound	Glaucoma, entropion, ectropion
Beagle	Glaucoma, cherry eye
Belgian sheepdog	Pannus
Belgian tervuren	Pannus
Bloodhound	Entropion, ectropion, cherry eye
Border collie	Anterior luxating lens
Boston terrier	Glaucoma
Bouvier des Flandres	Glaucoma
Boxer	Ectropion, corneal ulcers
Brachycephalic breeds	Corneal ulcers
Brittany spaniel	Anterior luxating lens
Bulldog (English)	Entropion, ectropion, cherry eye
Bull mastiff	Glaucoma, entropion, ectropion
Burmese mountain dog	Entropion
Cairn terrier	Glaucoma
Chesapeake Bay retriever	Entropion
Chinese Shar pei	Glaucoma, anterior luxating lens, entropion, cherry eye
Chow chow	Glaucoma, entropion
Clumber spaniel	Entropion, ectropion
Cocker spaniel	Glaucoma, entropion, ectropion, cherry eye
Dachshund	Pannus
Dalmatian	Glaucoma, entropion
English springer spaniel	Entropion
English toy spaniel	Entropion
Flat-coated retriever	Entropion
German shepherd	Pannus
Golden retriever	Glaucoma, entropion
Gordon setter	Entropion, ectropion

TABLE 22-2

Breed Predisposition for Ocular Disease—cont'd

Breed	Condition
Dogs	
Great Dane	Glaucoma, entropion, ectropion
Greyhound	Pannus
Irish setter	Entropion
Japanese chin	Entropion
Labrador retriever	Entropion, ectropion
Lhasa apso	Cherry eye
Mastiff	Entropion, ectropion
Newfoundland	Entropion, ectropion, cherry eye
Norwegian elkhound	Glaucoma
Old English sheepdog	Entropion
Pekingese	Entropion
Pomeranian	Entropion
Pug	Entropion
Rottweiler	Entropion
Saint Bernard	Entropion, ectropion
Samoyed	Glaucoma
Shih tzu	Entropion, ectropion
Siberian husky	Glaucoma, entropion
Smooth fox terrier	Glaucoma
Terriers	Anterior luxating lens
Tibetan spaniel	Entropion
Viszla	Entropion
Weimaraner	Entropion
Welsh springer spaniel	Glaucoma
Wire-haired fox terrier	Glaucoma, anterior luxating lens
Yorkshire terrier	Entropion
Cats	
Burmese	Corneal sequestrum, keratoconjunctivitis sicca (KCS)
Himalayan	Corneal sequestrum
Persian	Corneal sequestrum
Siamese	Corneal sequestrum

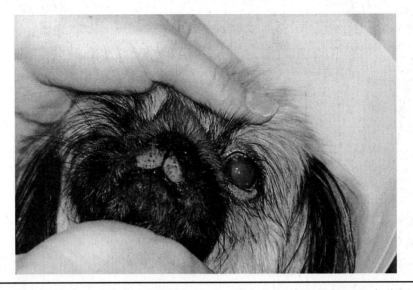

Fig. 22-3 A Pekingese with conjunctival hyperemia, with mucopurulent discharge in the left eye caused by a corneal ulcer.

Cornea

Corneal ulcers can cause epiphoria, blepharitis, mucopurulent discharge, and photophobia. Ulcers can be superficial, recurrent, collagenase, desmetocele, or viral; they occur when chemicals, foreign bodies, ectopic cilia, or trauma has irritated the cornea. Breed predisposition also can be a factor. Treatment varies according to the type of ulcer present. An Elizabethan collar should be placed and other necessary measures taken to prevent further trauma for all types of ulcers (Fig. 22-3, Color plate 5).

Superficial ulcers are commonly treated with an antibiotic solution or ointment (e.g., Gentocin ophthalmic solution or ointment or triple-antibiotic ointment). Recurrent erosions present as chronic ulcers that did not respond to previous therapies. Additional treatment or medication is needed, and a grid keratectomy usually is necessary. Topical and general anesthesia may be needed before the procedure. First, a cotton swab is used to débride the ulcer, then a 25-gauge needle is used to make a grid. This allows attachment of new epithelial cells to the cornea. A sodium chloride ointment (Muro 128 ophthalmic ointment) can be used to promote attachment of new epithelial cells.

Collagenase ulcers, or melting ulcers, are the most difficult to treat. Brachycephalic breeds are commonly affected. The cornea is made of collagen, and the ulcer produces a collagenase that eats through the cornea. Intensive medical therapy is necessary. Serum can be used from the patient (as an eye drop) to stop the collagenic activity. Acetylcysteine and Gentocin are also used hourly to stop collagenic activity in some cases. A nonsteroidal antiinflammatory drug (Voltaren) may be necessary if uveitis is present. Conjunctival grafting can be performed if the medical therapy fails.

Desmetocele is an ulcer that has progressed to the last layer of the cornea. The cornea will rupture if it progresses. Topical therapy may be indicated if blood vessels are present and no leakage occurs. Medical therapy must be attempted with caution. Sometimes just a sneeze will rupture the cornea. A topical antibiotic, acetylcysteine 10% (stops collagenic activity), and atropine 1% (dilates pupil and relieves pain) are commonly used for the medical treatment. Surgery is recommended to preserve vision and prevent rupture of the eye. Surgical correction may include conjunctival grafting or corneoscleral transposition.

Viral ulcers commonly occur in cats with a history of upper respiratory infection. Treatment includes a systemic antibiotic for a bacterial infection and topical antiviral medications (VIRA-A Ophthalmic Ointment, VIROPTIC Ophthalmic Solution).

KCS can cause purulent discharge, blepharitis, keratitis, and a dull cornea. Thickened eyelids may result from rubbing. Cats may have very mild signs, but Burmese cats are more susceptible. Cherry eye removal, conjunctivitis, congenital defects, anesthesia, drug therapy (i.e., sulfa drugs), and hypothyroidism can cause KCS. Treatment involves stimulating tear production with topical ointments (Optimmune) and maintaining moisture with artificial tears several times daily.

Keratitis can cause a cloudy or pigmented cornea and blepharitis; chronic exposure, KCS, virus, lagophthalmos, pannus, trichiasis, distichia, and facial nerve paralysis can cause this condition. The underlying problem must be determined and treated appropriately.

Pannus, the superficial vascularization of the cornea with infiltration of granulation tissue, is most common in certain breeds and believed to be an immune-mediated disease. Depigmenting of the third eyelid, granulation tissue, superficial blood vessels, and pigment on the cornea are common presenting signs. Optimmune ophthalmic ointment and corticosteroids are used to treat pannus.

A corneal foreign body can cause acute blepharospasm, epiphoria, and conjunctival hyperemia. The object usually can be removed with topical anesthetic. A small-gauge hypodermic needle or ophthalmic surgical forceps are used for this procedure. The ulcer is treated with topical antibiotics, and an Elizabethan collar is placed around the patient's head to prevent further damage. If the injury is deep, then acetylcysteine 10% may be needed.

Corneal sequestrum occurs when an area of the cornea has become sequestered. Brown or black areas can be seen on the cornea; epiphora and blepharospasm also can be observed. The animal usually has a history of corneal injury. It can also be caused by a virus or breed predisposition in cats. Topical therapy is used to prevent infection and lubricate the eye. Surgical excision is usually necessary to remove sequestered tissue.

Anterior Chamber

Uveitis, inflammation of the vascular layer of the eye, can cause blepharospasm, miosis, iritis, iris color change, photophobia, hypopyon, and epiphora. It can be idiopathic or caused by a virus, systemic illness, or trauma. Diagnosing and treating any underlying problems is important. Topical therapy can include nonsteroidal or steroidal antibiotics or a combination thereof.

Hyphema, blood in the anterior chamber, can cause blepharospasm, epiphora, and glaucoma. Trauma, retinal detachment, iris tumors, and ciliary body bleed are possible causes. Topical cortisone can be used if the cornea is intact. IV dexamethasone and intraocular injection of tissue plasmin activator is used to break up clots and reduce the chance of adhesion. Oral steroid therapy and topical therapy are continued until the clot is absorbed and the intraocular structures can be viewed.

Lens

Anterior lens luxation can cause corneal edema, blepharospasm, and lethargy. The resulting glaucoma causes severe pain in acute cases. Breed predisposition, trauma, and glaucoma are the most common causes of this condition.

IV mannitol 20% is administered (1 g/lb) over 30 minutes to relieve intraocular pressure. Mydriatics (Mydriacyl 1%, Murocoll-2 ophthalmic solution) can be used to dilate the pupil and allow the lens to fall behind the iris. Antiinflammatories and antiglaucoma medications also may be needed to control the pressure. It may be necessary to remove the lens to restore vision and relieve pressure and the inflammatory reaction in the acute cases.

Cataracts can cause epiphora, uveitis, blepharospasm, hypopyon, miosis, a white pupil, and vision loss in acute cases. Trauma, diabetes, and chronic uveitis are possible causes of this condition; cataracts can also be hereditary or age related.

The goal in acute onset is to control the reaction caused by the changing lens. Medications can control the reaction caused by the cataract but will not cure the condition. Topical steroids and nonsteroidal medications are used to control lens-induced uveitis. Mydriatics are used to dilate the pupil and prevent synechia. The cataract is removed once the lens-induced uveitis is controlled (Fig. 22-4, Color plate 6).

Nuclear sclerosis is the hardening of the nucleus; it may be confused with cataracts because it produces a graying of the lens. Depth perception and limited visual capabilities in various lighting may be observed. No treatment for this condition exists.

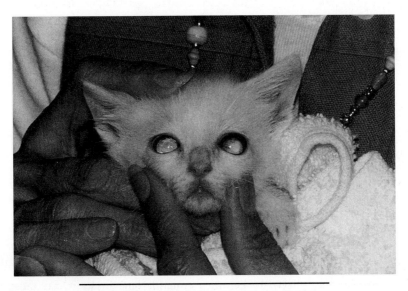

Fig. 22-4 A kitten with congenital cataracts in both eyes.

Conclusion

Determining the severity of an ophthalmic emergency over the phone is not easy. If the animal is experiencing pain around or on the surface of the eye (as evidenced by squinting, epiphora), then it must be seen. A mild infection can quickly turn into a severe problem if the animal rubs or scratches the area. Pain relief is important.

Many problems of the eye are a secondary sign of a primary infection. Other tests should be run to determine whether any other underlying medical problems exist.

The emergency facility must be equipped to deal with eye problems. Instruments used only for eyes should be stored in a separate pack; ointments and eyewash also should be available. Pain relievers and restraints are used to prevent the animal from damaging the eye after treatment. A variety of Elizabethan collars should be available to meet the needs of each patient.

Suggested Readings

Chrisman CL: *Problems in small animal neurology*, Malvern, Penn, 1991, Lea & Febiger.

Ocular disorders presumed to be inherited in purebred dogs, 1996, American College of Veterinary Ophthalmologists.

Physician's desk reference for ophthalmology, ed 27, Philadelphia, 1999, WB Saunders.

CHAPTER 23

Neurologic System Emergencies

Eric N. Glass, Marc Kent

With regard to the nervous system, emergencies fall into two general categories: (1) those situations in which the pet owner perceives there to be an emergency and (2) those that truly require emergency care. Both situations require attention. For example, almost every veterinarian and veterinary technician has experienced a frantic call from an owner whose healthy young pet has had its very first seizure lasting for less than 1 minute with a rapid return to normalcy. Although this may not constitute a life-threatening emergency, a veterinarian should see the pet the next morning. On the other hand, a seizure that lasts longer than 3 to 4 minutes or several seizures occurring within a short period of time truly is a veterinary emergency. In this case, immediate medical care at an emergency clinic is warranted. Prolonged or consecutive seizures can cause permanent neurologic damage and result in hyperthermia, disseminated intravascular coagulation (DIC), and death.

The distinction between these two situations is important when dealing with emergencies involving the nervous system—not only to help minimize the cost of veterinary emergency care to owners but also to provide appropriate attention to true emergencies. At this initial step the veterinary technician can play a major role in distinguishing these situations. The following chapter discusses common neurologic emergencies in which the veterinary technician can play an active role in triage, assessment, diagnosis, and treatment.

Clinical neurology relies heavily on the physical examination to help locate the anatomic portion of the nervous system with an abnormality. This is commonly referred to as *establishing a neuroanatomic diagnosis*. The ability to establish a neuroanatomic diagnosis from a physical examination alone is in stark contrast to diseases that affect other organ systems such as the liver, kidney, or blood, for which multiple ancillary laboratory or imaging procedures often are needed to determine the site of disease. This difference allows veterinarians to diagnose and treat neurologic emergencies rapidly.

The neurologic examination, the hallmark of clinical veterinary neurology, involves a systematic approach to evaluate the central and peripheral nervous system. The neurologic examination is outlined in Box 23-1. Accurate observations of patients with neurologic dysfunction are crucial in a busy emergency veterinary clinic; therefore veterinary technicians must understand not only how to perform a neurologic examination but also how to interpret the findings produced by it.

Seizures

Veterinary emergency clinics often deal with cats, dogs, and to a lesser extent other species such as ferrets and birds with seizure disorders. To help these patients rapidly, the ability to understand and recognize a seizure is essential. The veterinary literature includes excellent definitions of seizures. LeCouteur and Schwartz-Porsche have offered a contemporary definition, "The clinical manifestation of a paroxysmal cerebral disorder resulting from a transitory disturbance of brain function." The event "tends to appear suddenly out of a background of normality and then disappears with equal abruptness." This definition should be expanded to include the fact that seizures can originate from both the telencephalon (cerebral hemispheres) and the diencephalon (thalamus and hypothalamus), which together embryologically are called the *prosencephalon*.

Physiologically, seizures are thought to be associated with hyperexcitable neurons that suddenly depolarize in the prosencephalon. These neurons may have disturbed excitability caused by a structural abnormality, such as a brain tumor, brain trauma, inflammation, infection, or a congenital abnormality, or they may result from some metabolic or toxic disturbance in the cell or the surrounding parenchyma. The net result is a sudden uncontrollable electrical discharge of neurons. These neurons may then enlist surrounding neurons to recruit a larger portion of the brain into abnormal action.

As in human neurology, a great deal of effort has been devoted to classifying seizures in veterinary medicine. The location of the hyperexcitable neurons that spontaneously discharge determine the abnormal clinical signs seen during a seizure. Most often, clinicians recognize seizures by the motor movements that occur. As one can see, the observed manifestation of a seizure depends heavily on which aspects of the prosencephalon are affected; therefore what is observed during the seizure will vary considerably from patient to patient and even in the same patient during different seizures.

Very briefly, seizures have been divided into *partial* and *generalized seizures*. Partial seizures reflect a limited set of neurons being affected and sometimes are called *focal* or *local seizures*. For example, if the affected cells are located unilaterally in the motor cortex, then abnormal tonic-clonic movements may occur on the contralateral side of the body. A very common manifestation of a partial seizure is referred to as a *focal facial seizure* in which the motor movements are limited to the facial musculature. In addition to the motor movements that are observed, changes in the level of consciousness can also be appreciated during a partial seizure. Consciousness is difficult to discern in pets during a seizure; however, when no loss or alteration in consciousness occurs, the partial seizure is further categorized as a *simple, partial seizure*. When a loss of consciousness occurs (determined by the fact that the patient is unresponsive to stimuli such as being called to or being touched), the seizure is referred to as a *complex, partial seizure*.

In contrast, generalized seizures take place when synchronous electrical discharge of both sides of the prosencephalon occurs. In this case the pet will demonstrate tonic-clonic movement in all limbs. In this description, *tonic* refers to the increased muscular rigidity of the extensor muscles, whereas *clonic* refers to rhythmic jerking movements of the limbs. Additionally, the neck can be extended dorsally (i.e., opisthotonus). The facial muscles are often contracted. Chewing movements can be observed. Autonomic dysfunction such has hypersalivation, urination, and defecation can also occur in generalized seizures.

Unfortunately, this classification scheme, unlike the counterpart in human medicine, adds little to clinicians' understanding of the cause of a particular patient's seizure activity. In addition, in veterinary medicine this classification scheme does not appear to help in selecting the best anticonvulsant therapy or treatment for a particular patient.

Terms used by clients to describe a seizure are varied and include *epilepsy, fits,* and *convulsions*. The term *epilepsy* is somewhat problematic, because it has different meanings even among veterinary neurologists. Probably the most widely accepted definition of *epilepsy* is a nonprogressive, intracranial disorder that induces recurring seizures. Causes of epilepsy include genetically determined primary brain disorders and inactive, nonprogressive brain disorders that have resulted in a seizure focus. Idiopathic epilepsy is a disorder for which the exact cause or mechanism for the seizure is unknown; the disorder is not progressive.

Because owners recognize seizures by the motor movements that the patient exhibits, they are often confused with other clinical entities. The veterinarian and veterinary technician must accurately and quickly distinguish seizures from other diseases that occur episodically and suddenly. Some of the syndromes most commonly confused with seizures are listed in Box 23-2.

A systematic approach is imperative to identify the cause of seizures. A method to determine the cause of seizure activity is shown in Fig. 23-1. This method distinguishes patients with normal and abnormal neurologic examinations and takes

---

BOX 23-2

Episodic Syndromes Sometimes Confused with Seizures

Cataplexy and narcolepsy
Syncope
Behavioral abnormalities
  Obsessive-compulsive behaviors
Vestibular diseases
Myasthenia gravis
Pain
  Neck pain from intervertebral disc disease
Metabolic disturbances
  Polycythemia or hyperviscosity syndromes
  Portosystemic shunts
  Addison's disease
Polymyopathies and neuropathies

---

into consideration that most patients admitted to emergency clinics are having (or have just had) a seizure at the time of admission. The postictal period is the time after a seizure or group of seizures, during which the animal may be disoriented, unresponsive, confused, or restless. Many animals are temporarily blind. Some are very agitated or aggressive. Usually this transient period lasts for a few seconds to several hours after the seizure, but some dogs and cats have postictal periods can last for 1 to 2 days. The important thing to remember about the postictal period is that neurologic deficits identified during the neurologic examination may not represent the patient's true neurologic state. Many patients have abnormal findings during this period that do not persist once the animal has recovered from the postictal period. Importantly, deficits that are the result of seizures rather than the underlying cause are generally bilaterally symmetric. Patients demonstrating unilateral or asymmetrical deficits are more likely to have an underlying structural cause for their seizures; therefore definitive conclusions about the neurologic examination findings should not be made until after the patient has completely recovered from the postictal effects. Similarly, anticonvulsant medications used to stop seizures can influence the neurologic examination, primarily by altering the patient's sensorium (i.e., mental state). Conclusions about the cause of a seizure should be reached after the effects of anticonvulsant medications have worn off.

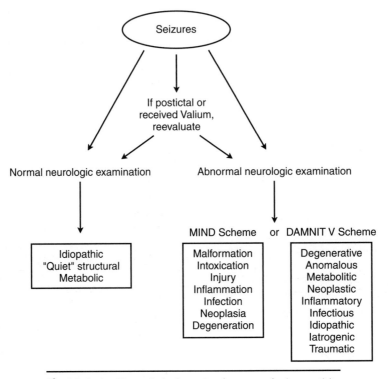

Fig. 23-1 Algorithm to help determine the cause of seizure activity.

When attempting to define causality for seizures, patients can be divided into those with and those without deficits noted on the neurologic examination. In Fig. 23-1, causes of seizures in a pet with a normal neurologic examination fall into three general categories: (1) metabolic and systemic disease, (2) quiet structural lesions of the brain, and (3) idiopathic epilepsy. Although most patients with metabolic diseases that result in seizures have an altered sensorium, occasionally, they may arrive for evaluation and be clinically normal. Animals with problems such as liver disease and hypoglycemia can have a normal neurologic examination. These diseases are identified through clinicopathologic testing such as complete blood count, chemistry profile, urinalysis, and specialized tests such as bile acid stimulation testing. Quiet structural causes of seizures are diseases that affect portions of the brain that do not have readily apparent abnormalities on the neurologic examination. For example, a brain tumor or a granuloma in the olfactory bulbs or frontal lobes of the brain can cause seizures without causing abnormalities in the neurologic examination. Quiet structural causes of

seizures often warrant further diagnostic procedures such as collection of cerebrospinal fluid and advanced imaging techniques such as computer-assisted tomography or magnetic resonance imaging. Finally, idiopathic epilepsy is a disease in which patients have recurrent seizures without an identifiable causality. It often occurs in dogs between 1 and 6 years of age. In some breeds of dogs a defined mode of inheritance has been identified. Patients with idiopathic epilepsy do not have neurologic deficits on neurologic examination. Similarly, these patients do not have clinicopathologic abnormalities, and magnetic resonance imaging and computed tomography reveal no abnormalities. Therefore idiopathic epilepsy is a diagnosis of exclusion.

If deficits are identified on the neurologic examination in a patient not in the postictal period and not having just received medication to stop seizures (e.g., valium), two acronyms are helpful to remind clinicians and technicians of broad categories of diseases that can cause seizures. The acronym *MIND* represents the following categories: malformation, intoxication, injury, inflammation, infection, neoplastia,

BOX 23-3

Treatment and Diagnosis in Patients Not Previously Diagnosed with a Seizure Disorder and those with Cluster Seizures or Status Epilepticus

1. Place IV catheter.
2. Draw blood for initial database to include the following:
   Blood glucose
   Electrolytes
   Packed cell volume and total protein
   Peripheral blood smear
   Complete blood cell count
   Chemistry profile
   Urinalysis
   Lead levels (if indicated)
   Serology for infectious diseases (if indicated)
3. Give IV drugs to stop seizures.
   Diazepam (Valium) (usually first choice)
   Dose: 0.25-1.0 mg/kg (repeat up to three times)
   Quick-dosing suggestions:
   • Small dog, 2.5-5.0 mg (repeat up to three times)
   • Medium dog, 5.0 mg (repeat up to three times)
   • Large dog, 10-20 mg (repeat up to three times)
   • Cats, 2.5 mg (repeat up to three times)

   Note: After the seizures stop, give the animal a constant rate infusion (CRI) of diazepam if necessary. Give the amount of diazepam used to stop the initial seizure in a solution of 1.2 ml lactated Ringer's solution/lb/hr.

   Pentobarbital (if not responsive to valium)
   • Dogs, 1-8 mg/kg IV (slow and to effect)
   • Cats, 1-4 mg/kg IV (slow and to effect)

   Note: It is not necessary to completely anesthetize the animal with pentobarbital as long as it stops the seizure. Anesthesia induced with pentobarbital may not totally stop seizure activity (as revealed by electroencephalogram), but it will prevent life-threatening hyperthermia and disseminated intravascular coagulation.

   Other drugs to consider include the following:
   • Propofol
   • Thiopental
4. Give maintenance anticonvulsant medications.
   Loading doses: The calculated doses needed to quickly achieve therapeutic serum concentrations.
   • Phenobarbital, 4 mg/kg IV, orally (PO), intramuscularly (IM), or rectally (PR) every 6 hr for 24 hr (total dose, 6 mg/kg) (can go as high as 30 mg/kg over the first 24 hr; stop loading if very groggy, especially in the cat)
   • Potassium bromide, 100-150 mg/kg every 12 hr for four doses or 2 days (can give PO or PR; can load much more rapidly by giving 300-600 mg/kg all at once if necessary; total loading dose should not exceed 600 mg/kg)
   Maintenance doses:
   • Phenobarbital, 1.0-4.0 mg/lb two to three times daily PO
   • Potassium bromide, 25-80 mg/kg/day

   Note: Use a higher dose if the animal is not on phenobarbital concurrently. Although unnecessary, a divided total dose usually can be given twice daily. Maintenance medication is essential in the anesthetized patient.

and degeneration. The acronym *DAMNIT V* stands for degenerative, anomalous, metabolic, neoplastic, inflammatory, infectious, idiopathic, iatrogenic, traumatic, and vascular (infarction).

Treatment and Diagnostic Procedures

Treatment of seizures in an emergency veterinary clinic should be directed at stopping seizure activity, then treating the secondary consequences of seizures. This treatment plan is paramount in patients with status epilepticus, a seizure lasting more than 5 minutes, or in patients having cluster seizures in which one seizure is followed by another seizure without a return to normal consciousness. Additionally, patients having more than 3 to 4 seizures in 30 to 40 minutes or a large number of seizures over a 12- or 24-hour period also need to be treated aggressively.

A specific treatment depends largely on whether the animal is taking antiepileptic drugs and usually has good seizure control or whether the patient is having seizures for the first time. Box 23-3 describes a step-by-step approach for the initial treatment and diagnosis for a first-time seizure.

The treatment protocol in Box 23-4 should be followed for patients in status epilepticus or with cluster seizures who have previously been on anticonvulsants and have a definitive cause for seizure activity, as well as for those who have been previously diagnosed with idiopathic epileptics. These patients usually do not need the extensive battery of blood tests that a patient who has just recently started to seizure needs. However, if it has been an extended period of time or a sudden change in the intensity or severity of the patient's seizures has occurred, then it may be necessary to repeat some of the blood work.

Monitoring and Care of Patients with Seizures

Once the seizure activity has been stopped, attention needs to be focused on the secondary effects of seizures. The majority of the effects of prolonged seizures are the result of extensive muscular activity. Hyperthermia is commonly encountered after prolonged seizures. Body temperatures can quickly rise above 105° F; therefore monitoring rectal temperatures is imperative. Active cooling should be initiated with body temperatures above 103.5° F. Once the body temperature returns to 102° F, active cooling should be discontinued, because extreme hyperthermia can affect normal abilities to thermoregulate; therefore body temperatures can easily drop below normal. Conditions like DIC, organ failures (e.g., renal, hepatic), and muscle necrosis can be a consequence of elevated body temperatures. Careful evaluation of venipuncture and venocatheter sites, as well as mucous membranes and less-haired regions of skin, can reveal petechial hemorrhages from thrombocytopenia or DIC. Likewise, dehydration and hypoglycemia can also occur after seizure activity. Finally, evaluation of the respiratory system is crucial. Occasionally, pulmonary edema, referred to as *noncardiogenic edema*, can develop after seizures. Animals who are in the early stages of noncardiogenic edema or are mildly affected will developed a rapid, shallow respiratory rate. In severe cases, dyspnea and cyanosis can result in severe hypoxia and even respiratory arrest. Thoracic auscultation can reveal respiratory crackles. Pulse oximetry or arterial blood gas analysis can identify hypoxemia. Chest radiographs reveal interstitial to alveolar lung patterns primarily in the caudal dorsal lung fields. If noncardiogenic pulmonary edema is identified, then administration of supplemental oxygen can be

---

BOX 23-4

Treatment and Diagnosis in Patients Previously Diagnosed with a Seizure Disorder and those with Cluster Seizures or in Status Epilepticus

1. Place IV catheter.
2. Draw blood for initial database to include the following:
   Blood glucose
   Electrolytes
   Packed cell volume and total protein
3. Give IV drugs to stop seizures.
   Diazepam (Valium) (usually first choice)
   Dose: 0.25-1.0 mg/kg (repeat up to three times)
   Quick-dosing suggestions:
   - Small dog, 2.5-5.0 mg (repeat up to three times)
   - Medium dog, 5.0 mg (repeat up to three times)
   - Large dog, 10-20 mg (repeat up to three times)
   - Cats, 2.5 mg (repeat up to three times)

Note: After the seizures stop, give the animal a constant rate infusion (CRI) of diazepam if necessary. Give the amount of diazepam used to stop the initial seizure in a solution of 1.2 ml lactated Ringer's solution/lb/hr.

Pentobarbital (if not responsive to diazepam)
- Dogs, 1-8 mg/kg IV (slow and to effect)
- Cats, 1-4 mg/kg IV (slow and to effect)

Note: It is not necessary to completely anesthetize the animal with pentobarbital as long as it stops the seizure. Anesthesia induced with pentobarbital may not totally stop seizure activity (as revealed by electroencephalogram), but it will prevent life-threatening hyperthermia and disseminated intravascular coagulation.

Other drugs to consider include the following:
- Propofol
- Thiopental
4. Continue with the maintenance drugs, usually phenobarbital or potassium bromide.
5. Consider starting other anticonvulsants if the maintenance drugs are not controlling the seizures adequately.
6. Obtain anticonvulsant blood levels to adjust dosing.

provided via face mask, nasal cannulas, or oxygen cages. Although controversial, furosemide (Lasix) administration may be beneficial.

After the initial emergency of cluster seizures or status epilepticus is resolved, an important aspect of seizure management involves continuing to give maintenance anticonvulsants despite recent administration of anticonvulsants to stop seizures. This treatment should be performed even with patients being administered anticonvulsants such as diazepam or propofol as a continuous rate infusion. The technician can administer maintenance anticonvulsants such as phenobarbital by different routes: IV, intramuscular (IM), orally (PO), or rectally (PR). Likewise, potassium bromide can be given either PO or PR.

Patients requiring anesthesia via a constant rate infusion (CRI) of diazepam or propofol to stop seizure activity need intensive nursing care and monitoring. Continued administration of maintenance anticonvulsants (phenobarbital and potassium bromide) can be performed by PR infusion. To do this, the technician should use a red rubber polyethylene feeding tube and large syringe, making sure to flush the catheter with water after administering the medication (to ensure that the patient receives the entire dose). A tomcat polyethylene catheter or teat cannula also can be used, but they are much shorter and the medication can spill from the anus.

The following also should kept in mind when treating an anesthetized patient:

- Monitoring respiratory rate and heart rate should be done hourly at a minimum. Ideally, using an electrocardiograph continuously can provide constant monitoring. When heart rates or respiratory rates fall below acceptable levels, lowering the CRI of anticonvulsants (or discontinuing it) should be done. Consider monitoring other physiologic parameters such as blood pressure, pulse oximetry, and arterial blood gas analysis.
- Monitoring of body temperature should be performed hourly. Active warming should be provided for hypothermic patients. Care must be taken not to induce thermal burning.
- Turning the patient every 6 hours, alternating the side of recumbency to prevent atelectasis and bed sores should be done.
- Lubricating the eyes to prevent corneal ulcers should be done.

- Expressing the urinary bladder manually should be performed two or three times daily to prevent overdistension of the bladder muscles. Consider placing a closed, indwelling urinary catheter.
- Maintaining IV access via an IV catheter should be done.
- Administering maintenance IV fluids should be performed.
- Giving anticonvulsants as indicated previously should be done.

Spinal Cord Trauma

Spinal cord trauma is very common in veterinary medicine. In general, spinal cord trauma is divided into intrinsic and extrinsic causes. Intrinsic causes include extrusion and protrusion of intervertebral disc material and fractures secondary to bone diseases such as congenital vertebral anomalies (atlantoaxial subluxation), neoplastic infiltration of vertebrae, or nutritional disorders leading to pathologic fractures. Extrinsic causes of spinal cord trauma include fractures, luxations, and subluxations secondary to traumatic events. This would include automobile accidents, gunshot wounds, and, much less commonly, animal abuse or bite wounds inflicted by another animal.

A schematic of the vertebral column is shown in Fig. 23-2. The diagram depicts three basic structures: (1) the bony vertebral column, (2) the intervertebral disc (between the ventral portions of two consecutive vertebrae), and (3) the spinal cord (between the dorsal and ventral portions of the bony vertebrae).

By far the most common cause of intrinsic trauma to the spinal cord is intervertebral disc disease. As shown in Fig. 23-2, the intervertebral disc is located between two consecutive vertebrae from the second cervical vertebrae through the caudal vertebrae of the tail. Under normal circumstances, the intervertebral disc acts as a cushion to absorb concussive energy along the vertebral column and provide structural integrity to the vertebral column. The intervertebral disc is composed of an outer fibrous material, the annulus fibrosus, and an inner gel-like material, the nucleus pulposus. The annulus fibrosus can rupture (because of external trauma or intrinsic factors), allowing the nucleus pulposus to extrude dorsally to impinge on the spinal cord or dorsolaterally to put pressure on the nerve roots. In certain breeds of dogs, chondrodystrophic breeds (e.g., dachshund, Lhasa apso, basset hound), the nucleus pulposus

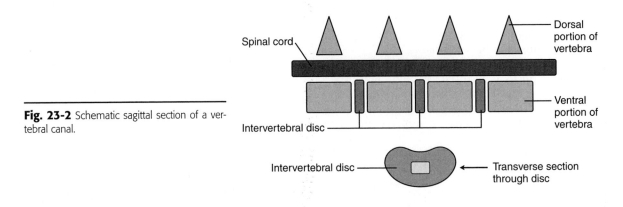

Spinal cord
Dorsal portion of vertebra
Ventral portion of vertebra
Intervertebral disc
Intervertebral disc
Transverse section through disc

Fig. 23-2 Schematic sagittal section of a vertebral canal.

degenerates and the annulus fibrosus weakens. When this occurs the disc can no longer absorb energy and ruptures through the annulus fibrosus, compressing the dorsally located spinal cord, even under minimal stress. In general, the nucleus pulposus displaces dorsally because the annulus fibrosus is thinnest dorsally, and the nucleus pulposus takes the path of least resistance. Intervertebral disc disease tends to occur in the thoracolumbar vertebral column approximately 85% of the time and approximately 15% of the time in the cervical vertebral column. In the thoracolumbar vertebral column, most herniations occur between the T10-L2 vertebras. The most common site to be affected is T13-L1 disc space. Several hypotheses have been proposed to explain this condition. Anatomically the dorsal longitudinal ligament is thinner in this region. In addition, no intercapital ligament exists between rib heads to provide extra support. Finally, greater mobility and less muscular support exist in this region than in the thoracic region. Figs. 23-3 and 23-4 illustrate the anatomic differences that can explain the increased frequency of disc extrusions at the T13-L1 intervertebral space. In the cervical vertebral column, disc herniation can happen at any site in the C2-C3 through C6-C7 disc space.

The types of injuries and forces on the vertebral canal most commonly associated with external trauma are shown in Fig. 23-5. Flexion alone usually results in extrusion of disc material into the spinal cord. The resulting clinical signs vary from mild paresis to complete paralysis and destruction of the spinal cord. A combination of compression and flexion forces, the type of injury most commonly seen in automobile accidents, usually results in a wedge fracture of the ventral portion of a vertebra. The compressive force occurs when the dog or cat tries to get

out of the way of the automobile. The vehicle hits the back end of the animal while the forelimbs are caught firmly on the ground. The majority of damage to the spinal cord occurs at the time of impact, and the resulting clinical signs vary. A third type of injury and force causing spinal cord trauma is that associated with concurrent flexion and rotation of the vertebral column. If rotation is the predominant force, then the resulting injury probably will involve a luxation and fracture of the vertebrae. If the majority of force is flexion of the vertebrae, then the injury probably will be luxation of the vertebral column. These types of injuries often are very unstable, and careful management is needed to prevent further damage to the spinal cord.

The site of the spinal cord injury must be localized accurately. Many times, even with severe vertebral fractures, the exact location of the injury is not obviously apparent on physical examination, especially in patients in which multiple organ systems are affected. Often in patients with fractures of the apendicular skeleton or those with thoracic injuries leading to dyspnea, neurologic signs may not be immediately apparent. Therefore a complete and thorough neurologic examination should be part of the assessment of every traumatized patient provided that the animal's cardiovascular system is stable. This examination is conducted not only to identify neurologic problems but also to prevent further injury to the spinal cord while providing other life-saving treatments or diagnostic procedures. In addition, examination helps to define specific sites to image (using radiography, myelography, or computed tomography) to further assess the nervous system.

For all practical purposes the spinal cord can be divided into four regions (Fig. 23-6). Spinal cord

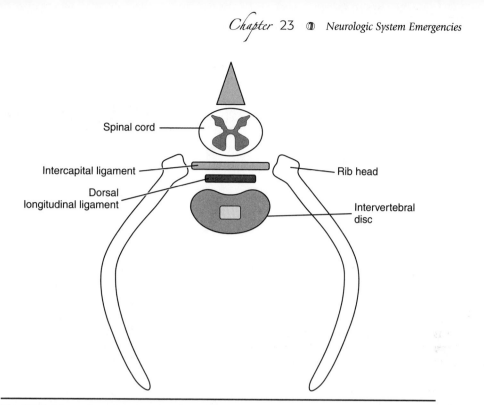

Fig. 23-3 Schematic transverse section through the T4-5 intervertebral space. The presence of intercapital ligament and thick dorsal longitudinal ligament should be noted.

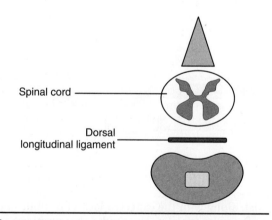

Fig. 23-4 Schematic transverse section through the T13-L1 intervertebral space. The very thin dorsal longitudinal ligament and the absence of rib heads and intercapital ligament should be noted.

injury alters the ability to conduct sensory imput to the brain and neuronal imput in terms of motor movements from getting to the limbs. The ascending sensory information regarding information about the location of the limbs and trunk in space is referred to as *general proprioception*. Descending upper motor neuron fibers from the brain that project down the spinal cord are responsible for tone, movement, and strength. Interference with these descending upper motor neuron fibers results in increased tone and hyperreflexia, as well as weakness referred to *spastic paresis* (weakness of neurologic origin in which increased tone in the limbs exists). The conduit of these descending upper motor neuron fibers from the spinal cord to the muscles of the limbs is the lower motor neuron system (nerves that project to the muscles and the muscles themselves). Injury of the lower motor system, from the cell body in the ventral gray horn of the spinal cord to the nerve root, peripheral nerve, neuromuscular junction, and muscle, results in decreased tone, hyporeflexia, and weakness (flaccid paresis; weakness with decreased muscular tone). The common clinical sequelae to a T13-L1 disc extrusion are shown in Fig. 23-6. Clinical signs are limited to the hind limbs and include paresis (weakness) or paralysis, hypertonia and hyperreflexia, and postural reaction deficits.

Some clinical exceptions to Fig. 23-6 should be noted. Spinal shock is a syndrome that is seen

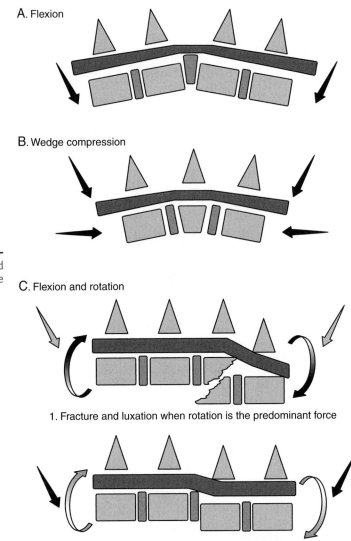

A. Flexion

B. Wedge compression

C. Flexion and rotation

1. Fracture and luxation when rotation is the predominant force

2. Luxation when flexion is the predominant force

Fig. 23-5 Types of injury and forces associated with trauma to the vertebral canal (arrows indicate direction of force).

with severe spinal cord trauma. Under most circumstances, when a spinal cord lesion is found at the T13-L1 spinal cord segments, the resulting clinical signs include hypertonia and hyperreflexia of the hind limbs. Occasionally a patient who arrives at a clinic within the first 12 hours of a severe spinal cord injury has the expected hyperreflexia. However, the hind limbs are hypotonic. The exact mechanism for this paradox is not known. Researchers believe that for a brief period a temporary lack of facilitators to the extensor muscles

exist, along with the expected lack of inhibition to the extensor muscles. The result is hypotonia in the hind limbs for the first 12 to 36 hours. The hypotonia is replaced by the expected hypertonia at the end of this period.

The second exception is Schiff-Sherrington syndrome. Most technicians working in a busy emergency clinic have seen examples of Schiff-Sherrington syndrome. Like spinal shock, this condition occurs when an animal experiences a very severe spinal cord injury (Fig. 23-7). Under these circumstances,

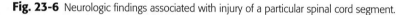

Spinal cord segment	C1-C6	C6-T2	T3-L3	L4-S1
Strength				
Fores	Paresis/Paralysis	Paresis/Paralysis	Normal	Normal
Hinds	Paresis/Paralysis	Paresis/Paralysis	Paresis/Paralysis	Paresis/Paralysis
Reflexes				
Fores	Hyper	Hypo	Normal	Normal
Hinds	Hyper	Hyper	Hyper	Hypo
Tone				
Fores	Hyper	Hypo	Normal	Normal
Hinds	Hyper	Hyper	Hyper	Hypo
Postural reactions				
Fores	Decreased	Decreased to normal	Normal	Normal
Hinds	Decreased	Decreased	Decreased	Decreased to normal

Fig. 23-6 Neurologic findings associated with injury of a particular spinal cord segment.

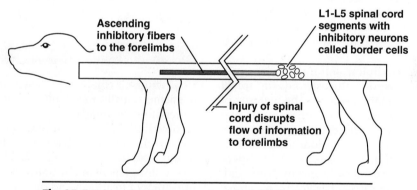

Fig. 23-7 Schematic of anatomic pathway for Schiff-Sherrington syndrome.

interference occurs to the ascending, inhibitory fibers from the L1-L5 spinal cord segments to the spinal cord segments innervating the forelimbs. These ascending fibers are inhibitors to the extensors of the forelimbs. Normally these fibers help the hind limbs and forelimbs coordinate movement. When severe spinal cord damage exists, this communication is interrupted. The result is severe extensor rigidity in the forelimbs.

Treatment

Treatment of a patient with a possible vertebral fracture begins before arrival at the hospital. If a patient must be transferred from one hospital to another, then it should be done with extreme care. When a client or referral veterinarian calls an emergency clinic, instructions should be given on how best to transport a patient with a possible vertebral injury.

This includes placing and carefully securing the patient on a flat board (e.g., door, piece of plywood) and warning owners that even the nicest pet may unexpectedly try to bite or scratch (because of severe pain associated with a spinal column injury). The patient can be secured in place with medical tape, belts, or even rope if necessary to ensure it remains still. Occasionally patients who are to be transferred from one hospital to another require sedation to keep them from causing further injury.

Once the injured patient arrives at the hospital, any unnecessary movement must be limited. The patient should receive a complete physical and neurologic examination before the possible vertebral fracture is addressed. Initial treatment is aimed at stabilizing the patient's respiratory and cardiovascular systems. If the animal is in pain, then opioid analgesics such as hydromorphone (0.05 to 0.1 mg/kg of body weight IV, IM, or subcutaneously [SQ]), butorphanol (0.2 to 0.4 mg/kg IV, IM, or SQ), oxymorphone (0.05 to 0.1 mg/kg IV or IM), morphine (0.5 to 2.0 mg/kg IV, IM, or SQ), or buprenorphine (0.01 to 0.15 mg/kg IV or IM) can be administered. Care must be taken to not compromise respiration with any medication in a patient who may have trauma such as a fractured rib or damaged lungs, because some these drugs can cause respiratory depression. In addition, diazepam (Valium) can be used as a sedative at a dose of 0.2 to 0.4 mg/kg IV if the patient is overly anxious or is flailing.

Little definitive clinical information is available about the use of corticosteroids in spinal cord injury in veterinary medicine. The majority of literature reports experimental studies in cats that received different types and doses of steroids and other antiinflammatory medications at the time of injury. The results of these studies vary with experimental procedure and often have conflicting findings. In human clinical studies involving spinal cord injury, methylprednisolone sodium succinate at a dose of 30 mg/kg at initial presentation, followed by 5.4 mg/kg/hr in a CRI for the next 23 hours has been shown to be beneficial if administered within 8 hours of the injury. Comparable studies have been done in veterinary medicine. Some neurologists and neurosurgeons use corticosteroids, whereas others do not. Similar dosing regimes for methylprednisolone sodium succinate have been used in veterinary medicine. Some veterinary neurologists use an initial dose of 30 mg/kg

methylprednisolone sodium succinate followed by two boluses of 15 mg/kg at 2 and 6 hours after the initial bolus. Care must be taken to administer the methylprednisolone slowly, over 5 to 10 minutes. Failure to administer this drug slowly can result in vomiting or hypotension.

Although commonly used in practice, little experimental and no clinical evidence shows that dexamethasone is effective in spinal cord trauma in veterinary medicine; therefore methylprednisolone sodium succinate should be used when available.

In the absence of methylprednisolone sodium succinate, dexamethasone can be tried at a dose of 0.5 to 1.0 mg/kg IV at initial presentation. Researchers believe that gastrointestinal side effects, such as gastrointestinal and colonic ulcers, are more common with dexamethasone than with methylprednisolone sodium succinate; if dexamethasone is used for spinal cord injuries, then concomitant gastroprotectant administration may be helpful.

Spinal cord injuries can be treated medically or surgically depending on the type and severity of the lesion. Medical management may involve a back or neck brace, cage rest, or drug therapy. Surgical intervention often involves some type of spinal cord decompression or vertebral column stabilization. Regardless of this decision, the initial emergency care is crucial for a positive outcome.

Head Trauma

Head trauma is common in the setting of emergency medicine, usually the result of being hit by a car. Other causes include blunt trauma from being hit by an object, falling from a height, or having an object fall on the animal. Regardless of the cause of the insult, head trauma results in the same pathophysiologic disorders as brain injury, so the same basic principles of treatment and care apply.

Initial Diagnosis

Most patients arrive at veterinary hospitals with a history of someone having seen the cause of trauma. Occasionally owners find their pets acting abnormally and have not witnessed the accident that caused the trauma. In this case one can surmise that a traumatic incident has occurred based on finding abrasions on the head and face, bleeding from the mouth or nose (epistaxis), blood in the ears or in and around the eyes, or asymmetric pupillary size (anisocoria).

Animals experience a wide variety of neurologic signs that depend on the area of the brain that is affected. Neurologic examination often is consistent with a disturbance of the prosencephalon. Most commonly, animals demonstrate an altered sensorium or state of mentation (e.g., dullness, stupor, coma). Other observations include circling; aimless, propulsive wandering; or seizures. Abnormal pupil size and symmetry can be seen as well. Occasionally, caudal fossa signs (cerebellum, pons, medulla, and caudal midbrain) predominate. In this situation, balance problems, abnormal eye movements (nystagmus), head tremors, or paralysis or paresis can occur.

Performing a thorough neurologic examination on admission to identify the location of lesions is critically important. These abnormalities can be monitored serially to detect improvement or deterioration in status. Based on sequential examinations, further diagnostics and treatments can be implemented. The frequency of monitoring depends on the critical nature of the patient and degree of impairment.

Pathophysiology

Injury that occurs with head trauma can be divided into two aspects: (1) primary brain injury and (2) secondary brain injury. Primary brain injury is mainly related to the concussive forces involved in the trauma and includes parenchymal lacerations related to shearing forces of the brain or from fractures of the calvaria (skull), as well as the resultant cerebral edema and intracranial hemorrhage that may be present. The intracranial hemorrhage can be epidural (i.e., between the calvaria and dura mater), subdural (i.e., between the dura mater and the arachnoid), subarachnoid (i.e., between the arachnoid and brain tissue), or intraparenchymal (i.e., within the brain tissue). In contrast to human patients, subdural hemorrhage is extremely rare in veterinary patients. Primary brain injury occurs at the time of the injury; therefore nothing can be done to lessen its effects. Consequently, treatment is directed at the secondary effects, secondary brain injury.

In people who suffer head trauma, this secondary injury is a major determinant of the outcome. Secondary brain injury can be divided into systemic or intracranial effects. Systemic secondary brain injury occurs as a result of ischemia (i.e., decreased perfusion or blood flow), hypotension (i.e., low blood pressure), hypoxia (i.e., low blood oxygen content), anemia, changes in blood glucose levels (either too high or too low), or acid-base or electrolyte disturbances. Intracranial secondary brain injury includes intracranial hypertension (i.e., raised intracranial pressure), cerebral edema, or a mass effect as a consequence of hemorrhage.

Serial Neurologic Monitoring

Integral to treatment is sequential monitoring. This monitoring allows the clinician to tailor treatment to the individual needs of the patient. Often technicians are relied on to evaluate the patient's changing mental status. The simplest parameter to evaluate that is often the most reflective of the patient's status is the patient's sensorium or mentation. Sensorium often is described as normal (i.e., alert and responsive), quiet, dull, stuporous (i.e., responsive only to noxious stimuli), or comatose (i.e., unresponsive to noxious stimuli). As the patient's condition deteriorates, mentation changes from normal to comatose.

In addition to mentation, pupil size and responsiveness to light must be evaluated. To fully understand the importance of anisocoria and pupillary light reactions (i.e., constriction of the pupil in response to light), an understanding of the neural control of the pupil is necessary. Pupil constriction begins with light stimulating the retina of the eye, resulting in stimulation of the optic nerve. This afferent limb (projecting to the central nervous system) of the reflex sends impulses through the thalamus to the midbrain, where the nervous control of the pupil is located (oculomotor neuron or cranial nerve III). The oculomotor nerve, after leaving the brain, stimulates the pupil to constrict in response to light. This reflex arc is under a degree of constant inhibition by nervous control from descending upper motor neurons from the prosencephalon.

Many patients with head trauma experience anisocoria. Changes in pupil size can be a result of trauma to the eye and surrounding structures, which often causes the pupil to be small (i.e., miotic) in response to pain or inflammation of the eye, whereas trauma to the brainstem, where the innervation to the pupil originates, results in a widely dilated (i.e., mydriatic) pupil that is unresponsive to light stimulation and does not constrict (pupillary light reflex).

Although anisocoria helps the clinician localize the traumatized region, evaluating pupillary changes from the initial status helps the clinician detect changes in intracranial pressure. As intracranial pressure increases, nerves that descend from the prosencephalon and inhibit the portion of the brainstem that causes pupillary constriction are inhibited. As a result, the oculomotor nerve is disinhibited and the pupils constrict. As pressure builds, the brain shifts inside the calvaria and begins to herniate, putting pressure on the origin of the oculomotor nerve in the brainstem and blocking its function. The pupils then become dilated and unresponsive.

One should remember that changes in pupil size and responsiveness can result from processes other than brain trauma and shifts in brain parenchyma. As mentioned previously, ocular trauma can also result in miotic pupils. Similarly, opioid medications administered for pain relief can cause the pupils to become miotic. Consequently, pupil size, symmetry, and responsiveness to light should not be the sole means with which to diagnose and monitor head trauma patients. Pupillary function should be evaluated in concert with other aspects of the neurologic examination such as mentation changes. A patient with severe brain trauma and brain herniation that results in mydriatic pupils, unresponsive to light, will also have a severely altered mentation.

Brain herniation is the final sequela to raised intracranial pressure. Brain herniation is a process by which intracranial pressure pushes the brain tissue out of its normal anatomic position. Brain tissue can herniate in several different ways, the most important of which is herniation out of the foramen magnum (a foramen of the calvaria through which the medulla oblongata transitions to the spinal cord). As the brain herniates out the foramen magnum, it puts pressure on the fibers that descend through the spinal cord and thereby causes paralysis. Animals undergoing this process assume a posture called *decerebrate, rigidity*. They are recumbent and opisthotonic (i.e., head and neck arched backward) and have both hind limb and forelimb extensor rigidity. In addition, the herniating brain tissue puts pressure on the nervous control centers for breathing and causes respiratory depression and eventual cessation of breathing. Here again, the posture of the patient should not be evaluated in a vacuum. Patients with severe brain herniation will also have severely affected mentation and an inability to ambulate. Alternatively, those patients who assume abnormal postures as a result of pain should be alert and responsive. Distinguishing these situations requires the critical evaluation of the entire neurologic examination.

Treatment

Although the primary brain injury has already occurred, the goal of treatment is to thwart the effects of secondary brain injury and the consequences of raised intracranial pressure. Treatment can be divided into brain-specific and nonspecific therapies. The most crucial aspect of treatment is to treat all the needs of the patient and not to concentrate on brain-specific therapies. In general, addressing the patient's systemic needs will additionally address the needs of the central nervous system. Secondary brain injury is the sequelae of hypotension, ischemia, and hypoxia. Therefore the aim of therapy is directed at normalizing such parameters. Hypotension has been shown to adversely affect outcome in people with head trauma. Hypotension results in cerebral ischemia (i.e., lack of blood flow). Mean arterial pressure is a major determinant of cerebral perfusion (i.e., blood flow). Cerebral perfusion equals the mean arterial pressure minus intracranial pressure. Therefore maintaining a normal mean arterial pressure ensures adequate cerebral perfusion and prevents cerebral ischemia. Appropriate IV fluid administration is crucial in treating hypotension. Fluid therapy can be provided through commonly used crystalloids (e.g., lactated Ringer's solution). In severely affected hypotensive patients, rapid correction of hypotension can be accomplished with hypertonic saline or hetastarch solutions. Equally as critical as correction of hypotension is avoiding hypertension. Blood pressure monitoring can aid in addressing hypotension and tailoring fluid administration. Mean arterial blood pressure should be kept greater than or equal to 90 mm Hg.

Similarly, hypoxia can result in secondary brain insult and thereby worsen outcome. Many patients with head trauma suffer concurrent trauma to other organ systems. Appropriate red blood cell mass should be evaluated with packed cell volume and serially monitored. Additionally, red blood cells should be given to maintain adequate red blood cell counts. Chest trauma also can contribute to hypoxia, because injuries such as pneumothorax, hemothorax, and pulmonary contusions impair ventilation and oxygenation. Patients with head trauma should always be evaluated for concurrent chest trauma.

Chest injuries must be treated adequately. Supplemental oxygen should be administered if necessary. Proper oxygenation is monitored by evaluating arterial blood gas analysis or pulse oximetry. Oxygenation saturation should be maintained between 98% and 100%.

Mannitol has long been used to reduce raised intracranial pressure and increase cerebral blood flow. It appears to work via two mechanisms: The first mechanism is by increasing intravascular volume and reducing blood viscosity, thereby increasing cerebral blood flow. This is accomplished immediately and seems to work best when mannitol is administered as a rapid IV bolus. In general, the infusion should not be given greater than 2 ml/kg/min bolus. The second mechanism of action is as an osmotic diuretic resulting in osmotic dehydration of the brain.

The duration of this effect varies from 90 minutes to 6 hours and is slightly dose dependent at doses ranging from 0.25 to 1.0 g/kg of a 25% solution. The duration of effect can be extended by addition of furosemide (Lasix) at 0.7 mg/kg approximately 15 minutes after mannitol administration. Mannitol administration can be repeated every 4 to 8 hours, with a maximum of three doses over 24 hours. Care must be taken when mannitol is given in the initial setting of resuscitation, because dehydration can precipitate hypotension. Additionally, monitoring should be performed to ensure that the patient does not become dehydrated. Mannitol administration should be avoided when known bleeding exists within the cranial vault. Administration of mannitol during active hemorrhage will result in increased blood outside of vascular structures, thereby increasing intracranial pressure. Like mannitol, furosemide should not be given to a dehydrated, hypovolemic, or hypotensive patient.

In cases of severe head trauma, mechanical ventilatory assistance sometimes is necessary. This is especially true in the setting of stupor or coma. Ventilation does require endotracheal intubation. Occasionally, sedation is needed when intubating patients with severe head trauma. In general, endotracheal intubation to ventilate patients is rarely done.

It has long been advocated that during mechanical ventilation, partial pressure of arterial carbon dioxide in arterial blood should be maintained between 25 and 30 mm Hg. End tidal carbon dioxide monitoring can be used in addition to blood gas analysis to serially monitor carbon dioxide. Hypocapnea induces cerebral vasoconstriction and a resultant reduction in intracranial pressure by reducing the total volume of blood in the cranial vault. However, prolonged hypocapnea can exacerbate cerebral ischemia. Prophylactic hyperventilation less than or equal to 35 mm Hg should thus be avoided.

Elevating the patient's head often is helpful in reducing the intracranial pressure by maximizing venous blood return from the brain to the heart. Placing a solid board under the patient and elevating the front 20 to 30 degrees can accomplish this. In addition, the team should be sure that no compression of the jugular veins occurs, thereby reducing venous return from the head.

Patients with head trauma may experience severe pain or altered mentation. This may result in the patient flailing around in the cage, causing further trauma and increased intracranial pressure. In these patients diazepam (Valium) should be used as a sedative at a dose of 0.2 to 0.4 mg/kg IV. In addition, opioid analgesics can be used to provide pain relief.

Steroids have been recommended in head trauma in the past. However, in people who suffer severe head trauma, steroids have been shown to lack efficacy and in some cases have been detrimental. Their use in human patients has been curtailed. In veterinary medicine, steroids are still used to a great extent; however, no convincing evidence shows that they are beneficial with head trauma in veterinary patients. Steroids can be used as a last resort or in severely traumatized patients. Methylprednisolone sodium succinate at an initial rate of 30 mg/kg IV is used in severe head trauma. Tapering doses of 15 mg/kg are given at 2 and 6 hours. Finally, head trauma must be approached with a standardized treatment regimen. Patients must be evaluated for central nervous system trauma and trauma to all other organ systems. Proper physiologic resuscitation is crucial. Brain-specific treatments must be supplemental to full resuscitation to all extracranial organ systems.

Vestibular Disorders

Veterinary emergency clinics often see patients with vestibular disorders. Luckily, these diseases rarely are life threatening at the time of presentation. Paramount to treating vestibular disorders is determining the location of the disturbance. For this reason, vestibular diseases are clinically divided into peripheral and central vestibular diseases. Peripheral vestibular

TABLE 23-1

Differences between Peripheral and Central Vestibular Disease

	Peripheral	Central
Postural reactions	Normal	Abnormal
Mental status	Normal	May be depressed
Cranial nerve deficits	7	5-12
Other nerves	Sympathetic	None
Nystagmus	Fast phase is opposite the side of the head tilt, either horizontal or rotary	Fast phase can be any direction; if vertical or if changes direction, then direction is usually central

disease implies that the neuroanatomic site is the vestibular portion of the vestibulocochlear (eighth) cranial nerve (located in the inner ear within the petrous temporal bone of the calvaria) and that no signs of a brainstem disturbance exist. In contrast, the anatomic site of central vestibular disease is the medulla, cerebellum, and pons. The vestibular signs associated with both peripheral and central vestibular disorders (i.e., head tilt and falling, leaning, or turning toward the side of the lesion) usually are identical. The other clinical signs are used to differentiate peripheral and central vestibular diseases. Table 23-1 indicates the clinical differences between peripheral and central vestibular disorders.

Differentiating between peripheral and central vestibular disease is important from a prognostic point of view. In general, central vestibular diseases carry a worse prognosis than peripheral vestibular diseases, but exceptions to this rule exist. For example, metronidazole toxicity and thiamine deficiency both are central vestibular diseases that have an excellent prognosis if recognized early. Similarly, a squamous cell carcinoma in the ear of a cat that causes peripheral vestibular disease has a very poor long-term prognosis. However, one should remember that central vestibular diseases have a poor prognosis and peripheral vestibular diseases have an excellent prognosis.

A few individual diseases should be mentioned. The first, idiopathic old dog (geriatric) peripheral vestibular disease, probably is the most common vestibular disease seen in an emergency clinic. This disease can affect dogs over the age of 8 years old. Dogs often have severe clinical signs including a head tilt with the fast phase nystagmus directed opposite the

side of the head tilt, a severe vestibular ataxia, and no postural reaction deficits all consistent with peripheral vestibular disease. Occasionally the patient is so severely affected that it is unable to ambulate. During the first 24 hours it may be difficult to distinguish between central and peripheral vestibular disease because of the severity of the vestibular ataxia. The most important thing to know about this disease is that the majority of patients improve with supportive care. Some dogs have a persistent head tilt, but the vestibular ataxia gradually improves over 2 to 6 weeks. The exact cause of this syndrome is unknown.

Feline idiopathic peripheral vestibular disease is another common vestibular syndrome. This is a disease of young to middle-aged indoor-outdoor cats. Indoor-only cats do not develop this syndrome. The majority of cats with this disorder are seen in July, August, and September. The disease is not recognized in large urban areas. As with the canine variety, all the clinical signs reflect involvement of the peripheral vestibular system. The exact cause of this syndrome is unknown. As with the dog, the majority of clinical signs in feline idiopathic vestibular disease resolve in 2 to 6 weeks.

Otitis media and otitis interna (i.e., ear infection) is a common syndrome causing peripheral vestibular disease in both cats and dogs. Ear infections occur as a primary infection or secondary irritation from ear mites or an allergen. Regardless of the cause, recognizing the neurologic signs associated with otitis media and otitis interna is important. These include findings consistent with peripheral vestibular disease, facial paralysis, and possibly Horner's syndrome. The latter findings are associated with damage to the seventh cranial nerve and the sympathetic nerve, respectively. Horner's syndrome is recognized by an elevated third eyelid; a small palpebral fissure, called *ptosis*; a sunken eye, called *enophthalmia*; and a small pupil, called *miosis*. If other cranial nerve abnormalities or postural reaction deficits are detected, then the cause of the vestibular disease cannot be just otitis media and otitis interna. Clinicians use a good otic examination or other imaging modalities such as radiographs, computed tomography, or magnetic resonance imaging to diagnose this syndrome.

No specific treatment generally is needed for vestibular disorders in an emergency clinic. Patients with vestibular disorders usually are stable, and immediate attention and treatments often are not warranted. Patients sometimes are started on maintenance fluids because they are too nauseated to drink or eat. It may be necessary to pad a cage with extra blankets to keep the animal from harming itself by rolling or flailing. In the case of ear infections, patients are started on broad-spectrum antibiotics. Occasionally medication is needed to sedate an animal with severe vestibular signs. Usually diphenhydramine at 2.2 mg/kg PO or IM twice daily is sufficient to cause sedation. Rarely, diazepam (Valium) may be necessary at 0.2 to 0.4 mg/kg IV or IM to gain the level of sedation needed. In general, steroids are not recommended for vestibular diseases in an emergency clinic setting for several reasons, including the ability of steroids to mask important clinical signs and laboratory findings necessary for an accurate diagnosis.

Occasionally steroids can exacerbate clinical diseases such as otitis media/interna. If a patient's clinical signs deteriorate dramatically and become life threatening, then it may be necessary to use steroids such as dexamethasone at an initial dose of 0.5 to 10 mg/kg IV or methylprednisolone sodium succinate at 30 mg/kg IV. Dexamethasone often is associated with adverse gastrointestinal signs, so a gastroprotectant may be helpful when using dexamethasone. Although many patients with vestibular disease are nauseated, specific antiemetic drugs usually are not necessary for treating vestibular diseases in animals.

Conclusion

A neurologic emergency can result from many factors. Seizures and trauma-related neurologic disorders are common in veterinary practice. Understanding how to examine and assess the neurologic small animal patient is crucial to successful treatment.

The goal in treating an animal with seizures is to stop all seizure activity. Monitoring must be continued once the seizure has stopped. Management may include caring for a fully anesthetized patient. Stabilizing the patient with spinal cord trauma begins where the injury occurred. The people transporting the animal must be aware that any movement may cause further damage. The emergency team can instruct the owners on how to protect themselves and the animal before transporting.

The site of the injury in spinal cord trauma or disease must be localized accurately once the animal arrives. This will allow the team to stabilize and perform necessary procedures without causing further injury. The small animal suffering from a neurologic disorder must be monitored closely during treatment. Adjustments in medication often are necessary to stabilize the animal. The veterinary technician must understand the degree of injury and record all findings accurately. Self-induced injury is common. Padding the cage and placing supportive blankets around the animal can prevent further injury.

Suggested Readings

Braund KG: *Clinical syndromes in veterinary neurology*, ed 2, St Louis, 1994, Mosby.

Chrisman CL: *Problems in small animal neurology*, ed 2, Philadelphia, 1991, Lea & Febiger.

de Lahunta A: *Veterinary neuroanatomy and clinical neurology*, ed 3, St Louis, 2006, WB Saunders.

Lorenz MD, Kornegay JN: *Handbook of veterinary neurology*, ed 4, St Louis, 2004, WB Saunders.

Mayhew I: *Large animal neurology: a handbook for veterinary clinicians*, Philadelphia, 1989, Lea & Febiger.

Summers BA, Cummings JF, de Lahunta A: *Veterinary neuropathology*, St Louis, 1995, Mosby.

Wheeler SJ: *Manual of small animal neurology*, ed 2, United Kingdom, 1995, BSAVA.

CHAPTER 24

Toxicologic Emergencies

Andrea M. Battaglia

Toxicity must be considered when an animal arrives at the clinic in an emergent state for an unknown cause. Clinical signs may include abnormal behavior, neurologic dysfunction, coagulopathies, lethargy, or gastrointestinal (GI) disorders. Diagnosis of poisoning usually is made by a confirmation from the owners that the animal was exposed to the toxin, as well as by clinical signs exhibited by the animal and chemical analysis. Possible underlying disease processes must be ruled out. Animals with metabolic diseases can have many of the same clinical signs as a poisoned animal. Clinical signs cannot be the final factor in diagnosing toxicity.

Toxicity can result from ingestion, inhalation, injection, ocular, cutaneous, or topical exposure. Ingestion is the most common and occurs accidentally, when the animal eats something or when uninformed owners give an animal a toxin in the form of food or an over-the-counter medication. Occasionally toxicity may occur at a hospital when a drug dose is miscalculated (Boxes 24-1 and 24-2).

In cases of toxicity the animal should be brought to the veterinary hospital immediately. Owners should not treat the animal at home because of the increased risks to the owner and the animal. Time cannot be wasted. For topical exposures, the owner can wash the animal (if stable) in a mild dishwashing detergent before bringing it into the hospital.

Equipment list:

- The basics (IV catheters and wrap materials, IV fluids, electrocardiograph, oxygen, crash cart)
- Emetics
- Activated charcoal
- Stomach tubes of various sizes
- Valium and other muscle relaxants

Treatment

The goals of treating the poisoned animal are to treat the patient, evaluate its condition, and stabilize vital signs. This includes checking the airway, breathing, and circulation. These patients may arrive in various

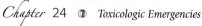

stages of toxicity and have very mild clinical signs (e.g., anxiety) or very serious clinical signs (e.g., seizure, coma).

The technician should attempt to get a thorough history from the owners. This may be difficult if a recreational drug is involved, because owners may be embarrassed or fear that law enforcement agencies will become involved. However, the technician must be told what was ingested or what toxin the animal was exposed to for the best possible treatment plan and prognosis. Many times treatment begins based on clinical signs because the toxin cannot be identified.

The veterinary team is at risk when treating the poisoned animal. For example, what has been ingested can convert to poisonous gases. When emesis is induced, the gas is emitted. Zinc phosphide (used in rodenticides, most commonly in gopher baits) is converted to phosphine gas when ingested. Therefore, these animals should be treated in a well-ventilated area.

The team must protect themselves from coming into contact with topical exposures by wearing gloves and protective clothing. Protective eyewear is highly recommended before bathing the animals to

avoid the spread of contaminants should they shake during the bathing procedure.

Toxins can cause behavioral abnormalities and hypersensitivity. The team must be focused on the patient to avoid any unnecessary injury.

Preventing Further Absorption

Ocular Exposure

The eyes should be rinsed with large amounts of physiologic saline for 20 to 30 minutes. For chemical burns, the eyes can be treated with lubricant ointments and lid closure techniques. Corticosteroids may be beneficial and used only if the corneal epithelium is intact. The severity of ocular damage that can occur depends on the type of chemical that was in the eye and how quickly it was treated.

Topical Exposure

The animal who has been exposed to a toxin topically should be bathed only in a mild liquid dishwashing detergent (detergent made for use in sinks, not dishwashers). Solvents can disperse chemicals and increase the exposed area of the skin. In addition, they change skin permeability. Topical ointments also should be avoided because they can enhance absorption of the chemical.

The person bathing the animal should wear protective clothing, including a mask and goggles, to avoid contamination. Bathing should continue until all toxin has been removed, rinsing frequently with large amounts of water. If the substance is a powder, then the animal should be vacuumed before bathing. Ingestion must also be considered in animals who arrive with a topical poisoning because of the grooming instinct.

Ingested Toxins

Inducing emesis, performing gastric lavage, and administering adsorbents, cathartics, and enemas can decontaminate the animal who has ingested a toxin.

Rapid dilution of the toxin with large amounts of milk or water is not recommended because it may enhance the absorption of toxins into the GI tract. Dilution is considered only for animals who may have ingested a corrosive substance.

Inducing emesis involves introducing a technique or substance to the animal so that it will vomit. This procedure is preferred over gastric lavage for removing stomach contents. Vomiting removes 40% to 60% of the chyme (i.e., semifluid mass of partially digested food passed from the stomach to the duodenum).

Several emetic substances are available. Emetics work by two different mechanisms: (1) local gastric irritation or (2) central nervous system (CNS) stimulation. Some work by both mechanisms. Emetics are most effective when administered quickly and some food is in the stomach.

The most common emetics include syrup of ipecac, hydrogen peroxide, salt, liquid dishwashing detergent, and apomorphine.

Syrup of ipecac is obtained from plant roots and contains active alkaloids, emetine, and cephaeline, which act by local gastric irritation and stimulate the chemoreceptor trigger zone. Water should be given after administration. The recommended dose is 0.5 to 1 teaspoon per 10 lb orally in the dog or 1 teaspoon orally for average-sized cat. Cats find the taste very objectionable, and diluting the dose 50:50 with water may assist in administration. Vomiting should occur within 30 minutes. Side effects have been observed most commonly when the fluid extract was used (which is no longer available) or with chronic use. Side effects include cardiotoxicity, hemorrhagic diarrhea, and skeletal muscle weakness. Activated charcoal absorbs ipecac well and can be used if any side effects are observed.

Hydrogen peroxide (3%) induces emesis by gastric irritation. The recommended dose is 1 tablespoon per 20 lb and can be repeated if emesis has not occurred within 10 minutes. This product is not a reliable emetic.

Salt acts as a pharyngeal stimulator and is not recommended because of the risk of sodium toxicity. Salt is also unreliable as an emetic.

Dishwashing detergent has been used primarily in humans and only in dogs experimentally. The recommended dose for humans is 3 tablespoons of detergent in 8 oz of water; the dose is not adjusted by size. Dishwashing detergent is not recommended because of it questionable efficacy and potential for side effects.

Apomorphine is considered the most reliable emetic in the clinical setting and is a morphine derivative that stimulates dopamine receptors in the chemoreceptor zone (which activates the vomiting center). The recommended dose for apomorphine is 0.04 mg/kg IV or 0.08 mg/kg intramuscularly (IM). The dose for topical conjunctival or subcutaneous (SQ) application is 0.03 mg/kg. Apomorphine is poorly absorbed after oral administration. If using apomorphine topically on the conjunctiva, then the conjunctiva should be rinsed thoroughly with physiologic saline after the animal vomits to alleviate some of the irritation that will occur. Side effects that can occur with apomorphine include lethargy or restlessness and protracted vomiting. Vomiting usually occurs within 10 minutes of IV injection and within 20 minutes of administration via other routes. Some consider apomorphine use in cats to be contraindicated.

Xylazine hydrochloride is an α_2-agonist that has sedative, analgesic, and muscle relaxant properties and is commonly used as an emetic for cats. The dose for cats is 0.44 mg/kg IM or SQ. For dogs the recommended dose is 1.1 to 2.2 mg/kg IM or SQ or 1.1 mg/kg IV. The animal must be monitored closely when this drug is used because of the possibility of increased respiratory depression and bradycardia. Vomiting usually occurs within a few minutes.

Vomiting should not be induced during a seizure or if the animal is comatose, dyspneic, hypoxic, or lacking normal pharyngeal reflexes. It also is contraindicated if the animal has ingested a caustic substance or a CNS stimulant. Caustic substances can permanently damage the mucosa of the GI system. If the toxin is a CNS stimulant, then inducing vomiting may increase the risk of seizures. The technician should not

BOX 24-3

Technical Tip: Gastric Lavage Technique

- A large-bore stomach tube and large amounts of tepid water are necessary for the lavage.
- The animal is lightly anesthetized so intubation with a cuffed endotracheal tube is possible; this reduces the patient's risk of aspirating any of the fluid.
- The tube is premeasured from the tip of the nose to the xiphoid cartilage, lubricated, then introduced into the stomach. The stomach tube must be passed with care, and the lavage should be done with very little pressure. The toxin may weaken the stomach wall, and lavaging could push the toxin into the duodenum.
- Once the lavage has been completed, activated charcoal should be given.
- The tube should be kinked at the end before removal to prevent excess fluid from running into the mouth, which increases the risk of aspiration.

attempt to induce vomiting in rabbits or rodents, because they lack the natural ability to vomit.

Gastric lavage is the act of washing out the stomach (Technical Tip Box 24-3). Gastric lavage is most reliable and efficient when performed 2 to 4 hours after ingestion; however, the technique is not recommended for animals who have ingested a caustic substance or are having seizures.

A gastrotomy or endoscopy should be considered in animals who have ingested metal objects (e.g., pennies, lead weights), which can be confirmed radiographically.

Activated Charcoal

Activated charcoal acts as an adsorbent. An adsorbent is a drug that inhibits GI absorption of drugs, toxins, or chemicals by attracting and holding them to its surface. Activated charcoal decreases the amount of toxin released into the circulation because it contains large-bore molecules to which toxins bind. Although activated charcoal does not inactivate the toxin by changing its chemical composition, it prevents further absorption.

Several types of activated charcoal are available. The type chosen should be vegetable or petroleum in origin. Animal-based charcoal should not be used. Charcoal is available in suspension, paste, tablet, and powder form. Highly activated charcoal made from petroleum (SuperChar Vet, Gulf Biosystems) has better adsorbent qualities than activated charcoal.

The suspension forms (Toxiban, Vet a Mix) can be administered orally or through a stomach tube. Toxiban with sorbitol also is available in suspension form. The sorbitol acts as a cathartic (charcoal treatment can cause constipation).

Activated charcoal compressed in tablet form (B.C. Crowley and Requa Manufacturing) was found to be approximately 25% less adsorptive than powders or suspension but sometimes is preferred because of its ease of administration. The powdered form must be made into a slurry before administration. The recommended dilution is 1 g activated charcoal in 5 to 10 ml water.

The dose is 2 to 8 g charcoal per kilogram of body weight. It may be beneficial to administer the activated charcoal three to four times a day for 2 to 3 consecutive days for some intoxications.

Dairy products and mineral oil are known to decrease the adsorbent properties of activated charcoal. Mixing other types of food with activated charcoal can either enhance or reduce the efficiency of the charcoal (it can prevent the charcoal from interacting with the toxin or allow more time for the charcoal and drug to interact by decreasing gastric emptying). Many factors determine the effects that food may have on the charcoal. The amount and time of food ingestion and the amount and physical characteristics of the charcoal must be considered. In general, charcoal should not be mixed with food.

Some animals will willingly eat the charcoal. The technician should offer it to them in a bowl before attempting to administer it with a syringe.

Administering charcoal can be a very messy procedure. Creating a bib for the animal, placing the animal in a tub, and wearing protective clothing such as a mask, cap, and gown can save cleanup time.

Cathartics

Cathartics are used in conjunction with activated charcoal to assist in the elimination of the toxin and the toxin-bound charcoal. Cathartics can also decrease the incidence of charcoal-induced constipation. They should be used 30 minutes after activated charcoal treatment or charcoal with a cathartic is administered once (to avoid excessive fluid loss).

Sodium sulfate is the preferred cathartic because of its efficiency in evacuating the bowel. A recommended dose is 250 to 500 mg/kg orally in the dog and 200 mg/kg orally in the cat. Cathartics containing magnesium have been reported to result in hypermagnesemia and CNS depression. Cathartics should not be used if the animal has diarrhea or if the toxin that has been ingested may cause diarrhea. Precautions must be taken in using cathartics in very old and very young animals.

What To Do with Toxins Already Absorbed

Most toxins that are absorbed are excreted through the kidneys. Increasing kidney function through the use of diuretics has been suggested for animals who have severe clinical signs, those who have ingested a potentially lethal dose, and those whose condition continues to deteriorate. The most common diuretics used are mannitol and furosemide. When monitoring renal function, the technician notes urine output and performs regular laboratory tests to ensure proper hydration is maintained throughout treatment. If urine output is below normal, then peritoneal dialysis must be considered.

Ion Trapping

Ion trapping increases the excretion rate of the toxin. Most drugs are weak acids or weak bases. Many drugs cannot pass through a cell membrane unless they are in a nonionized form. The pH of a drug combined with the pH of the environment the drug is in determines how well the drug is ionized and absorbed. Weakly acidic drugs placed in an acidic environment do not ionize readily and absorb well. Weakly basic drugs absorb well in an alkaline environment. If a mildly acidic drug is in an alkaline environment or a mildly alkaline drug is in an acidic environment, then the drug is readily ionized and unable to be absorbed (which is what traps it in its environment). The animal who has ingested a toxin that is reabsorbed by the kidneys can benefit from ion trapping by changing the pH of the urine. This helps prevent toxin reabsorption into the distal tubules. Urinary alkalinizers, sodium bicarbonate, increase elimination of the weak acids, and urine acidifiers

(i.e., ammonium chloride) increase elimination of weak bases.

Gastrotomy

A gastrotomy or gastric endoscopy may be indicated if the animal has ingested metal objects such as pennies or lead weights.

Supportive Care

Supportive care depends on many factors, including the type of toxin, the amount of toxin, and the success of the initial stabilization and treatment. Supportive care can range from observing the animal for the night to assisting ventilation or controlling seizure activity by anesthetizing the patient.

Most animals will receive an IV catheter and supportive fluid therapy. Visual monitoring will be continuous to note any changes including further decompensation.

Specific Types of Toxicities

Methylxanthines

Methylxanthines stimulate the heart and respiratory muscles and cause minor diuresis. Caffeine, theobromine, and theophylline can be found in coffee, tea, stimulants, medications, and chocolate.

Chocolate (Theobromine Toxicity). Theobromine is found in cocoa beans, cocoa bean hulls, chocolate, colas, and tea. The cocoa bean contains three methylxanthine compounds: (1) caffeine, (2) theophylline, and (3) theobromine. Theobromine is toxic to dogs and cats. Cats are less likely to experience this type of toxicity because of their selective eating habits. The toxic dose of theobromine is 250 to 500 mg/kg. Milk chocolate contains 44 mg/oz theobromine, and baking chocolate contains 390 mg/oz theobromine.

Clinical signs include anxiousness, vomiting, diarrhea, tachycardia, cardiac arrhythmias, urinary incontinence, ataxia, muscle tremors, abdominal pain, hematuria, seizures, cyanosis, coma, and sudden death caused by cardiac arrhythmia.

Diagnosis is based on the history and clinical signs and the presence of xanthenes in serum, plasma, tissue, urine, or stomach contents. Theobromine is stable in serum and plasma for 7 days at room temperature.

Treatment includes inducing vomiting (if not contraindicated), gastric lavage, charcoal, and cathartics. It may be beneficial to induce vomiting even if the ingestion occurred more than 2 hours earlier, because chocolate melts and forms a semisolid mass in the stomach. Diazepam may be necessary to control seizure activity, as well as antiarrhythmics to control arrhythmias. Catheterizing the bladder frequently is also recommended, because methylxanthines can be reabsorbed from the urinary bladder.

Caffeine. Caffeine can be found in coffee, tea, chocolate, colas, and stimulant drugs. The lethal dose is 140 mg/kg. The clinical signs include vomiting, diuresis, restlessness, and hyperactivity. Tachypnea and tachycardia may be present. Ataxia, cyanosis, cardiac arrhythmias, and seizures also may be observed. Death is not common in caffeine toxicity but can result from cardiac collapse. Diagnosis and treatment are the same as for theobromine toxicity.

Rodenticides

Anticoagulants include warfarin, pindone, bromadiolone, brodifacoum, chlorphacinone, difethialone, diphacinone, coumafuryl, dicoumarol, and difenamarol, which are sold under various names and a variety of formulations.

These anticoagulants bind the vitamin-K factor, which then inhibits the synthesis of prothrombin (factor II), as well as factors VII, XI, and X. The depletion of these factors slows all coagulation pathways. This effect can occur within 6.2 to 41 hours in a dog and is very dependent on the type of anticoagulant ingested.

The various types of anticoagulant rodenticides are classified as first-generation or second-generation rodenticides. The categorization is based on the rodenticide's ability to kill warfarin-resistant rats. A few first-generation rodenticides include warfarin, pidone, diphacinone, and chlorophacinone. They can depress the clotting factors for 7 to 10 days. The second-generation rodenticides (capable of killing warfarin-resistant rats) include brodifacoum and bromadiolone. These can depress the clotting factors for 3 to 4 weeks.

Animals usually are poisoned by directly ingesting rodenticides, but delay toxicosis also can occur (in which poisoning is induced when an animal eats something that has died from eating a rodenticides). Although it has been noted in cats or other animals who regularly consume rats and animals who may already be hypoprothrombic because of another disease process, the problem is uncommon.

The lethal dose varies with many factors, including the species of the animal who has been exposed, age, preexisting disease conditions such as renal failure or liver failure, number of ingestions, and concurrent drug (e.g., aspirin) use.

Clinical signs occur after the depletion of active clotting factors, which usually occurs 1 to 2 days after ingestion. Clinical signs include lethargy, vomiting, anorexia, ataxia, diarrhea, hemorrhage, melena, dyspnea, epistaxis, scleral or subconjunctival hemorrhage, bruising, and pale mucous membranes. Sudden death may result from hemorrhage into the pericardium, thorax, mediastinum, abdomen, or cranium.

Diagnosis is based on the history of exposure to the toxin, prolonged bleeding times, and the response to vitamin-K therapy, which usually occurs 24 to 48 hours after the initiation of therapy. Dye-colored feces may be present if a rodenticide has been ingested.

Treatment includes inducing vomiting (if not contraindicated) and administering activated charcoal and cathartics. Whole blood transfusions may be necessary to replace clotting factors and red blood cells if the patient is anemic. Fresh frozen plasma (10 to 20 ml/kg) can be used for animals in need of the clotting factors but not red cells. Vitamin K (3 to 5 mg/kg) should be administered every 24 hours until toxic concentrations of the anticoagulant are no longer in the animal. Vitamin K will begin the synthesis of new clotting factors 6 to 12 hours after administration. Clotting factors should return to normal within 24 to 36 hours. Oral administration with canned dog food is the preferred route unless the clinician is concerned about GI dysfunction or if activated charcoal has been administered. The fat in the dog food will increase the absorption rate. SQ administration is the next best route unless animal is hypovolemic. IV administration may cause anaphylaxis, and IM injections may cause hemorrhage.

The animal who arrives with a packed cell volume of more than 30% and mild clinical signs should be given vitamin K and observed.

Animals who have ingested brodifacoum or diphacinone (second-generation anticoagulants) should remain on vitamin K therapy for 21 days.

Cholecalciferol. Cholecalciferol is an active vitamin-D_3 derivative used in the rodenticides Quintox, Rampage, and Rat-Be-Gone. The baits contain 0.075%

active ingredient and usually are in a cereal or pellet form. The mechanism of action is calcium reabsorption from the bone and intestine into the blood; then increased calcium absorption by the kidneys occurs. Hypercalcemia (more than 11.5 mg/dl) is the result. If not treated appropriately, then it will result in soft tissue calcification and nephrosis. Death is caused by hypercalcemic cardiotoxicity. The toxic dose can range from 1 g/kg to 100 g/kg.

Clinical signs usually occur 12 to 36 hours after ingestion and include anorexia, vomiting, muscle weakness, and constipation. Signs can progress to hypertension, ventricular fibrillation, seizures, polyuria, and polydipsia. Calcium deposits can be found on postmortem examination in soft tissues, aorta, tendons, and muscle if long-term exposure has occurred.

The diagnosis is based on the history of exposure and the clinical signs (most often discovered when a routine serum chemistry panel is performed and the serum calcium concentration is greater than 12 mg/dl).

Inducing vomiting and administering activated charcoal and cathartics are recommended if ingestion has occurred within 2 hours of presentation. Correcting the electrolyte balances with IV physiologic saline (not lactated Ringer's solution, because it contains calcium) is also recommended. The following drugs are commonly used to reduce and prevent hypercalcemia. Furosemide (5 mg/kg IV followed by 2.5 mg/kg orally three or four times a day) increases calcium excretion from the kidneys. Prednisone (2 to 3 mg/kg orally once or twice a day) helps decrease calcium reabsorption from the bone and intestines. Calcitonin also is administered (4 to 6 IU/kg SQ every 2 to 3 hours initially) until serum calcium levels stabilize (less than 11.5 mg/dl) and is a peptide hormone that functions in hypercalcemia to lower the calcium concentration. Decreasing the calcium and phosphorus mobilization from bone and increasing phosphate movement into the bone from extracellular fluid accomplishes this. Calcitonin also increases renal calcium and phosphorus excretion. Furosemide and prednisone treatment is continued for 2 to 4 weeks, and a low-calcium diet is recommended.

Bromethalin. Bromethalin is found in rodenticide (i.e., Assault, Vengeance, Trounce) and is a pellet (usually green or tan) sold in 0.75 to 1.5 oz packages. Bromethalin is an uncoupler of oxidative phosphorylation in the CNS. Cerebral edema and an increase in cerebrospinal fluid pressure results in decreased nerve impulse conduction, paralysis, and death. The toxic dose in dogs is 4.7 mg/kg; in cats the toxic dose is 1.8 mg/kg.

In a high-dose toxicity, clinical signs usually appear within 24 hours of exposure, including excitement, tremors, and seizures. In a low-dose toxicity, clinical signs can be observed 1 to 5 days after ingestion. Tremors, depression, and ataxia are more common signs. The diagnosis depends on the history of exposure to the toxicant and the clinical signs on presentation.

Treatment includes decontaminating the intestinal tract if recent ingestion has occurred. Once the clinical signs have appeared, the effectiveness of treatment is questionable. Mannitol and glucocorticoids have been used to decrease and control cerebral edema. Diazepam or phenobarbital is recommended for seizure control. The animals who have the greatest chance for survival are those who have ingested small amounts and have been treated aggressively with supportive care. Improvement may occur within 2 to 3 weeks in these cases.

Rodenticides are available in many different concentrations, formulations, and packaging. Many appear to be very similar because of their color and pellet or cereal property. The clinician must determine the trade name, the chemical name of the rodenticide ingested, the concentration of the active ingredient, the largest amount the animal may have ingested, and the time interval since exposure before a proper treatment regimen can be determined.

Acetaminophen

Acetaminophen is a common over-the-counter medication used for analgesia and is available in capsules, tablets, and liquid. The common strengths of the drug in tablet form are 80 to 160 mg/dose for children and 500 to 1000 mg/dose for adults. In most species, acetaminophen is biotransformed. Cats cannot biotransform acetaminophen because of reduced ability to form the specific enzyme glucuronyl transferase, which is needed to conjugate acetaminophen to glucuronic acid. The glucuronic acid binds to the drug, changing it to a nontoxic form. A toxic dose for dogs is 160 to 600 mg/kg; a toxic dose for cats is 50 to 60 mg/kg. If a cat is given two doses within 24 hours, then death is almost inevitable. The most common cause of intoxication is owner administration.

Clinical signs can be observed 1 to 2 hours after ingestion. In cats they include vomiting, salivation, facial and paw edema, depression, increased respiratory rate, dyspnea, and pale mucous membranes. Cyanosis is another common clinical sign (usually observed 4 to 12 hours after acetaminophen ingestion) and occurs because of the methoglobinemia. Prognosis in cats is guarded to poor.

Dogs can experience lethargy, anorexia, vomiting, and abdominal pain. Dogs can recover spontaneously within 48 to 72 hours in moderate toxicity. More severe toxicity may result in hepatic necrosis, icterus, weight loss, hemolysis, and hemoglobinuria. Death usually occurs within 2 to 5 days after the presentation of clinical signs.

Diagnosis includes the history and presentation of clinical signs. Treatment of acetaminophen toxicity involves restoring the depleted glutathione stores and converting methemoglobin back to hemoglobin.

Initially, vomiting should be induced if ingestion has been within 2 hours. Activated charcoal with sorbitol is recommended because it decreases the absorption of acetaminophen from the GI tract. This stage of therapy is followed immediately with the antidote, *N*-acetylcysteine. *N*-acetylcysteine is a glutathione stimulator that helps protect the liver. Oxygen should be administered to cyanotic patients.

N-acetylcysteine is given at an initial loading dose of 140 to 280 mg/kg orally or IV, then given at a maintenance dose of 70 mg/kg orally or IV four times a day for 2 to 3 days. IV *N*-acetylcysteine is available in a sterile 10% to 20% solution. It should be diluted with saline or sterile water before IV administration. Treatment is most effective if administered within 8 hours of acetaminophen ingestion.

Ascorbic acid (30 mg/kg orally four times a day) is used for methemoglobinemia in affected cats. Blood transfusions also may be necessary to treat animals with a packed cell volume less than 15% or to aid in the treatment of methemoglobinemia. Supportive care including fluid therapy is necessary. Clinical response should be seen within 36 to 48 hours.

Metals

Lead is a common toxicity in companion animals. Cats are less likely to have this toxicity than dogs because of their selective eating habits. Lead toxicity is more common in dogs and cats less than 6 months of age because of their chewing habits and because the blood-brain barrier can be penetrated easily in immature animals.

The most common source for lead poisoning is lead-containing paint, which was used before the 1950s. Other sources include batteries, linoleum, plumbing supplies, ceramic containers that were not glazed properly, lead pipes, fishing sinkers, and shotgun pellets. Lead poisoning usually results from a recent exposure but can result from chronic exposure and accumulation. The most common signs involve the GI and nervous systems.

Anorexia, vomiting, abdominal pain, diarrhea, megaesophagus, and constipation usually are observed before the neurologic signs. These signs are more commonly observed with high-level toxicity. Anxiousness, behavioral changes (e.g., whining, barking, continuous running, snapping), tremors, seizures, ataxia, opisthotonus, and blindness also are seen.

Diagnosis begins with a history and clinical signs. Blood smears containing large numbers of nucleated red blood cells, with increased numbers of cells with basophilic stippling and a packed cell volume of 30% or more supports the possibility of lead poisoning. To confirm the diagnosis, whole blood is submitted for lead levels. Concentrations of 35 µg/dl or more is supportive, but a concentration of 60 µg/dl is diagnostic.

Treatment includes removing any lead from the GI tract, which may be accomplished through a magnesium or sodium sulfate cathartic, or surgery may be indicated if the object is made of lead. The following chelators are commonly used to treat lead poisoning. Thiamine is given IM or SQ at 2 mg/kg to alleviate the clinical signs; however, it can cause muscle soreness at the injection site. Commercial calcium ethylenediaminetetraacetic acid (EDTA) is used to help remove lead the body stores. The drug is given IV or SQ 100 mg/kg/day divided into four daily doses for 2 to 5 days (10 mg EDTA in 1 ml 5% dextrose). This drug can cause renal toxicity and should not be used in anuric patients. Hydration must be maintained throughout this treatment to promote renal function and the proper excretion of the chelated lead. D-penicillamine is another drug commonly used as a chelation treatment in animals less severely affected by the lead poisoning or as a treatment after the calcium EDTA therapy. The recommended dose is 110 mg/kg/day divided into three or four oral doses given 30 minutes before feeding for 1 to 2 weeks. Adverse side effects include vomiting, anorexia, and lethargy. If this occurs, then the animal can be premedicated with dimenhydrinate (Dramamine), or the dose can be reduced to 55 mg/kg/day orally divided into three or four doses.

Zinc toxicosis most commonly occurs after the ingestion of pennies, galvanized metal, and zinc oxide ointment. This toxicity is most common in dogs. Zinc oxide is used in many products, including diaper rash ointment, cosmetics, soaps, rubber, textiles, and electrical equipment. An animal with an acute toxicity after zinc oxide ingestion may have severe vomiting, CNS depression, and lethargy. Subacute or chronic toxicity from elemental zinc may cause hemolysis, regenerative anemia, renal failure, vomiting, lethargy, diarrhea, pica, icterus, spherocytosis, and an inflammatory leukogram.

Diagnosis is based on the history of exposure and clinical signs. Foreign objects may be discovered by an abdominal radiograph. Serum zinc levels above the normal range of 0.06 to 0.2 mg/dl would confirm the diagnosis.

Treatment includes removing any metal object endoscopically or surgically. Stabilization and supportive care may include blood transfusions and fluid therapy. Chelation therapy with the use of calcium EDTA also should be implemented.

Ethylene Glycol

Ethylene glycol is one of the most common causes of poisonings in companion animals. It can be found in antifreeze used for automobile radiators, color film–processing solutions, and other heat exchange fluids. The most common form ingested is drained radiator solution from automobiles. Animals like the sweet taste. The minimal lethal dose of the undiluted product for the cat is 1.5 ml/kg. The minimal lethal dose of undiluted product for the dog is 6.6 ml/kg. Ethylene glycol is converted in the liver into several metabolites that cause severe metabolic acidosis and acute renal failure.

The most common clinical signs observed within 12 hours after ingestion include CNS depression (the animal may appear intoxicated), vomiting, ataxia, lethargy, polydipsia, polyuria, seizures, coma, and death. Tachypnea and tachycardia may be observed 12 to 24 hours after ingestion. Severe lethargy, vomiting, diarrhea, oliguria, isosthenuria, azotemia, uremia, and death usually are observed 12 to 24 hours after ingestion.

Diagnosis begins with the history and presentation of clinical signs. An increase in serum osmolality, hypocalcemia, a high ion gap, and metabolic acidosis are considered a strong indication of ethylene glycol poisoning.

Ethylene Glycol Poison Test (a.k.a Antifreeze Poison Test) is a one step 8 minute test, available to veterinarians that will test for the presence of ethylene glycol poisoning in both cats and dogs. Kacey in Asheville, NC (828-258-1482) is the company that manufactures this test.

Calcium oxalate monohydrate crystals can be observed on a urinalysis but cannot confirm ethylene glycol poisoning unless clinical signs exist. This type of crystal also can be found in the urine of normal dogs and cats. More commonly, these crystals are seen in dogs that have been poisoned with ethylene glycol than in cats.

Treatment includes inducing emesis and administering adsorbents if ingestion occurred within 3 hours of presentation. Sodium bicarbonate may be necessary to correct metabolic acidosis, and fluid therapy will be needed for diuresis and maintaining hydration. Ethanol and 4-methylpyrazole are used to inhibit ethylene glycol metabolism and prevent or reduce the effects of the renal phase.

A limited study showed that 4-methylpyrazole is effective in preventing renal failure in cats. Researchers used 125 mg/kg IV at 1, 2, 3 hours after ethylene glycol ingestion, then 31.25 mg/kg IV 12, 24, and 36 hours after the ingestion with fluid therapy.

The ethanol dose in dogs is 5.5 ml 20% ethanol/kg IV every 4 hours for five treatments, then every 6 hours for four treatments.

The ethanol dose in cats is 5 ml 20% ethanol/kg IV every 6 hours for five treatments, then every 8 hours for four more treatments. The goal is to give enough alcohol to cause CNS depression but not semicoma. Animals treated with ethanol must be monitored closely; it reduces body temperature and can cause death if overdosed.

The 4-methypyrazole dose for dogs is 20 mg/kg IV as a 5% solution for the first dose, then 15 mg/kg at 12 hours, 10 mg/kg at 24 hours, and 5 mg/kg at 36 hours. It has been shown to be more effective in dogs than ethanol and does not cause the negative side effects (as does ethanol therapy).

Peritoneal dialysis may also be necessary and beneficial in removing ethylene glycol and its metabolites from the body, especially if the animal is oliguric or anuric.

Snail Bait

Metaldehyde and methiocarb are two types of snail or slug killers. The baits are very palatable to dogs and cats. Metaldehyde's mechanism of action is unknown; methiocarb is a carbamate and parasympathomimetic. Both cause a rapid onset of severe neurologic symptoms that include hypersalivation, incoordination, muscle fasciculations, hyperesthesia, tachycardia, and seizures. Hyperthermia and severe acidosis also are common, and cats have nystagmus. Bradycardia, respiratory and neurologic depression, and pulse irregularities may be noted in severely affected animals.

Diagnosis is based on the history and presentation of clinical signs. The odor of acetaldehyde (resembles formaldehyde) in the stomach contents may be noted.

The treatment includes inducing emesis and administering adsorbents. Pentobarbital or other muscle relaxants may be necessary to control CNS hyperactivity. Supportive care includes correcting acidosis.

Garbage Toxicity

Garbage toxicity is more common in dogs, and those allowed to roam freely are at greatest risk. Enterotoxemia can occur if the animal ingests decomposed food, carrion, or compost. The small bowel pH may rise above 6, which results in an absence of hydrochloric acid (achlorhydria). Hydrochloric acid promotes normal digestion and prevents multiplication of bacteria. Achlorhydria increases the risk of enterotoxemia. Common enterotoxin-producing bacteria associated with enterotoxicosis include *Streptococcus*, *Salmonella*, and *Bacillus* species.

Clinical signs can begin within minutes to a few hours after ingestion. The signs include anorexia, lethargy, vomiting, diarrhea, ataxia, tremors, and anxiousness. This can progress to endotoxic shock and death. The tremors can be mild to severe.

Diagnosis is based on the history and clinical signs. Treatment includes fluid therapy, broad-spectrum antibiotics, and intestinal protectants. Muscle relaxers or Valium may be necessary to control the tremors. Cordicosteriods should be administered in large doses if endotoxic shock is present.

Insecticides

Pyrethrins and Pyrethroids. Pyrethrins are extracted from the *Chrysanthemum cineriaefolium* and other related plant species. They are commonly used in pet sprays, dips, shampoos, dusts, foggers, premise sprays, and yard and kennel sprays to control flea and tick infestation in dogs and cats.

Pyrethroids are synthetic compounds that vary significantly in structure and potency. They are most commonly found in pet sprays, dips, foggers, premise sprays, and yard and kennel sprays.

If these products are used according to the instructions on the labels, then toxicity is uncommon. When they are used frequently in heavy applications or used on sensitive animals (more common in cats than dogs) or when an ingestion occurs, toxicity can result.

Common clinical signs include hypersalivation, vomiting, diarrhea, tremors, hyperexcitability, or lethargy in the early phase of the toxicity. Clinical signs can progress to dyspnea, tremors, and seizures.

Diagnosis is based on the history and clinical signs. Treatment includes bathing the animal in a mild soap for topical exposures. Inducing vomiting and administering activated charcoal and cathartics is recommended for ingestion. Diazepam (0.5 to 1 mg/kg IV, 5 to 10 mg to effect) may be necessary to control mild tremors but is ineffective for severe neuromuscular activity. Atropine (0.02 to 0.04 mg/kg IM or SQ) can be used to control hypersalivation and bradycardia.

Methocarbamol, a skeletal muscle relaxant, is very effective in controlling tremors at 55 to 220 mg/kg IV. One third to one half of the dose is administered as a bolus IV until the desired relaxation occurs, then the remainder is given to effect; injections can be repeated not exceeding 330 mg/kg in 24 hours.

Organophosphates. Organophosphates and carbamate insecticides inhibit cholinesterase activity. This interferes with autonomic nervous system function. These insecticides are highly fat-soluble and are well absorbed from the skin and GI tract. Carbamates are found in dusts, sprays, shampoos, and flea and tick collars. Organophosphates are commonly found in dips, pet sprays, dusts, yard and kennel sprays, premise sprays, and systemics. Toxicity usually occurs after one of these preparations have been applied to the animal's skin or if the animal has licked the preparation off during grooming. Cats, animals who have been previously exposed to an anticholinesterase insecticide, and animals who are malnourished are more susceptible to this toxicity.

Clinical signs of carbamate and organophosphate poisoning may include excessive salivating, vomiting, diarrhea, muscle twitching to fasciculations, and miosis. Signs can progress to seizures, coma, respiratory depression, and death. Diagnosis is based on the history and clinical signs. The response to a dose of atropine (0.2 mg/kg) also supports the diagnosis.

Treatment of this toxicity includes washing the animal in a mild detergent if a topical exposure has occurred and administering activated charcoal if ingestion has occurred. Atropine also is recommended to control the muscarinic signs at a dose rate of 0.2 to 0.4 mg/kg, half IV and half IM or SQ. This dose can be repeated; however, caution must be taken not to induce an atropine intoxication, signs of which include tachycardia, ataxia, and lethargy. Pralidoxime chloride is recommended for organophosphate poisoning; it reactivates cholinesterase that has been inhibited. The dose is 20 mg/kg IM twice a day for several days or until clinical signs of the toxicity are no longer observed. Exposure to another anticholinesterase insecticide should be avoided until 4 to 6 weeks after recovery.

Plant Toxicity

Plant ingestion is most common in confined animals and juvenile animals. Most toxicity occurs with the ornamental plants that are kept indoors. The severity of toxicity is very dependent on the type of plant, the part of the plant, and the amount that has been ingested. A sample of the plant assumed to have been ingested by the animal should be identified by its scientific name if possible. Many ornamental plants contain different types of toxins, which can cause different clinical signs with varying degrees of severity. Many references can be accessed for this information. A local greenhouse, florist, or garden store may be able to assist in the identification if necessary.

The most common plants ingested by companion animals are from the Araceae family (i.e., dumb cane and split-leaf philodendron). These plants contain calcium oxalate crystals and histamine releasers. Common clinical signs include hypersalivation, oral mucosal edema, and local pruritus. More severe signs may be observed if a large amount of the plant has been ingested and can include vomiting, dysphagia, dyspnea, abdominal pain, vocalization, hemorrhage, gastritis, and enteritis.

The oral cavity should be rinsed with milk or water to remove the calcium oxalate crystals, and GI decontamination and supportive care may be necessary. The prognosis for this toxicity usually is very favorable.

Another type of ornamental commonly used for landscaping known to cause more severe toxicity in dogs and cats is the grayanotoxin-containing plants. The family *Ericaceae* contains the commonly known plants *Rhododendron* (rhododendron, azalea), *Kalmia* (lambkill, mountain laurel, bog laurel), and *Pieris* (Japanese pieres).

Clinical signs occur within 2 to 6 hours after ingestion and can include vomiting, diarrhea, abdominal pain, CNS depression, weakness, dyspnea, tachypnea, hypotension, and pulmonary edema. Animals who have ingested these plants often are found dead. Occasionally, seizures are observed before death.

Treatment includes inducing emesis (if not contraindicated), activated charcoal administration, gastric lavage, and supportive care.

Conclusion

Animals are exposed to many toxins each day. This chapter covers a few of the most common toxicities observed in veterinary practice. Many good reference materials focus on specific toxins, signs commonly observed, and treatments; these texts should be available in every practice.

Poison control center numbers also should be posted. The ASPCA National Animal Poison Control Center is a 24-hour service staffed by veterinarians and board-certified veterinary toxicologists. They can provide updated information on many species-specific responses to poisons and treatment protocols. For more information, call 1-888-426-4435 (a fee is charged for these calls).

Veterinary technicians must educate owners during routine visits about the dangers of potential toxicity. The animals at greatest risk are juveniles and those allowed to roam without supervision. Preventive information can be provided through handouts or newsletters.

Suggested Readings

Aronson L, Drobatz K: Acetaminophen toxicosis in 17 cats, *J Vet Emerg Crit Care* 6(2):65, 1996.

Bailey EM, Garland T: Toxicologic emergencies. In Murtaugh R, Kaplan P: *Veterinary emergency and critical care medicine*, St Louis, 1992, Mosby.

Beasley VR, Dorman DC: Management of toxicosis. In Beasley VR: *Veterinary Clinics of North America. Small animal practice: toxicology of suspected pesticides, drugs and chemicals,* Philadelphia, 1990, WB Saunders.

Dibartola S: *Fluid therapy in small animal practice,* Philadelphia, 1992, WB Saunders.

Dorman DC: Anticoagulant, colecalciferol and bromethalin based rodenticides. In Beasley VR: *Veterinary Clinics of North America: small animal practice (toxicology),* Philadelphia, 1995, WB Saunders.

Dorman DC: Diagnosing and treating toxicosis in dogs and cats, *Vet Med* 92(3):171, 1997.

Firth A: Treatment of snail bait toxicity in dogs: literary review, *J Vet Emerg Crit Care* 2(1):25, 1992.

Forrester SD: Diseases of the kidney and ureter. In Leib M, Monroe W: *Practical small animal internal medicine,* Philadelphia, 1997, WB Saunders.

Garland T, Bailey M: Toxic ornamental and garden plants. In Bongara JD, Kirk RB: *Kirk's current veterinary therapy,* ed 12, Philadelphia, 1995, WB Saunders.

Gfeller RW, Messonier SP: *Small animal toxicology and poisonings,* ed 2, St Louis, 2004, Mosby.

Hansen S: Management of adverse reactions to pyrethrin and pyrethroid insecticides. In Bongara JD, Kirk RB: *Kirk's current veterinary therapy,* ed 12, Philadelphia, 1995, WB Saunders.

Knight M, Dorman D: Selected poisonous plant concerns in small animals, *Vet Med* 92(3):260, 1997.

Kore A: Over-the-counter analgesic drug toxicosis in small animals, *Vet Med* 92(2):158, 1997.

Monroe W: Diseases of the parathyroid gland. In Leib M, Monroe W: *Practical small animal internal medicine,* Philadelphia, 1997, WB Saunders.

Murphy M: *A field guide to common animal poisons,* Ames, Iowa, 1996, Iowa State University Press.

Murphy M: Toxin exposures in dogs and cats: pesticides and biotoxins, *J Am Vet Med Assoc* 205(3):414, 1994.

Nicholson S: Toxicology. In Ettinger S, Feldman E: *Textbook of internal medicine,* Philadelphia, 1995, WB Saunders.

Oliver J, Lorenz M, Kornegay J: Systemic and multifocal signs. In *Handbook of veterinary neurology,* Philadelphia, 1997, WB Saunders.

Owens JG, Dorman DC: Common household hazards for small animals, *Vet Med* 92(2):140, 1997.

Owens J, Dorman D: Drug poisoning in small animals, *Vet Med* 92(2):149, 1997.

Plumlee KH: *Clinical veterinary toxicology,* St Louis, 2004, Mosby.

Talcott PA, Dorman DC: Pesticide exposures in companion animals, *Vet Med* 92(2):167, 1997.

Thrall MA et al: Ethylene glycol. In Peterson ME, Talcott PA, editors: *Small animal toxicology,* Philadelphia, 2001, WB Saunders.

Wanamaker BP, Pettes CL: *Applied pharmacology for the veterinary technician,* ed 3, St Louis, 2004, WB Saunders.

25

Avian and Exotic Emergencies

EDWARD L. SPINDEL, TANYA JACKSON

Exotic species are becoming increasingly popular as companion animals. Owners frequently form strong emotional bonds with these pets and will go to great lengths to treat them. Exotic species provide an exciting challenge in emergency medicine, because the clinical syndromes they have are often unique to each species.

The following overview discusses exotic animal emergencies commonly encountered by the general practitioner and veterinary technician. This chapter is a compilation of selections from the literature and notes from the authors' personal experiences. Sections include common avian, rabbit, rodent, ferret, and reptile emergencies. Techniques, including restraint and venipuncture, are followed by diagnostic and treatment methods. Each section concludes with a chart of basic emergency drugs and drug doses.

Avian Emergencies

Supplies

- Avian mouth speculum (or paper clips and hemostat)
- 25-gauge and 27-gauge needles
- Intraosseous (IO) catheters (22-gauge 1½-inch and 20-gauge 2½-inch spinal needles) (If the previous sizes are not available, then a 25-gauge 1½-inch needle can be inserted as a stylet inside a 20-gauge 1-inch needle.)
- Microtainer blood tubes
- Incubator cage (heated)
- Oxygen (O_2) cage
- Nebulizer
- Feeding tubes, assorted sizes (approximately 8 French, parakeet; 14 French, African grey; 16 to 18 French, large macaw).
- Emeraid or exact hand-feeding mixture
- Basic emergency drugs (Tables 25-1 and 25-3).

TABLE 25-1

Avian Physiologic Facts

Life span	Budgerigar 10-16 yr	Cockatiel 15-20 yr	African grey 45-50 yr	Large Macaw (blue and gold) 70-75 yr
Average adult weight	30 g	90 g	500 g	1000 g
Age at sexual maturity	6-9 mo	6-12 mo	4-6 yr	5-7 yr

Techniques

Restraint. The key to good avian restraint is to accomplish procedures as quickly and easily as possible to reduce stress on the patient. Many birds are well trained and will step up to their owners when out of the cage. The bird can then be taken from the owner. If it becomes necessary to remove a bird from its cage, perform the following:

- Take out all perches and bowls that can be easily removed.
- Place the cage in a closed, dimly lit room if any chance exists that the bird may escape.
- Use a paper towel for small birds such as budgerigars and towels for larger birds.
- Slowly enter the cage, and attempt to immobilize the head first.
- Bring the bird out of the cage, gently but firmly keeping control of the head and gaining control of the wings with the other hand.

Note: To hand off a bird to another staff member, one should allow the other person to gain control of the head by placing the thumb under the mandible and elevating the head; then the other hand should be used to gain control of the wings (Fig. 25-1).

Venipuncture. The jugular vein is the authors' preferred site for blood collection. The jugular vein is largest on the right side of the neck and is located in a featherless tract in the right jugular groove. The cutaneous ulnar vein, more useful in larger species, crosses a featherless tract at the ventral surface of the elbow joint. This site tends to bleed longer after blood collection and is a fragile area where any compromise results in significant damage to surrounding tissues. The medial metatarsal vein (useful primarily in birds such as pheasants, ducks, chickens, and geese) crosses the medial surface of the leg just above the tarsal (hock) joint. At all the previously mentioned sites, and especially at the ulnar vein site, applying pressure immediately after blood draw is necessary because hematomas will quickly form (because of the thin skin and muscle covering the vein).

All materials should be ready before beginning so that the procedure is quick and stress is minimized. One should restrain the bird as shown in Fig. 25-1. The technician holds the bird, feet facing the technician and head toward the doctor (or vice versa, depending on who is drawing). The technician's right hand restrains the bird's feet and wings, in a towel if necessary, holding the head with the left hand. The doctor (or technician, if drawing) takes the bird's head with his or her left hand (thumb under the neck, holding firmly so as not to be bitten), and the bird's jugular vein is occluded near the thoracic inlet with the left thumb. The crop is mobile in this area and can be positioned so that the vein is superficial. The doctor draws the blood with his or her right hand (Fig. 25-2).

Immediately after withdrawing the needle, the thumb moves up to hold off the vein and the bird is held in an upright position until clotting occurs.

Key Point: It is safe to draw up to 1% of the bird's body weight in grams. For example, in a 450 g Amazon parrot, it is safe to draw about 4.5 ml (450 × .01), although this volume is rarely necessary (Table 25-2).

Tube Feeding. Tube (or gavage) feeding is used only if the bird needs supplemental feeding and will not eat on its own. The decision to tube feed a critically ill avian patient must be weighed against the potential stress of the tube-feeding procedure. Subcutaneous (SQ) administration of 5% dextrose may be a better choice in some cases.

Key Point: In avian medicine, *less* is often *best*.

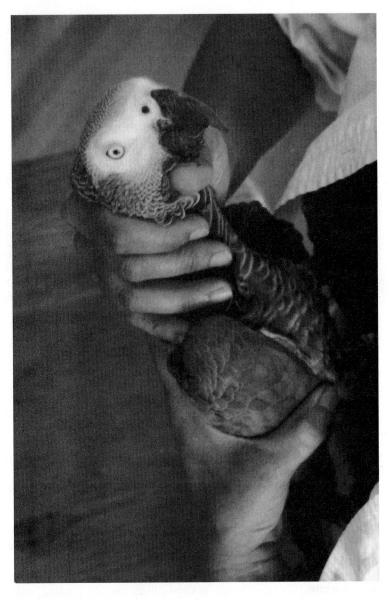

Fig. 25-1 Proper avian restraint.

Products such as Emeraid (Lafeber), Exact (Kaytee), or homemade formulas can be tube fed. The clinician should mix the formula to remove lumps so that the solution will pass easily through the tube; then it should be warmed to baby bottle temperature. Formulas fed too hot can result in serious crop burns.

Key Point: Approximately 5% of the bird's body weight (in grams) can be fed at one time. For example, a 30 g budgerigar can be fed 1.5 ml; a 100 g cockatiel can be fed 5 to 6 ml. Because individual requirements may vary, one should always pay close attention during the procedure.

A feeding tube size should be chosen that will minimize the chance of tracheal intubation. For example, an 8-French red rubber feeding tube works well for a parakeet or Quaker parrot; a 14 French for an African grey; and a 16 to 18 French for a large macaw.

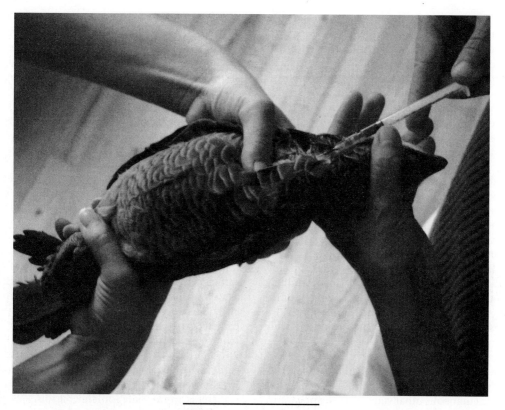

Fig. 25-2 Avian venipuncture.

TABLE 25-2

Useful Facts for Common Avian Medical Procedures

Procedure/Therapy	Guidelines
Amount of blood safely drawn (ml)	1% of body weight in grams
Volume of fluid bolus given IV or IO (ml)	1% of body weight in grams
Daily fluid volume (maintenance)	40-50 ml/kg/day
Amount of each tube feeding (ml) (approximate)	5% of body weight in grams (Weigh daily to ensure that the caloric density is being met)
Amount of food/day (ml)	Previously mentioned amount fed twice to three times a day (bid-tid)

The bird's mouth should be carefully opened with the feeding tube, with a speculum (an opened paper clip works well in smaller birds), or with a loop of gauze. The clinician should locate and avoid the glottis, which opens on the base of the tongue. The esophagus opens caudal to the glottis and to the right of the trachea. The tip of the feeding tube should be lubed and the red rubber or rigid avian feeding tube passed over the roof of the mouth and gently from the right side of the bird's mouth into the crop. Palpate the feeding tube and the trachea as two distinct tubes in the bird's neck to ensure proper placement of the feeding tube. The tube can also be seen and felt in the crop area when moved in and out at the mouth. The formula should be fed slowly and the oral cavity watched. If the formula backs up in the mouth, then the clinician should stop, kink and remove the tube, and release the bird so that it can cough out the excess. The more swiftly this is done, the more likely the bird will clear any formula from the airway. The patient should be fed two to three times daily.

Fluid Administration. The decision to administer fluids and the route chosen depend on the condition of the patient and the degree of dehydration. IV fluids can be supplied to birds in shock or to those suffering significant blood or fluid loss. SQ fluids may be administered to moderately dehydrated patients. A fairly large volume may be give SQ, and the slow absorption rate makes cardiac overload unlikely. Oral fluid supplementation alone is reserved for the noncritical patient but is the preferred route if the patient is able to stand, swallow, and is in the condition to metabolize food.

Assessment of Dehydration. Calculate the degree of dehydration by examining skin fold elasticity, volume of the cutaneous ulnar vein, and the appearance of the eyes. Minor loss of skin elasticity indicates approximately 5% dehydration. A definitely noticeable loss of skin elasticity, along with dry mucous membranes and a dry appearance to the eyes, indicates about 7% to 10% dehydration. When the skin fails to move back when tented, the mucous membranes are tacky, the extremities are cool and possibly muddy in color, and the eyes appear sunken, dehydration has reached 10% to 12%.

Key Point: Fluid volume should always be estimated conservatively. Volume overload is a frequent complication when fluids are administered too rapidly. The patient can always be reevaluated in 1 or 2 hours, and more fluids administered at that time if necessary.

Catheter Placement. IO catheters are generally the most useful type of catheters in avian patients. IO catheters can be placed in the proximal or distal ulna, as well as the proximal tibiotarsus. The authors' preferred site is the proximal ulna, which allows the bulky catheter cap to rest over the bird's back rather than being exposed at the distal ulna (i.e., carpal joint) (Figs. 25-3 and 25-4). Spinal needles can be used as IO catheters. A 22-gauge 1½-inch catheter is appropriate for Quakers and cockatiels, and a 20-gauge 2½-inch catheter is appropriate for large parrots.

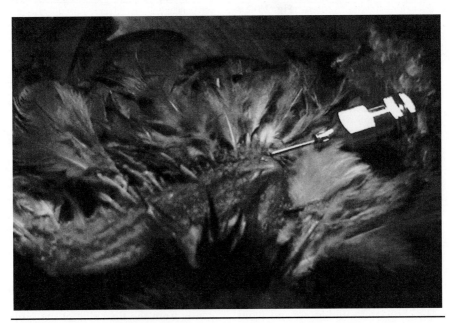

Fig. 25-3 IO catheter placement in the ulna. The reader should note placement in the proximal versus distal ulna.

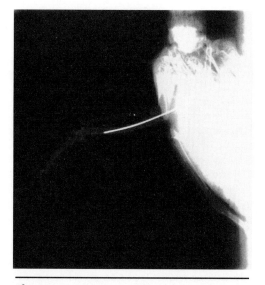

Fig. 25-4 Radiograph of the IO catheter in Fig. 25-3.

BOX 25-1

Technical Tip: Suggested Intravenous and Intraosseous Bolus Volumes

- Budgerigar, 1-2 ml
- Cockatiel, 1-2 ml
- Cockatoo, 12 ml
- African grey/Amazon, 8-10 ml
- Large Macaw, 15-25 ml (Olsen, Orosz)

BOX 25-2

Technical Tip: Avian Daily Fluid Requirement Calculation

- Total amount of fluids to be administered/day = daily maintenance + one-half fluid deficit
- Daily maintenance = 40-50 ml/kg/day
- Fluid deficit (ml) = body weight (grams) × percent dehydration

    For example, a 500 g African grey is 10% dehydrated:

    Maintenance = 50 ml/kg × 0.5 kg = 25 ml
    Fluid deficit = 500 × 0.10 = 50 ml
    Administer one half of fluid deficit = 25 ml
    Total volume to be administered on day 1 = 50 ml

IV catheters are rarely used except in moribund patients. They are far more difficult to manage in avian patients than are IO catheters.

Key Point: Never place an IO catheter in the avian humerus or femur. The humerus and often the femur (depending on the species) are pneumatic bones with direct communication to the air sacs. Fluid administration into a pneumatic bone can result in the drowning of an avian patient.

Disadvantages of IO catheters include risk of bone contamination and difficulty maintaining the catheter. However, IO catheters do offer quick placement and excellent fluid absorption.

Key Point: An initial IV or IO fluid bolus of (1% of the body weight in grams) may safely be given to a critical avian patient. For example, a 100 g cockatiel is given the following:

1% × 100 g = 1 cc (Technical Tip Box 25-1)

Key Point: SQ fluids may be given at 2% of body weight in grams per dose. Locations for SQ fluid administration include the wing web, the thigh web, and the skin over the spine. The air sac extension that may be just caudal to the thoracic inlet should be avoided.

Fluids may be supplied primarily by tube feeding in the noncritical patient. If the patient is being fed a slurried diet, then the clinic may provide approximately 100% of the fluid requirement by the oral (PO) route (Technical Tip Box 25-2).

The volume of fluid administered can generally be decreased as the hydration approaches normal and especially as the bird begins eating and drinking on its own.

Types of fluids commonly used include lactated Ringer's (for shock or dehydration), normal saline (for shock or hypercalcemia), and hypertonic saline (for hypovolemic shock or sepsis). Solutions of 5% dextrose provide energy for birds that have been off feed for 24 hours.

Anesthesia. Isoflurane or sevoflurane are the anesthetic gases of choice for avian patients. Very small birds may need to be maintained via masks, which can be fashioned from plastic syringe cases. Larger birds can be intubated, allowing for assisted ventilation if necessary.

To intubate open the mouth with gauze loops or a mouth speculum, and visualize the glottis at the base of the tongue. A noncuffed endotracheal tube should be placed gently into the trachea and rolled gauze put in the bird's mouth to keep it from biting off the end of the endotracheal tube. The tube should be taped in place.

It is important to monitor avian patients carefully during induction and maintenance of anesthesia. Keeping the avian patient on the lightest possible plane of anesthesia is necessary, because attempts at resuscitation are usually futile. Useful monitoring parameters include movement in response to stimuli, positive palpebral and corneal reflexes, jaw tone, rate and depth of respiration, and heart rate. Electrocardiograph monitors are useful in examining trends during anesthesia. Signs of arrest include pupillary dilation and feather erection.

Discussion

Blood Feathers. As new feathers grow in, they contain a vascular shaft that regresses as the feather matures. If this new pin or blood feather breaks along the vascular shaft, then a significant amount of blood can be lost; however, bleeding is rarely sufficient enough to cause death (Fig. 25-5). The bleeding feather should be grasped with a hemostat and pulled out in the direction of the feather follicle to reduce the chance of skin laceration. If some bleeding occurs after the feather is pulled, then pressure can be applied to the area until the bleeding stops.

Avian Dystocia and Egg Binding. Egg binding is a very common avian emergency, especially in small birds (e.g., Quakers, lovebirds, cockatiels, finches). Clinical signs include depression (e.g., puffed bird on the bottom of the cage), straining (often with obvious tail bob), dyspnea, and occasionally paresis of the pelvic limbs.

Diagnosis is often possible by palpation of the cloacal area, which may reveal a firm, rounded mass (egg) distending the area. Radiography often reveals one (and sometimes two) obvious calcified eggs within the abdomen.

Treatment depends on condition of the patient and size and position of the egg. Initially, attempts are made to deliver the egg medically. The patient should be treated with fluid therapy, high humidity (e.g., steam vaporizer, moist towels in 90° F

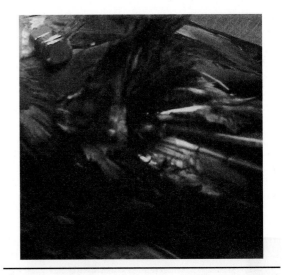

Fig. 25-5 Blood feather. The reader should note the blood-filled feather shaft, which has been broken at its base.

incubator), and lubrication of the cloacal area. Calcium may be administered if indicated.

If the egg is not delivered within a few hours, or if the patient's condition begins to deteriorate at any time, then the bird should be masked with isoflurane or sevoflurane and attempt to deliver the egg manually. Plenty of lube should be placed in the cloacal area around the egg; gentle, firm manual pressure placed behind the egg may be sufficient to expel it from the cloaca. Because these eggs are often abnormal in shape, size, and shell thickness, they may break during manipulation. Remove as much of the shell and contents as possible and return the bird to an incubator.

Egg-bound birds can become critical very quickly, and surgical intervention may become necessary to remove the egg to prevent shock and death. If surgery is undertaken, then anesthesia must be very carefully monitored and the patient kept at the lightest plane possible.

Toxins. Some of the most common toxins in caged birds include toxic gases, heavy metals, and toxic plants. The main key to treating toxicities in birds is to *stabilize them first*. Many toxic patients arrive at the clinic in a critical state and should be stabilized with heat, O_2, and fluids as indicated. Because no antidote exists for most of the common toxins, the patient must be treated symptomatically and with supportive care.

Ingested Toxins. *Chocolate.* The ingestion of even a small amount of chocolate can cause toxic effects. Chocolate contains theophylline and caffeine, which can induce hyperexcitability, cardiac arrhythmias, seizures, vomiting, diarrhea, and death. Treatment of chocolate toxicity includes supportive care and crop gavages with activated charcoal to delay continued absorption of the toxin. Cathartics such as Epsom salts (magnesium sulfate, 1 g/kg PO) or Metamucil (psyllium hydrophilic mucilloid) can be mixed with the charcoal to aid in removal of the toxins from the lower gastrointestinal (GI) tract.

Avocados and Other Plants. Although the toxicity of the avocado is still controversial, certain varities of avocados do appear to have varying toxic potential. Simply avoiding them altogether is wise. Avocado toxicity has been described in budgerigars and canaries, with clinical signs including anorexia, fluffed feathers, respiratory dyspnea, and death. Postmortem findings often include pulmonary congestion. Treatment is primarily supportive, but activated charcoal and use of a diuretic may be indicated.

Other plants known to have toxic potential in birds include the poinsettia, rhododendron, yew, clematis, dieffenbachia, and parsley. Although studies in budgerigars have shown these and other plants to have toxic potential, wide individual and species variation to plant toxicity exist. The most common clinical signs in plant toxicoses include lethargy, diarrhea, and regurgitation.

Treatment is primarily supportive, including activated charcoal or fluid therapy if indicated.

Mycotoxins. Moldy foods such as seeds, pelleted foods, and millet can be potential sources of mycotoxin toxicity. Treatment is symptomatic, but this toxicity can be severe and even acutely fatal.

Alcoholic Beverages. Because of such small body size, consumption of relatively small amounts of alcohol can lead to ataxia and death in avians. Treatment is supportive and symptomatic, including activated charcoal gavage.

Nicotine Ingestion. Ingestion of nicotine from chewing on cigarettes or cigarette butts can result in signs ranging from depression and cyanosis to hyperexcitability, vomiting, diarrhea, seizures, and acute death. Treatment is purely symptomatic.

Heavy Metal Ingestion (Lead and Zinc). The two most common heavy metals causing toxicosis in birds are lead and zinc. Lead may be encountered via ingestion of costume jewelry, solder, batteries, lead-based paints, linoleum, as well as a variety of other sources. In wild birds such as ducks and geese, lead shot is a common incidental finding on radiographs. Ingestion of lead shot is a common cause of clinical lead toxicity in waterfowl.

Signs of lead toxicity may be acute or chronic and include lethargy, depression, anemia, and GI signs (e.g., regurgitation, diarrhea). Neuromuscular weakness may also be present, seen as wing droop, ataxia, and leg paresis. Chronic symptoms include emaciation, blindness, seizures, and death.

Radiography often reveals metallic densities in the GI tract. Blood lead levels greater than 20 µg/dl are suggestive of lead toxicity; levels above 50 µg/dl are diagnostic of lead toxicity.

Treatment includes symptomatic and supportive care such as fluid therapy, assisted feeding, antibiotics, surgical removal of the metallic foreign body if indicated, and chelation therapy. Calcium disodium ethylenediamine tetraacetate or D-penicillamine are the most common chelating agents in use. Calcium disodium ethylenediamine tetraacetate is dosed at 35 mg/kg twice a day (bid) intramuscularly (IM) for 5 days, then off for 3 to 4 days as needed until cessation of clinical signs. D-penicillamine can be administered PO at 55 mg/kg bid for 3 to 6 weeks. Alternatively, calcium disodium ethylenediamine tetraacetate and D-penicillamine can be combined for a few days until clinical signs cease (and D-penicillamine continued for the 3 to 6 weeks). Gavage with a peanut butter slurry may be used to promote passage of heavy metal from the GI tract (and continued daily until objects are gone). The passage of heavy metals should be monitored with radiography.

Zinc may be encountered in galvanized wire and wire clips, in pennies minted after 1982 (96% zinc), and in Monopoly game pieces (98% zinc). Signs of zinc toxicity include polyuria and polydipsia, weight loss, GI symptoms, weakness, anemia, seizures, and death. Treatment is similar to that for lead toxicity (discussed previously).

Inhaled Toxins. Birds have a very unique respiratory system, allowing for two passes of air through the respiratory tract with each respiration. They are therefore highly sensitive to air-borne chemicals, including many household cleaners.

Teflon and other nonstick cookware surfaces, including self-cleaning ovens, when overheated, can release polytetrafluoroethylene gas. Clinical signs of polytetrafluoroethylene toxicity range from depression, weakness, wheezing, and dyspnea to seizures and death. The first line of treatment is fresh air (in an O_2 cage, if possible). Stress and excitement should be avoided. Steroids, antibiotics, diuretics for pulmonary edema, and supportive care may also be helpful.

Key Point: Any odor (e.g., gasoline, fuel oil, kerosene, paint) detected by a client is potentially harmful to a bird. Therefore the bird should be removed from the premises immediately and good ventilation ensured.

Respiratory Emergencies. Avian respiratory emergencies are some of the most difficult to treat, because patients often arrive at the clinic in such a fragile state. In addition, diagnosis can be difficult because a wide range of conditions can result in respiratory signs.

The first step to take with a dyspneic bird is to assess whether the patient is near agonal in its respiratory state. Because manipulation of these patients may result in death, they should immediately be placed in an incubator cage with O_2. After 15 to 30 minutes, assess the possibility of examining the bird. By this time the bird's respiratory rate should have decreased, and its skin color should reflect improved oxygenation of blood. Any bird in severe respiratory distress should be handled with extreme care. The added stress of a simple examination can result in such a patient dying in their hands. Therefore he or she should attempt to stabilize the patient first, preferably in a quiet, dark O_2 cage at 90° F.

Differentials for upper respiratory signs include granulomas; vitamin-A deficiency; bacterial, viral, and fungal infections; foreign bodies; and neoplasia.

Lower respiratory signs can be the result of all of the previously mentioned causes, as well as immune-mediated diseases, infections, abdominal effusion, abdominal masses, and a variety of other conditions.

If the initial assessment indicates that the patient can withstand a brief examination then take the following four steps:

1. Check the oral cavity for any masses, foreign bodies, or other obstructions (e.g., fungal plaques, granulomas).
2. Auscult the chest for crackles or wheezes. Auscultation can often best be accomplished in small birds with the unaided ear, listening over the bird's back. Larger birds (e.g., greys, Amazons) can be auscultated with a stethoscope over the back and on each side of the chest.
3. If necessary, cannulate the patient by introducing an IV catheter into the caudal air sac. The area caudal to the last rib should be prepared and the catheter gently introduced just through the very thin skin and musculature into the air sac. Positive pressure ventilation at 15 mm Hg or simply turning on the O_2 flow can aid in oxygenation.
4. Deliver medications directly to the compromised respiratory tract via nebulization when indicated. When appropriate, this approach results in the most rapid improvement in respiratory signs (Table 25-3).

Ferret Emergencies

Supplies

- 24-gauge ¾-inch IV catheters
- Fluid pump or buretrol
- Syringe-case anesthesia masks (Tables 25-4 and 25-5)

Techniques

Restraint. Most pet ferrets are very tractable and can easily be examined with minimal restraint. For ferrets with a tendency to bite or wiggle, a firm hold on the scruff gives good control and stimulates the relaxation reflex. For SC injections and other procedures, ferrets can be scruffed with one hand and injected with the other hand. The stretch technique, or scruffing with one hand and extending the rear legs with the other hand, is also a useful immobilization technique.

Venipuncture. The jugular and cephalic veins are the most useful sites for venipuncture in the ferret. For jugular venipuncture the ferret should be restrained as one would restrain a cat (with head elevated and legs pulled straight down over the edge of the table). A 22-gauge needle and 3-ml syringe are usually appropriate. Cephalic veins are useful for catheter placement but offer a very limited amount of blood for collection (e.g., for a blood glucose measurement). The ferret should be restrained the same for cephalic venipuncture as one would restrain a cat—scruffing the ferret with one hand and holding off the cephalic vein with the opposite thumb.

TABLE 25-3

Basic Avian Emergency Drugs

Daily fluid requirement	40-50 ml/kg/day
Bolus IV fluid volume	1% of body weight in grams
Tube feeding ml/feeding	5% of body weight in grams
Baytril	Cockatiel: 5-10 mg/kg orally (PO) twice a day (bid) Grey: 15-30 mg/kg PO bid
Gentamicin/nystatin	Crop infections: Gentocin (100 mg/ml) 0.1 ml/100 g PO bid with Nystatin oral suspension 100,000 U/ml; (Alpharma) 0.03 cc/10 g PO once a day to three times a day (sid-tid)
Sulfamethoxazole with trimethoprim	50 mg/kg PO bid (oral suspension, cherry flavor); 200 mg/40 mg per 5 ml (Hi-Tech; Pharmacal)
Nebulizing medications	Gentocin 1 ml/tylosin 1 ml/saline 1 ml in nebulizer cup (also can add dexamethasone as needed); nebulize for 15-20 min tid

TABLE 25-4

Ferret Physiologic Facts

Rectal temperature	100°-104° F (<103° F is average)
Heart rate	180-250 beats per minute
Average adult weight	750 g
Life span	5-8 yr

Catheter Placement. Key Point: The cephalic vein is most commonly used for placing indwelling IV catheters in ferrets. A 24-gauge ¾-inch catheter works well for most ferrets, and animal should be restrained as for cephalic venipuncture.

Ferrets are notorious for removing catheters, so adequate taping is essential. A T-port should be attached to the catheter, taped with a butterfly, and then taped around the leg. The turned up IV line should be included in another round of tape and the entire catheter wrapped in Vet-Wrap (leaving the port exposed). Close monitoring is important to prevent the ferret from becoming tangled in or kinking the IV line.

IO catheterization and fluid administration is an option (often the sole option) in shock conditions.

IO catheters can be placed in the proximal femur in ferrets (as placed in a kitten).

Fluid Therapy. Always calculate required daily fluids, then administer them. The daily maintenance fluid requirement for ferrets is thought to be approximately 30 to 40 ml/lb/day plus loss. The IV or IO route is preferred for very sick or dehydrated ferrets. Ferrets can be easily overhydrated because of their small body size. A fluid regulator or Buretrol device (Baxter Health) aids in preventing too rapid an administration of calculated fluids. When using a Buretrol, the total daily fluid volume can be divided into two (or optimally three) slow bolus doses. Types of IV fluids used in ferrets are similar to those used in dogs and cats.

SC fluids can be administered in the loose dorsal scapular skin. Two or three SC boluses can be given to meet daily fluid requirements.

Urethral Catheterization. Urethral obstruction in ferrets may arise from adrenal disease causing secondary prostatomegaly or from urethral calculi. Although relatively uncommon, urethral obstruction is a definite medical emergency. Urethral catheterization in male ferrets can be challenging because of the small size of the urethral opening and the hooked shape of the os penis. If passage of a urinary catheter in a blocked

TABLE 25-5

Common Ferret Medical Procedures

Amount of blood safely drawn	0.5% of body weight in grams (e.g., can withdraw 5 ml in 1 kg ferret) Usually need 1.5-2.0 ml for full blood work
Amount to syringe feed per feeding	Offer Nutri-Cal frequently Syringe Purina CV or Hill's a/d at ≈10 ml/kg three times a day (tid) Monitor weight daily to evaluate whether caloric demand is being met Adjust as indicated by weight gain or loss Calculate caloric requirement and necessary amount of selected food to meet requirement
Daily fluid requirement	30-40 ml/lb/day plus loss

ferret is not possible, then cystocentesis or emergency cystotomy may be performed with attempts to flush the urethra normograde from the bladder.

Discussion

Adrenal disease and insulinoma are the two most common diseases seen in ferrets in the United States. Other common problems include foreign bodies, *Helicobacter mustelae* infection, and coronaviral diarrhea (i.e., green slime disease).

Adrenal Disease. Adrenal disease is a chronic syndrome. Ferrets will frequently arrive at the emergency department with adrenal disease caused by secondary complications (including prostatomegaly) that result in urethral obstruction, weakness, anorexia, and dehydration.

A large percentage of ferrets over the age of 3 years will develop adrenal disease, most commonly in the form of benign adrenal hyperplasia and adrenal adenoma. Adrenal neoplasia occurs less commonly (approximately 15% are carcinomas). Symptoms of adrenal disease usually begin with alopecia at the tip of the tail, which progresses to symmetrical truncal alopecia. Intense pruritus may accompany or precede the alopecia.

A ferret with adrenal disease showing signs of debilitation should first be stabilized symptomatically. Treat with fluids, antibiotics, and/or syringe feeding if necessary. Diets such as Hill's a/d, Purina CV, or meat-based baby foods can be offered or syringe fed.

Adrenalectomy is the authors' treatment of choice for ferrets less than 5 years of age. In ferrets over 5 to 6 years of age, Leuprolide (Depot Lupron TAP)

can be administered at 100 µg/kg IM monthly until remission of clinical signs. Injections are repeated as needed (in response to the return of clinical signs). Repeating injections every 3 to 6 months is usually required. Lupron does not affect or reduce adrenal tumor size and is a palliative treatment for clinical signs of adrenal disease.

Insulinoma. Insulinomas are extremely common in ferrets over 3 to 4 years old. The classic presentation is a weak, lethargic ferret, occasionally ataxic, drooling, or in hypoglycemic seizures. Attempt to document the hypoglycemia with a blood glucose level. The normal blood glucose in ferrets is greater than 80 mg/dl. Blood glucose below this is an indicator of possible insulinoma; blood glucose less than 60 mg/dl is diagnostic. Ferrets who are weak, salivating, or both often have glucose levels of 20 to 40 mg/dl.

Emergency treatment of a hypoglycemic episode involves rubbing Karo or other high-sucrose syrup on the ferret's gums. Diluting Karo syrup 50:50 with tap water eases administration. For ferrets that do not respond or are in status epilepticus, administer 50% dextrose as a slow IV bolus until the ferret responds. IV fluids and corticosteroids at shock doses (Dex SP 4 to 8 mg/kg IM, IV) can be added for prolonged seizure activity or moribund, unresponsive ferrets.

Once the ferret is responsive, try to initiate frequent meals of high-protein ferret food. Prednisolone syrup or 1 mg prednisone tablets can be administered at 0.5 mg/kg, gradually increasing to 2 mg/kg as needed to control clinical signs. Surgical debulking of medically uncontrollable hypoglycemia secondary to insulinoma is very rewarding. Adding diazoxide may assist long-term maintenance.

TABLE 25-6

Basic Ferret Drugs and Doses

Drug	Dose
Prednisolone syrup (15 mg/5ml) (Hi-Tech, Pharmacal)	0.5 mg/kg orally (PO) twice a day (bid)
Amoxicillin	10-20 mg/kg PO bid
Amoxicillin with interferon	Mix 0.15 cc interferon with 10.85 ml water to equal 11 ml; add to 15 ml bottle of Amoxidrops and dose as previously mentioned
Sucralfate	Carafate suspension 1 g/10 ml (Aventis) 0.5 ml PO bid
Bismuth subsalicylate (Pepto Bismol)	0.25 ml/kg PO q4-6h
Metronidazole	15-20 mg/kg PO bid
Lupron	100 µg/kg intramuscularly (IM) q4wk until remission of signs
Clavamox	12.5 mg/kg PO bid

Helicobacter Mustelae **Gastritis and Enteritis.** Clinical illness occurs in stressed young ferrets 12 to 20 weeks of age and in older ferrets exposed to newly acquired carriers that are shedding. History invariably supports this exposure.

Clinical signs include lethargy, anorexia, weight loss, and diarrhea (often with dark, tarry stools) (melena). Histopathologic lesions of clinical *H. mustelae* infection include mucous depletion, a leukocytic infiltrate in the gastric wall, gastric ulceration, and hemorrhagic gastric erosions.

Definitive diagnosis is possible by fecal culture, or polymerase chain reaction of combined oral, stomach, and rectal swabs.

Treatment has traditionally involved triple therapy with amoxicillin, metronidazole, and bismuth subsalicylate. However, a newer enrofloxicin and bismuth subcitrate (Omeprazole) combination may be more successful at clearing the organism.

Hydration and colonic issues should always be addressed with appropriate calculated supportive care.

Coronaviral Diarrhea Syndrome. Veterinarians treating ferrets have long known of a typical diarrhea syndrome of ferrets commonly known as *green slime disease*. Recently this syndrome has been connected with a coronaviral infection in ferrets. Clinical signs include diarrhea that becomes green and mucoid (turning to melena in severe cases), anorexia, weakness, dehydration, and emaciation. Treatment is purely supportive, with fluid therapy and feeding of slurried food via syringe if necessary. IV catheter placement and administration of IV fluids via fluid regulator or buretrol is optimal. SQ fluids may be substituted if vasoconstriction makes catheter placement impossible, but this method is less effective. Antibiotics such as amoxicillin (the authors add interferon), Baytril, or metronidazole appear to expedite recovery. Syringe feeding of easily digestible foods such as Purina EN may also be necessary until the ferret is eating on its own.

Foreign Bodies. Ferrets are famous for their curiosity, which includes the desire to play with and taste new objects. Rubber objects (e.g., pencil erasers and toys) are often favorite materials to chew.

Clinical signs of foreign body ingestion include anorexia, lethargy, weakness, and diarrhea. If the owner reports regurgitation, vomiting, or both, then a foreign body should be highly suspect. Foreign bodies in the small intestine may be palpable, with localized pain or discomfort on palpation. Diagnosis is based on history, clinical signs, and radiography.

Treatment is usually surgical. An IV catheter is placed and the patient stabilized before surgery. Surgery should be performed as soon as possible, because these patients can become quickly debilitated. Most ferrets recover rapidly after foreign body removal and are able to eat on their own within 24 hours of surgery (Table 25-6).

Rabbit and Rodent Emergencies

Supplies

- IO catheters (22-gauge 1½-inch spinal needles *or* a 25-gauge 1½-inch needle used as a stylet inside a 20-gauge 1-inch needle).
- IV catheters (24-gauge ¾-inch *or* 22-gauge 1-inch needle)
- Otoscope cone dedicated for oral examination use
- Blender for preparation of syringe feeding slurry (Tables 25-7 and 25-8)

Techniques

Restraint. Rabbits are built for springing with their hind legs and will often attempt to do so during restraint. The handler should always support a rabbit's back and rear legs during restraint or transport, because the act of kicking off without a firm surface to push against can result in spinal fractures.

TABLE 25-7

Rabbit Physiologic Facts

Rectal temperature	101.3°-104.0° F
Heart rate	130 to 325 beats per minute
Respiratory rate	30-60 breaths per minute
Adult weight	2-5 kg (Species-dependent)
Life span	5-6 yr (up to 15 yr) (Species-dependent)
Age of sexual maturation	4-10 mo (Species-dependent)
Gestational length	29-35 days

TABLE 25-8

Common Rabbit Medical Procedures

Syringe feeding in ml/lb	2-3 ml/lb fed 2-3 times daily
Maintenance fluid requirement	60-100 ml/kg/day

Covering the rabbit's eyes and face with one hand can both calm the rabbit and prevent it from jumping forward during a physical examination. For transport, the rabbit's front legs may be supported and held with one hand, with a finger between the feet and its hindquarters tucked under the elbow while the other hand supports the rear legs. Alternatively, the rabbit can be placed in a football hold, with the head tucked under one elbow and the rabbit's scruff held with the other hand. To examine the belly or for sexing, the rabbit can be cradled on its back like a baby in the technician's arm, with one hand supporting the rear legs.

Venipuncture. Several sites are available for venipuncture in rabbits. The jugular veins yield the largest volume, but the cephalic and saphenous veins are also useful. Jugular venipuncture can be accomplished by holding the rabbit with head elevated and legs pulled over the edge of the table, similar to positioning for feline jugular venipuncture. The medial saphenous vein can be accessed by restraining the rabbit in later recumbency and holding off the vein above the hock.

Catheter Placement. IV catheters are most easily placed and stabilized in the cephalic vein. In most rabbits a 24-gauge ¾-inch or 22-gauge 1-inch over-the needle catheter can be used. The catheter should be taped and secured in place as one would for a feline catheter.

IO catheters can be placed in rabbits when shock or severe dehydration makes peripheral catheterization difficult. The greater trochanter of the femur is easily accessible for IO catheterization. A 22-gauge 1½-inch spinal needle can be used (if this size is not available, then a 25-gauge 1½-inch needle placed as a stylet inside a 20-gauge 1-inch needle can be used). The technician should clip and prepare the area, and insert the needle with a clockwise twisting motion. The device should be capped with a male-end catheter cap and secured with tissue glue if necessary. The long bones of rabbits are fragile and prone to shattering; therefore IO catheters should be placed with care. Ear veins should be avoided, because a high chance for thrombosis, necrosis, and sloughing of ear tissue exists. Stabilizing the catheter comfortably is difficult.

Anesthesia can safely and effectively be accomplished by premedication with Torbugesic at 0.1 to 0.5 mg/kg IV, followed by mask induction with either isoflurane or sevoflurane.

Discussion

Hairballs and Gastric Stasis.
One of the most common presentations in pet rabbits is the anorexic rabbit who has not defecated in several days. Very often, this history is indicative of gastric stasis, or hairball syndrome. If this syndrome is caught early, then the rabbit is generally bright and alert and physical examination is fairly normal. However, once this syndrome has progressed, the rabbit may become severely dehydrated, lethargic, and weak.

Some causes of gastric stasis include inappropriate fiber in the diet (Timothy hay), hairballs in the stomach (sometimes secondary to low fiber), and GI infections.

Treatment involves rehydration, improving gastric motility, and syringe feeding until feces become normal and the patient is eating well on its own. Pineapple juice blended with rabbit pellets is thought to be beneficial for improving gastric motility (and potentially for beneficially decreasing the gastric pH). The rabbit should be syringe fed at approximately 2 ml/lb two to three times daily. SQ fluids should be given if indicated. Critical patients require IV fluids. Metoclopramide, cisapride, or both may be helpful to increase gastric motility, as long as gastric outflow is not obstructed. Antibiotics (e.g., enrofloxacin, trimethoprim-sulfa) should be given to reduce bacterial overgrowth. Rabbits have poor pain tolerance, so analgesics such as Torbugesic may be very useful for reducing abdominal discomfort.

During recovery, feces will at first be very small, dry, and scant. Over time, feces should increase in size, number, and consistency until normal. The rabbit should be offered fresh greens such as Romaine lettuce, carrots, and Timothy hay to get it eating on its own. Syringe feeding should be continued until the rabbit is eating alfalfa pellets well and feces are completely normal.

Continued deterioration over the first 24 hours of hospitalization is an indication for surgical intervention. Successful recovery from surgery requires committed nursing care for 2 to 12 weeks.

Bacterial Enteritis.
Enterotoxemia (caused by clostridial bacteria) and colibacillosis (caused by pathogenic *Ehrlichia coli*) are the two most common causes of bacterial enteritis in rabbits. Clinical signs of enteritis include soft stool to watery diarrhea containing blood or mucous, sepsis, severe dehydration, and sometimes death. Underlying causes of bacterial overgrowth include stress, lack of adequate fiber in the diet, or antibiotic therapy resulting in changes in gut flora. In mild cases of enteritis, simply eliminating all treats and adding hay to increase dietary fiber may correct the problem. Diagnosis of bacterial enteritis in rabbits is based on clinical signs and fecal culture.

Treatment should be started while fecal cultures are pending. The patient should be treated empirically with enrofloxacin or metronidazole. In mild cases of enteritis, eliminating all treats and adding hay to increase dietary fiber may correct the problem. In cases of clostridial overgrowth, treatment consists of aggressive fluid therapy IV or IO if necessary, coupled with efforts to normalize gut flora and decrease numbers of pathogenic bacteria. Antibiotic therapy in such cases may only add to the decrease in numbers of normal bacterial flora. Metronidazole has been found to be helpful at 20 mg/kg q12h. Clearance of pathogenic bacteria may be aided by the addition of metoclopramide or cisapride, as well as a high-fiber diet.

Colibacillosis, on the other hand, should be treated with appropriate antibiotics based on culture and sensitivity results. Most *Ehrlichia coli* strains are sensitive to enrofloxacin or trimethoprim-sulfa. The clinic staff should be aggressive with fluid therapy and administer a high-fiber diet via syringe feeding if necessary. These syndromes should be treated until the rabbit is eating well on its own and producing normal feces.

Cystic Calculi and Cystitis.
Cystic calculi are relatively common in rabbits and guinea pigs. Clinical signs include depression, weight loss, stranguria, hematuria, hunched stance, and depression. Discreet calculi may be palpable in the bladder. Radiography is useful to identify calculi that may be cystic, urethral, ureteral, or renal in location.

Key Point: When performing radiography of the rabbit's bladder, do not confuse calcium sediment (radiodense sand) with cystic calculi. Calculi will appear as discreet, radiodense stones (Figs. 25-6 and 25-7).

Key Point: Normal urinalysis in the rabbit may be characterized by calcium oxalate crystalluria and sometimes a pink or orange discoloration of the urine. A dipstick can be used to differentiate hematuria from normal pigment coloration.

Hematuria usually indicates the presence of cystic calculi. Rabbits with either calcium sludge or calcium carbonate calculi usually have excessive dietary calcium intake.

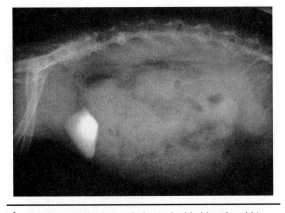

Fig. 25-6 Normal calcium sludge in the bladder of a rabbit, not to be confused with a true cystic calculus, as seen in Fig. 25-7.

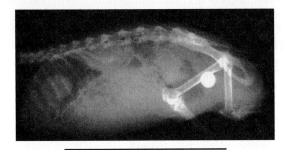

Fig. 25-7 Guinea pig cystic calculus.

Cystitis (rare) should be treated with a 2- to 3-week course of antibiotic therapy. Trimethoprim-sulfa is usually effective.

Treatment of cystic calculi may be possible by retropulsion via repeated flushing of the bladder with saline. Usually treatment is surgical. The patient should be stabilized as indicated with IV fluids and antibiotics before cystotomy (and the calculi submitted for quantitative analysis).

Respiratory Infections and *Pasteurella.* Upper and lower respiratory infections are very common in rabbits. *Pasteurella multocida* infection, commonly known as *snuffles*, is the most common causative agent in upper respiratory disease of rabbits. Other causative agents of upper respiratory disease include *Moraxella* and *Bordetella bronchiseptica.*

Clinical signs of pasteurellosis in rabbits include rhinitis and sinusitis, with nasal exudates and often excessive tearing from the eyes (i.e., epiphora), as well as conjunctivitis and often a snuffling or snoring sound audible during respiration. Sequelae of *Pasteurella* infection include otitis (when infection has spread from the nares to the middle ear), erosion of the nasal turbinates, and hematogenous spread resulting in bacteremia, fever, and acute death. *Pasteurella* pneumonia, pleuritis, and pericarditis are also possible sequelae of chronic infection.

Definitive diagnosis is by culture; however, the organism may be difficult to grow, and several culture attempts may be necessary. Treatment is based on long-term antibiotic therapy of typically 45 days or longer because of the invasive nature of the disease. Antibiotics generally effective against *Pasteurella* infection include enrofloxacin (5 to 10 mg/kg PO q12h) and chloramphenicol (50 mg/kg PO q12h). Antiobiotics should be started immediately and therapy adjusted based on the results of culture and sensitivity. The patient should be treated supportively with fluids and syringe feeding as indicated.

Dental Disease. Every anorexic rabbit should receive a thorough dental examination. The incisor teeth and cheek teeth should be examined for overgrowth and resulting malocclusion. Overgrowth of incisor teeth is very common in rabbits; even when overgrowth is corrected, recurrence is likely. Owners may elect to have incisors extracted in cases in which frequent trimming is necessary.

Overgrown incisors can be trimmed with small wire nippers or dental instruments. A Dremel is useful for filing the edges. Cheek teeth can be examined with a dedicated otoscope head. The cheek teeth should be flat on the occlusal surface, without obvious raised ridges on either the lingual or buccal surfaces. Malocclusion of cheek teeth is common, with obvious deviation of the overgrown teeth either medially or laterally. Anesthesia may be required to evaluate these teeth and is necessary when trimming the overgrown cheek teeth. In severe cases of malocclusion, incisors may penetrate soft tissues around the jaw, and molars may overgrow to penetrate and cause abscesses in the maxillary or mandibular bone or surrounding soft tissue. These severe cases usually require surgical extraction and aggressive supportive care, including fluid and antibiotic therapy.

Abscesses. Any fluctuant or firm growth on a rabbit is an abscess until proven otherwise. Pus in rabbits is solid, white, and caseous, and abscesses must be surgically excised with clean margins. When excision is not possible, such as with foot or facial abscesses, the area should be well débrided and kept open until

TABLE 25-9

Rabbit and Rodent Drugs and Doses

Drug	Dose
Sulfamethoxazole	Rabbit: 15 mg/kg orally (PO) twice a day (bid) Guinea pig, chinchilla: 15 mg/kg PO
Baytril	Rabbit: 5-20 mg/kg PO bid Rodent: 2.5-5.0 mg/kg PO bid
Metoclopramide	0.2-0.4 mg/kg PO three times a day (tid)
Cisapride	0.5 mg/kg PO q8-24 hrs
Nebulizing meds: Gentocin, tylosin, saline (Dex)	Place 1 cc of each medication as needed in nebulizer cup
Fresh pineapple juice	Mix with blenderized pellets for syringe feeding
Torbugesic (Butorphanol tartrate)	0.05-0.4 mg/kg SQ or IM q 8-12 hrs PRN

healed. Marsupialization is the surgical procedure of choice to permit long-term flushing of the abscess pocket. Recurrence of abscesses is not uncommon.

Common pathogens causing rabbit abscesses include *Pseudomonas multocida*, *P. aeruginosa*, and *Staphylococcus* species. Good empiric antibiotic choices include enrofloxacin and trimethoprim-sulfa. Choice of antibiotics is optimally based on culture and sensitivity.

Uterine Adenocarcinoma. Uterine adenocarcinoma is very common in unspayed rabbits over 4 years of age. In the authors' practice, attempt to explain this risk to rabbit owners and advise spaying at 4-5 months of age. The most common clinical sign of uterine adenocarcinoma noted by owners is hematuria, or frank blood at the end of urination. Other clinical signs include depression, anorexia, and dehydration. Metastasis to the lungs, liver, or bone may occur within the first year of the disease (or later).

Ovariohysterectomy is the treatment of choice. The rabbit should be stabilized with IV or IO fluids and antibiotics before surgery if possible. Prognosis is good if metastasis has not yet occurred (Table 25-9).

Reptile Emergencies

Supplies

- Spinal needles, for use as IO catheters (20-gauge 2½-inch needles for adult iguanas)
- Red rubber feeding tubes (various sizes)
- Incubator cage
- Prepared reptile foods or alfalfa pellets for syringe feeding
- Blender (Tables 25-10 and 25-11)

Techniques

Restraint. When working with lizards, the technician should move slowly and ascertain the amount of restraint necessary. Many domestic lizards are very tame and will require minimal restraint, which will put the owner at ease.

The head and tail ends of large lizards must be simultaneously restrained to prevent bites and whiplash from the tail. The head should be held with one hand firmly just caudal to the mandible, while surrounding both the hind legs and the tail with the other hand. To examine the oral cavity, the technician should hold the maxilla with one hand while pulling down gently but firmly on the dewlap with the other. Care must be taken to prevent being bitten; all human bites should be treated as serious events.

Venipuncture. The ventral abdominal vein and the ventral tail vein are the most accessible sites for venipuncture in lizards. For tail venipuncture, the lizard can be gently restrained, standing normally with the tail extended over the edge of the table. (Iguanas restrained in lateral or dorsal recumbency will invariably struggle and thrash.) The needle should be introduced midventrally near the base of the tail and advanced until the flash of blood is seen. If bone is

TABLE 25-10

Reptile Physiologic Facts

Approximate adult weights	Green iguana, 3 kg Bearded dragon, 500 g Jackson's chameleon (male), 40 g
Life span	Green iguana, 12 yr Bearded dragon, 10 yr Jackson's chameleon, 8 yr
Sexual maturity (first clutch) (approximate)	Green iguana, 3-4 yr Bearded dragon, 1-2 yr Jackson's chameleon, 1 yr
Gestation and incubation lengths	Green iguana, ≈73 days Bearded dragon, ≈60 days Jackson's chameleon, 90-180 days
Preferred environmental temperature (varies with species)	Approx. 85° F
Environmental humidity	Approx. 70% (varies dramatically species to species)

TABLE 25-11

Common Reptile Medical Procedures

Amount to syringe feed per feeding	25-30 ml/kg orally (PO) Weigh daily to assess need for adjustments
Bolus amount of IV or IO fluids	1% of body weight per gram
Daily maintenance fluid volume	40-50 ml/kg/day

hit, the clinician should slowly back out the needle while aspirating until the flash of blood is seen. For ventral abdominal venipuncture, the lizard should be restrained in dorsal recumbency and the needle introduced about one third of the way up from the vent, midventrally at a 10-degree angle. The needle should be popped through the skin and thin abdominal musculature while aspirating for the flash of blood.

Catheters. IO catheters are relatively simple to place and very effective for fluid therapy in lizards. The femur is most often used and can be approached either from the greater trochanter or from the distal femur at the stifle joint. The authors typically prefer advancing the catheter from the stifle, up through the intercondylar area of the femur, with the leg flexed 90% at the stifle. A 20-gauge 2½-inch spinal needle is optimal for an adult green iguana. Alternatively, a 25-gauge 1½-inch needle can be used as a stylet within the lumen of a 20-gauge 1-inch needle. The stifle is scrubbed and the needle aseptically introduced and advanced up the marrow cavity with a clockwise twisting motion. The needle is first aligned with the femoral shaft; once inside the marrow cavity, the needle can be drawn caudally to account for the caudal curvature of the femoral shaft. Once in place, the stylet is withdrawn and the catheter flushed with 0.6% saline (i.e., reptilian saline). The IO catheter will usually not need to be additionally secured to remain in place. A light wrap can be placed to prevent the catheter from being bumped or bent.

Alternative catheter sites include the ventral abdominal and cephalic veins, but cutdowns are usually necessary to access these veins. These veins also tend to be fragile, necessitating careful securing with tissue glue, tape, and suture to prevent kinking or damaging the vein.

Fluid Therapy. Fluids can be administered to reptiles by slow bolus via IO catheters or by SQ injection. Reptiles have a normal serum salinity of 0.6%, versus the normal 0.9% salinity of mammalian serum. The authors therefore routinely dilute the normal saline to 0.6% for reptile administration. Mammalian saline solutions may benefit the lizard in shock because of their hypertonic nature in reptiles.

Bolused fluids can be administered at approximately 1% of the animal's body weight in grams. Several daily boluses should be administered to meet the maintenance plus rehydration daily fluid requirement.

Tube Feeding. Tube feeding is relatively simple in lizards and can be readily taught to most clients when necessary. Approximate feeding tube sizes include 8-French Bard infant feeding tubes for very small juveniles, 14-French red rubber feeding tubes for medium-sized juveniles, and 18-French red rubber feeding tubes for adults. A mouth speculum can be fashioned from a syringe case by cutting off the narrow end. The feeding tube is marked buy measuring from the lizard's nose to the last rib. The feeding tube is prefilled with the desired food to account for dead space. The tube is lubricated and passed gently over the glottis (located at the base of the tongue) and down the esophagus to the premarked site.

The slurry should be administered slowly. If food starts to back up into the oral cavity, then stop administration, withdraw the tube, and put the reptile down immediately to permit its adjustment to material in the oral cavity. Be sure to feed the animal the correct amount (generally 20 to 30 ml/kg) of Emeraid or, when the patient is able to handle it physically, a mixture of Emeraid and slurried reptile food.

Injections. SQ injections can be administered by tenting the skin in the dorsal scapular or femoral areas. IM injections should be administered in the front legs to prevent the concentrated exposure of the kidneys to any potentially nephrotoxic compound.

Anesthesia. Anesthesia can be difficult in lizards because of their ability to breath-hold, especially when confronted with noxious substances such as anesthetic gas. Masking with isoflurane or sevoflurane is adequate for most procedures. Intubation can be accomplished in the larger lizards. The tube can be taped around the lizard's head. Ketamine injection can be used safely alone or in combination with inhalants.

Discussion

Metabolic Bone Disease. Metabolic bone disease (MBD) is a common problem seen in reptiles in most practices. Common causes include low calcium diets, a negative dietary calcium/phosphorous ratio in the diet, and possibly lack of appropriate exposure to ultraviolet light. Ultraviolet light is also important for appetite stimulation. In adult reptiles other causes of MBD include egg production, renal disease, and septicemia. Affected adults are usually hypocalcemic, with total serum calcium levels less than 8.0 mg/dl.

Clinical signs of classic MBD include weakness, anorexia, fibrous osteodystrophy (often with laterally bowed mandibles), and osteomalacia (rubber jaw). Pathologic fractures and folding fractures of weakened bone are common (Fig. 25-8). Limbs and extremities may be swollen. Hypocalcemic lizards may exhibit weakness, muscle twitching, or seizure activity.

Diagnosis is by history, clinical signs, and radiography if possible. Radiography often reveals a generalized loss of bone density, poor contrast between bone and soft tissue, and the presence of folding fractures or pathologic fractures of the vertebrae, long bones, or both. Plasma calcium and phosphorus levels are also useful, especially when measuring response to treatment. In early stages, reptiles may be normocalcemic; however, in the later stages of MBD many reptiles will be hypocalcemic, with elevated serum phosphorus levels.

Treatment of MBD initially involves force-feeding a balanced diet, administration of calcium, and providing an ultraviolet light source. If the patient is anorectic, tube feed a slurried, easily digestible food such as Emeraid II or blended iguana food, supplied at approximately 15 to 25 ml/kg PO. Feeding should begin at a low volume and increase as the patient is able to handle and digest larger volumes. Calcium glubionate (Neo-Calglucon, Sandoz; Calcionate Syrup, Rugby) should be administered at 10 mg/kg (or 1 ml/kg) PO once a day (sid) to bid until the patient is eating well on its own. For critical patients, IO catheter placement with administration of balanced fluids may be necessary. Severe cases should receive calcium at 100 mg/kg IO or IM until tremors,

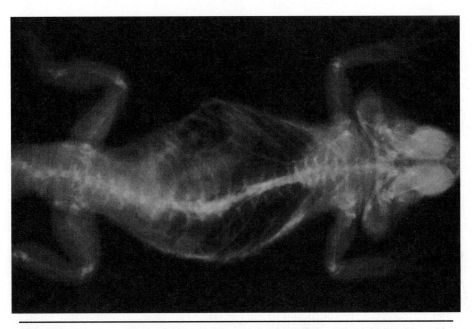

Fig. 25-8 Severe metabolic bone disease (MBD) in a bearded dragon. The reader should note the presence of both the pathologic and the folding fractures, as well as the generalized lack of bone density. This beardie was unable to raise off the cage floor.

seizures, or both resolve. Calcium delivered PO or IV may be substituted when signs have resolved. Rep-Cal can also be sprinkled on the food. Vitamin D_3 can be administered at 1000 IU/kg IM q7d for two treatments to permit calcium absorption from the GI tract.

Prognosis depends on severity of the case and willingness of the owner to treat the patient at home (often for prolonged periods). Without treatment, patients with MBD will invariably die. Severe cases may not respond well to treatment. If caught early enough and treated aggressively, however, then MBD can be successfully treated.

Reptile Dystocia and Egg Binding. A very gravid lizard will often go off feed and therefore needs to be on an adequate plane of nutrition, including adequate calcium intake, prior to laying her clutch. Appropriate environmental conditions also need to be met, with an ambient temperature of approximately 85° F and provision of an appropriate nesting area. The nest box should be large enough for the lizard to enter and turn around in and contain moist sand at least 2 inches deep. If any of the previously mentioned conditions are not met, then

the lizard may become egg-bound (i.e., unable to lay her eggs).

Hypocalcemia may precede and be an underlying cause of egg binding, or the egg-bound condition itself can result in a hypocalcemic state. The typical egg-bound lizard initially arrives at the clinic anorectic and lethargic. In the later stages, egg-bound lizards may demonstrate profound weakness, dehydration, muscular twitching, and sometimes overt seizures due to hypocalcemia.

Diagnosis is based on history, clinical signs, and usually radiography. Although chelonians have eggs that appear similar to avian eggs on a radiograph, lizards have soft-shelled eggs with almost soft tissue density (Fig. 25-9).

Critical patients should first receive medical treatment. Start with providing an appropriate environment, warm-water soaks, rehydration, and calcium supplementation. Critical or very ill patients will likely require surgical salpingectomy. The patient should be stabilized before surgery with SQ or IO fluids, warmth, and calcium supplementation.

Abscesses. Lizards form caseous abscesses that often appear as firm, raised swellings. These abscesses

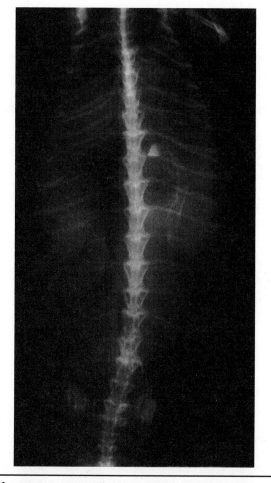

Fig. 25-9 Egg-bound iguana. The reader should note the soft tissue density of the intraabdominal eggs.

are usually traumatic in origin and can be found anywhere on the body, most commonly on the face.

Treatment consists of aggressive surgical excision of the abscess, followed by copious flushing with antibacterial solution such as chlorhexidine (Nolvasan). The abscess should be left open to heal by second intention. In the authors' experience, even widely extensive areas of excision and débridement (up to half a reptile's face in some instances) have healed and granulated in with little evidence of previous infection.

Otitis media and otitis externa is common in aquatic turtles. A large, elliptic incision through the tympanic membrane is required to gain access to the

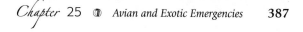

TABLE 25-12

Basic Reptile Drugs and Doses

Drug	Dose
Amikacin	5 mg/kg intramuscularly (IM) first dose, then 2.5 mg/kg q72h IM
Baytril	5-10 mg/kg q24h orally (PO), IM, or subcutaneously (SC)
Sulfamethoxazole	30 mg/kg once a day (sid)
Calcium	Calcionate Syrup (Rugby) 1.8 g/5 ml Give 1 ml/kg PO twice a day (bid) Neo-Calglucon (Calcium glubionate, Sandoz) Give 100 mg/kg IM, SC

caseous plug. Aggressive flushing and removal of debris is necessary for resolution of symptoms.

Optimally, antibiotic therapy should be based on culture and sensitivity results. Some of the more common bacterial pathogens isolated from reptile abscesses include *Pseudomonas*, *Pasteurella*, and other gram-negative aerobe species, as well as many species of anaerobes. Amikacin and Baytril are good choices for empiric treatment until culture and sensitivity results can be obtained (Table 25-12).

Foreign Bodies. Foreign body ingestion is not uncommon in lizards who are allowed to roam freely around the home. Wood chips and other indigestible bedding material can also cause potential GI blockage. The authors have removed a variety of foreign items from lizards, ranging from rocks and other bedding material to metal items and even a man's cotton athletic sock.

Foreign bodies should be on the "rule out list" for any anorectic lizard. Anorexia and lack of fecal production may be the only clinical signs of blockage early in the condition. Progressive dehydration, emaciation, and profound weakness will develop in later stages.

Radiography is often diagnostic; treatment of obstructive foreign bodies is surgical. IO catheterization for fluid support is advisable in more advanced cases. Antibiotics such as amikacin may be indicated in cases in which abdominal contamination from GI leakage is suspected.

Renal Failure. Renal failure in reptiles mimics the clinical picture of MBD. Symptoms include dehydration, lethargy, anorexia, and often secondary osteomalacia. Diagnosis is possible with radiography and evaluation of blood calcium, phosphorus, and uric acid. On radiographs, the renal silhouette will often be enlarged and radiodense, and dystrophic mineralization of tissues may be visualized.

Treatment includes IO fluids, supplementation of calcium if loss has occurred, and oral phosphate binders if hyperphosphatemia is present.

Suggested Readings

Carpenter JW et al: *Exotic animal formulary*, ed 2, St Louis, 2001, WB Saunders.

Mader DR: *Reptile medicine and surgery*, St Louis, 2006, WB Saunders.

Olsen GH, Orosz SE: *Manual of avian medicine*, St Louis, 2000, Mosby.

Quesenberry KE, Carpenter JW: *Ferrets, rabbits, and rodents: clinical medicine and surgery*, ed 2, St Louis, 2004, WB Saunders.

Ritchie BW et al: *Avian medicine: principals and application*, Lake Worth, FL, 1994, Wingers Publishing.

26

Disaster Medicine

AMY N. BRETON

Introduction

Disaster medicine has been a topic in veterinary medicine for the past 25 years. However, after the terrorist attacks in the United States on September 11, 2001 (often referred to as *9/11*), disaster medicine was a topic that was pushed to the forefront. Before that event, most of veterinary disaster medicine was focused on natural disasters. The veterinary community trained and planned for what to do in the event of a hurricane, tornado, flood, or earthquake. After 9/11, the focus shifted to how the industry should deal with artificially created disasters. but Hurricane Katrina showed the veterinary community what horrific devastation can occur from a natural disaster. The PETS Act was signed into law by President Bush on October 6, 2006. The PETS Act requires local and state emergency preparedness authorities to include in their evacuation plans how they will accommodate household pets and service animals in case of a disaster. Local and state authorities must submit these plans in order to qualify for grants from the Federal Emergency Management Agency (FEMA).

Fifty-six percent of Americans own a pet; therefore when a disaster strikes, animals usually are involved. Today veterinarians and technicians are considered first responders (Fig. 26-1, *A-C*). The recent years' disasters have shown that veterinary professionals are not prepared for the animals in their communities.

Disaster medicine can appear vastly different from the medicine that veterinary professionals practice every day. Even during the busiest times, such as when working in an emergency department, some control of the situation is possible. During a disaster, the situation can quickly become out of control at any moment. Technicians should understand what types of disasters they might experience and how to handle different disaster situations. In addition, all veterinary hospitals should have an established disaster plan. Being prepared before a disaster helps prevent the veterinary hospital from becoming a victim during a disaster.

Disaster medicine is vastly different from other disciplines of veterinary medicine. A disaster occurs when community resources become overwhelmed, causing the inability to function normally. This type of situation is unpredictable, whether it is artificially or naturally created.

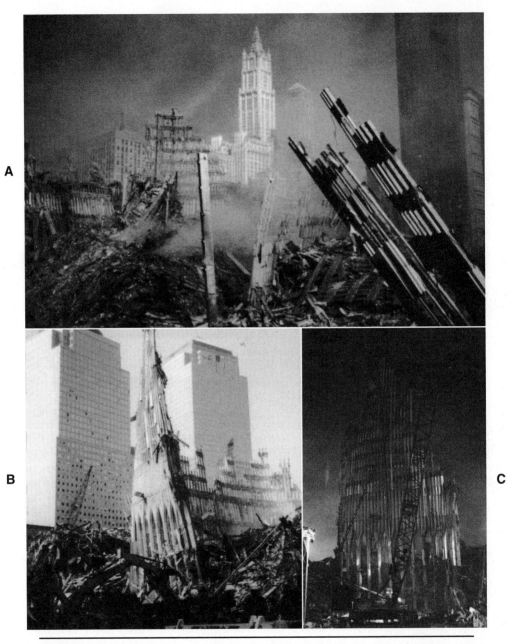

Fig. 26-1 A-C, Scenes from New York City World Trade Center after the terrorist attack of September 11, 2001.

Artificially created disasters include terrorism events, fires, and hazardous material spills. Examples of natural disasters include fires, hurricanes, tornados, tsunamis, earthquakes, and droughts.

Working as a technician during a disaster is vastly different from working as a technician in a clinic setting. Stress, working conditions, types and numbers of animals involved, and the legal issues of working during a disaster all contribute to making it a unique and challenging situation.

Stress is a common feature in the daily life of an emergency critical care veterinary technician. Multiple traumas, fast-paced environment, and rarely taking breaks are all considered routine, and the stress experienced is multifaceted. Most technicians who become involved in a disaster situation reside near or in the town where the disaster has occurred. The local veterinary hospital may be the only functioning veterinary hospital in town; therefore the amount of responsibility for those who work at the hospital can become enormous during a disaster, and the clinic may become overwhelmed with people and their pets. Individuals assisting during the crisis should care for their family members and themselves first—only then will they be able to remain truly focused on the needs of others.

The conditions (Fig. 26-2) encountered during a disaster are different from those found in a regular clinic setting and can contribute to an already stressful situation. Working outdoors, with limited supplies, unfamiliar people, and different organizations is considered common. Mosquitoes, gnats, flies, and other insects may be numerous. Keeping patients clean and dry may be very difficult, and surgery may not be a possibility.

Even the smallest things that were taken for granted may become luxuries. For example, electricity and running water may not be available. A clinic that is affected by a disaster must look at its capabilities in the aftermath of the disaster. Members of the clinic should fully assess what they *can* offer versus what they *cannot* offer to the public. Looking at the entire situation and assessing what would be most beneficial for the clinic and the clients is important.

Locating a fully functioning veterinary hospital (outside of the devastated area) to which clients can be referred is critical. Hospitals that are not fully functioning may be used as boarding facilities. The staff needed for boarding animals is minimal in comparison to a staff needed to medically treat animals and will therefore allow staff members to have more time to deal with personal problems caused by the disaster. Creating an individual and community veterinary hospital disaster plan will help alleviate some of the stress associated with assisting in a artificially created or natural disaster (Box 26-1).

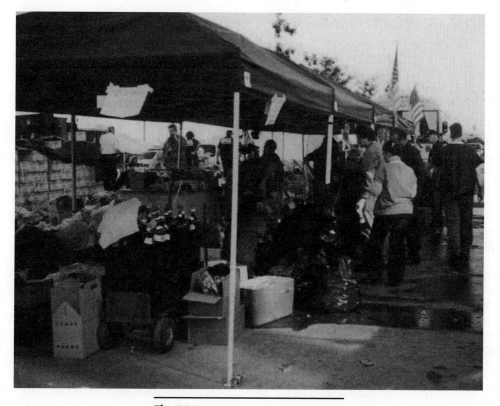

Fig. 26-2 Outside veterinary field hospital.

BOX 26-1

Veterinary Clinic Disaster Plan Details

- Basic responsibilities

Come up with the incident command system (ICS) for the clinic.

Keep current contact information for all employees.

- Information to be kept offsite

Insurance papers

Inventory of everything (with cost)

Written business plan

Copy of computer records (updated and replaced every week)

Pictures of and receipts for items used in the clinic

Pictures of the clinic (interior and exterior)

List of suppliers, contact numbers, and delivery schedule

- Explanation of the clinic's role during a disaster
- Policies created before the disaster

Will the clinic accept wildlife?

Will the clinic accept farm animals?

Will the clinic function as a kennel for strays?

- Charging clients during disasters

Will the clinic work for free, at a discount, or remain closed?

Will the clinic donate goods and services to those in need?

- Establishing a community veterinary disaster plan

Talk to colleagues and get phone numbers.

Develop an agreement before the disaster occurs.

  Decide if profits are shared.

  Decide to use another clinic for a certain percentage of patients.

  Determine what equipment is available for use at other clinics.

  Decide if personnel can be exchanged to help at other clinics.

Find a clinic outside an affected area that may be able to help. If all clinics are down, find out if a larger facility out of the area.

Find an off-site location where clinics can pool resources.

Compile a verbal stockpile system for pharmaceuticals.

Discover if a facility is available for isolating animals.

  Animals with bite wounds (possible rabies)

  Animals with the same disease (if in large numbers)

- Maintaining accurate records of animals seen

  Have a form in duplicate ready to use.

  Take a photograph to document the animal.

  Place identification bands on all animals.

- Supplies for the clinic (to be kept in a secure and separate area)

Generators

Tarps

Rope

Wet-dry vacuum

Leashes

Cardboard cat carriers

Disposable isolation gowns

Disposable medical gloves

Masks

Set of muzzles

Set of wildlife gloves

Caution tape

Orange cones or flags

Polaroid camera and film

Duct tape or other heavy-duty tape

Portable floodlights

Flashlights

- Training for the clinic disaster team

Hazardous materials (two people should take level-one course)

ICS system (two people should take level-one course)

Online training (provided by Federal Emergency Management Agency [FEMA])

On-site training (provided by Humane Society of the United States [HSUS] throughout the year [includes hands-on training])

Have someone become familiar with posttraumatic stress disorder (PTSD), and have contact numbers on hand for organizations that provide help for PTSD.

- Additional considerations

Have everyone become trained on how to triage mass casualties.

  Agree on a triage method.

  Use role-playing techniques.

Have everyone become familiar with the medical forms used during a disaster.

Gather all important contact numbers, including the following:

  Wildlife experts

  PTSD help numbers

  Grief-counseling numbers

  Poison control

  Local/state/federal official numbers

The types of animals needing assistance during a disaster may be numerous. The area veterinary hospitals involved must know their limitations. A protocol should be created for employees to follow. Local farmers, wildlife rehabilitators, park rangers, game wardens, zookeepers, and members from the United States Fish and Wildlife Service can be used as a resource; they can assist in developing the protocols and training the support staff on handling different species.

Legal Issues

Veterinary professionals who help in a disaster must be clear on the legal issues involved in the situation. Injuries to the support staff, animals, and owners must be understood and addressed. The following questions should be asked before a staff member or other person is allowed to participate:

- Do you have health insurance?
- What will happen if you become injured and cannot work?
- Will your job allow you to take time off to help with disaster relief?

Worker's compensation does not apply when someone is injured outside of his or her job. An employer is not required to keep a staff person's position if they volunteer and become injured during a disaster. Addressing these concerns and talking to the employer before accepting a volunteer is important.

Most responders fall under the protection of the Good Samaritan laws. In each state the Good Samaritan laws regarding animals may vary. The clinic staff should know if the state in which they are working has a written Good Samaritan animal law that protects individuals who volunteer to help during a disaster.

The American Animal Hospital Association took a stand regarding veterinarians and technicians when they published their position,

Currently there is no legal duty in North America for veterinarians in private practice to provide emergency care to animals. However, under most circumstances, the American Animal Hospital Association supports the provision of humane or emergency care. To encourage veterinarians and veterinary technicians to assist with emergency veterinary care, the American Animal Hospital Association recommends the adoption of the following Uniform Good Samaritan Law by all states and provinces:
A veterinarian or veterinary technician who, on his or her own initiative or other than at the request of the owner, gives humane or emergency treatment without fee to a sick or injured animal shall not be liable for civil damages as a result of his or her acts or omissions in the absence of gross negligence. The veterinarians may euthanize the animal as a humane act to relieve suffering.
Any licensed veterinarian or veterinary technician who in good faith provides emergency care at the scene of an emergency to the human victim(s) shall not be liable for any civil damages as a result of any acts or omissions by such persons providing the emergency care (http://www.aahanet.org/About_aaha/About_Position.html#samaritan., November 1994).

Types of Disasters

- Terrorism: Search and rescue (S&R) dogs with burned or lacerated feet are common. Smoke or other toxic gas inhalation may cause the dogs to become very sick. Dehydration from overwork and heat is common. Stress diarrhea may also occur. Animals may be trapped inside nearby buildings and arrive at the clinic stressed, dehydrated, and emaciated.
- Foreign animal disease: Veterinarians working with large animals are usually the first to diagnose foreign animal disease. Veterinarians should carry with them a list of whom to contact if a foreign animal disease is suspected. Typically the United States Department of Agriculture is notified immediately. The clinician should research the disease to better explain the illness to owners. He or she should also expect to deal with questions such as, "Can my dog get mad cow disease?" Volunteers from the veterinary community may be needed to help perform physicals on animals or to deal with questions from the general public in a large-scale epidemic.
- Fire: During a wildfire animals often run scared and relocate themselves in yards and barns where they do not belong. House pets may be abandoned and brought in by local rescue groups. Dehydration, stress, and anorexia can be common. The proper authorities such as the United

States Fish and Wildlife Service or local wildlife rehabilitators should ideally handle wildlife. Clients may bring burned or injured birds and squirrels to the veterinary hospital in the area. The clinic should post a list of contact numbers of those individuals equipped to deal with wildlife before the disaster.

- Hurricanes and tornadoes: Wildlife may be relocated to unexpected places. Snakes, spiders, and birds may end up in places that are not desirable. Often times, house pets are abandoned. Dehydration, stress, and anorexia can be common. Clients may be calling with questions on how to get snakes or birds out of their homes. The clinic should have telephone numbers of wildlife removal companies that can deal with such questions.

- Floods: Often house pets are abandoned during floods. Dehydration, stress, anorexia, and near drowning can be common. Pets may end up in towns far away from their homes. Owners may not think to call veterinary hospitals to look for their pets.

Triaging

The term *triage* comes from the French word that means *to sort*. During a disaster, patients must be triaged in a way that will benefit the most animals. Having to triage mass casualties and many different species at once is common.

When triaging animals during a disaster, thinking "outside" of the disaster is important. Several scenarios may give a false sense of the patient's condition. Preexisting illnesses may be present in several patients. Animals may start to acquire new illnesses that are not related to the disaster. For example, the dog that initially arrived at the clinic with a large laceration comes back because of pancreatitis, or the cat that came in for hypothermia develops pyelonephritis. The hospital that is dealing with the animals affected by the disaster should transfer these patients to a hospital that is not affected and able to see patients for nonemergencies. Attempting to function as a "regular" emergency hospital *and* a "disaster" hospital often does not work well for the staff or for the pets. The hospital must choose whether it will accept and treat all animals affected by the disaster or only the recovery and return of regular patients. If the hospital chooses to deal with disaster animals only, then clients should be informed that the hospital's focus is on helping only those animals. Most clients will understand this policy, and their devotion to the clinic will only grow stronger because of the dedication shown by staff members in helping those animals affected by the disaster.

Having an organized approach will help ensure that the most patients possible are triaged appropriately. A method must be designed for dealing with numerous patients at once.

Two methods can be used to efficiently triage during a disaster: (1) START (Simple Triage And Rapid Treatment) and (2) SAVE (Secondary Assessment of Victim Endpoint). Both methods were developed for triaging human casualties during war and disasters. To date, no similar method has been specifically designed for triaging animals; however, both START and SAVE are widely accepted in the veterinary community as efficient triage methods for dealing with nonhuman patients.

START Method

With the START method, each animal is quickly assessed for respiration, alertness, and perfusion status. This is also known as their *RAP status*. Using this system, animals are color-coded and moved to their color-coded areas. Animals should be marked with the appropriate color. Owners can be given cards for their animals, and unowned animals can be marked with identification bands. The date, time, who triaged, initial problem, and color should all be listed. As a base, animals that are walking are considered *green*. These are animals that have minimal injuries and are considered stable enough to wait for medical treatment. Having every staff member in the clinic become familiar with the color-coded system helps decrease confusion if and when disaster strikes. Using the START method, animals can be quickly assessed and brought to appropriate treatment areas to receive the treatment needed. Areas should be set up and staffed to deal with that particular color animal. Animals may need to be reassessed as time passes. Reassessment times should be agreed upon so that animals will not be forgotten. An animal's status may change, and it may be given a different color depending on the current condition (Table 26-1).

TABLE 26-1

Start Color Code System

Color	Type of Injury
Red	Critical—The patient must receive simple life-saving procedures to ensure survival.
Yellow	The patient should survive as long as simple care is given within a few hours.
Green	Minor injuries—The patient can wait for treatment and still survive.
Black	Dead or dying—The patient's injuries are very severe, and the patient is unlikely to survive regardless of the treatment received.

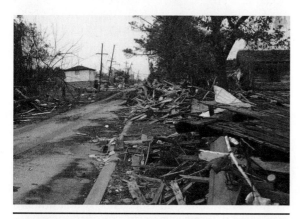

Fig. 26-3 Areas affected by disasters must be considered dangerous areas. Special precautions must be taken.

SAVE Method

The SAVE method is much faster than the START method and works well when resources and personal are limited. It will help to conserve the resources and personal by focusing them on patients who have the best chance of survival. Using the SAVE method, patients are divided into three categories:

1. Those who will die regardless of the treatment
2. Those who will survive regardless if treated or not
3. Those who will benefit if medical intervention occurs immediately

Only those that fall in groups two and three are given care. Group number two is put on "hold" while group number three is treated. After group number three has been dealt with, group number two can be reassessed and treated. Placing an animal in one of the groups is a judgment call and can be difficult at times. Decisions must be made quickly to save the most patients possible.

In one six hour period over 300 animals were triaged by a veterinary staff of ten mainly using the SAVE method during Hurricane Katrina. Veterinarians and technicians were able to complete thorough exams once the selection process was completed.

Owner in the Disaster

Dealing with pet owners can be very stressful during a disaster. Their houses may have been destroyed, family members may be missing or injured, and all of their personal belongings may be gone. Their pets may be all they have left. Stray animals should not be euthanized because the numbers have exceeded resources. All organizations must work together to find the pets home. The pet may be the only hope for the owners for recovery after a disaster. It is also important to avoid judging the owners that left the animal behind. They may not have been aware of how severe the situation was and thought the animal would be safer at home. Government agencies may also be limiting their ability to bring their pets with them in order to expatiate the rescue attempts of humans. Compassion and understanding qualities that one must have if they are going to assist during a disaster (Fig 26-3).

Finding assistance for clients often will be as important as helping their pets. These clients may not be equipped to deal with their pets' conditions, and their decisions may not be rational. Understanding posttraumatic stress disorder (PTSD) will assist everyone in this situation. The clinic should have numbers available for owners of local specialists who deal with PTSD. Grief counseling can also be suggested.

Owners, kennel owners, breeders, zookeepers, and farmers all know how to handle their animals well. In most disasters, *the more hands the better* method holds true. Certainly not every owner can help during a disaster. Many of these owners may be distraught and unable to deal with the situation at hand. Every situation is unique and must be considered on an individual basis.

Self-Protection

Self-protection during a disaster is important. The rate and severity of bites and scratches increases during a disaster. Preventing injury to the handlers and medical support staff is a priority (Box 26-2).

Shelter animals may exhibit behaviors during a disaster which they would not normally show under normal circumstances. There is an increase of aggression during times of disasters and it is important to be careful when dealing with these animals. Using appropriate tools to protect staff is imperative.

All stray animals should be handled with gloves. Vaccine and disease history is unknown. Many animals may arrive with various substances on their skin. What may appear to be dirt and oil could also be a caustic substance. Any animal with a signs of a possible contagious disease should be isolated immediately.

Location and surroundings in and around a disaster area are often unpredictable and dangerous. Any disaster is considered a *hazardous working environment*. During an average day in an emergency clinic, bumping into a cabinet or tripping over a rolled up piece of carpet is something we attempt to avoid. However, during a disaster, walking into a puddle of water where a live wire fell or reaching into the bottom of drawer to find a rattlesnake could be a deadly mistake; therefore veterinary professionals must remain alert during a disaster Fig 26-4.

Marking dangerous areas with cones or caution tape will help decrease the amount of injuries. A safety officer should be appointed to help make staff aware of the dangers. A briefing should occur before each new shift, and a safety officer should speak to the group about concerns. During a disaster, a safety officer should always be on duty to monitor the situation.

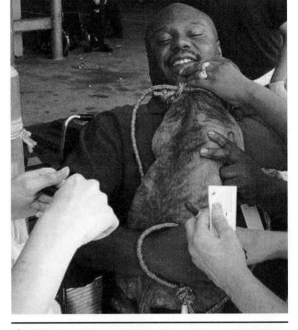

Fig. 26-4 All efforts must be made to reunite victims of disasters with their pets.

Common Emergencies

Even though a disaster is occurring, animals that arrive at the clinic as emergencies should still be considered just emergencies. One of the biggest differences seen during an emergency is that animals may come without owners and no identification—this is when the Good Samaritan Laws apply.

The clinic should not overtreat the patient. Ear mites and matted fur can be uncomfortable but certainly are not an emergency. During a disaster, treating animals should be done using appropriate judgment, understanding that time and resources are limited.

Disasters create many types of conditions and emergencies. The topics discussed have ranged from radiation exposure, weapons of mass destruction, biologic warfare, chemical warfare, explosives, and foot and mouth disease. Listed following are emergencies that have occurred during disaster situations in the United States.

Shock

Shock is a very common emergency during a disaster. Most of the time an injury has caused the shock, but certainly some animals can go into shock because of stress. Before treating the shock in the animal, the team should assess the animal's overall condition and decide whether reversing the shock will give the animal a good chance for survival.

Orthopedic and Soft Tissue Injuries

Orthopedic and soft tissue injuries are common during a disaster. Not all orthopedic and soft tissue injuries are emergencies. Being able to refer nonemergency patients to a clinic that is not affected by the disaster may be the best option. Most orthopedic and soft tissue injuries are not life threatening, but they certainly can be painful. Providing pain relief by administering an analgesic and stabilizing the affected area by placing a bandage (if appropriate) can be done quickly before referring the patient elsewhere.

Wounds

Wounds of all types are common during a disaster. Certainly a dog can live with a minor laceration to its pad. It may be painful, but it will live. However, a stick impaled through the abdomen is a wound that is an emergency. Being able to stabilize the patient may be a possibility, but surgery may not be an option. Euthanasia may be the only option, unless the patient can be transferred to a fully functional hospital.

Neurologic Injuries

Neurologic injuries can occur for varying reasons during a disaster. Smoke inhalation may cause an animal to arrive in an altered state. Being thrown around the yard during a tornado and suffering spinal trauma is another scenario. Performing a complete neurologic assessment of the patient is necessary. Some patients who suffer head trauma or other neurologic disorders may take a long time to recover. Most neurologic patients require constant monitoring. During a disaster, cage space and staff may be limited. Waiting a week or more to see if the patient recovers from head trauma may not be an option.

Hyperthermia and Hypothermia

Hyperthermia and hypothermia are very common during disaster. Knowing where and how the patient was rescued is important. Rushing to warm up the patient may not be beneficial. Although hyperthermia or hypothermia always has a cause, the clinician may not discover it during the time of the disaster. However, considering all possibilities and determining what the overall prognosis is for that patient is important.

Smoke and Burn Injuries

Animals that have been involved in a fire or have been burned smell like smoke, have whiskers or hair that has been singed, are covered in soot, or have visible burns. Oxygen should be immediately given to these patients even if respiratory signs are not apparent. Providing oxygen will help with carbon monoxide elimination and tissue hypoxia. Clinical signs will often worsen for up to 48 hours after exposure. Once admitted, the animal's condition can become life threatening.

Near Drowning

The true definition of a near-drowning victim is "survival for at least 24 hours after underwater submersion." If the patient dies before 24 hours, then the animal is considered a drowning victim. During a flood or hurricane, near-drowning victims are common. Symptoms of near drowning may include respiratory signs, hypothermia, pulmonary edema, and vomiting. Respiratory changes may be delayed by up to 48 hours after the incident because of infection from contaminated water. Neurologic signs may include lethargy, stupor, coma, or seizures as a result of the cerebral acidosis, electrolyte changes, and increased intracranial pressure. Providing oxygen, antibiotics, intravenous fluids, and heat therapy may be indicated. Long-term prognosis varies based on how much water was aspirated, how long the patient was submerged, the patient's age, and any other preexisting conditions. It may also be possible for a patient to fall into water contaminated with a toxic substance such as bleach.

Search and Rescue Canines

Any medical condition in a S&R dog is an emergency. S&R teams vary and can be state, private, or federally formed. The federally recognized teams are categorized as task forces, with most states having one or more. State and federal laws protect many of these

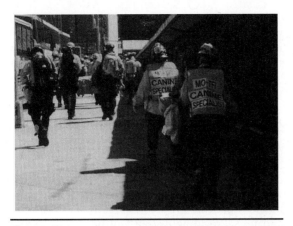

Fig. 26-5 Missouri Task Force One going to work during 9/11.

dogs. During a disaster, S&R dogs must get back to working status as quickly as possible.

In most cases the handler of a S&R dog will want to be present for any treatment performed on the dog. Sometimes it may be mandatory that the handler is present. Canine police dogs are better handled with their owners there to provide commands. Some police dogs are dual trained for both police work and S&R work. Understanding that the dog is the handler's partner and team member is important; the person cannot help with disaster relief if he or she does not have a working dog.

Occasionally S&R dogs encounter unique hazards that cause them harm. In the aftermath of the 1995 Oklahoma City bombing and the 9/11 attack in New York, dogs used to search the rubble for survivors were exposed to inhalant toxins while working. Several routes of exposure exist:

- Respiratory exposure: Dogs cannot wear gas masks. Substances like fiberglass or halogenated gases may cause symptoms of pulmonary edema or respiratory tract irritation.
- Dermal exposure: Corrosive agents may burn or injure the skin.
- Oral exposure: Ingestion of materials is a potential hazard for any dog. Detergents, acidic toxins, and other materials may be licked or ingested on purpose or by accident.
- Ocular exposure: During 9/11, many dogs arrived at the field hospital with red, injected sclera. Liquids splashing into eyes or even debris blowing onto the eyes can cause serious eye injuries.

If a toxin is suspected, animal poison control center is called for advice. Having book references on hand is an important back-up in case phone lines are not functional. After 9/11 veterinarians wrote many toxicology reports regarding S&R dogs, and the national poison centers have all that information. Injuries will be different for every disaster.

The 9/11 terrorist attacks inspired one of the largest showings of S&R dogs in the history of the United States (Fig. 26-5). Hundreds of S&R dogs were called into action. Experiences gained from working with so many S&R dogs provided a wealth of knowledge for future disasters involving working dogs.

Several medical conditions were common for S&R dogs during 9/11. S&R dogs were more susceptible to dehydration because they worked long shifts in the heat. During a disaster, a clinic may become the "checkpoint" for the medical evaluation of S&R dogs before and after each shift. Offering this service to S&R teams is a great way to help out during a disaster, because most S&R teams do not have staff veterinarians. During 9/11 most S&R dogs were given subcutaneous fluids after each shift to help combat dehydration. Handlers who had fluids given to their dogs noticed a dramatic improvement in energy level and attitude. Because S&R dogs love to work and are driven to perform, the handler may never see any signs of dehydration until the animal is too ill to recover. Severe dehydration can lead to hypovolemia. These dogs must then be hospitalized until they are stable. Handlers should be instructed on ways to prevent dehydration. Taking more frequent and longer breaks and ensuring dogs drink an appropriate amount of water is key to preventing dehydration.

Stress diarrhea was found to be common in dogs that work for long hours under stressful conditions. If diarrhea is severe enough, then it can lead to dehydration. In severe cases the diarrhea became hemorrhagic. Keeping a close eye on S&R dogs and addressing diarrhea as soon as it begins is an important factor in keeping these dogs working.

During 9/11 several dogs had hemorrhagic cystitis. All dogs responded to supportive care, and no evidence of toxicosis or infectious disease was ever found. Minor skin infections also occurred. Bathing the dogs and putting them on antibiotics helped with most skin infections. Other issues of S&R dogs included minor lameness, minor lacerations, ear infections, and eye infections.

Most S&R dogs did not wear booties while working during the crisis, because booties tended to

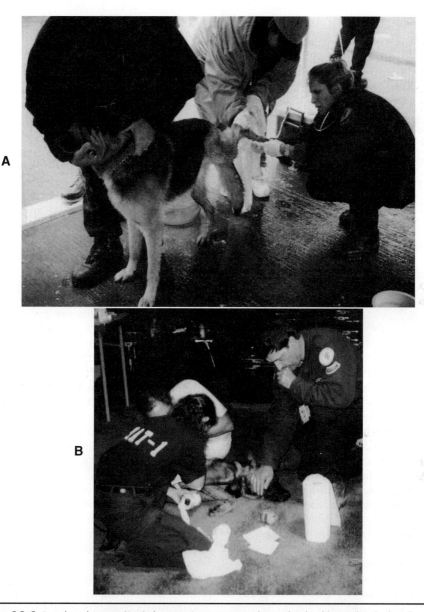

Fig. 26-6 Search and rescue (S&R) dogs receive treatment. The reader should note that the handlers are present to help restrain the dogs.

decrease traction and inhibit their ability to walk. Despite their feet being unprotected, a remarkably low occurrence of injuries to the pads was reported. Thousands of booties for dogs were donated and initially given out to handlers, but after weeks went by with limited injuries, the handlers found it best to work their dogs without the booties (Fig. 26-6).

Decontamination

Decontamination of animals became critical during 9/11 and Hurricane Katrina (Fig. 26-7). S&R dogs during 9/11 were arriving at the field hospitals covered in dirt and grime. To humans the air around the smoldering World Trade Center site was painful to

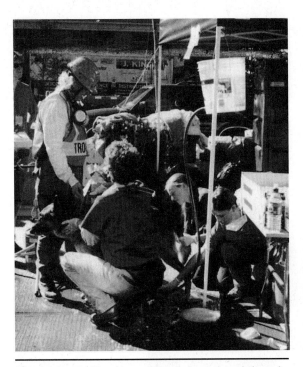

Fig. 26-7 Search and rescue (S&R) dog is hosed down for decontamination.

inhale. The S&R dogs were working with their noses close the ground and without gas masks. Reports of asbestos and toxic gases were everywhere. The effects of inhaling such gases are still not known and will probably not be fully discovered for upwards of 50 years after the attack. A large continuous study by the University of Pennsylvania Veterinary School is being conducted to monitor the overall health of dogs involved in searching during that time.

One of the biggest treatments administered during 9/11 was decontamination of the S&R dogs. Washing them down and trying to remove any hazardous materials after they were done searching was extremely important. Most information compiled on decontamination of animals has been adapted from human medical research.

First and foremost, veterinary staff must protect themselves. Vomit, urine, and feces of S&R dogs may contain hazardous materials. Wearing gloves, disposable gowns, and even eye protection is a required. S&R dogs should be assessed for any life-threatening ailments first. The clinician should remember that symptoms from a toxic substance may not appear until long after exposure. Keeping track of S&R dogs'

symptoms is key to helping with a diagnosis. For example, if a few of the S&R dogs brought to a clinic begin to cough and the clinician suspects that the coughing is the result of exposure to an airborne toxic substance, then all S&R dog handlers should be notified so that precautions can be taken to prevent further toxicosis.

Dermal absorption of hazardous materials during 9/11 and Hurricane Katrina was a big concern. Decontamination baths were set up to help minimize any problems in the S&R dogs. Bathing with a detergent soap (e.g., Dawn, GOJO) and water became routine when dogs were dog searching the World Trade Center areas. This helped to remove any oil-based contaminants that the dogs may have encountered. Flushing of the eyes and nostrils with saline can help remove any irritants. Changing gloves and gowns between patients is ideal. Animals brought to Lamar-Dixon and other facilities were hosed down and washed with Dawn liquid dish soap. All people washing the animals needed to wear gloves, apron and boots.

Using extra precaution when dealing with animals during a disaster is important, because they have the potential to be covered in corrosive materials that can be damaging to the veterinary staff. Protecting oneself first and then treating the patient is the safest way to handle a potential exposure to a toxic substance.

Surgery

Taking a patient to surgery during a disaster should only occur in an emergency, if the patient's prognosis will benefit from it, and if the clinic has the resources to safely perform the procedure. Appropriate cautions must still be taken to ensure the patient's safety.

Patients who are stable should be referred to another clinic that is fully functioning. Fractures, major lacerations, most ocular injuries, and some hemoabdomens are surgeries that are not emergencies and should be done only under pristine conditions.

Performing surgery requires more staff, uses more resources, and ties up cage space for an extended period of time. Taking a patient to surgery may decrease the number of other patients who can be seen and treated at the hospital. Considering the overall effects that taking a patient to surgery during a disaster will have to the entire clinic, staff, and other patients is important.

Record Keeping

One of the most important tasks in emergency medicine is the ability to keep accurate records. During a disaster, having premade forms ready for use to keep accurate records is important. During 9/11 this became one of the biggest challenges that Veterinary Medical Assistance Teams (VMAT) faced. When VMAT personnel arrived on the scene, they immediately started treating S&R dogs. Because of the large number of working canines being seen and the overwhelming state of the disaster, complete records were not kept during the first couple of days. Handlers that returned to the field hospital a few days later had to communicate what had been done to their dogs during the previous visit. No computers were available and electricity was limited at the field hospital. The team had established a command center in a building nearby that had computers, copy machines, and paper. Realizing that they had no information on the handlers or the dogs they were treating, they quickly created forms. The forms were not in duplicate and therefore posed a problem when things had to be handwritten twice so that the owners could have a copy. When over 6000 animals overwhelmed Lamar-Dixon during hurricane Katrina the record keeping system failed. Organizations such as Petfinder.com were brought in to help with the enormous task of logging and keeping track of that many animals.

Even during a disaster, maintaining accurate records is important. This is especially true if no owner is present. If an animal's owner is eventually found, then he or she will want to know how the pet was treated during the separation period—hence accurate records are needed. A medical record is a legal document. For example, if it was deemed that a pet should be euthanized and an owner is later found, being able to provide a record describing why the pet was euthanized is important. All veterinary clinics should have printed forms (created in duplicate) for use in disasters. Multiple copies should be made in advance and stored away in the event they are needed. Forms should be fast and easy to use; checking boxes and circling answers is the easiest way to record basic information.

Having a Polaroid or other instant camera ready with some film stored away is very useful to take pictures of unowned animals. If an animal must be euthanized and an owner comes to identify it, then a photograph is important. Stapling the pictures to the patient's record will provide quick access to the picture if an owner is trying to locate their pet.

The Humane Society of the United States (HSUS), Petfinder.com, and other rescue organizations have computer systems that form a list of animals that have no owners. Since Hurricane Katrina even more emphasis has been placed on record keeping. When taking in and treating an unknown animal, the clinic staff should find the local group that is handling rescue and placement of animals so that the animal can be added to the database. Owners may not think to look for their pets at veterinary clinics and may only go to the rescue organization for assistance.

Recheck Appointments

Plans should be made for postdisaster care of each animal that enters the hospital. The client should be encouraged to return to the regular veterinarian for follow-up care. However, if the client's hospital is closed for an extended time, then a recheck appointment at the facility should be set up.

Providing owners with enough medication is also another consideration. The clinician should limit the amount dispensed to avoid running out of stock supplies. Clients should be instructed to follow up with their regular veterinarians once they are open for business. Local veterinary hospitals should put together a verbal and written "stockpile" system before the disaster strikes. Accurate records should be maintained so that hospitals can be reimbursed after the disaster subsides.

Helping the Local Veterinary Infrastructure

Talking to other local clinics before a disaster occurs and creating a support team will help the clinician's facility and the local community. Being able to share equipment and even personnel can be a huge benefit to multiple clinics during a disaster. Talking to local shelter groups and letting them know what services you can provide them can be a huge benefit. Making contact before a disaster always helps during a disaster.

Veterinarians should not act as shelters without the supervision of another organization. The primary role for a veterinarians and their team is to provide medical care for the stray animals. The veterinary team and shelter need to work together to help each other during a disaster. Groups like the Humane Society of the United States and other local shelter organizations help with the sheltering and placement of animals during a disaster. These groups understand the legal issues with taking in stray animals and usually boast large databases necessary for finding the owners.

Communication before a disaster will help to expedite things during a disaster. If all local veterinarians had each other's contact numbers, then when a disaster struck they could easily communicate with each other to assess damage, determine what clinics could function, and decide who needed help. Ultimately the goal of any disaster is to get the local community functioning by itself again. Once that occurs, the situation stops being a current disaster (Box 26-3).

Personal Recovery after the Disaster

Being aware of PTSD is very important. All responders, no matter what the magnitude of the disaster, have the potential to suffer PTSD. A "debriefing" should be done at the end of each day that someone has worked in a disaster. This should include asking how tired the person is, what bothered the person the most, how he or she is dealing with the disaster, and if the person wants to return to help the next day. Realizing that each person deals with stress differently is important. Creating opportunities for each person to talk and share feelings is equally important. Ideally a couple of people in the clinic should not be directly involved in dealing with veterinary medicine during the disaster. These individuals can include administrators or receptionists. Sometimes just having someone who will listen will make all the difference when dealing with the stress of the disaster. If someone appears to be suffering from PTSD, then seeking appropriate help is important.

People who were involved in rescue efforts or who were victims of a disaster may suffer from PTSD. This syndrome was initially diagnosed in people who served in the military during war times. It has been now recognized in anyone who has been involved with a disaster or traumatic event. The National Center for Post-Traumatic Stress Disorder (www.ncptsd.va.gov) has a wide variety of information for anyone affected by a disaster. The National Center for PTSD say that 8% of men and 20% of women will experience PTSD symptoms. Roughly 30% of those

---

| BOX 26-3 | ⓜ |

Personal Disaster Kit for Disaster Responders

- Flashlight
- Batteries for flashlight and all electronics
- Small battery-operated radio
- Medications
  Personal prescription drugs
  Over-the-counter drugs
- One week of clothing
- Garment bag
- Immunization record
- Medical record
- Important documents
  Homeowner's policy
  Health insurance policy and identification cards
  Credit card numbers
  Bank numbers
- Current contact number list of family members and friends
- Laundry detergent
- First aid kit
- Travel size shampoo/conditioner/soap/toothpaste
- Extra toothbrush
- Extra towel
- Duct tape
- Trash bags (multiple sizes)
- Sunscreen
- Bug repellent
- Candles
- Toilet paper
- Water bottles

---

afflicted will suffer from a chronic form for the rest of their lives. The definition used by the National Center for PTSD is:

Post-Traumatic Stress Disorder, or PTSD, is a psychiatric disorder that can occur following the experience or witnessing of life-threatening events such as military combat, natural disasters, terrorist incidents, serious accidents, or violent personal assaults like rape. People who suffer from PTSD often relive the experience through nightmares and flashbacks, have difficulty sleeping, and feel detached or estranged, and these symptoms can be severe enough and last long enough to significantly impair the person's daily life (http://www.ncptsd.va.gov/facts/general/fs_what_is_ptsd.html).

The National Center for Post-Traumatic Stress Disorder's website contains some valuable links to other websites that provide help for those suffering from PTSD.

Relaxing after a disaster can be very difficult. Usually people push themselves to their limits by working 16- to 18-hour days. They never stop to think of themselves and feel that more needs to be done, at the clinic or at home. After the disaster is over and life starts to return to normal, it can become very difficult to relax, because the body and mind have a difficult time slowing down.

Continuing to eat well, taking regular breaks, and having periods of scheduled "down time" to avoid burnout is vital. Everyone must care for himself or herself before offering care to others.

Becoming Involved

Often disasters strike without warning. One of the largest issues during Hurricane Katrina was the number of people that came to help. Managing and dealing with the thousands of people that showed up became very difficult and hindered the relief efforts of many teams. Much discussion has occurred about implementing rules and regulations against volunteers without any training in disasters. Some states are working on those laws and regulations now. An organization that is already on the scene runs with a set of rules and regulations that the public usually does not understand.

Involvement may not be voluntary; it may be mandatory. Disasters occur all the time. Unless individuals are part of the organization already on the scene, they must remember to follow their rules and guidelines or leave when asked.

Preparing oneself for a disaster will assist in recovery efforts immensely. This is the first step in becoming involved with disaster relief efforts. A small disaster pack of personal items and disaster pack for pets located in a designated area can be prepared before a disaster strikes (see Box 26-3; Box 26-4).

Today many organizations allow individuals to volunteer to assist outside of their local areas.

The American Veterinary Medical Association formed VMAT in 1994. Their mission is to "assist the local veterinary community with the care of animals and to provide veterinary oversight and advice concerning animal related issues and public health during a disaster or after a request from an appropriate agency."

BOX 26-4

Pet Disaster Kit for Pet Owners

Items to be packed up and stored away in bag:

- Current medical records including vaccinations
- Extra leash and collar
- Identification tags for all collars or harnesses
- Current photographs and written descriptions of pets
- Extra bowls
- Small bag of cat litter and small cat litter box
- Can opener
- Number of veterinarian
- Extra towels

Items on checklist that must be brought if disaster occurs:

- Two-week supply of any medications needed (should always be kept in the house)
- Carrier
- Two-week supply of food (should always be kept in the house)
- Pet beds
- Pet toys
- Three-day supply of water

(www.vmat.org. VMAT Mission Statement). The VMAT teams are part of the National Disaster Management System that fall under the Federal Emergency Management Agency (FEMA). When called into action, these highly trained veterinarians and technicians are considered to be part-time employees of FEMA. FEMA will activate the team, giving them as little as 12 hour's notice that they are going to be deployed. Members can be deployed up to 14 days. The team is self-sufficient and can establish a fully functioning (including minor surgery) veterinary hospital (where technicians can use their medical skills during a disaster) (Fig. 26-8). Members are required to fulfill training requirements before they are considered deployable. If activated, then the team members are paid a salary and are covered by federal worker's compensation. They are also protected under the Federal Tort Claims Act against any personal liability during deployment and are exempt from licensure, certification, and registration requirements outside of the state in which they are registered.

The HSUS has developed Disaster Animal Response Teams. The teams consist of animal care professionals, volunteers, and other disaster professionals. Typically their focus is rescue and placement of animals. As an education leader, the HSUS also helps local communities and individuals plan and prepare for a crisis. For example, they provide brochures on how pet owners can keep pets safe during and after a disaster.

The Emergency Animal Rescue Service is another large organization that was formed in 1988 to deal with fires, floods, hurricanes, and other natural disasters. Since then, the group has grown to more than 2000 volunteers in the United States. The Emergency Animal Rescue Service is part of the United Animal Nations—an organization devoted to the care and protection of all animals. Similar to Disaster Animal Response Teams, the Emergency Animal Rescue Service has the capability to set up shelters and work with the rescue of animals.

Some cities and towns have established their own animal disaster teams. Typically, these teams are available only to the community if a local disaster strikes. Some states have even formed their own state animal disaster teams. North Carolina, for example, offers one of the most impressive State Animal Response Teams (SART) in the country (formed after Hurricane Floyd devastated the state in 1999). It was such a large-scale animal disaster that no one knew how to deal with appropriately. Over 3 million domestic and farm animals were lost. After the disaster subsided, a team of people got together and talked about how the disaster could have been handled more successfully. Since then, North Carolina's SART system has been the model for many other states' animal response teams, which establish complete disaster plans for their states. Currently, teams in Massachusetts, Maine, Connecticut, Pennsylvania, Colorado, and Maryland have been (or are in the process of being) formed.

Disaster Training

Training is needed in any disaster situation. The two main requirements are (1) training for personal protection and (2) training for the actual disaster.

Becoming certified in a level-one hazardous materials (i.e., hazmat) course is a must for at least one member of the clinic's disaster team. Most animal disaster teams require a level-one hazmat course. Local fire departments often offer such courses throughout the year. Online training is available through FEMA (www.fema.gov/about/training). In most cases these courses are free. Courses focus on how to read hazardous materials signs and the basics of what to look for when entering a disaster scene. Certain websites (e.g., www.saferesponse.com) also offer a free online hazmat course. Taking a hazmat course will help out any disaster responder.

The incident command system (ICS) has become a universal system for those dealing with any type of disaster. It was developed by a California fire department in the 1970s. Since then, local, state, and federal branches all use the ICS system (Fig. 26-9). The ICS is designed to have certain key people fill specific duties and establish a chain of command. Many local fire departments, as well as FEMA, offer ICS training courses.

One person in the veterinary hospital should familiarize himself or herself with the ICS system to make it easier to communicate with local, state, and federal responders during a disaster. The ICS system can be applied to the smallest of veterinary hospitals. If each clinic appoints key members using ICS before the disaster happens, then it will be easier to function if one does occur. Using the ICS system, a person would be designated as the *Incident Commander* or *Administrative Officer*.

Training for individual disasters can vary. The myriad of disasters that can occur require flexible skills. Thinking "outside of the box" when dealing with certain situations is common. For example,

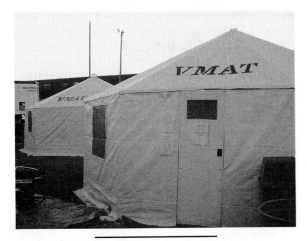

Fig. 26-8 VMAT field tents.

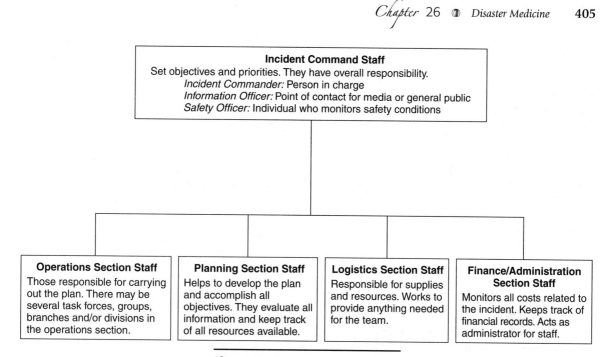

Incident Command Staff
Set objectives and priorities. They have overall responsibility.
Incident Commander: Person in charge
Information Officer: Point of contact for media or general public
Safety Officer: Individual who monitors safety conditions

Operations Section Staff
Those responsible for carrying out the plan. There may be several task forces, groups, branches and/or divisions in the operations section.

Planning Section Staff
Helps to develop the plan and accomplish all objectives. They evaluate all information and keep track of all resources available.

Logistics Section Staff
Responsible for supplies and resources. Works to provide anything needed for the team.

Finance/Administration Section Staff
Monitors all costs related to the incident. Keeps track of financial records. Acts as administrator for staff.

Fig. 26-9 Incident Command Staff graph.

BOX 26-5

Animal Disaster Teams Organizations

Veterinary Medical Assistance Teams (VMAT): www.vmat.org

Emergency Animal Response Service: www.uan.org/ears

Humane Society of the United States (HSUS): www.hsus.org

---

having a clean, sterile environment to do a laceration repair may not be feasible. Placing a large sterile drape under the patient may be the best solution. Lack of intravenous poles may require innovative ideas on how to hang fluid bags.

Many veterinary conferences have started to include disaster medicine as a topic. The International Veterinary Emergency and Critical Care Conference, held once a year, has had disaster medicine as a topic since 1998. The National Disaster Medical System offers a conference once a year specifically geared toward the National Disaster Medical System teams, which include topics in veterinary disaster medicine presented by members of VMAT. The HSUS hosts a National Conference on Animals in Disasters once a year which is meant to bring local, state and federal agency together to facilitate talk about how to help animals in disaster more effectively.

Joining an animal disaster team is another great way to become involved. It takes time and commitment to join one of the teams. Speaking to team members and visiting websites will provide more in-depth information and help one decide if a particular team is the right choice (Box 26-5).

Many organizations (government and private) are devoted to disaster medicine (Box 26-6). Organizations like the FEMA offer online disaster training. For example, FEMA offers free courses on the ICS and livestock in disasters through their Emergency Management Institute. Many of the organizations listed in Box 26-6 also will provide brochures and other written materials on disaster medicine. The American Veterinary Medical Association offers a great guide to pet owners on how to prepare for a disaster. The HSUS provides a free online manual for the general public and animal care providers on preparing for and dealing with animals in disasters. Many of the courses and literature offered by these organizations are provided at little or no cost.

Very few books have been published on veterinary disaster medicine, and most published before

BOX 26-6

Sites That Contain Information on Disaster Training

National Disaster Medical System: www.ndms.dhhs.gov

Federal Emergency Management Agency (FEMA): www.fema.gov

Department of Homeland Security: www.dhs.gov

American Veterinary Medical Association: www.avma.org

American Animal Hospital Association: www.aahanet.org

American Veterinary Medical Foundation: www.avmf.org

9/11 contain outdated material. A large number of publications were printed after 9/11 dealing with human health and disasters. There are many books currently being written on animals in disasters. However, much of the material on humans in disasters can be adapted for use in veterinary medicine. Going to the library or searching the Internet will provide a list of publications covering human disaster medicine; most of the information regarding veterinary disaster medicine has been presented at conferences or in magazines and journals. Several veterinary emergency books have started to include chapters on disaster medicine.

Clinicians should realize that some of the best information is obtained through personal experience. Becoming distracted during a disaster is easy to do; therefore veterinary professionals must maintain their focus on critically ill or injured patients while using the life-saving skills they have learned throughout their careers.

Conclusion

Disaster medicine is an evolving field of veterinary medicine. Becoming involved may not be a choice; therefore being prepared before a disaster is important. Veterinary hospitals can create a plan and to expedite patient care during a disaster. In addition, veterinary professionals should become educated and know what resources are available during a disaster so that they can provide the best care possible.

Suggested Readings

Gwaltney-Brant S, Murphy L, Wismer T et al: General toxicologic hazards and risks for search and rescue dogs responding to urban disasters, *Proc The Long Island Veterinary Medical Association Toxicology and Search and Rescue Dogs*, 2003, pp 1-4.

Heath S: *Animal management in disasters*, St Louis, 1999, Mosby.

Murphy L: Decontamination and treatment techniques for SAR dogs in an urban disaster area, *Proc The Long Island Veterinary Medical Association Toxicology and Search and Rescue Dogs*, 2003, pp 27-28.

Otto C: Case study: 911 at the World Trade Center—care of SAR canines, *Proc 8th Ann Mtg IVECCS*, 2002, pp 150-153.

Otto C, Franz M, Kellogg B et al: Field treatment of search dogs: lessons learned from the World Trade Center disaster, *Proc The Long Island Veterinary Medical Association Toxicology and Search and Rescue Dogs*, 2003, pp 43-52.

Text taken from *www.avma.org/disaster/vmat/default.asp*, 2005.

Wingfield W, Lanman L. In Winfield W, Raffe M: *The veterinary ICU book*, Jackson Hole, WY, 2002, Teton New Media, pp 1226-1246.

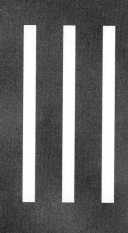
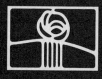

PRACTICE MANAGEMENT

Maintaining a 24-hour emergency critical care team is very challenging, but it can be done successfully using proper scheduling techniques. Proper scheduling includes considering how changing schedules or rotating workers will affect their lives personally and physically.

This section describes how using different rotations and maintaining a routine to optimize sleep can help alleviate the stress of working overnights or rotations.

Veterinary personnel need to understand the liability risks that they take when assuming responsibility for the medical care of critically ill or injured patients. Many times the owners are extremely distraught and may be unable to make a decision that will be beneficial for all individuals involved.

Veterinary personnel need to be able to identify and minimize risks to themselves while still being able to provide the immediate care for patients. The importance of informed consent, documentation, and communication are discussed.

CHAPTER 27

The Art of Scheduling

ANDREA M. BATTAGLIA

One common reason why technicians leave a position in emergency or critical care is because of the inconsistency of a schedule or the inability to continue working a specific shift or rotation. In 1952 researchers from the University of Minnesota began looking at how biologic rhythms dictate human desires, moods, and abilities. They began to study every feature of metabolism, growth, injury, and illness. Chronobiology was developed, and the advances in this area have been very helpful in determining how to best help those people involved with shift work. People responsible for scheduling a team of 24-hour emergency or critical care veterinary technicians must consider many factors: how changing a specific person's shift may affect his or her personal, physical, and emotional well-being; whether rotations are necessary; and what schedule best fits the needs of the hospital. The manager of the schedule should communicate and reevaluate each veterinary technician's progress during training periods and when a change in shifts is necessary.

Shift lag is the term used for the negative effects of shift work. Manifestations of these effects can be emotional and physical. Managers may receive complaints that one of the veterinary technicians has been very moody and irritable lately. This behavior may be out of character for the individual, and when approached with the concern, the person may become very emotional and upset. Shift lag may be the problem and should be considered.

Reports of an increase of dose calculation errors or forgotten treatments during a shift also can manifest if someone is having difficulties handling his or her hours. Other problems associated with shift lag include sleep-awake disorders, gastrointestinal disorders, and cardiovascular disorders. Sleep deprivation has been considered the main cause of shift lag.

Sleep Deprivation

The light of the sun and the darkness of the night reset the internal biological clock, or circadian rhythm, each day. Those who work the late shift (also called the *graveyard shift* or *night shift* [e.g., 11 PM to 6 AM]) are at the greatest risk, because around 3 AM the body is at its lowest ebb and the daily biological clock is reset. This conflict is called *circadian dysrhythmia*. Those who work evenings and nights are continually readjusting this clock. The majority of people soon revert to a daytime schedule. Some individuals work very well at night and have been labeled as "night owls." These people are able to sleep well during the day and adjust hours of sleep without any problem. Their individual genetic makeup allows them to adjust easily.

The most common complaint of people working various shifts is sleep deprivation. The average person needs 7.5 to 8.5 hours of sleep each day. The veterinary technician who works the night shift averages 5 to 7 hours less sleep per week than the person who works the day shift. Over time this leads to serious physical problems.

Sleep-deprived people are more susceptible to colds, flu, and gastrointestinal problems. People who work nights are more prone to heart disease, accidents, and obesity.

Women who work rotating shifts may have more difficulty conceiving. Two European surveys found that women working irregular shifts were twice as likely to experience delays in conceiving. Miscarriages and low birth weights also were higher in women with unstable work schedules.

Depression and chronic fatigue also are common among night workers. If poor morale is affecting the staff, then fatigue may be the cause.

Weight gain commonly affects shift workers because of the tendency to snack on unhealthful foods. Attaining a standard mealtime is difficult during these hours. Research has also suggested that sleep-deprived people have larger appetites. Boredom also can increase snacking during these hours.

Many studies have been done over the years to determine how to help people adapt to shift work. Twenty percent of all workers in the United States are involved in shift work (26% if part-time employees are included). Law enforcement, news publishing, emergency services, hospitals, food, printing, military, airlines, paper production, and railroads are just some of the industries affected. It is clear that many lives depend on people who are fully functional while the majority of the population is sleeping.

Creating the Optimal Shift for Employees

Scheduling is one of the greatest challenges a manager faces. What works for one person may not work for the others—a schedule that meets the needs of the employees may not meet the needs of the hospital.

To create a successful schedule, the manager should begin by determining what person is best suited for what shift. Each veterinary technician should be interviewed to determine what would work best for him or her. The staff should be allowed to submit their own ideas. They should know that their preferences may not be possible, but the manager is willing to consider all possibilities. Open and frequent communication promotes teamwork.

The manager should discuss possible scenarios that may occur on different shifts to determine which veterinary technicians may be able to handle specific shift expectations. Allowing the applicants to shadow during different shifts will allow them to interact with veterinary technicians who work nights and ask questions they may have about working the different hours.

Most procedures and activities will occur during the day. The person who works during the day is someone who enjoys the busy pace, as well as working with many people (and occasionally different services).

The person scheduled to work the second shift assists in bridging the gap between the two shifts. This person also enjoys the busy pace and communicates well with coworkers. The hours tend to be very busy for emergency clients.

The overnight shift requires someone who is experienced and works well independently. His or her ability to observe and interpret observations should be excellent. Many times the overnight veterinary technician is the primary caregiver and needs to be able to relay important information over the phone to the doctor. The person should be able to communicate well not only to the professional staff but also to the clients. The overnight shift is a time when communication is necessary, and it must be very clearly stated and as detailed as possible. Most people this individual will be communicating with are people whose sleep cycle has been disrupted.

The manager should overlap the staff for at least 1 to 2 hours. The combined team from the two different shifts is able to work closely together to complete procedures or treatments before the previous shift leaves. Overlapping shifts promotes a team effort to accomplish the same goal; it also gives the team time to complete thorough case reviews and updates and answer any questions that arise once the relief shift begins to assess patients' conditions.

The overlap also gives the combined team time to interact with coworkers and help eliminate the feeling of isolation that sometimes occurs among veterinary technicians who work nights.

Consistency is extremely important. The ideal situation would be to eliminate shift rotation schedules (because it sometimes takes days for the body to adjust to a new schedule). The clinic should have a pool of part-time people to cover for vacations, holidays, personal days, and sick leave. This reduces the number of times regular staff people must rotate shifts and increases the consistency of the schedule.

Finding people who are interested in working only nights is difficult, so rotations have become part of the system.

A variety of rotations have been developed. Some rotations are more beneficial to the normal body rhythms; others are detrimental to them. Optimized shift rotation schedules are schedules designed specifically to meet the normal daily rhythms or circadian cycles of human physiology.

The most beneficial rotations are slow rotations in which each person stays on a specific shift 5 to 14 days. Two weeks on a specific shift is best. Slow rotation by phase advance is the rotation night to afternoon to morning; this rotation method is considered to be physiologically and emotionally harmful.

Slow rotation by phase delay is the rotation from morning to afternoon to night and is considered to be the ideal shift rotation. When the veterinary technician rotates through this shift structure, he or she gains 8 hours of sleep.

Rapid rotations also occur, which are shifts that rotate the veterinary technician through several shifts during 1 week. Rapid rotations are considered the worst type of schedule. The daily rotation disrupts the body rhythms, making it very difficult for the veterinary technician to be productive.

The next category is the dedicated shift, in which the veterinary technician is assigned to a single shift during his or her stay with the practice. This is preferred to any rotation but in many cases is not an option.

Shift schedules should be evaluated routinely. Employees working night shifts should be monitored for productivity and for the physical and emotional effects of the schedule. This will help prevent employee turnover and accidents caused by fatigue. In addition, sleep schedules should be posted so that the staff can avoid calling sleeping employees, if possible. The supervisor of the veterinary technician working nights should avoid encroaching on employees' sleep time when scheduling mandatory meetings or performance reviews.

The manager responsible for the schedule should remember that not every schedule will work for every team, and what is currently working may need to be adjusted depending on the needs of the hospital. Many options are available to choose from; involving those who will be directly affected by any shift structure is important.

Helpful Hints for Day Sleeping

Emergency and critical care veterinary technicians must make an extra effort to take care of themselves to be efficient and productive workers during all hours. Applicants for positions in a 24-hour unit must understand that they may be expected to work different shifts. Many people agree to these arrangements without understanding how such schedules can affect them.

A new veterinary technician working nights can try taking a 3-hour nap before the shift begins and sleeping right after the shift is over. The goal is to increase the sleep time after the shift and decrease it before the shift. This gradual change has worked for many.

The veterinary technician working nights can become a successful day sleeper; he or she should keep the routine as consistent as possible. When trying to establish a healthy sleep pattern, the technician also should do the following:

- Go to bed immediately after work—Resist the temptation to do anything because this stimulates the body clock to go into the day mode. Exercise should be planned after sleep.
- Exercise at least five times a week for emotional and physical well-being.
- Seek total darkness—This can be accomplished by using dark, heavy drapes or black plastic garbage bags over the windows to block any sunlight. A blindfold may be a good investment.
- Be vocal about the need for peace during these hours—Inform friends about sleep schedules, put a "Do Not Disturb" sign on the door, and wear earplugs if necessary.
- Use white noise—White noise has been used as a sleep inducer and has been found to be very

successful for some people. White noise is acoustic or electrical noise in which the intensity is the same at all frequencies. Fans and bubbling fish filters are two examples. Tapes and machines made specifically for white noise also are available.

- Keep the environment cool—Many people sleep better in a cooler environment. Adjust the thermostat to a comfortable temperature.
- Avoid using sleep inducers—Melatonin supplements are commonly used to help travelers avoid jet lag, get some sleep, and reset their body clocks. Melatonin is the sleep-inducing chemical released in the brain during the hours of darkness. The synthetic form may be helpful in assisting the body to adjust to the first few days of night shift work, but no studies have been done to evaluate the safety of chronic use.
- Do not use sleeping pills—Sleeping pills are not recommended because of the psychologic addiction that may occur. Any such drugs should be used in moderation. It may be best to use them only on the first day after the first night back on the night shift.

It takes extra effort for the night worker to arrange a sleep schedule, but doing so is worth it. In the book *Restful Sleep*, Deepak Chopra writes, "The purpose of sleep is to allow the body to repair and rejuvenate itself. The deep rest provided during sleep allows the body to recover from fatigue and stress and enlivens the body's own self repair and homeostatic, or balancing, mechanisms."*

Working the Night Shift

To become as productive, efficient, and healthy as possible when working the night shift, emergency and critical care veterinary technicians should do the following:

- Drink plenty of water—Dehydration was noted to be very common among people who work at night.
- Avoid caffeinated beverages after midnight during the shift—Caffeine remains in the body for an average of 6 hours and can interfere with sleep

and cause indigestion. One should cut back on caffeine slowly if accustomed to consuming large quantities. Withdrawal symptoms include headaches and nausea.

- Plan to eat the biggest meal of the day during the lunch break on the night shift—Doing this will help limit snacking throughout the shift.
- Bring plenty of healthful snacks for late-night cravings.
- Exercise during the night shift—Exercising during the night shift has been proven to increase alertness and ability to sleep during the day. Take at least 20 minutes to do some aerobic exercise. Walking the animals during the shift may not be enough unless the caseload of ambulatory animals is high. Walking up stairs or around the hospital may be necessary.

Veterinary technicians should also remember that bright light therapy for night workers is becoming very popular. It helps the body clock shift to an active mode by suppressing the secretion of the nighttime hormone melatonin. Bright lights also may enhance the effectiveness of serotonin and other neurotransmitters, which shift the circadian rhythm (10,000 lux therapy is the intensity suggested, which is 20 times the intensity of average indoor light). Spending 3 to 6 or more hours under bright lights increases alertness during the night shift and the ability to sleep during the day. Practices can install these light sources, or light boxes can be purchased individually.

After the Shift

After a shift, limiting exposure to sunlight and avoiding eating a breakfast-type meal is best. Dark sunglasses can be used on the ride home.

If a person cannot adjust to the night shift, the only other solution may be a day shift. People in their middle 40s to early 50s have greater difficulty adjusting to these shifts.

Conclusion

The veterinary technician who chooses to work in an emergency and critical care unit may be asked to work a variety of shifts during his or her employment. The shift worker and the employer must

---

*From Chopra D: *Restful sleep*, New York, 1994, Harmony Books.

understand the physical and psychologic strain this type of work can cause. Once this is understood and accepted, the people involved with shift work can take the necessary steps to prevent shift lag. The person responsible for scheduling and the shift workers must act as a team. The veterinary technician must be committed to making an extra effort to obtain a restful sleep. The person responsible for scheduling the shift workers must be committed to providing optimal rotations to prevent disruption to the workers' normal body rhythms.

Maintaining a 24-hour emergency critical care team is very challenging. The schedule must be reassessed and changes made as needed.

Suggested Readings

Anderson-Parrado P: Energizing ourselves naturally with some good old-fashioned shut eye, *Better Nutrition* 59(3):28, 1997.

Campbell S: Effects of timed bright-light exposure on shift work adaptation in middle-aged subjects, *Sleep* 18(6):408-416, 1995.

Chopra D: *Restful sleep*, New York, 1994, Harmony Books.

Czeisler CA: Rotating shift work schedules that disrupt sleep are improved by applying circadian principles, *Science* 217:460, 1982.

Czeisler CA, Johnson MP, Duffy JF et al: Exposure to bright light and darkness to treat physiologic maladaptation to night work, *N Engl J Med* 322(18):1254, 1990.

Dearholt SL, Feathers CA: Self-scheduling can work, *Nurs Manage* 28(8):47, 1997.

Ehret CF: Future perspectives for the application of chronobiological knowledge in occupational work scheduling, *Invited testimony for the Investigations and Oversight Subcommittee of the Committee on Science and Technology*, Washington, DC, U.S. House of Representatives, March 24, 1983.

Ehret CF: New approaches to chronohygiene for the shift worker in the nuclear power industry. In Reinberg A et al: *Advances in the biosciences: night and shift work biological and social aspects*, New York, 1981, Pergamon.

Goodkind M: Night shifts can be easier, Stanford University Medical Center News Bureau, *Health Tips*, January 1996.

Lewy AJ: Treating chronobiologic sleep and mood disorders with bright light, *Psychiatr Ann* 17(9):664, 1997.

Orlock C: *Inner time*, New York, 1993, Birch Line Press Book.

Slon S: Night moves, *Prevention* 49(6):106, 1997.

Weight gain on the night shift, *Tufts University Diet and Nutrition Letter* 14(8):1, 1996.

28

Risk Management and the Emergency Veterinary Technician

Marcie Marshall

As society becomes increasingly litigious, veterinary professionals find themselves in a more precarious position than ever before in the history of the profession. Lawyers seeking to find new niches for themselves look to veterinarians and veterinary staff to provide them with an entirely new clientele. As consumers, clients are more educated and demand a consistently higher level of competence and accountability. The veterinary industry, seeking to raise the level of care owners are willing to provide to their pets, promotes the human-animal bond and by using terms such as *pet parent*. Unfortunately, this sets up veterinary professionals as targets for litigation when and if mistakes or misunderstandings happen. Litigation can be anything from a day in small claims court to an investigation by the Attorney General's office to civil court cases that require payment for damages. Outcomes vary from loss of time to exorbitant attorney's fees and suspension or loss of licensure.

Risk management, for the purposes of this chapter, involves understanding the liability risks that veterinary personnel take when they assume responsibility for the medical care of patients, as well as implementing systems to reduce these risks as much as possible. Risk management is more than preventing obvious negligence or malpractice; it must be part of everyday practice. Risk management involves identifying and minimizing risks to ourselves and to ensuring the ability to carry on in the profession.

As licensed, registered or certified technicians, veterinary professionals can be held liable for their mistakes (up to and including fines and loss of professional licensure). It behooves everyone involved in every aspect of patient care to learn how to practice good medicine while protecting themselves and their colleagues. How can veterinary technicians protect themselves, their veterinarians, and their practices without compromising care? Quite simply, by practicing smart. From the moment that the client and the patient walk through the door to the time the case is resolved, veterinary professionals must remain diligent about communication and documentation.

Triage and Risk Management

Triage in emergency hospitals is a fundamental part of managing risk by offering immediate assessment of patients, communicating with owners to ease their tension, and bridging the communication gap from "front" to "back." Triage starts the moment the pet walks through the door. A well-trained emergency receptionist can immediately distinguish between an animal that is apparently stabile and one that needs to be whisked to the treatment room for immediate life-saving care. He or she is also able to sooth anxious owners with supportive words, while taking control of the situation and initiating the appropriate paperwork and consent for emergency treatment. Short of profuse bleeding, obvious seizure activity, or other easily visible life-threatening emergencies, receptionists should *not* be relied upon to assess level of emergency, or in the case of busy weekends and potentially long waits, the order of examinations. This task should be reserved for the licensed or certified veterinary technician or licensed veterinarian. Only a staff member with specialized, professional training should assess the minutia involved with triage. A clear and systematic triage program is one of the first steps in managing risk and providing high-quality emergency patient care.

One example of why receptionists should not be required to triage patients happened at an emergency and specialty hospital. An angry client called to complain and request a refund of money spent at the hospital. The client was upset because the doctor misdiagnosed the pet's problem. Upon investigation it was found that the client presented the pet during a busy weekend and said the pet was lethargic and not eating. As the receptionist took more information, the client explained that this was how the dog acted previously when it had an ear infection. The receptionist paraphrased what the client said on the examination form by writing, *cc: ear infection?* The busy doctor entered, did an examination, and questioned the client about previous ear infections. The client described the dog's lethargy, shaking head, and scratching, and the doctor did a physical examination, took a swab of the ear, and found yeast on cytology. The dog was sent home with ear medication.

The next day the dog was brought to the regular veterinarian and diagnosed with a serious case of pancreatitis. The owners were angry that doctor did no blood work and no further diagnostics than ear cytology.

Upon verbal discussion with the doctor, he had no recollection of the case. Very little was documented on the file to indicate any discussion the doctor had with the client. Thus the clinic did not serve the patient well and potentially could have had a much worse case on its hands had the pet not been quickly diagnosed by the regular veterinarian. Unfortunately, the situation created a negative impression of the clinic for both the client and the regular veterinarian.

In emergent situations, emotions run high and clients feel helpless. They will do whatever they feel they can to comfort their pets and alleviate their suffering. This is also the time when the pet is at its most vulnerable, fearful, and painful, and the chances for injury to the owner are high. Owners should never restrain their own pets! Veterinary professionals can be held liable for damages if a client is injured while they are providing care for a pet. A gentle explanation to the distressed client who insists on holding his or her pet during a procedure may include the following: "Mrs. Brown, I understand that you are very worried about Buffy, but you must allow us to restrain her so that we may provide the care she needs quickly and safely. We are professionals and will take care of her like she was our own."

Informed Consent

Informed consent is a practice-wide responsibility, the single-best method of managing risk, and essential for veterinary practices. Obtaining informed consent should be a mandate in every practice as a basic means of risk management. However, informed consent is one of the most misunderstood and underused risk management tools in practices today. Informed consent is the process by which veterinary professionals assess the patient, make a plan for diagnostics and treatments based on accepted standards of care, inform the client of the assessment and plan (as well as the potential risks involved and cost of treatment), and obtain permission from the client to proceed. Whenever major changes in the treatment plan or further diagnostics are necessary that are not included in the initial plan, clients must be notified and given the opportunity to accept or decline continued care. Therefore it benefits all involved to be as clear as possible with the clients during the initial visit, before hospitalization. This clarity sets a precedent for expectations on the part of the hospital and the client.

Roles in Obtaining Informed Consent

Informed consent in the emergency practice begins on the telephone. When the client calls to get directions to the hospital, the receptionist courteously informs him or her of the emergency examination cost, that all diagnostics and treatments are additional, and that payment is expected when service is rendered. Upon arrival the client is required to complete an information form that asks for personal information, pet information, and reason for the visit. The client should be informed that the medical record information is protected and the practice will communicate with no one other than those indicated by the client. Thus the client must indicate (by signature) if he or she wants the practice to share records with the regular veterinarian. The client information form should explain billing policies and deposit and payment requirements, including any service charge or monthly billing fee on any unpaid balance. The wording of the form should be reviewed by the clinic's attorney for legitimacy. Because this form is the first document the client sees (even before meeting with the veterinarian), it should *not* include wording that authorizes diagnostics and treatments. This is not appropriate because the client has no way of understanding what he or she is authorizing without completing the process of informed consent; therefore the legitimacy of the document is depreciated.

Next (or concurrently depending on timing and urgency) the technician triages the pet to determine immediate status and level of medical need. If the patient can be triaged in an isolated area from the rest of the waiting room (e.g., examination room, triage room, triage area) in which the conversation between the technician and the client can be private, this will help alleviate some stress on the part of the client. Privacy may also encourage the client to be more forthcoming with history or financial details, because the risk of embarrassment is reduced. Triage information must be documented at this time (i.e., temperature, pulse, respiration (TPR), level of consciousness (LOC) reason for visit). The technician communicates pertinent information with the receptionist, and the file is completed for the examination.

Next the veterinarian does the examination in a systematic way according to the accepted practices and standards set forth by federal, state, and individual hospital standards. From a risk management standpoint, the veterinarian should require the full attention of the owner (i.e., no cell phones) and to learn to verbalize his or her examination. One of the most frustrating questions from a client who does not want to pay for an examination is, "Why should I pay for an examination when all the veterinarian did was look at him?" This sometimes occurs after the veterinarian has spent considerable time and effort quietly assessing all systems while the client is distracted by noisy children or constant cell phone interruptions.

From the examination and history, the veterinarian determines if further diagnostics are needed. Once a plan is made, the client is presented with an estimate for the cost of diagnostics and treatment. The person presenting the estimate should not be the veterinarian. Nothing reduces the client's perception of the veterinarian's motivation faster than when the veterinarian starts discussing money. A seasoned receptionist is probably best equipped to present an estimate, because he or she is the most accustomed to delicate discussions about finances and payment options. Simple questions can easily be answered by the receptionist, who was briefed on the situation when the doctor gave him or her the travel sheet for the estimate. However, complicated medical questions involving the necessity of certain tests or treatments may require the veterinarian or a technician to revisit the client. Once an estimate has been finalized, it must be signed by the client and a separate form completed that authorizes the hospital to perform the medical plan. This form should include wishes for cardiopulmonary resuscitation and reiterate payment obligations.

If the practice does not regularly "x-ray pocketbooks" but offers top-notch care to all clients at each visit, then it will encounter clients who simply cannot afford the level of care proposed at the first estimate. The clinic must have "Plan B" ready in case the first plan is rejected (and make sure that "Plan A" is declined by the client by a signature indicating his or her wishes to *not* pursue that level of care).

For example, a client arrives at the clinic with an unvaccinated puppy that is lethargic, vomiting, and has diarrhea. The client authorizes a parvovirus test that is positive. The doctor (or the technician) discusses the seriousness of the disease and explains that because of the puppy's physical condition, he should be hospitalized for a few days on supportive care to prevent dehydration and death. The owner is presented with an educational pamphlet that describes parvovirus and express concern over the cost. The receptionist presents the owner with an estimate for $2500 to $4000 for 3 to 5 days in isolation and medical care. The owner cannot afford this treatment.

Plan B is for 24 hours in isolation with a plan to transfer the animal to the referring veterinarian on Monday, because hospitalization may be less costly there. The owner still cannot afford treatment. Against medical advice, the owner elects to take the puppy home and try to give supportive care there. The puppy is given two injections and a bolus of fluids; the owner is strongly encouraged to follow up with the referring veterinarian on Monday. The medical record should include a declined estimate for the 3 to 5 days hospitalization plan, a declined estimate for the 24-hours plan, an accepted estimate for the fluids and injections given, and a signed *against medical advice form* that states the client is going against the advice of the veterinarian by taking the puppy home. Further, the file should have documented client communications indicating the client was verbally informed and given a pamphlet that describes parvovirus, its route of transmission, and the seriousness of the disease.

Imagine that the owners were breeders of rottweilers. They recently bought a male and a female and decided to get into breeding, despite the fact that they have little knowledge of the breed, intestinal parasites, and diseases. This is their first litter, and they have had many people in and out of their home looking at the puppies. They have three puppies left, and one puppy became ill (they brought it to the hospital on a Sunday morning). Because the clinic was extremely busy on Sunday morning, the veterinary team did not have time to deal with all the paperwork involved in keeping good records and risk management. The clients did not want to hospitalize their pet, but they did allow the technician to provide some care and took the puppy home. They were given the parvovirus handout and advised to see their regular veterinarian on Monday (although the technician felt the puppy would probably die). Two months later, the veterinarian received a letter from a lawyer informing him that the client is suing him and everyone involved in the case, as well as the managers and hospital owners for negligence. The client claims that he was not properly informed of the seriousness of the disease and offered only to treat the puppy on outpatient because the clinic was obviously very busy. The client claims that not only did they lose that puppy but also the other two puppies in the litter. The dam who was not well vaccinated became ill and aborted the litter she was carrying at the time with a potential loss of $1200 per puppy. Now the breeder's reputation has been damaged and customers who had expressed interest in buying a puppy from them have reneged. If the team practiced good risk management

procedures, all the documentation would allow the clinic to demonstrate that the client was fully informed and made an informed decision *not* to treat the pet. The lesson is this: If good risk management procedures are not practiced, the clinic will have a difficult time disproving false claims by clients.

Keeping the Client Informed

Veterinary technicians are increasingly required to act as liaisons between doctors and clients. The technician must remember that clients are very nervous and afraid of what their beloved pet is experiencing, as well as what the future may hold in terms of long-term prognosis. Thus it may seem that clients are being difficult when they call five times daily and visit their pets as often as possible. The emergency veterinary technician may become frustrated with these clients and begin to avoid contact with them. On the contrary, clients should be allowed to be part of their pet's health care team. The more the client is kept "in the loop," the greater the chance for an overall positive experience for all involved, despite the outcome. The client is the one who, if not kept informed, perceives a lack of communication or, worse, deception on the part of the veterinary staff; this results in the client becoming confused, angry, and litigious. An ounce of prevention, in the form of appropriate client communications and updates, is worth a pound of cure in the form of legal fees and liability insurance coverage.

Documenting Medical Records

Medical records are legal documents (McWay, 2003). They are the possession of the hospital, but a copy must be provided to the client upon written request. Thus everyone who touches the medical record must do so with the understanding that it may be read by the client or a judge some day. For the sake of remaining true to the spirit of this chapter, the author limits the discussion of medical records as it pertains to client communications.

Any and all communications with a client regarding the care of a pet must be documented in the medical record. Electronic medical records are preferred by most clinics because most people are familiar with keyboards. Electronic medical records eliminate errors caused by poor handwriting and simply look more professional than paper records. Electronic medical records are almost never lost or misplaced, and they are accessible wherever a computer terminal is found (thus eliminating errors or missed documentation as the result of having to wait to document something until after someone else is done with the record).

What to Say

In documenting medical records (i.e., client correspondence) it is important to be complete, objective, and concise. The date, time, names of individuals involved in the conversation, and the route of conversation must be identified as follows:

"8/10/2005, 13:40, Called 555-222-1234 Spoke with Mrs. Jones re: Fluffy's response to treatment thus far. Explained that Fluffy is progressing—however, more slowly than we had hoped. May need 1 to 2 more days of hospitalization and treatment before we know more about her long-term prognosis. Offered transfer back to the regular veterinarian or keep here. Explained I spoke with Dr. Smith and she would prefer that Fluffy stay here because they have no overnight staffing, but would be willing to take Fluffy during the day and transfer back here for overnights. Mrs. Jones questioned bill so far. Put Sara on with Mrs. Jones to explain invoice thus far and go over estimate for next 24 to 48 hours care and treatment. When I got back on with Mrs. Jones, she stated she wanted to leave Fluffy here for duration of treatment. Thanked me for calling her with the update, and stated she will be in at 8 PM (20:00) to visit Fluffy and put more deposit on her account for increased estimate. Explained to Mrs. Jones that I would not be here when she visits tonight, but Dr. Brown will receive rounds from me and will be updated on Fluffy's condition and continued plan for treatment.—Dr. Green"

What Not to Say

The previous documentation summarizes a conversation in a very objective, concise, and complete way. All parties are identified, and the doctor did not actually discuss costs or money with the client. However, she was informed of the costs of continued treatment by Sara (the receptionist), who is better equipped to discuss sensitive financial issues with clients because of her training.

The following is what not to say in the medical record:

"8/10/2005 13:40 Mrs. Green called (for the fourth time since 8 AM this morning!) to check on Fluffy. Explained that Fluffy is not doing as well as I thought she would, and I am not sure what to do with her. We could try more fluids and keep her for another day or so to see what happens, or she could go back to her regular veterinarian. But they will not be there overnight, so she will have to run her back and forth from us to them. Mrs. Jones wanted to know how much the bill was so far. I told her I did not know, that I doubt we have gone past her estimate yet, and if Fluffy stays for 2 more days, then we will need more money for a deposit. Mrs. Jones was a bit huffy with me and started to get an attitude. She said she would stop by later today to visit. I told her I would not be here when she came in.—Dr. Green"

The same individuals, the same patient, and the same condition were involved in both examples; however, the differences in communication style and documentation between the first and second examples are quite evident. Unlike the first situation, the second situation is already "brewing" discontent. The client has called several times, but the doctor seems unsure of the treatment plan. He is not proactive in answering Mrs. Jones' question about the bill or providing an estimate for next 1 to 2 days of care. Dr. Green adds an interpretation of the client's attitude.

In the first scenario, regardless of the outcome of Fluffy's case, a positive interaction between the hospital and the client is established and maintained. In the second scenario, even when Fluffy goes home well, the client still has a negative impression about the care she and her pet received from the hospital. If Fluffy dies—look out!

Mission, Standards, and Protocols

Every well-managed veterinary hospital should establish and abide by its mission, standards, and protocols. A mission statement is a simple statement that the hospital makes about why it exists. Decisions about everything in the practice, large or small, should be made with consideration of the mission of the practice. Clients and team members should be able to sense the practice's mission. If the phrase *high-quality medical care* is included in the mission statement, then all patients should have the opportunity to receive that care. If a clinic's mission is to offer that kind of care to all patients, it should not become mired in the dichotomy of the client's ability to afford that care vs. his or her ability to pay for it. If a client can only afford Plan B, then the clinic will deliver the care outlined in Plan B to the best of its ability.

Standards of care are a collection of absolutes that affect daily practices. A clinic's standards are a set of statements that it makes about the care and treatment clients and patients can expect at the hospital. For example, a standard in an emergency veterinary hospital could be, "All patients will be triaged by a certified veterinary technician within 5 minutes of arrival," *or* "All hospitalized patients with an intravenous catheter in place will receive full catheter care every 24 hours according to the protocol defining catheter care at the XYZ Emergency Hospital."

A hospital's standards are derived from its mission. They are not simply statements about the care it *hopes* to provide for patients but the care that the hospital is dedicated to providing. Every member of the emergency team must know and subscribe to the clinic's standards of care.

Protocols are detailed instructions on how to maintain the clinic's standards of care and ultimately its mission. Emergency hospital protocols can be grouped into five different categories: (1) administrative, (2) nursing, (3) medical, (4) cleaning and maintenance, and (5) safety. The protocols within a hospital can be as detailed or as broad-ranged as necessary for each situation. For example, an administrative protocol for dealing with angry clients can be somewhat flexible based on that client's specific situation. However, the protocol should include who deals with angry clients and what manner of communication is required. If the client simply needs to "vent" about a situation and is apparently dealing with a large amount of grief, then the team would not direct the client to the clinic's insurance carrier. Instead the doctor or hospital manager would likely handle the situation with tact and skill. However, a client making serious accusations regarding malpractice or negligence and seeking financial restitution would be handled much differently. However, nursing protocols such as those for catheter care, intravenous fluid administration, animal handling, and surgical assisting are relatively cut and dry.

Protocols should be written, kept updated, and located in an area that is accessible at all times. Some practices have all protocols in one large binder or bound manual. Some have separate manuals for each category. Administrative protocols include receptionist protocols, documentation of medical records, as well as other administrative issues such as handling of pet remains and discharging patients from the hospital. Nursing protocols include treatment responsibilities, protocols on triage, radiology, intravenous catheter placement, and fluid administration. Safety protocols include all information regarding Occupational Safety and Health Association (www.osha.gov) regulations (e.g., personal protective equipment for each task, reporting workplace injury or illness, emergency evacuation procedures). Medical protocols include specific hospital protocols for administering anesthesia, surgery, and pain management. Cleaning and maintenance protocols include dilution rates for disinfectants and cleaners, protocols for cleaning cages, for sweeping and mopping, and for laundry, as well as daily, weekly, and monthly cleaning and maintenance checklists.

Protocols are an essential part of a successful, well-managed emergency veterinary hospital for several reasons: they allow for the consistent training of new employees, they provide a resource for existing doctors and team members, they allow for consistency in the care and treatment of all patients, and they help employees to subscribe to the clinic's standards and mission.

Consistency in care and treatment of team members, patients, and clients is an essential aspect of risk management in the emergency veterinary hospital. Inconsistency in treatment of team members leads to confusion and discontent, and ultimately to turnover. Inconsistency in care and treatment of patients leads to negligence, and inconsistency in treatment of clients leads to miscommunication and litigation.

Risk management in the emergency veterinary hospital is important to the licensed, registered or certified veterinary technician. The technician is frequently the "hub" of the veterinary medical team and can be the facilitator of appropriate triage, informed consent, client communications and documentation, and overall standards and protocols—all essential facets of appropriate risk management. During the process of implementing appropriate risk management techniques and protocols, the veterinary technician inevitably raises the level of care and service the clinic provides to patients and clients. In addition, the technician sets an example for referring veterinarians and ultimately raises the level of professionalism within the industry.

Suggested Reading

McWay DC: *Legal aspects of health information management,* Clifton Park, NY, 2003, Thomson Learning.

Index